THROMBOLYTIC THERAPY FOR PERIPHERAL VASCULAR DISEASE

THROMBOLYTIC THERAPY FOR PERIPHERAL VASCULAR DISEASE

ANTHONY J. COMEROTA, MD

Professor of Surgery
Chief, Section of Vascular Surgery
Temple University School of Medicine
Philadelphia, Pennsylvania

WITH 47 CONTRIBUTORS

J. B. LIPPINCOTT COMPANY
Philadelphia

Acquisitions Editor: Lisa McAllister
Sponsoring Editor: Paula Callaghan
Indexer: Textbook Writers Associates
Cover Designer: Mark James
Production Manager: Janet Greenwood
Production Editor: Mary Kinsella
Production Service: Textbook Writers Associates
Prepress: Jay's Publishers Services
Printer/Binder: Quebecor/Kingsport

6 5 4 3 2

Library of Congress Cataloging-in-Publication Data

Thrombolytic therapy for peripheral vascular disease/[edited
    by] Anthony J. Comerota; with 47 contributors.
        p.   cm.
    Includes bibliographical references and index.
    ISBN 0-397-51343-7
    1. Peripheral vascular disease—Chemotherapy.
    2. Thrombolytic therapy.   I. Comerota, Anthony J.
    [DNLM: 1. Peripheral Vascular Disease—drug therapy.
    2. Thrombosis—drug therapy.   3. Thrombolytic
Therapy.   WG 610
    T5352 1994]
    RC694.T48   1994
    616.1'31061—dc20
    DNLM/DLC
    for Library of Congress   94-18164
                                                        CIP

The authors and publisher have exerted every effort to ensure
that drug selection and dosage set forth in this text are in accord with current recommendations and practice at the time
of publication. However, in view of ongoing research, changes
in government regulations, and the constant flow of information relating to drug therapy and drug reactions, the reader is
urged to check the package insert for each drug for any change
in indications and dosage and for added warnings and precautions. This is particularly important when the recommended
agent is a new or infrequently employed drug.

TO MY PATIENT AND UNDERSTANDING WIFE,
ELSA,

AND MY CHILDREN,
ANTHONY, MAYA, AND MARK.

CONTRIBUTORS

KENNETH M. ALFIERI, MD
Assistant Professor
Department of Radiology
University of Missouri-Kansas City School
    of Medicine
Truman Medical Center
Kansas City, Missouri

SURESH AMBLE, MD
Vascular and Interventional Radiologist
Columbia Hospital
Chicago, Illinois

JEFFREY L. ANDERSON, MD
Professor of Medicine
University of Utah
Chief, Division of Cardiology
Latter Day Saints Hospital
Salt Lake City, Utah

WILLIAM R. BELL, MD
Edyth Harris Lucas-Clara Lucas Lynn Professor
    in Hematology
Professor of Medicine
Radiology and Nuclear Medicine
Johns Hopkins University School of Medicine
Baltimore, Maryland

JOSEPH J. BOOKSTEIN, MD
Professor of Radiology
University of California, San Diego
School of Medicine
University of California San Diego Medical
    Center
San Diego, California

MARK A.H. COHEN, MD
Diagnostic Radiology Fellow
Division of Radiology
The Cleveland Clinic Foundation
Cleveland, Ohio

ROBERT W. COLMAN, MD

Sol Sherry Professor of Medicine and Professor
 of Physiology
Director, Sol Sherry Thrombosis Research Center
Chief, Hematology Division
Temple University School of Medicine
Philadelphia, Pennsylvania

GREGORY J. DEL ZOPPO, MD

Department of Molecular and Experimental
 Medicine
The Scripps Research Institute
Staff Physician
Division of Hematology/Medical Oncology
Scripps Clinic and Research Foundation
La Jolla, California

EDWARD M. DRUY, MD, FACR

Professor of Radiology
George Washington University Medical Center
Chief, Section of Special Procedures
 and Interventional Radiology
George Washington Hospital
Washington, DC

JANETTE D. DURHAM, MD

Assistant Professor of Radiology
University of Colorado Health Science Center
Denver, Colorado

WILLIAM R. FLINN, MD

Professor and Chief
Section of Vascular Surgery
University of Maryland
Baltimore, Maryland

CHARLES W. FRANCIS, MD

Associate Professor of Medicine
University of Rochester School of Medicine
 and Dentistry
Attending Physician
Strong Memorial Hospital
Rochester, New York

JUERGEN FROEHLICH, MD

Clinical Scientist
Genentech, Inc.
South San Francisco, California

VALENTIN FUSTER, MD, PHD

Director, Cardiovascular Institute
Mount Sinai Medical Center
Arthur M. and Hilda A. Master Professor
 of Medicine
Mount Sinai Medical Center
New York, New York

GEOFFREY A. GARDINER, JR., MD

Associate Professor of Radiology
Jefferson Medical College
Director, Division of Cardiovascular
 and Interventional Radiology
Thomas Jefferson University Hospital
Philadelphia, Pennsylvania

SAMUEL Z. GOLDHABER, MD

Associate Professor of Medicine
Harvard Medical School
Staff Cardiologist
Brigham and Women's Hospital
Boston, Massachusetts

VICTOR GUREWICH, MD

Associate Professor of Medicine
Harvard Medical School
Director, Institute for the Prevention
 of Cardiovascular Disease
Deaconess Hospital
Boston, Massachusetts

EDGAR HABER, AB, MD, AM (HON), MA
 (OXON)

Elkan R. Blout Professor of Biological Sciences
Harvard School of Public Health
Professor of Medicine
Harvard Medical School
Physician, Massachusetts General Hospital
Senior Physician, Brigham and Women's
 Hospital
Boston, Massachusetts

JACK HENKIN, PHD

Adjunct Assistant Professor
Chicago Medical School
Section Head, Thrombolytics Discovery
Abbott Laboratories
North Chicago, Illinois

JACK HIRSH, MD, FRCP(C)

Professor of Medicine
McMaster University
Director, Hamilton Civic Hospitals Research
    Centre
Hamilton, Ontario
Canada

RUSSELL D. HULL, MD

Department of Medicine
The University of Calgary Health Sciences
Calgary, Alberta
Canada

IK-KYUNG JANG, MD

Assistant Professor of Medicine
Harvard Medical School
Assistant in Medicine, Cardiac Unit
Massachusetts General Hospital
Boston, Massachusetts

BARRY T. KATZEN, MD, FACR, FACC

Clinical Professor of Radiology
University of Miami School of Medicine
Medical Director
Miami Vascular Institute at Baptist Hospital
Miami, Florida

DAVID A. KUMPE, MD

Professor of Radiology and Surgery
University of Colorado Health Sciences Center
Director of Interventional Radiology
University Hospital
Denver, Colorado

WALTER J. MCCARTHY, MD

Assistant Professor
Northwestern University Medical School
Active Staff
Northwestern Memorial Hospital
Chicago, Illinois

THOMAS O. MCNAMARA, MD

Professor of Radiological Sciences
University of California, Los Angeles
School of Medicine
Chief of Cardiovascular and Interventional
    Radiology
Co-Director of Endovascular Therapy
University of California, Los Angeles Medical
    Center
Los Angeles, California

HERBERT I. MACHLEDER, MD

Professor of Surgery
University of California, Los Angeles
School of Medicine
University of California, Los Angeles Hospital
Los Angeles, California

PATRICK A. MARCOTTE, PHD

Thrombolytics Discovery
Abbott Laboratories
Abbott Park, Illinois

VICTOR J. MARDER, MD

Professor of Medicine and Pathology
Associate Chair of Academic Affairs
Chief, Hematology Unit
Department of Medicine
University of Rochester School of Medicine
    and Dentistry
Rochester, New York

SHIRLEY M. OTIS, MD

Senior Consultant, Division of Neurology
Director, Vascular Laboratories
Associate Clinical Professor of Neurology
University Hospital
Chief of Staff, Green Hospital
San Diego, California

JOSEPH F. PIETROLUNGO, DO, MS

Interventional Fellow
Department of Vascular Medicine
Cleveland Clinic Foundation
Cleveland, Ohio

GRAHAM F. PINEO, MD, FRCP(C), FACP

Professor of Medicine
University of Calgary
Director, Clinical Trials Unit
Calgary General Hospital
Calgary, Alberta
Canada

A. KONETI RAO, MD

Professor of Medicine
Thrombosis Research and Pathology
Temple University School of Medicine
Philadelphia, Pennsylvania

GARY E. RASKOB, MD

Assistant Professor
Department of Medicine, College of Medicine
Department of Biostatistics and Epidemiology
College of Public Health
University of Oklahoma Health Sciences Center
Associate Scientist
Veterans Administration Medical Center
Oklahoma City, Oklahoma

KENNETH C. ROBBINS, PHD

Research Professor
Northwestern University Medical School
Division of Hematology/Oncology
Department of Medicine
Chicago, Illinois

ANNE C. ROBERTS, MD

Associate Professor of Radiology
University of California, San Diego
Chief of Radiology
University of California, San Diego Medical
    Center
Thornton Hospital
San Diego, California

RONALD N. RUBIN, MD

Professor of Medicine
Temple University School of Medicine
Chief of Clinical Hematology
Temple University Hospital
Philadelphia, Pennsylvania

ARTHUR A. SASAHARA, MD

Senior Venture Head
Thrombolytics Research
Abbott Laboratories
Abbott Park, Illinois
Professor of Medicine, Emeritus
Harvard Medical School
Boston, Massachusetts

SOL SHERRY, MD, DSC (HON) (DECEASED)

Distinguished Professor of Medicine Emeritus
Temple University School of Medicine
Philadelphia, Pennsylvania

MICHAEL B. SILVA, JR., MD

Division of Vascular Surgery
New Jersey Medical School
University of Medicine and Dentistry
    of New Jersey
Newark, New Jersey

JOHN C. SOBOLSKI, MD, PHD

Vice President for Medical and Regulatory Affairs
Nitromed
Boston, Massachusetts
Assistant Professor of Medicine
Department of Medicine
Chicago Medical School
Chicago, Illinois

DAVID L. STUMP, MD

Senior Director
Clinical Research
Genentech, Inc.
South San Francisco, California

ERIC J. TOPOL, MD

Chairman, Department of Cardiology
Director, Center for Thrombosis and Arterial
    Biology
Professor of Medicine
Ohio State University
The Cleveland Clinic Foundation
Cleveland, Ohio

FONG Y. TSAI, MD, FACR
Professor and Chairman
Department of Radiology
University of Missouri, Kansas City
School of Medicine
Truman Medical Center
Kansas City, Missouri

KARIM VALJI, MD
Assistant Professor of Radiology
University of California, San Diego
Head, Division of Vascular and Interventional
 Radiology
University of California, San Diego Medical
 Center
San Diego, California

MARC VERSTRAETE, MD, PHD, FRCP(EDIN),
 FACP(HON)
Professor of Surgery
Center for Molecular and Vascular Biology
University of Leuven
Belgium

JOHN V. WHITE, MD
Associate Professor of Surgery
Temple University School of Medicine
Philadelphia, Pennsylvania

PREFACE

The use of thrombolytic agents for patients with thrombotic and embolic problems encompasses many and diverse specialties involved with the care of patients with thromboembolic disorders. Thrombolytic therapy often reflects a degree of sophistication in the art and science of caring for patients with thrombotic and embolic disorders. Many physicians would intuitively prefer to eliminate the pathologic thrombus or embolus; however, both acute and long-term benefits have been questioned in light of associated risks and increased cost. During the past decade, data have emerged demonstrating both acute and long-term benefits to patients treated for myocardial infarction, pulmonary embolism, venous thrombosis, arterial and graft occlusion, and stroke.

Concepts are changing and advances ongoing at the clinical and developmental level. *Thrombolytic Therapy for Peripheral Vascular Disease* is designed to provide a current review of the application of thrombolytic agents for patients presenting with the spectrum of vascular diseases. I have been fortunate in recruiting the leaders in the field as contributors, who have provided the most current information in a clinically applicable fashion.

Thrombolytic Therapy for Peripheral Vascular Disease is intended to be comprehensive yet practical. Introductory chapters review the normal mechanisms of hemostasis and the physiology and pathophysiology of the fibrinolytic system, as well as the pathogenesis of thrombosis. These chapters establish the foundation for the remainder of the text.

Four chapters cover the currently available thrombolytic agents and are followed by a section addressing the use of thrombolytic therapy for specific clinical disorders. Four chapters are dedicated to venous thromboembolic disease. The current data from prospective trials are included in the chapter on pulmonary embolism. Modern concepts of therapy for acute deep venous thrombosis are covered, along with separate chapters for primary and secondary axillosubclavian vein thrombosis.

The next section addresses intraarterial and catheter-directed thrombolytic therapy for arterial and graft occlusion. An overview of catheter-directed lytic therapy includes a brief discussion of the recently completed and ongoing trials of catheter-directed thrombolysis for arterial and graft occlusion. Separate chapters specifically address acute limb ischemia, chronic arterial occlusion, and therapy for occluded bypass grafts. Technical developments in drug delivery systems have improved the results of catheter-directed techniques, and are also included in this section. A review of intraoperative, intraarterial thrombolytic therapy and thrombolysis used to salvage occluded dialysis access grafts round out this section.

Thrombolytic therapy has been most extensively studied in patients with acute myocardial infarction, which is comprehensively reviewed, including the results of the recently concluded GUSTO trial. The use of thrombolytic therapy for acute stroke and cerebrovascular occlusion is addressed in the final two clinical chapters. The last section of this book reviews the hemorrhagic complications, the appropriate use of anticoagulants for arterial and venous thromboembolic disorders, newer antithrombotic agents, and future forms of thrombolytic therapy.

The most important concept in the development of this text was to anticipate the needs of clinicians, residents, and students involved in the care of patients with thromboembolic vascular disease, and provide the information necessary, in a single volume, to provide state-of-the-art care.

I am personally indebted to each of the contributors for their dedicated efforts in providing timely submissions and current information. I thank J.B. Lippincott for its confidence in me, specifically Lisa McAllister and Paula Callaghan for their friendly persuasion, persistence, and patience. Finally, I am most grateful to my loving wife and children, to whom this book is dedicated.

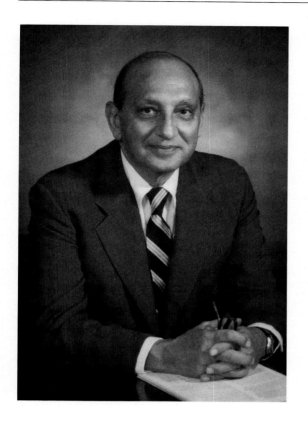

IN MEMORY OF
SOL SHERRY, MD, DSC (HON)

It is fitting that we take a moment to remember Sol Sherry, MD, one of the pioneers in the field of thromboembolic disease, a superior researcher, dedicated teacher and a talented physician. Doctor Sherry is recognized as "the father of thrombolytic therapy." After graduating from New York University School of Medicine, he spent the early part of his career in the laboratories of William S. Tillett, MD, who was studying the properties of the Streptococcus. Dr. Sherry's insightful basic studies of fibrinolysis and his clinical observations led to the application of thrombolytic therapy to acute myocardial infarction. His seminal contributions laid the foundation and forged the future of thrombolytic therapy.

Doctor Sherry continued his work in fibrinolysis at the Barnes Hospital in St. Louis, Missouri, and established his reputation as an excellent administrator and teacher in the finest tradition of academic medicine. This was followed by a sixteen year tenure at Temple University School of Medicine, where he was Chairman of the Department of Medicine and established one of the finest internal medicine residency programs in the country, founded the Temple University Thrombosis Research Center which now bears his name, and ultimately was named Dean of the Temple University School of Medicine.

Doctor Sherry's organizational skills led to the founding of the International Society of Thrombosis and Hemostasis, The Council on Thrombosis of the American Heart Association, and the Scientific Council on Thrombosis of the International Society of Cardiology.

Doctor Sherry has left an indelible mark on each of us. We who have been stimulated by his teaching and writings, who have been enlightened by his discussions, comforted by his compassion, and amused by his sense of humor, will miss him.

CONTENTS

1

REVIEW OF NORMAL HEMOSTASIS

Robert W. Colman

Hemostasis is the process by which blood is maintained in a fluid state under physiologic conditions, which allows reactions to vessel injury to stem blood loss by sealing the defect. Thrombosis may occur if the capacity of the natural anticoagulant mechanisms is overwhelmed by the intensity of the stimulus. Because of the recent advances in modern medicine, patients usually survive the hemostatic challenge of major surgery and trauma but are left vulnerable to venous thrombosis. Alternatively, diet, smoking, and other environmental insults may lead in the genetically susceptible individual to atherosclerotic vessels which predispose to arterial thrombosis.

The normal vascular endothelium maintains blood fluidity by inhibiting blood coagulation and platelet aggregation and promoting fibrinolysis. The endothelial cell monolayers represent a protective barrier which separates blood cells and plasma proteins from highly reactive components in the deeper layers of the vessel wall. Such elements include von Willebrand factor and collagen, to which platelets adhere, and tissue factor, a membrane protein located in fibroblasts in the adventitia and in macrophages in the atherosclerotic plaque, which initiates blood coagulation (Fig. 1-1). When the vessel is severed, injury disrupts the endothelial barrier, and blood is exposed to these subendothelial structures. When platelets are stimulated by subendothelial collagen, they expose and/or assemble membrane glycoproteins IIb and IIIa, which can then bind von Willebrand factor (vWF), responsible for platelet adhesion and fibrinogen required for aggregation. Secretion of coagulant proteins from alpha granules is mediated by synthesis of thromboxane A_2, phosphorylation of cytosolic and membrane proteins, and translocation of intracellular calcium. Protein procofactors, such as factor V, secreted by platelets, or factor VIII, derived from plasma, assemble enzyme complexes on the platelet surface which catalyze, respectively, factor X and prothrombin activation. The result is factor Xa and thrombin formation, which markedly augment their own production manyfold by converting factors V and VIII into activated cofactors, factor Va and VIIIa. This explosive cellular and molecular reaction is modulated

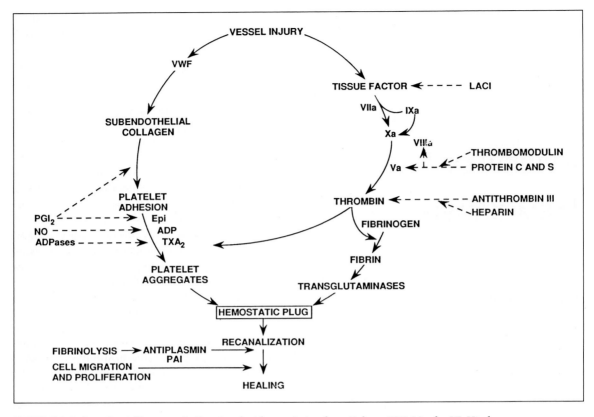

FIGURE 1-1. Overview of hemostasis. Reprinted with permission from Colman RW, Marder VJ, Hirsh J, Salzman EW: Overview of hemostasis. In Colman RW, Marder VJ, Hirsh J, Salzman EW (eds): Hemostasis and Thrombosis: Basic Principles and Clinical Practice, 3d ed. Philadelphia, JB Lippincott, 1994.

by endothelial cell elaboration of antithrombotic compounds, such as prostaglandin I_2 (PGI_2) and nitric oxide (NO), and by exposure of thrombomodulin and heparan. Plasma protease inhibitors, which are important regulators, include antithrombin III (AT III) for factors IXa, Xa, and thrombin; C1-inhibitor for the contact system enzymes, factor XIIa, factor XIIf, and kallikrein; and α_1-antitrypsin for factor XIa. The activated proteins C and S also limit coagulation by degrading factors Va and VIIIa.

Thrombin cleaves fibrinogen, which forms fibrin monomers that then undergo spontaneous polymerization to form the fibrin clot. Covalent cross-linking of the fibrin by factor XIIIa, itself activated by thrombin, increases the mechanical stability of the clot and renders it more resistant to fibrinolysis. Plasminogen is converted to plasmin by plasminogen activators elaborated by endothelial cells. Plasminogen activator inhibitors and α_2-antiplasmin regulate the fibrinolytic process. Thrombin is protected from inhibition by AT III when bound to the fibrin clot; similarly, plasmin bound to the fibrin clot is protected from α_2-antiplasmin inhibitor. Fibrinolysis thus occurs, releasing fibrin degradation products in the process. Lysis of the clot is required for the orderly deposition of collagen, fibrous tissue, and subsequent wound healing.

VESSEL WALL

Endothelial cells maintain the fluidity of the blood by synthesis of inhibitors of blood coagulation and modulators of platelet activation, by regulating vascular tone and permeability, and by forming a protective barrier that separates blood components from reactive subendothelial components. Endothelial cells synthesize and secrete the extracellular matrix, which contains collagen, fibronectin, laminin, and vWR, all of which promote cellular adhesion. Blood coagulation is inhibited on the endothelial cell surface by thrombomodulin and heparan sulfate. Fibrinolysis is first stimulated by the endothelial cell secretion tissue plasminogen activator (t-PA) and is then blocked by plasminogen activator inhibitor 1 (PAI-1). Endothelial cells, by releasing PGI_{2} and NO, produce vasodilation and inhibit platelet aggregation but also can synthesize endothelins, which induce vasoconstriction (Fig. 1-2).

Vessel injury can lead to hemorrhage if the endothelial barrier permeability increases, if the vasoconstriction is impaired because of vessel wall or extravascular matrix abnormalities, or if t-PA secretion is not balanced by PAI-1 production. Endothelial injury may be mediated by immune complexes[1] or viruses.[2] Neutrophil elastase released in inflammatory states perturbs endothelial cells[3] and cleaves connective-tissue proteins,[4] which may contribute to hemorrhage in vasculitis. Attenuation and fenestration of the endothelial cell monolayer may contribute to the hemorrhage in immune thrombocytopenia purpura and

explain the prompt response to prednisone therapy before a detectable rise in platelet count.[5]

The nonthrombogenic properties of endothelial cells are lost when they are stimulated by thrombin, interleukin 1 (IL-1), tumor necrosis factor (TNF), DDAVP, and endotoxin. Synthesis of tissue factor and PAI-1 is induced and the concentration of surface-bound thrombomodulin is reduced by endotoxin, IL-1, and TNF, while DDA VP results in the release of high-molecular-mass vWF multimers which augment platelet adhesion to the injured endothelium.[6,7] Endothelial cells contain receptors, termed *integrins*,[8] that allow binding of fibronectin, collagen, laminin, and vitronectin. Endothelial cells also contain intercellular adhesion molecules (ICAMS)[9] and endothelial adhesion molecules (ELAMS),[10] which act as counterreceptors for leukocyte adhesions.

Endothelial cells vary in function with their anatomic site. Converting enzyme is synthesized principally by aortic endothelium and not by cardiac microvessel endothelium, while thromboxane A_{2} is synthesized predominantly in pulmonary arterial endothelium. Endothelial cell turnover increases at sites of hemodynamic stress and injury. Endothelial cells contain stress fibers involved in cell attachment and maintenance of endothelial junctional apposition. Macromolecules pass across the endothelium into the vessel

FIGURE 1-2. *Thromboresistant properties of endothelium. The endothelial cells synthesize prostacyclin (PGI_{2}), thrombomodulin, heparan, and plasminogen activators, all of which inhibit hemostasis (and thrombus formation) and contribute to the maintenance of vascular patency. Reprinted with permission from Colman RW, Marder VJ, Hirsh J, Salzman EW: Overview of hemostasis. In Colman RW, Marder VJ, Hirsh J, Salzman EW (eds): Hemostasis and Thrombosis: Basic Principles and Clinical Practice, 3d ed. Philadelphia, JB Lippincott, 1994.*

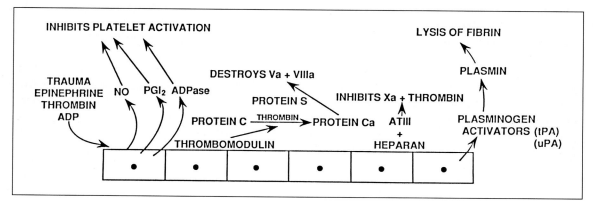

wall through open intercellular junctions, by endocytosis, and via transendothelial pores. Vessel permeability and subsequent hemorrhage are increased by vasodilation (e.g., bradykinin), by severe thrombocytopenia, and by high doses of heparin.

PGI$_2$, synthesized and released from endothelial cells close to the site of hemostatic plug formation, could inhibit platelet aggregation.[11] Thrombomodulin[12] and heparan sulfate[13] bound to endothelial cells can modulate thrombin action and thus limit fibrin formation beyond the confines of the hemostatic plug. Heparan sulfate activates AT III and so catalyzes the inhibition of thrombin and factor Xa. Thrombomodulin binds to thrombin and inhibits its ability to cleave fibrinogen, stimulate platelets, and activate factors V and VIII while markedly enhancing the ability of thrombin to catalyze the formation of active protein C. This enzyme, in turn, inactivates factors Va and VIIIa and enhances fibrinolysis, probably by binding an inhibitor of plasminogen activators.[14] Protein C activity is controlled by protein C inhibitor[15] and stimulated by protein S, a cofactor.[16] Protein S is, in turn, controlled by C4-binding protein, which complexes with it,[17] thus preventing its action. Thus the binding of thrombin to thrombomodulin alters its specificity, resulting in the loss of coagulant activity and in an increase in its ability to activate protein C and, therefore, to act as an anticoagulant. The synthesis of PGI$_2$ by endothelial cells is stimulated by epinephrine and mechanical trauma.[18] Other agonists, including histamine, ATP, and acetylcholine, stimulate endothelial cell synthesis of NO. Thus endothelial cells exposed to appropriate stimuli synthesize and release two distinct mediators of vasodilation and inhibition of platelet function. Stimulated endothelial cells also synthesize a group of peptides, known as *endothelins,* which have counterregulatory properties, including vasoconstriction.[19,20] Endothelial cells also elaborate plasminogen activators which, in the presence of fibrin, promote fibrinolysis and hemorrhage. PAI-1 is also elaborated with a different time course and in response to different stimuli.[21] Deficiency of α$_2$-antiplasmin or PAI-1 causes a bleeding tendency, an indication that unopposed

physiologic fibrinolysis disrupts the hemostatic balance.

Perturbed endothelial cells mount a procoagulant response[6] characterized by an increased synthesis and release of PAI-1, release of vWF,[22] synthesis and expression of tissue factor, and reduction of thrombomodulin. The postoperative fibrinolytic shutdown is associated with increased synthesis and release of PAI-1[21] and is mediated by cytokines elaborated as a response to tissue damage. Although these changes protect the newly formed hemostatic plug from premature dissolution, the alteration may contribute to the increased risk of postoperative venous thrombosis.

All these vascular processes are coordinated with similarly complex processes in the platelet and in plasma coagulation, fibrinolytic, and inhibitor pathways to maintain normal hemostasis. However, when the hemostatic response is excessive, intravascular thrombosis may result.

ROLE OF PLATELETS

Reactions of platelets involved in hemostasis include adhesion to the cut end of a blood vessel; spreading of adherent platelets on the exposed subendothelial matrix; secretion of stored platelet ADP, serotonin, calcium, coagulant proteins, and granule factors; and formation of large platelet aggregates. In addition, platelet membrane sites become available for binding of coagulant proteins which accelerate coagulation, resulting in formation of a fibrin network that forms a scaffold for the fragile platelet plug. The platelet-fibrin clot subsequently retracts into a compact mass.

Platelets adhere to points of endothelial disruption, e.g., at the cut end of a divided blood vessel. The binding sites are vWF, which attaches to platelet glycoprotein (GP) Ib-IX complex, and fibrinogen, as well as fibronectin, through GPIIb-IIIa.[23] These adhesive proteins form a bridge from subendothelial proteins to platelets. Bernard-Soulier disease, in which patients lack GPIb-IX, and von Willebrand's disease, in which vWF is decreased or defective, both predispose to hemorrhage. At high shear rates, such as those found in arteries, plasma vWF is required for normal adhesion of platelets to subendothelium.[24] However, at low shear rates, such as in veins, adhesion of platelets to subendothelial adhesive proteins is normal. Thus other proteins can substitute for the action of vWF. For example, collagen can interact with platelet GPIV or the integrin GPIa-IIa complex.[25] Abnormalities in either of these platelet receptors for collagen may predispose to hemorrhage.

Platelets spread on the extracellular matrix and recruit additional platelets, which adhere first to the adherent platelets and then to each other, forming platelet aggregates. Alteration in the arrangement of surface membrane glycoproteins, GPIIb-IIIa, is required to bind fibrinogen, as well as vWF, fibronectin, and vitronectin. Fibrinogen, a divalent molecule, can bridge from platelet to platelet, thereby mediating aggregation. Several other integrins, such as the vitronectin receptor, are present on the surface of both blood cells and endothelial cells and can act as receptors for adhesive proteins. Fibrinogen forms a bond only with GPIIb-IIIa on stimulated platelets, while vWF and collagen can bind to resting platelets. Glanzmann thrombasthenia, a genetic disorder in which the GPIIb-IIIa complex is deficient, presents with a severe hemorrhagic diathesis.[27] Congenital afibrinogenemia also exhibits bleeding, in part due to the abnormality in platelet aggregation. Platelet aggregation is enhanced by fibronectin and thrombospondin, which also bind to integrins.

Platelets are stimulated by multiple agonists in vitro, including physiologic compounds[28] such as thrombin, adenosine diphosphate (ADP), collagen, arachidonic acid, and epinephrine, and each has its specific receptors on the platelet surface for these agonists (Fig. 1-3). The receptor-agonist complexes couple in the platelet membrane with G proteins, which hydrolyze guanosine triphosphate (GTP). G proteins, in turn, are linked to protein kinases, which phosphorylate other proteins or the receptor protein itself. Morphologic changes accompanying these biochemical events include disappearance of the microtubules that normally maintain the platelet's discoid shape, storage granule centralization, and pseudopod formation. Agonists, such as thrombin, lead to activation of phospholipase C (PLC),

which cleaves phosphatidylinositol bisphosphate (PIP_2) to form inositol-trisphosphate (IP_3) and diacylglycerol (DAG). The latter stimulates protein kinase C (PKC),[29] and IP_3 leads to an increase of ionized calcium in the cytoplasm concentration.[30] Calcium-dependent processes include phosphorylation of the light chain of myosin by a specific kinase and hydrolysis of arachidonic acid from membrane phospholipids by phospholipase A_2.[31]

Arachidonic acid is first converted to prostaglandin endoperoxides by cyclooxygenase and then to the potent platelet agonist thromboxane A_2. Aspirin alkylates a reactive serine in cyclooxygenase, resulting in permanent inactivation of the enzyme. After thrombin stimulation, high concentrations of intracellular calcium lead to activation of a calcium-dependent neutral cysteine protease (calpain), which participates in proteolysis of cytoskeletal proteins and hydrolysis of receptor proteins.[32] DAG, like IP_3, a product of the action of PLC, activates a ubiquitous enzyme, PKC, in platelets. One of the substrates for PKC is plekstrin, a 47-kDa protein. Its function has not been established, but it may be a phosphatase that reduces ionized calcium[33] by hydrolyzing IP_3. DAG may be responsible for calcium-independent reactions associated with activation of platelets or may potentiate the activation of PKC by Ca^{2+}, thus stimulating secretion.[34]

Platelets exhibit three types of granules forming intracellular compartments, namely, dense bodies (housing serotonin, ATP, ADP, pyrophosphate, and calcium), alpha granules (storage site for fibrinogen, vWF, factor V, high-molecular-weight kininogen, fibronectin, α_1-antitrypsin, β-thromboglobulin, platelet factor 4, and platelet-derived growth factor), and lysosomes (composed of acid hydrolases). Stimulation of platelets results in activation of the platelet cytoskeletal contractile apparatus, which leads to granule centralization. Receptor-mediated stimulation results in elevated cytoplasmic calcium, polymerization of filamentous actin, and myosin light chain phosphorylation. Fusion of the granular envelope with the lining membranes of intracellular canaliculi allows external secretion of the contents of each type of granule.

ADP reacts with two receptors. One, aggregin

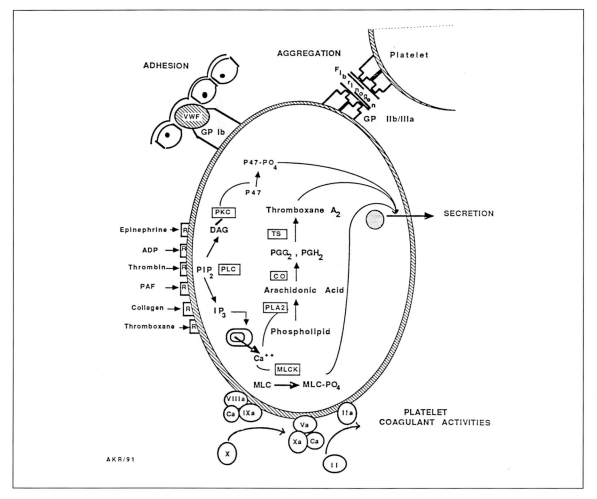

FIGURE 1-3. Platelet function (supplied by Dr. A. Koneti Rao). Adhesion to endothelial cells is mediated by glycoprotein Ib (GPIb), which binds von Willebrand factor (vWF) on the endothelial cells. Aggregation is mediated by glycoproteins IIb-IIIa (GPIIb-IIIa) bridged to GPIIb-IIIa on another platelet by fibrinogen. Various agonists such as adenosine diphosphate (ADP), platelet-activating factor (PAF), etc. are pictured as interacting with specific receptors and activating phospholipase C, probably through G proteins. This enzymes catalyzes the cleavage of phosphatidyl inositol bisphosphate (PIP$_2$) to inositol triphosphate (IP$_3$), which mobilizes Ca^{2+} from the dense tubular system to activate myosin light chain kinase (MLCK), which phosphorylates myosin light chain (MLC). Ca^{2+} also activates phospholipase A$_2$ (PLA$_2$) to release arachidonic acid from phospholipids, which is in turn converted by cyclooxygenase (CO) to PGG$_2$ and PGH$_2$ and then by thromboxane synthetase (TS) to thromboxane A$_2$. The other product of the cleavage of PIP$_2$ is diacylglycerol (DAG), which stimulates protein kinase C (PKC) to phosphorylate the intracellular protein P47 to P47-PO$_4$. The latter, thromboxane A$_2$ and MLC-PO$_4$ together stimulate secretion or products of the dense alpha and lysosomal granules. Platelet coagulant activity is generated by coagulation factors shown in Roman numerals from "tenase" (VIII, IXa, Ca^{2+}) and "prothrombinase" (Va, Xa, Ca^{2+}) on the platelet external membrane phospholipid to convert prothrombin (II) to thrombin (IIa). Reprinted with permission from Colman RW, Marder VJ, Hirsh J, Salzman EW: Overview of hemostasis. In Colman RW, Marder VJ, Hirsh J, Salzman EW (eds): Hemostasis and Thrombosis: Basic Principles and Clinical Practice, 3d ed. Philadelphia, JB Lippincott, 1994.

(100 kDa), mediates shape change and aggregation; the second (45 kDa) decreases stimulated adenylate cyclase activity and reduces platelet cyclic AMP.[35] The latter receptor is blocked by clopidogrel, an analogue of ticlopidine.[36] Epinephrine interaction with platelets proceeds through an α_2-adrenergic receptor that has been cloned and sequenced.[37] The primary structure of the human platelet thromboxane A_2 receptor has been established.[38] The mechanism by which these receptor-agonist interactions result in unmasking of fibrinogen binding sites is unknown.

Following activation, platelets expose receptors for specific plasma coagulant proteins, e.g., factors Va and VIIIa. The former may be either secreted or expressed by the platelet, while the latter is bound from plasma. These "acquired" receptors, in conjunction with anionic phospholipids exposed on activated platelets, function as binding sites, respectively, for factors Xa and IXa and thus provide an efficient catalytic environment for the conversion of prothrombin to thrombin by factor Xa[39] and activation of factor X to Xa by factor IXa.

Cyclic 3′,5′-adenosine monophosphate (cyclic AMP) is the most important negative regulator of platelets.[40] Platelets contain adenylate cyclase, the enzyme that converts ATP to cyclic AMP. Arachidonic acid products prostaglandin D_2 (PGD_2) in platelets and PGI_2 (prostacyclin) in endothelial cells stimulate this enzyme, increasing cyclic AMP. Cyclic nucleotide phosphodiesterases that hydrolyze cyclic AMP to AMP decrease intracellular cyclic AMP concentration.[41] Protein kinase A is stimulated by cyclic AMP and, in turn, by an ATP-dependent calcium pump which results in a decrease in cytosolic Ca^{2+}. Cyclic AMP inhibits all functions of platelets, including aggregation, secretion, shape change, and adhesion. Endothelial cells modulate platelet activation using surface-associated proteins, including an ADP-destroying ectoenzyme (ADPase), and thrombomodulin, a powerful thrombin inhibitor. Endothelial cells, when perturbed by exposure to ATP, produce NO, a potent vasodilator that inhibits platelet function by raising platelet cyclic GMP.[42] Platelets synthesize NO from L-arginine, which results in an increase of cyclic GMP,

which is a powerful down-regulator of platelet activity.[43] Cyclic GMP either may directly inhibit platelet activation or may competitively inhibit low-K_m cAMP phosphodiesterase.[44]

BLOOD COAGULATION

The traditional division of the coagulation system into intrinsic and extrinsic pathways has been supplanted because tissue factor–factor VIIa complex has been shown to be a potent activator of factor IX as well as factor X. The critical component is tissue factor, an intrinsic membrane protein composed of a single polypeptide chain that functions as a cofactor and therefore is analogous to the contact system cofactor HK, to the intrinsic system cofactor factor VIII, and to the "final common pathway" cofactor factor V (Fig. 1-4). Tissue factor pathway inhibitor (TFPI) is a protein which, in the presence of factor Xa, inhibits the tissue factor–factor VII complex.[45] Macrophages[46] and endothelial cells[47] synthesize tissue factor when exposed to endotoxin or IL-1.[48]

Factor VII, one of a group of vitamin K–dependent proteins (including factors IX and X, prothrombin, and protein C), is the only plasma protein unique to the extrinsic pathway. All five of these proteins are synthesized as prozymogens and are activated to serine proteases by limited proteolytic hydrolysis. The sixth family member, protein S, is the only vitamin K–dependent protein that is a cofactor rather than a zymogen. The unique γ-glutamyl carboxyl acid (Gla) residues at the N-terminal end of each molecule require vitamin K for their postribosomal formation. Gla residues are required for calcium binding; one calcium chelates with the two carboxyl groups of a Gla residue. The calcium ion then bridges to the phosphate residues of phospholipid in the cell membrane. Factor VII coagulant activity is increased by factor XIIa of the contact system, factor IXa, or factor Xa (both substrates); the more active form is designated factor VIIa. The zymogen factor VII is also capable of slow autoactivation in the presence of tissue factor. The factor VIIa–tissue factor enzyme complex, which assembles on the activated monocyte or perturbed endothelial cell, has two principal substrates, factor IX, an intrinsic pathway protein, and factor X, of the common pathway. Both factors Xa and IXa remain membrane-bound in part by its Gla residues.

The required cofactor for factor IXa to catalyze the conversion of factor X to factor Xa is factor VIII, which exists in plasma in a noncovalent complex with vWF. Hemophilia A and hemophilia B, which produce identical hemorrhagic states, are due, respectively, to decreased or dysfunctional factors VIII or IX. The clinical similarity results from a lack in each case of a proper "tenase" complex that is critical for factor X activation (see Fig. 1-4). The most severe clinical syn-

FIGURE 1-4. The clotting cascade. The central precipitating event is considered to involve tissue factor (TF), which under physiologic conditions is not exposed to the blood. With vascular and/or endothelial cell injury, TF acts in concert with activated factor VIIa and phospholipid (PL) to convert factor IX to IXa and factor X to Xa. The "intrinsic pathway" includes "contact" activation of factor XI by the factor XIIa–activated high-molecular-weight kininogen (HKa) complex. Factor XIa also converts factor IX to factor IXa, and factor IXa in turn converts factor X to factor Xa, in concert with factors VIIa and PL (the "tenase" complex). However factor Xa is formed, it is the active catalytic ingredient of the "prothrombinase" complex, which includes factor Va and PL, and converts prothrombin to thrombin. Thrombin cleaves fibrinopeptides from fibrinogen, allowing the resultant fibrin monomers to polymerize, and converts factor XIII to XIIIa, which cross-links (XL) the fibrin clot. Thrombin accelerates the process (interrupted lines) by its potential to activate factors X, VIII, and XIII, but continued proteolytic action also dampens the process by activating protein C, which degrades factors Va and VIIIa. Natural plasma inhibitors tend to retard clotting by neutralizing factor XIIa (C1-inhibitor), factor VIIa-TF (tissue factor pathway inhibitor), and factors IXa and Xa and thrombin (antithrombin III). (Arrow = active enzymes; open rectangles = cofactors or substrates; filled rectangles = sites of inhibitor action; and dashed lines = feedback reactions.) Reprinted with permission from Colman RW, Marder VJ, Hirsh J, Salzman EW: Overview of hemostasis. In Colman RW, Marder VJ, Hirsh J, Salzman EW (eds): Hemostasis and Thrombosis: Basic Principles and Clinical Practice, 3d ed. Philadelphia, JB Lippincott, 1994.

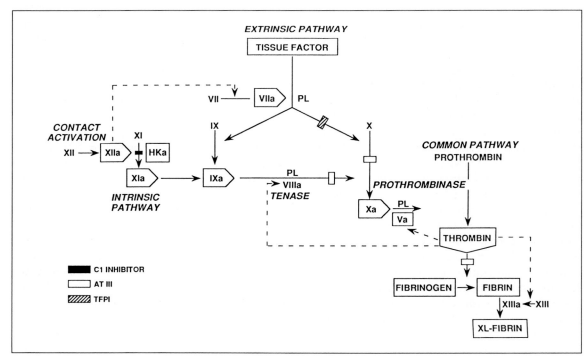

drome, manifested by spontaneous joint hemorrhage (hemarthroses), occurs with levels of 0% to 1% (factors VIII or IX). At factor levels of 5% to 30%, symptoms may be mild, except in serious trauma such as surgery. Coagulant activity above 30% of normal usually suffices for normal hemostasis. Since carriers (mean 50%) are usually asymptomatic, one can deduce that clotting proteins are usually present in excess. Deficiency in factors VII and X results in a hemorrhagic syndrome. A clinical deficiency in tissue factor has not been described.

The intrinsic system of coagulation initiated by components entirely contained within the vascular system results in the activation of factor IX by a novel dimeric serine protease, factor XIa (see Fig. 1-4), providing a pathway independent of factor VII for blood coagulation. The events in surface activation provide a paradigm for the understanding of plasma proteolytic cascades. However, the role of the contact system proteins in initiation of the intrinsic pathway of coagulation in physiologic hemostasis is unlikely; only a deficiency of factor XI is associated with a hemorrhagic tendency. A possible explanation for this paradox is that thrombin can activate factor XI.[49,50] Although this occurs in a purified system, in plasma, competing substrates such as high-molecular-weight kininogen and fibrinogen block this reaction.[51] Contact proteins participate in the initiation of the inflammatory response, complement activation, fibrinolysis, and kinin formation.[52] Factor XII (Hageman factor) binds to negatively charged surfaces and undergoes autoactivation, thus serving as the initiating protein. Activated factor XII (XIIa) has been cleaved at a single bond inside a disulfide bridge, revealing the catalytic site. Specific amino acids on the heavy chain of factor XII are responsible for binding to the surface, allowing a large increase in local concentration of the enzyme. This facilitates cleavage of its substrates, prekallikrein and factor XI, to form kallikrein and factor XIa. Further cleavage of factor XIIa results in the liberation of factor XII fragment (factor XIIf), which can activate the first component of complement as well as prekallikrein in the fluid phase. The factor XIIa heavy chain contains a kringle, an epidermal growth factor domain, and fibronectin-like binding domains.

Both prekallikrein and factor XI exist in a noncovalent bimolecular complex[53] with high-molecular-weight kininogen (HK), which, by attaching to surfaces, facilitates the reactions of factor XIIa on its substrates. The molecular assembly of cofactor, enzyme, and substrate (a recurrent theme in blood coagulation) results in maximal efficiency and speed of the molecular reactions. A negatively charged surface is involved for the contact system proteins, while for later reactions in the clotting cascade (see Fig. 1-4) a phospholipid or cell membrane provides the surface. The process of positive feedback, which is repeated elsewhere in the coagulation system, is illustrated by the action of kallikrein on its substrates, factor XII and HK. Kallikrein cleaves factor XII to convert it to factor XIIa, thereby accelerating contact activation. Kallikrein cleaves HK to liberate the nonapeptide bradykinin, which may mediate in part the hypotension in septic shock. Activated HK (HKa) binds at least 10-fold better to the surface than to the intact procofactor,[54] thereby allowing more prekallikrein or factor XI to associate with the activating surface. The conversion of factor XIIa to factor XIIf by kallikrein, an effect that switches off surface-bound coagulation, is an example of negative-feedback regulation. Another example is factor XIa cleavage of the light chain of HK, which contains the coagulant activity, thus destroying its cofactor activity.[55]

The lack of any of the three proteins involved in the contact system pathway, namely, factor XII (Hageman factor), prekallikrein, and HK, results in slow generation of thrombin and a prolonged in vitro clotting time or partial thromboplastin time. However, only a deficiency of factor XI may result in a hemostatic disorder. Thus there may be an unknown reaction that may bypass the first three contact proteins and directly activate factor XI. For example, platelets may participate in the activation of factor XI in a factor XII–independent reaction. However, factor XI deficiency only results in a mild disorder of hemostasis in half the affected individuals. Thus blood coagulation in vivo is probably initiated by factors IX or X through the extrinsic pathway.

Factor Xa slowly converts prothrombin to thrombin. Prothrombin has a distinct functional domain (Gla residues) responsible for calcium binding to phospholipid, a domain similar to epidermal growth factor containing β-hydroxyaspartic acid, which can bind Ca^{2+}, a region for cofactor (factor V) interaction, an activation peptide region, and a portion containing the catalytic center. Cleavage of prothrombin by factor Xa results in removal of the N-terminal Gla portion, and the resulting two-chain thrombin molecule detaches from the phospholipid surface. The interaction of the four components of the prothrombinase complex (factor Xa, factor V, phospholipid, and calcium) provides a markedly increased rate of prothrombin activation—more than 300,000-fold over that achievable with only the enzyme (factor Xa) and substrate (prothrombin). Factor V is probably supplied as a result of its secretion from platelet alpha granules or fusion with the plasma membrane, where it serves as a "receptor" for factor Xa binding to the activated platelet.[56] Thus the bleeding manifestations of factor V deficiency may resemble those of qualitative platelet disorders.

Plasma proteolytic inhibitors serve to limit and control the extent and speed of both blood coagulation and fibrinolytic reactions (Table 1-1). C1 inhibitor accounts for 95% of the plasma inhibitory capacity for factor XIIa and more than 50% toward kallikrein[57]; however, hereditary deficiency of C1 inhibitor results in angioedema rather than bleeding. The major inhibitor of factor XIa[58] is α_1-antitrypsin, but its major role is its inhibition of neutrophil elastase, unopposed effects of elastase in the lung alveoli, resulting in emphysema. The major inhibitor of factors IXa and Xa and thrombin is AT III. A decrease in AT III to 40% to 50% predisposes to thrombotic disorders. The striking increased risk of venous thromboembolism indicates that AT III plays a major regulatory role and that a delicate balance exists between the procoagulant and anticoagulant forces. The arginine in the active center of AT III reacts with the catalytic site, serine, in the enzymes to form covalent inactive complexes. The inhibition produced by AT III is markedly potentiated by heparin, a sulfated polysaccharide and close relative to the heparan sulfate that exists on the endothelial surface (see Fig. 1-2). Heparin binds to lysine-containing sequences in AT III and to thrombin to increase the inactivation rate. Once thrombin is bound to fibrin,[59] it is resistant to AT III and even more so to AT III–heparin complex. Heparin factor II[60] is a second inhibitor that selectively inactivates thrombin in the presence of heparin and also in the presence of dermatan sulfate.

α_2-Macroglobulin is a "back up" inhibitor for most plasma coagulant and fibrinolytic enzymes. α_2-Macroglobulin–enzyme complexes may serve as repositories of enzymatic activity because enzymes trapped in the "cage" structure of this inhibitor exhibit some enzymatic activity. In addition, the caged enzymes are protected from other inhibitors. Severe α_2-macroglobulin deficiency has not been described, and mild deficiency is asymptomatic. α_2-Antiplasmin is the primary inhibitor of plasmin.[61] The reaction prevents systemic fibrinogenolytic response to physiologic agonists, limiting the fibrinolytic response to thrombi to the affected region and allowing hemostatic plugs to remain intact. In the absence of α_2-antiplasmin, hemostatic plugs dissolve before healing has occurred, and a hemorrhage results.[62] A deficiency in PAI-1 also results in bleeding.[63] Protein C inhibitor is also a serpin that can inactivate protein C and plasminogen activators[64]

TABLE 1-1. Plasma Protease Inhibitors
of Coagulation and Fibrinolysis

Inhibitor	Major Enzymes Inhibited
C1 Inhibitor	Factor XIIa, factor XIIf, kallikrein
α_1-antitrypsin	Factor XI, elastase
Antithrombin III	Factor IXa, factor Xa, thrombin
α_2-macroglobulin	Kallikrein, thrombin, plasmin
α_2-antiplasmin	Plasmin
Heparin cofactor 2	Thrombin
Plasminogen activator inhibitor 1	t-PA, urokinase
Protein C inhibitor	Protein C, t-PA, urokinase

Reprinted with permission from Colman RW, Marder VJ, Hirsh J, Salzman EW: Overview of hemostasis. In Colman RW, Marder VJ, Hirsh J, Salzman EW (eds): Hemostasis and Thrombosis: Basic Principles and Clinical Practice, 3d ed. Philadelphia, JB Lippincott, 1994.

and thus function as a potential procoagulant molecule.

FIBRIN FORMATION AND FIBRINOLYSIS

Thrombin acts on multiple substrates, including fibrinogen, factor XIII, factors V and VIII, protein S, and protein C, as well as on platelet and endothelial cell proteins (Fig. 1-5). Thrombin plays a pivotal role in the process of hemostatic plug formation, influencing its form, rate of formation, and limitation. Thrombin action on factors VIII and V produces an increase in the "tenase" and "prothrombinase" complexes (see Figs. 1-4 and 1-5) and results in rapid fibrin strand formation. Thrombin bound to a thrombus,[65] extracellular matrix,[66] cell surface, or artificial surface is particularly effective. Not only is it localized to sites of needed coagulation, but it is also protected against inhibitors. Paradoxically, thrombin can limit the hemostatic response by combining with thrombomodulin, an endothelial cell membrane protein, thus altering its specificity. Thrombin then cannot clot fibrinogen but gains the capacity to efficiently activate the anticoagulant proteins C and S.[14] Thrombin also induces the release of t-PA, initiating local fibrinolysis, a reaction enhanced by the presence of fibrin.[67]

The final steps in hemostasis are fibrin formation and cross-linking, which, together with the primary platelet aggregate, comprise the hemostatic plug. Fibrinogen is present in high concentration in both plasma (200 to 300 mg/dL) and platelet granules and interacts with multiple hemostatic proteins, including factor XIII, fibronectin, vWF, α_2-plasmin inhibitor, PAI-1, plasminogen, and tissue plasminogen activator (t-PA). Thrombin binds to fibrinogen and liberates fibrinopeptides A and B,[68] exposing new polymerization sites[69] and resulting in fibrin monomer and polymer formation. The clot-to-plasmin degradation is influenced mainly by cross-linking, mediated by factor XIIIa.[70] In addition, by linking α_2-plasmin inhibitor to fibrin, factor XIIIa may protect the clot against fibrinolysis.[71] Factor XIII exists in plasma as a four-chain precursor molecule,[72] and after thrombin activation, the enzyme induces cross-linking of the fibrin polymer, forming covalent isopeptide bonds between lysine

FIGURE 1-5. *The multitude of actions of thrombin, resulting in procoagulant tendencies, potentiation of ongoing react feedback inhibition, or limitation of clotting. Reprinted with permission from Colman RW, Marder VJ, Hirsh J, Salzman EW: Overview of hemostasis. In Colman RW, Marder VJ, Hirsh J, Salzman EW (eds): Hemostasis and Thrombosis: Basic Principles and Clinical Practice, 3d ed. Philadelphia, JB Lippincott, 1994.*

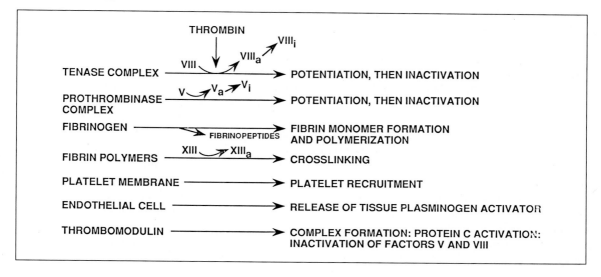

donors and glutamine receptors.[73] The two γ chains are cross-linked rapidly to form γ-γ dimers, while α chains are cross-linked more slowly to form a network.[74]

The platelets are approximated by the fibrin mesh, which also contributes to their attachment to the vessel wall. The hemostatic plug is stabilized by interactions with other adhesive proteins such as thrombospondin and fibronectin released from the platelet. These proteins may bridge the plasma proteins and the platelet interior, as well as link the fibrin fibers and the subendothelial matrix. Fibronectin is cross-linked by factor XIIIa to fibrin,[75] and its binding site for collagen could serve as an attachment site linking fibrin to the vessel wall.[76] vWF also serves as a bridge between the platelet membrane[76] and the subendothelium.[77] The Arg-Gly-Asp sequence in thrombin and the β15–42 sequence of fibrin may contribute to clot stability by inducing endothelial cell cytoskeletal changes.[78] The platelet membrane GPIIb-IIIa complex could join plasma fibrinogen (or platelet fibrinogen) to intracellular actin, thereby mediating clot retraction.[79]

Hemorrhage or thrombosis may result from derangements in fibrinogen function or concentration or with its interaction with thrombin or factor XIII. Such dysfunctional fibrinogen may manifest as a poorly polymerizing protein, as decreased liberation of a fibrinopeptide, or as inadequate cross-linking of fibrin. A deficiency or an abnormality in factor XIII may contribute to both a hemorrhagic condition and inadequate wound healing. The most common acquired disorder of fibrinogen, disseminated intravascular coagulation (DIC), is caused by systemic coagulation and/or proteolytic degradation of plasma fibrinogen by plasmin and can result in hemorrhage or thrombosis.

Hemostasis is controlled and localized by rapid vascular flow and hemodilution, by plasma protease inhibitors, by localized activation on the endothelium of an inhibitory enzyme (protein C), and by fibrinolysis. Rapid blood flow can detach small clumps of platelets from the vessel wall. Thrombin present in the hemostatic plug first contributes to its formation by activating the procofactors factors V and VIII but ultimately generates activated protein C, which inactivates these same cofactors. Factor Xa or thrombin, which diffuse away from the clot, are bound to inhibitory plasma proteins that decrease their coagulant potential. The most important inhibitor is AT III, which forms a tight complex with both factor Xa and thrombin. However, the catalytic site of thrombin is inaccessible to the inhibitor, while the enzyme is bound to fibrin. Thrombin may retain the ability to cleave fibrinopeptides even in the presence of heparin.[59] Thrombin on the endothelial cell surface binds to a specific receptor, thrombomodulin. The thrombin-thrombomodulin complex serves as an activator for protein C (see Fig. 1-2), which is released from the endothelial cell surface. After interaction with the cofactor protein S, activated protein C cleaves with factors Va and VIIIa to destroy their coagulant properties. Genetic deficiencies of protein C, protein S, and AT III predispose to pathologic thromboembolic disease.

Fibrinolysis is the most effective mechanism for limiting clot formation. Fibrinolysis involves a cascade mechanism similar to clotting factor activation with features such as zymogen-to-enzyme conversion, feedback potentiation and inhibition, and a critical balance with inhibitors. Plasminogen is the major zymogen present in plasma at twice the molar concentration of the major inhibitor of plasmin, α_2-plasmin inhibitor. Thrombin stimulates endothelial cells to release plasminogen activators and their inhibitors in a precise sequence that serves to facilitate fibrin formation.[80] Both tissue plasminogen activator and prourokinase have the capacity to convert plasminogen to plasmin.[81] Plasmin exerts positive feedback by cleavage of an activation peptide from plasminogen, rendering it more susceptible to surface binding and subsequent activation by plasminogen activators. Plasminogen bound to fibrin by lysine binding sites located on its "kringle" structures renders it a superior substrate for activated. Two proteins, lipoprotein (a), with multiple kringles,[82] and histidine-rich glycoprotein,[83] inhibit plasminogen binding to fibrin. The small proportion of plasma plasminogen bound to fibrin during clot formation is sufficient to influence subsequent physiologic fibrinolysis.[84]

However, α_2-plasmin inhibitor is also cross-linked to fibrin at the locus of factor XIIIa action,[71] while PAI-1 in the matrix[80] is bound to vitronectin.[85] The balance between profibrinolytic molecules and antifibrinolytic inhibitor molecules determines the timing and degree of clot lysis. For example, plasminogen[86] and t-PA and urokinase[87] bind to specific receptors on endothelial cells and convert Glu- to Lys-plasminogen.[88] In contrast, IL-1[89] and lipoprotein (a)[9] stimulate expression of PAI-1 on endothelial cells, favoring thrombosis. Tumor necrosis factor contributes to hemorrhage by inducing endothelial cells to produce t-PA, which activates plasminogen to plasmin, thereby converting prourokinase to urokinase, which proteolyzes the extracellular matrix.[91] Bleeding occurs when plasminogen inhibitors are deficient. Thrombosis occurs when plasminogen molecules are defective[92] or when PAI-1 is increased in the experimental transgenic mouse model.[93]

The neutral serine protease (elastase) released from neutrophil lysosomal granules by C5a or kallikrein also may contribute to local fibrinolysis.[94] Solubilized fibrin degradation products are liberated into the circulation, including unique cross-linked derivatives such as D-dimer that can be distinguished from fibrinogen degradation products[95] and which can be assayed in blood samples. D-dimers serves as a diagnostic marker of thrombin and/or factor XIIa plus plasmin action and reflects both prior clot formation and ongoing fibrinolysis. A small but significant amount of active thrombin is associated with fibrin or its derivatives that could serve to propagate the coagulant process elsewhere in the circulation.[59] Active plasmin molecules released into the circulation during fibrinolysis are extremely susceptible to inhibitor neutralization by α_2-plasmin inhibitor, thereby limiting lysis to the microenvironment of the clot. In patients with defective hemostatic plug formation, naturally occurring fibrinolysis may aggravate bleeding, and the use of fibrinolytic inhibitors such as epsilon amino caproic acid may promote hemostasis locally.

Endothelial cells and platelets, clotting factors and adhesive protein, and inhibitory mechanisms of clotting, fibrinolysis, and platelet aggregation all form an integrated system to promote the right balance and location of hemostasis. This highly developed system allows an efficient hemostatic response to hemorrhage but avoids a thrombogenic response distant from the site of injury or persisting beyond the initial stimulus and its consequences. Imbalance of this intricate process may result in a hemorrhagic or thrombotic disorder. Therapeutic intervention such as thrombolytic therapy must be prescribed carefully to correct a defect without producing its own hemostatic derangement.

Acknowledgments

I wish to acknowledge the expert manuscript preparation by Rita Stewart. This review was supported in part by grants from NHLBI, HL45486 (SCOR in Thrombosis) and HL46341, as well as a grant from NIDDK, DK43735.

REFERENCES

1. Cines DB, Tomaski A, Tannenbaum S. Immune endothelial-cell injury in heparin-associated thrombocytopenia. N Engl J Med 1987;316:581.
2. MacGregor RR, Friedman HM, Macarak EJ, Kefalides NA. Virus infection of endothelial cells increases granulocyte adherence. J Clin Invest 1980;65:1469.
3. LeRoy EC, Ager A, Gordon JL. Effects of neutrophil elastase and other proteases on porcine aortic endothelial prostaglandin I$_2$ production, adenine nucleotide release, and responses to vasoactive agents. J Clin Invest 1984;74:1003.
4. Janoff A, Sloan B, Weinbaum G, et al. Experimental emphysema induced with purified human neutrophil elastase: tissue localization of the instilled protease. Am Rev Respir Dis 1977;115:461.
5. Kitchens CS. The anatomical basis of purpura. Prog Hemost Thromb 1982;5:211.
6. Nawroth PP, Handley DA, Esmon CT, Stern DM. Interleukin 1 induces endothelial cell procoagulant while suppressing cell-surface anticoagulant activity. Proc Natl Acad Sci USA 1986;83:3460.
7. Schleef RR, Bevilacqua MP, Sawdey M, et al. Cytokine activation of vascular endothelium: effects on tissue-type plasminogen activator and type 1 plasminogen activator inhibitor. J Biol Chem 1988;263:5797.
8. Hynes RO. Integrins: a family of cell surface receptors. Cell 1987;48:549.

9. Dustin ML, Garcia Aguilar J, Hibbs ML, et al. Structure and regulation of the leukocyte adhesion receptor LFA-1 and its counterreceptors, ICAM-1 and ICAM-2. Cold Spring Harb Symp Quant Biol 1989;54(pt 2):753.

10. Hession C, Osborn L, Goff D, et al. Endothelial leukocyte adhesion molecule: I. Direct expression cloning and functional interactions. Proc Natl Acad Sci USA 1990;87:1673.

11. Weksler BB, Marcus AJ, Jaffe EA. Synthesis of prostaglandin I$_2$ (prostacyclin) by cultured human and bovine endothelial cells. Proc Natl Acad Sci USA 1977;74:3922.

12. Esmon CT, Owen WG. Identification of an endothelial cell cofactor for thrombin-catalyzed activation of protein C. Proc Natl Acad Sci USA 1981; 78:2249.

13. Lollar P, Owen WG. Clearance of thrombin from circulation in rabbits by high-affinity binding sites on endothelium: possible role in the inactivation of thrombin by antithrombin III. J Clin Invest 1980;66:1222.

14. Esmon NL, Owen WG, Esmon CT. Isolation of a membrane-bound cofactor for thrombin-catalyzed activation of protein C. J Biol Chem 1982;257:859.

15. Heeb MJ, Espana F, Geiger M, et al. Immunological identity of heparin-dependent plasma and urinary protein C inhibitor and plasminogen activator inhibitor-3. J Biol Chem 1987;262:15813.

16. Walker FJ. Regulation of activated protein C by protein S: the role of phospholipid in factor Va inactivation. J Biol Chem 1981;256:11128.

17. Dahlback B. Inhibition of protein Ca cofactor function of human and bovine protein S by C4b-binding protein. J Biol Chem 1986;261:12022.

18. MacIntyre DE, Pearson JD, Gordon JL. Localization and stimulation of prostacyclin production in vascular cells. Nature 1978;271:549.

19. Warner TD, Mitchell JA, de Nucci G, Vane JR. Endothelin-1 and endothelin-3 release EDRF from isolated perfused arterial vessels of the rat and rabbit. J Cardiovasc Pharmaco 1989;13(suppl 5): S85.

20. MacCumber MW, Ross CA, Glaser BM, Snyder SH. Endothelin: visualization of mRNAs by in situ hybridization provides evidence for local action. Proc Natl Acad Sci USA 1989;86:7285.

21. Wiman B, Chmielewska J, Ranby M. Inactivation of tissue plasminogen activator in plasma: demonstration of a complex with a new rapid inhibitor. J Biol Chem 1984;259:3644.

22. Ribes JA, Francis CW, Wagner DD. Fibrin induces release of von Willebrand factor from endothelial cells. J Clin Invest 1987;79:117.

23. Pytela R, Pierschbacher MD, Ginsberg MH, et al. Platelet membrane glycoprotein IIb/IIIa: member of a family of Arg-Gly-Asp–specific adhesion receptors. Science 1986;231:1559.

24. Weiss HJ, Turitto VT, Baumgartner HR. Effect of shear rate on platelet interaction with subendothelium in citrated and native blood: I. Shear rate–dependent decrease of adhesion in von Willebrand's disease and the Bernard-Soulier syndrome. J Lab Clin Med 1978;92:750.

25. Staatz WD, Rajpara SM, Wayner EA, et al. The membrane glycoprotein Ia-IIa (VLA-2) complex mediates the Mg^{++}-dependent adhesion of platelets to collagen. J Cell Biol 1989;108:1917.

26. Lam SC, Plow EF, DSouza SE, et al. Isolation and characterization of a platelet membrane protein related to the vitronectin receptor. J Biol Chem 1989;264:3742.

27. Nurden AT, Caen JP. The different glycoprotein abnormalities in thrombasthenic and Bernard-Soulier platelets. Semin Hematol 1979;16:234.

28. Colman RW. Platelet receptors. Hematol Oncol Clin North Am 1990;4:27.

29. Nishizuka Y. The role of protein kinase C in cell surface signal transduction and tumour promotion. Nature 1984;308:693.

30. Feinstein MB. The role of calcium in blood platelet function. In: Weiss GB, ed. Calcium in drug action. New York: Plenum Press, 1978:197.

31. Pickett WC, Jesse RL, Cohen P. Initiation of phospholipase A2 activity in human platelets by the calcium ion ionophore A23187. Biochim Biophys Acta 1976;486:209.

32. Colman RW, Hoffman I. Calpains and hemostasis. In: Mellgren R, Murachi T, eds. Intracellular calcium-dependent proteolysis. Boca Raton, FL: CRC Press, 1990:211.

33. Berridge NJ. Inositol trisphosphate and diacylglycerol as second messengers. Biochem J 1984;220: 345.

34. Rink TJ, Sanchez A, Hallam TJ. Diacylglycerol and phorbol ester stimulate secretion without raising cytoplasmic free calcium in human platelets. Nature 1983;305:317.

35. Mills DC, Figures WR, Scearce LM, et al. Two mechanisms for inhibition of ADP-induced platelet shape change by 5'-p-fluorosulfonylbenzoyladenosine: conversion to adenosine, and covalent modification at an ADP binding site distinct from that which inhibits adenylate cyclase. J Biol Chem 1985;260:8078.

36. Mills DC, Puri R, Hu CJ, et al. Clopidogrel inhibits the binding of ADP analogues to the receptor mediating inhibition of platelet adenylate cyclase. Arterioscler Thromb 1992;12:430.

37. Kobilka BK, Matsui H, Kobilka TS, et al. Cloning, sequencing, and expression of the gene coding for the human platelet alpha 2-adrenergic receptor. Science 1987;238:650.

38. Hirata M, Hayashi Y, Ushikubi F, et al. Cloning and expression of cDNA for a human thromboxane A$_2$ receptor. Nature 1991;349:617.

39. Hoyer LW, Colman RW, Wyshock EG. Coagulation cofactors: factors VIII and V. In: Colman RW, Hirsh J, Marder VJ, Salzman EW, eds. Hemostasis and thrombosis: basic principles and clinical practice. 3rd ed. Philadelphia: JB Lippincott, 1993: 109.

40. Haslam RJ, Davidson MM, Fox JE, Lynham JA. Cyclic nucleotides in platelet function. Thromb Haemost 1978;40:232.

41. Grant PG, Colman RW. Purification of cAMP phosphodiesterase from platelets. Methods Enzymol 1988;159:772.

42. Rapoport RM, Murad F. Endothelium-dependent and nitrovasodilator-induced relaxation of vascular smooth muscle: role of cyclic GMP. J Cyclic Nucleotide Protein Phosphor Res 1983;9:281.

43. Radomski MW, Palmer RM, Moncada S. An L-arginine/nitric oxide pathway present in human platelets regulates aggregation. Proc Natl Acad Sci USA 1990;87:5193.

44. Grant PG, Colman RW. Purification and characterization of a human platelet cyclic nucleotide phosphodiesterase. Biochemistry 1984;23:1801.

45. Rao LV, Rapaport SI. Studies of a mechanism inhibiting the initiation of the extrinsic pathway of coagulation. Blood 1987;69:645.

46. Edwards RL, Rickles FR. Macrophage procoagulants. Prog Hemost Thromb 1984;7:183.

47. Colucci M, Balconi G, Lorenzet R, et al. Cultured human endothelial cells generate tissue factor in response to endotoxin. J Clin Invest 1983;71: 1893.

48. Bevilacqua MP, Pober JS, Majeau GR, et al. Interleukin 1 (IL-1) induces biosynthesis and cell surface expression of procoagulant activity in human vascular endothelial cells. J Exp Med 1984;160: 618.

49. Gailani D, Broze GJ Jr. Factor XI activation in a revised model of blood coagulation. Science 1991; 253:909.

50. Naito K, Fujikawa K. Activation of human blood coagulation factor XI independent of factor XII: factor XI is activated by thrombin and factor XIa in the presence of negatively charged surfaces. J Biol Chem 1991;266:7353.

51. Scott CF, Colman RW. Fibrinogen blocks the autoactivation and thrombin-mediated activation of factor XI on dextran sulfate. Proc Natl Acad Sci USA 1992;89:11189.

52. Colman RW. Surface-mediated defense reactions: the plasma contact activation system. J Clin Invest 1984;73:1249.

53. Mandle RJ, Colman RW, Kaplan AP. Identification of prekallikrein and high-molecular-weight kininogen as a complex in human plasma. Proc Natl Acad Sci USA 1976;73:4179.

54. Scott CF, Silver LD, Schapira M, Colman RW. Cleavage of human high-molecular-weight kininogen markedly enhances its coagulant activity: evidence that this molecule exists as a procofactor. J Clin Invest 1984;73:954.

55. Scott CF, Silver LD, Purdon AD, Colman RW. Cleavage of human high-molecular-weight kininogen by factor XIa in vitro: effect on structure and function. J Biol Chem 1985;260:10856.

56. Miletich JP, Jackson CM, Majerus PW. Properties of the factor Xa binding site on human platelets. J Biol Chem 1978;253:6908.

57. Schapira M, Scott CF, Colman RW. Protection of human plasma kallikrein from inactivation by C1 inhibitor and other protease inhibitors: the role of high molecular weight kininogen. Biochemistry 1981;20:2738.

58. Scott CF, Schapira M, James HL, et al. Inactivation of factor XIa by plasma protease inhibitors: predominant role of alpha 1-protease inhibitor and protective effect of high-molecular-weight kininogen. J Clin Invest 1982;69:844.

59. Hogg PJ, Jackson CM. Fibrin monomer protects thrombin from inactivation by heparin–antithrombin III: implications for heparin efficacy. Proc Natl Acad Sci USA 1989;86:3619.

60. Tollefsen DM, Majerus DW, Blank MK. Heparin cofactor II: purification and properties of a heparin-dependent inhibitor of thrombin in human plasma. J Biol Chem 1982;257:2162.

61. Moroi M, Aoki N. Isolation and characterization of alpha$_2$-plasmin inhibitor from human plasma: a novel proteinase inhibitor which inhibits activator-induced clot lysis. J Biol Chem 1976;251:5956.

62. Koie K, Kamiya T, Ogata K, Takamatsu J. Alpha$_2$-plasmin-inhibitor deficiency (Miyasato disease). Lancet 1978;2:1334.

63. Schleef RR, Higgins DL, Pillemer E, Levitt LJ. Bleeding diathesis due to decreased functional activity of type 1 plasminogen activator inhibitor. J Clin Invest 1989;83:1747.

64. Suzuki K, Deyashiki Y, Nishioka J, et al. Characterization of a cDNA for human protein C inhibitor: a new member of the plasma serine protease inhibitor superfamily. J Biol Chem 1987;262:611.

65. Francis CW, Markham RE Jr, Barlow GH, et al. Thrombin activity of fibrin thrombi and soluble plasmic derivatives. J Lab Clin Med 1983;102:220.

66. Bar Shavit R, Eldor A, Vlodavsky I. Binding of thrombin to subendothelial extracellular matrix: protection and expression of functional properties. J Clin Invest 1989;84:1096.

67. Levin EG, Marzec U, Anderson J, Harker LA. Thrombin stimulates tissue plasminogen activator release from cultured human endothelial cells. J Clin Invest 1984;74:1988.

68. Blomback B, Blomback M. The molecular structure of fibrinogen. Ann NY Acad Sci 1972;202:77.

69. Pandya BV, Gabriel JL, OBrien J, Budzynski AZ.

Polymerization site in the beta chain of fibrin: mapping of the B beta 1–55 sequence. Biochemistry 1991;30:162.

70. Robbins KC. A study on the conversion of fibrinogen to fibrin. Am J Physiol 1944;142:581.

71. Sakata Y, Aoki N. Cross-linking of alpha 2-plasmin inhibitor to fibrin by fibrin-stabilizing factor. J Clin Invest 1980;65:290.

72. Schwartz ML, Pizzo SV, Hill RL, McKee PA. Human factor XIII from plasma and platelets: molecular weights, subunit structures, proteolytic activation and cross-linking of fibrinogen and fibrin. J Biol Chem 1973;248:1395.

73. Folk JE, Finlayson JS. The epsilon-(gamma-glutamyl)lysine cross-link and the catalytic role of transglutaminases. Adv Protein Chem 1977;31:1.

74. McKee PA, Mattock P, Hill RL. Subunit structure of human fibrinogen, soluble fibrin, and cross-linked insoluble fibrin. Proc Natl Acad Sci USA 1970; 66:738.

75. Mosher DF. Action of fibrin-stabilizing factor on cold-insoluble globulin and alpha$_2$-macroglobulin in clotting plasma. J Biol Chem 1976;251:1639.

76. Ruoslahti E, Pekkala A, Engvall E. Effect of dextran sulfate on fibronectin-collagen interaction. FEBS Lett 1979;107:51.

77. Wagner DD, Urban Pickering M, Marder VJ. Von Willebrand protein binds to extracellular matrices independently of collagen. Proc Natl Acad Sci USA 1984;81:471.

78. Bar Shavit R, Sabbah V, Lampugnani MG, et al. An Arg-Gly-Asp sequence within thrombin promotes endothelial cell adhesion. J Cell Biol 1991;112:335.

79. Nachmias V, Sullender J, Asch A. Shape and cytoplasmic filaments in control and lidocaine-treated human platelets. Blood 1977;50:39.

80. Schleef RR, Podor TJ, Dunne E, et al. The majority of type 1 plasminogen activator inhibitor associated with cultured human endothelial cells is located under the cells and is accessible to solution-phase tissue-type plasminogen activator. J Cell Biol 1990;110:155.

81. Lijnen HR, Collen D. Interaction of plasminogen activators and inhibitors with plasminogen and fibrin. Semin Thromb Hemost 1992;8:2.

82. Mao SJ, Tucci MA. Lipoprotein (a) enhances plasma clot lysis in vitro. FEBS Lett 1990;267:131.

83. Lijnen HR, Hoylaerts M, Collen D. Isolation and characterization of a human plasma protein with affinity for the lysine binding sites in plasminogen:

role in the regulation of fibrinolysis and identification as histidine-rich glycoprotein. J Biol Chem 1980;255:10214.

84. Alkjaersig N, Fletcher NP, Sherry S. The mechanism of clot dissolution by plasmin. J Clin Invest 1959;38:1086.

85. Preissner KT, Grulich Henn J, Ehrlich HJ, et al. Structural requirements for the extracellular interaction of plasminogen activator inhibitor 1 with endothelial cell matrix-associated vitronectin. J Biol Chem 1990;265:18490.

86. Hajjar KA, Harpel PC, Jaffe EA, Nachman RL. Binding of plasminogen to cultured human endothelial cells. J Biol Chem 1986;261:11656.

87. Hajjar KA, Hamel NM. Identification and characterization of human endothelial cell membrane binding sites for tissue plasminogen activator and urokinase. J Biol Chem 1990;265:2908.

88. Hajjar KA, Nachman RL. Endothelial cell-mediated conversion of Glu-plasminogen to Lys-plasminogen: further evidence for assembly of the fibrinolytic system on the endothelial cell surface. J Clin Invest 1988;82:1769.

89. Nachman RL, Hajjar KA, Silverstein RL, Dinarello CA. Interleukin 1 induces endothelial cell synthesis of plasminogen activator inhibitor. J Exp Med 1986;163:1595.

90. Etingin OR, Hajjar DP, Hajjar KA, et al. Lipoprotein (a) regulates plasminogen activator inhibitor-1 expression in endothelial cells: a potential mechanism in thrombogenesis. J Biol Chem 1991;266:2459.

91. Niedbala MJ, Picarella MS. Tumor necrosis factor induction of endothelial cell urokinase-type plasminogen activator mediated proteolysis of extracellular matrix and its antagonism by gamma-interferon. Blood 1992;79:678.

92. Aoki N, Moroi M, Sakata Y, et al. Abnormal plasminogen: a hereditary molecular abnormality found in a patient with recurrent thrombosis. J Clin Invest 1978;61:1186.

93. Erickson LA, Fici GJ, Lund JE, et al. Development of venous occlusions in mice transgenic for the plasminogen activator inhibitor-1 gene. Nature 1990;346:74.

94. Plow E: Leukocyte elastase release during blood coagulation: a fibrinolytic system. J Clin Invest 1982;69:564.

95. Kopec M, Teisseyre E, Dudek-Wojciechowska G. Studies on "double D" fragment from stabilized bovine fibrin. Thromb Res 1973;2:283.

Anthony J. Comerota (Ed.). *Thrombolytic Therapy for Peripheral Vascular Disease.* Copyright © 1995 J. B. Lippincott Company.

2

PATHOGENESIS OF THROMBOSIS

Ik-Kyung Jang

Valentin Fuster

PATHOGENESIS OF ATHEROMATOUS PLAQUE

Vascular injury is divided into three types depending on the severity of the damage[1] (Fig. 2-1). Type I consists of functional alterations without obvious morphologic changes; it initiates spontaneous atherosclerosis in the vessel wall. Type II consists of endothelial denudation and intimal injury without penetration into internal elastic lamina; it is usually caused by spontaneous plaque rupture and also occurs following venous bypass graft. Type III is a deeper injury involving both intima and media; it often results from percutaneous transluminal angioplasty. In the development of spontaneous atherosclerosis, intimal injury of various degrees (type I) seems to occur continuously as a result of turbulent blood flow and motion and contraction of the artery.[2,3] The denuded areas rapidly become covered with mural thrombi consisting mainly of platelets and fibrin (type II). Platelets and thrombin in the thrombi enhance the lipid uptake of macrophages and thereby lead to foam cell formation and atherosclerosis. At the same time, platelets and thrombin stimulate smooth muscle cell proliferation and migration, thereby accelerating the progression of atherosclerotic plaques.[4–6] Smooth muscle cells and fibroblasts also synthesize connective tissue and incorporate lipid into the cells. All these processes lead to the formation of a fibromuscular lesion or fibrous capsule of a lipid-rich plaque that can be ruptured leading to type III injury with thrombus formation.

Macrophages play an important role in these processes. Macrophages, originated from circulating monocytes, lipid-laden smooth muscle cells, and extracellular lipid, contribute to atherogenesis by enhancing transport and oxidation of low-density lipoprotein, secreting mitogenic factors, and generating toxic products such as free radicals.[7–10] In addition, macrophages release proteases, such as elastase and collagenase, thereby forming an abscess that makes the plaque prone to rupture.[11] Furthermore, macrophages may release tissue factor and plasminogen activator inhibitor 1 and promote local thrombosis.[12]

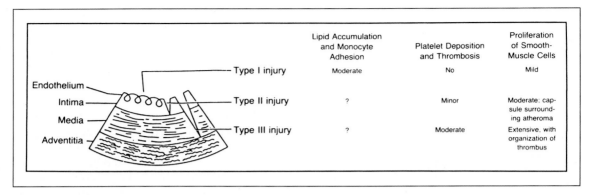

FIGURE 2-1. Three types of vascular injury and vascular response. (Adapted with permission from Fuster et al. The pathogenesis of coronary artery disease and the acute coronary syndrome. N Engl J Med 1992;326:242.)

PLAQUE RUPTURE AND THROMBOSIS

When atheromatous plaque ruptures, thrombus is formed at the site of rupture.[13] This thrombus may embolize distally, causing distal limb ischemia, or progressively encroach the lumen, resulting in proximal limb ischemia. The exact mechanism of plaque rupture is unknown. It may include mechanical tear by high shear forces, changes in vascular tone or turbulence at the site of stenosis, or disruption of ingrown vasa vasorum causing intraplaque hemorrhage and plaque expansion.[14] It may just be an incidental event during the evolution of atheromatous plaque, which occurs when the cap has thinned to the extent that normal hemodynamic stresses may fragment it. Enzymes may be released by macrophages that digest collagen and elastin of the fibrous cap of atheromatous plaque. When rupture occurs, several events may follow: (1) the contents of the plaque may discharge and embolize distally, (2) blood pressure may extend the tear and cause intraplaque hemorrhage, and (3) platelets may begin to aggregate at the site of rupture, resulting in partial or complete obstruction of the lumen or distal embolization.[14–16] The ratio of platelets to fibrin of the intraluminal thrombus formed in association with plaque rupture depends on several factors. These include the geometry of plaque, the mechanism of rupture, the presence of side branches or collaterals, and the degree of residual lumen. In any case, the core of

the thrombus always consists of platelet-rich material, and the above-mentioned factors determine the ratio of platelets to fibrin.

Activation of Platelets

Platelets may be activated by several different pathways. When plaque ruptures, subendothelium exposes collagen on the bottom of the plaque. The collagen, in conjunction with thrombin generated locally from the coagulation system, stimulates phospholipase C on platelet membrane phosphatidylinositol and releases calcium from the dense granules into the cytoplasm. Calcium induces platelet contraction, with a further release of arachidonate, serotonin, and adenosine diphosphate. Adenosine diphosphate, released from red blood cells and platelet-dense granules, induces platelet-platelet interaction in the presence of calcium and fibrinogen by exposure of binding receptors such as IIb-IIIa to fibrinogen and von Willebrand factor, resulting in platelet aggregation. Another pathway is initiated by arachidonate from the platelet membrane (Fig. 2-2). Arachidonate is converted to thromboxane A_2 by cyclooxygenase and thromboxane synthetase. Thromboxane A_2 is not only a strong agonist for platelet aggregation but also a strong vasoconstrictor. It exposes occult fibrinogen and von Willebrand factor binding sites in the glycoprotein IIb-IIIa complex by mobilizing intracellular calcium.[17,18]

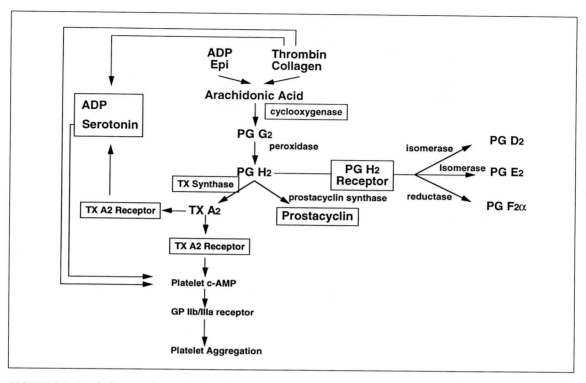

FIGURE 2-2. *Arachidonic acid cascade shows different steps to induce platelet aggregation (ADP, adenosine diphosphate; c-AMP, cyclic adenosine monophosphate; Epi, epinephrine; GP, glycoprotein; PG, prostaglandin; TX, thromboxane).*

When platelets become activated, membrane receptors, such as Ib, Ia, and IIb-IIIa, are exposed. In the arterial system with a high shear rate, both glycoprotein Ib and IIb-IIIa appear to play an important role in platelet-subendothelium interaction (platelet adhesion) through von Willebrand factor[19,20] and fibrinogen. The relative importance of von Willebrand factor to fibrinogen in platelet adhesion has been tested using various models and antibodies.[21–25] These studies invariably showed that von Willebrand factor is more important than fibrinogen in platelet-subendothelium interaction. Glycoprotein Ia is important in platelet adhesion through collagen.[26] Platelet-platelet interaction (aggregation) is mainly mediated by the glycoprotein IIb-IIIa receptor. Fibrinogen has been thought to play a major role in platelet aggregation, because defective platelet aggregation in thrombasthenia patients was ascribed to fibrinogen. However, recent studies have shown

that von Willebrand factor or other adhesive proteins may be more important than fibrinogen. In patients with afibrinogenemia, platelet aggregation was preserved,[27,28] and even when antibody to fibrinogen was added to the blood of patients with afibrinogenemia to remove even a trace of fibrinogen, platelet aggregation, even though reduced, was still preserved to some extent.[29] In addition, a specific monoclonal antibody against glycoprotein IIb-IIIa that blocks von Willebrand factor and other adhesive proteins but not fibrinogen decreased platelet aggregation, suggesting that von Willebrand factor or other adhesive proteins blocked by this antibody also might be important in platelet aggregation.[30]

Activation of the Coagulation System

When the plaque ruptures, both intrinsic and extrinsic coagulation systems become activated by

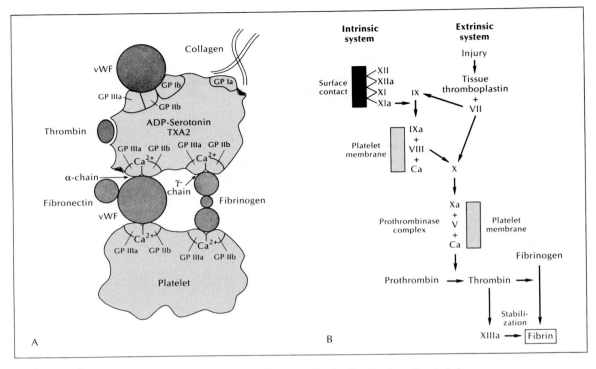

FIGURE 2-3. (**A**) *Platelet membrane receptors and adhesive molecules for platelet-subendothelium and platelet-platelet interaction.* (**B**) *Intrinsic and extrinsic coagulation pathways.*

collagen and tissue factor exposed in the subendothelium (Fig. 2-3). Factors IX, VIII, X, and V are activated on the platelet membrane. Tissue factor activates not only the extrinsic system by binding factors VII and VIIa in the presence of calcium but also the intrinsic system by activating factors IX and X[31,32] and thereby plays a major role in the whole coagulation system. The final product, thrombin, catalyzes fibrinogen to fibrin, stabilizes fibrin through the cross-linking by factor XIII, and stimulates new thrombin generation by stimulating factors V and VIII. In addition, thrombin is a strong agonist for platelet aggregation.[33–35] Activated platelets increase prothrombinase activity,[36,37] which further promotes thrombin production from prothrombin. Thrombin, when generated in the circulation, is rapidly inhibited by antithrombin III. However, fibrin-bound thrombin is partially protected from circulating antithrombin III and thus continues to produce fibrin and activate platelets.

Role of Thrombus in Atherogenesis

Thrombus plays an important role not only in the development of new atheromatous plaques but also in the progression of plaques. There seems to be continuous plaque fissuring and healing by organization of thrombus on the plaque surface. Pathologic studies have shown evidence of recurrent fissures on the plaque surface, which gradually lead to vascular obstruction.[14,15] Indeed, recent studies revealed the presence of platelet- and fibrin-related products inside the plaque using antibodies specifically directed to platelet, fibrin, fibrinogen, and fibrin or fibrinogen degradation products.[38,39] The mechanism of fibrotic organization of thrombus is not known. Platelets may play a key role by releasing substances such as platelet-derived growth factor and transforming growth factor β. This hypothesis is supported by animal experiments in rabbits and pigs. In rabbits with thrombocytopenia, intimal hyperplasia was significantly reduced following balloon injury as compared with that in control rabbits with normal platelets.[40,41] von Willebrand factor is an important protein for platelet adhesion and aggregation. Pigs lacking this protein (those with von Willebrand's disease) had significantly less mural thrombus and atherosclerosis.[42,43] All this in vitro and in vivo evidence supports the role of thrombus in the generation and growth of atheromatous plaques.

ACUTE OCCLUSION

When the lumen is totally occluded, thrombus propagates both proximally and distally and forms "head" and "tail" parts that consist mainly of fibrin and red cells due to blood stasis.[16,44,45] The ratio of platelets to fibrin is clinically important because platelet-rich thrombus is much more resistant to thrombolytic therapy than fibrin- and erythrocyte-rich clot[46] and therefore requires a strong antiplatelet regimen in conjunction with fibrinolysis.

RISK FACTORS FOR THROMBOSIS

The development, progression, and duration of local thrombosis following plaque rupture depends on local factors as well as systemic thrombogenic risk factors (Table 2-1). Some of these risk factors can be modified by preventive or therapeutic measures and thereby may alter the clinical course.

Local Factors

The depth of plaque disruption is important to the extent and the stability of thrombus. Using a pig extracorporeal-perfusion model, Badimon et al.[47] showed that on the vessel wall with superficial damage, platelet thrombus reached a peak at

TABLE 2-1. *Local and Systemic Thrombogenic Risk Factors*

Local factors
    Degree of plaque disruption (i.e., collagen, tissue factor)
    Degree of stenosis (i.e., change in geometry)
    Residual thrombus (i.e., thrombin)
Systemic factors
    Epinephrine levels (i.e., stress, circadian variation, smoking)
    Cholesterol and lipoprotein (a) levels
    Fibrinogen and factor VII levels

5 to 10 minutes after exposure and then embolized distally, suggesting that the thrombus was not stable. The exposure of collagen type I (mimicking a deep vessel injury) on the perfusion system produced a dense platelet thrombus that did not embolize spontaneously. In the clinical setting, superficial injury to a plaque leads to a transient occlusive thrombus, causing reversible limb ischemia. Deep injury to a plaque exposes collagen, tissue factor, and other vessel components, leading to persistent thrombotic occlusion and infarction. This process may be partially altered by antiplatelet therapy such as aspirin.

The degree of residual stenosis determines the shear rate and local platelet activation. Lassila et al.[48] demonstrated that platelet deposition parallels the degree of stenosis. Although this may not be as important as the degree of plaque disruption in the initiation of thrombosis, the degree of residual lumen may be the most important factor for reocclusion following spontaneous or pharmacologic thrombolysis. Balloon angioplasty is a widely used modality for this purpose.

Residual thrombus appears to be the most thrombogenic stimulus.[49] The degree of platelet deposition is increased two to four times on a residual thrombus as compared with a deeply injured arterial wall. After partial lysis of a thrombus, thrombin bound to fibrin may become exposed to circulating blood and stimulate both platelets and the coagulation system. Complete thrombolysis with a potent thrombolytic agent during a sufficient period of time should be able to reduce reocclusion following a successful thrombolysis.

Systemic Risk Factors

Several systemic factors may be important in a primary hypercoagulable or thrombogenic state of circulation. Catecholamines may stimulate platelet aggregation and enhance thrombin generation. There is evidence to support their role in arterial thrombosis; arterial thrombosis appears to be related to emotional stress,[50,51] circadian variation,[52,53] and cigarette smoking,[54] which also may be related to the release of catecholamines.

Other important risk factors are hypercholesterolemia[55] and lipoprotein (a).[56] Lipoprotein (a) is similar to plasminogen in structure, resulting in competitive inhibition of the fibrinolytic properties of plasminogen[57] and predisposing patients to thrombotic complications. Other coagulation factors, such as fibrinogen and factor VII, have been implicated as thrombogenic risk factors. Several studies have shown that high plasma fibrinogen concentrations are also independent risk factors for cardiovascular disease.[58,59] It is difficult to modify some of the systemic thrombogenic risk factors (stress, fibrinogen, and coagulation factor VII). However, intense effort should be delivered to alter some of the risk factors that can be changed, such as smoking and hypercholesterolemia.

Summary

Thrombosis plays a crucial role in the development, progression, and acute exacerbation of peripheral vascular disease. Following spontaneous intimal injury, platelets begin to adhere to and aggregate at the site of injury, forming a mural thrombus. Organization of the thrombus and smooth muscle cell proliferation, migration, and hyperplasia lead to the development of atheromatous plaques. This process occurs repeatedly, and as a consequence, atheromatous plaques are formed. When the plaque separating the atheromatous lipid pool from the arterial lumen ruptures, both coagulation system and platelets become activated by tissue factor, thrombin, and collagen. This leads to formation of a larger thrombus which may encroach the lumen and cause clinical symptoms such as limb ischemia and/or necrosis.

Conclusion

When atheromatous plaque ruptures, both the coagulation system and platelets become activated by exposed tissue factor, thrombin, and collagen in the subendothelium. This results in the formation of a mural thrombus, which may grow into the lumen, causing a proximal limb ischemia, or may embolize distally, causing a distal ischemia. Activated platelets also release vasoactive substances, such as thromboxane A_2 and serotonin, and cause vasospasm, which promotes further local platelet aggregation. Local and systemic thrombogenic risk factors have been identified. Modification of these risk factors may abort or attenuate clinical events.

References

1. Fuster V, Badimon L, Badimon JJ, Chesebro J. The pathogenesis of coronary artery disease and the acute coronary syndrome. N Engl J Med 1992; 326:242.
2. Davies MJ, Woolf N, Rowles PM, Pepper J. Morphology of the endothelium over atherosclerotic plaques in human coronary arteries. Br Heart J 1988;60:459.
3. Davies MJ, Bland MJ, Hartgartner WR, et al. Factors influencing the presence or absence of acute coronary thrombi in sudden ischemic death. Eur Heart J 1989;10:203.
4. Schwartz CJ, Valente AJ, Kelly JL, et al. Thrombosis and the development of atherosclerosis: Rokitansky revisited. Semin Thromb Hemost 1988;14: 189.
5. Cunningham DD, Farrell DH. Thrombin interaction with cultured fibroblasts: relationship to mitogenic stimulation. Ann NY Acad Sci 1986; 485:240.
6. Shuman MA: Thrombin-cellular interactions. Ann NY Acad Sci 1986;485:288.
7. Steinberg D, Parthasarathy S, Carew TE, et al. Beyond cholesterol: modifications of low-density lipoprotein that increase its atherogenicity. N Engl J Med 1989;320:915.
8. Schwartz CJ, Valente AJ, Sprague EA, et al. The pathogenesis of atherosclerosis. Clin Cardiol 1991; 14(suppl 1):I-1.

9. Mitchinson MJ, Ball RY. Macrophages and athero-genesis. Lancet 1987;2:146.

10. Gown AM, Tsukada T, Ross R. Human atherogen-esis: II. Immunocytochemical analysis of the cellu-lar composition of human atherosclerotic lesions. Am J Pathol 1986;125:191.

11. Richardson PD, Davies MJ, Born GVR. Influence of plaque configuration and stress distribution on fissuring of coronary artery atherosclerotic plaques. Lancet 1989;2:941.

12. Drake TA, Morrissey JH, Edgington TS. Selective cellular expression of tissue factor in human tis-sues: implications for disorders of hemostasis and thrombosis. Am J Pathol 1989;134:1087.

13. Falk E. Unstable angina with fatal outcome: dy-namic coronary thrombosis leading to infarction and/or sudden death: autopsy evidence of recur-rent mural thrombosis with peripheral emboliza-tion culminating in total vascular occlusion. Cir-culation 1985;71:699.

14. Davies MJ, Thomas AC. Plaque fissuring: the cause of acute myocardial infarction, sudden is-chemic death, and crescendo angina. Br Heart J 1985;53:363.

15. Falk E. Plaque rupture with severe pre-existing stenosis precipitating coronary thrombosis: char-acteristics of coronary atherosclerotic plaques underlying fatal occlusive thrombi. Br Heart J 1983;50:127.

16. Friedman M, Van den Bovenkamp GJ. The patho-genesis of a coronary thrombus. Am J Pathol 1966;48:19.

17. Shattil SJ, Brass LP. Induction of the fibrinogen re-ceptor on human platelets by intracellular media-tors. J Biol Chem 1987;262:992.

18. Coller BS. Activation affects access to the platelet receptor for adhesive glycoprotein. J Cell Biol 1986;103:451.

19. Sakariassen KS, Nievelstein PF, Coller BS, Sixma JJ. The role of platelet membrane glycoproteins Ib and IIb/IIIa in platelet adherence to human artery subendothelium. Br J Haematol 1986;63:681.

20. Weiss HJ, Turitto VT, Baumgartner HR. Effect of shear rate on platelet interaction with subendo-thelium in citrated and native blood: I. Shear rate–dependent decrease of adhesion in von Wille-brand's disease and the Bernard-Soulier syndrome. J Lab Clin Med 1978;92:750.

21. Ruggeri ZM, Bader R, de Marco L: Galnzmann thrombasthenia: deficient binding of von Wille-brand factor to thrombin-stimulated platelets. Proc Natl Acad Sci USA 1982;79:6038.

22. Sakariassen K, Bolhuis PA, Sixma J. Human blood platelet adhesion to artery subendothelium is me-diated by factor VII–von Willebrand factor bound to the subendothelium. Nature 1979;279:636.

23. Badimon L, Badimon JJ, Turitto VT, Fuster V. Platelet deposition in von Willebrand factor defi-cient vessel wall. J Lab Clin Med 1987;110:634.

24. Badimon L, Badimon JJ, Turitto VT, Fuster V. Platelet interaction to vessel wall and collagen: study in homozygous von Willebrand's disease as-sociated with abnormal collagen aggregation in swine. Thromb Haemost 1989;61:57.

25. Badimon L, Badimon JJ, Turitto VT, Fuster V. Role of von Willebrand factor in mediating platelet–vessel wall interaction at low shear rate: the im-portance of perfusion conditions. Blood 1989;73:961.

26. George JN, Nurden AT, Phillips DR. Molecular de-fects in interaction of platelets with the vessel wall. N Engl J Med 1984;311:1084.

27. Cattaneo M, Kinlough-Rathbone R, Lecchi A, et al. Fibrinogen-independent aggregation and deaggre-gation of human platelets: studies in two afibrino-genemic patients. Blood 1987;70:221.

28. Soria J, Soria C, Borg JY, et al. Platelet aggregation occurs in congenital afibrinogenemia despite the absence of fibrinogen or its fragments in plasma and platelets, as demonstrated by immunoenzy-mology. Br J Haematol 1985;60:503.

29. Weiss HJ, Hawiger J, Ruggeri ZM, et al. Fibrino-gen-independent interaction of platelets with sub-endothelium mediated by glycoprotein IIb-IIIa complex at high shear rate. J Clin Invest 1989;83:288.

30. Lombardo VT, Hodson E, Roberts JR, et al. Inde-pendent modulation of von Willebrand factor and fibrinogen binding to the platelet membrane gly-coprotein IIb/IIIa complex as demonstrated by monoclonal antibody. J Clin Invest 1985;76:1950.

31. Nemerson T. The reaction between bovine brain tissue factor and factor VII and X. Biochemistry 1966;5:601.

32. Osterud B, Rapaport SI. Activation of factor IX by the reaction product of tissue factor and factor VII: additional pathway for initiating blood coagula-tion. Proc Natl Acad Sci USA 1977;74:5260.

33. Hanson SR, Harker LA. Interruption of acute platelet-dependent thrombosis by the synthetic antithrombin D-phenylalanyl-L-prolyl-L-arginyl chloromethyl ketone. Proc Natl Acad Sci USA 1988;85:3184.

34. Heras M, Chesebro JH, Penny WJ, et al. Effects of thrombin inhibition on the development of acute platelet-thrombus deposit or during angioplasty in pigs: heparin vs hirudin, a specific thrombin in-hibitor. Circulation 1989;79:657.

35. Jang IK, Gold HK, Ziskind AA, et al. Prevention of platelet-rich arterial thrombosis by selective thrombin inhibition. Circulation 1990;81:219.

36. Miletich JP, Jackson CM, Majerus PW. Interaction of coagulation factor Xa with human platelets. Proc Natl Acad Sci USA 1977;74:4033.

37. Rosing J, van Rijn JL, Bevers EM, et al. The role of activated human platelets in prothrombin and factor X activation. Blood 1985;65:319.

38. Bini A, Fenoglia JJ Jr, Mesa-Tejada R, et al. Identification and distribution of fibrinogen, fibrin, and fibrin(ogen) degradation products in atherosclerosis: use of monoclonal antibody. Arteriosclerosis 1989;9:109.

39. Smith EB, Kean A, Grant A, Stirk C. Fate of fibrinogen in human arterial intima. Arteriosclerosis 1990;10:263.

40. Cohen P, McComb HC. Platelets and atherogenesis: II. Amelioration of cholesterol atherogenesis in rabbits with reduced platelet counts as a result of ^{32}P administration. J Atheroscler Res 1968; 8:389.

41. Friedman RJ, Stemerman MB, Werz B, et al. The effect of thrombocytopenia on experimental arteriosclerotic lesion formation in rabbit. J Clin Invest 1977;60:1191.

42. Fuster V, Bowie JW, Lewis JC, et al. Resistance to atherosclerosis in pigs with von Willebrand's disease: spontaneous and high cholesterol diet-induced arteriosclerosis. J Clin Invest 1978;61: 722.

43. Fuster V, Fass DN, Kaye MP, et al. Arteriosclerosis in normal and von Willebrand pigs: long-term prospective study and aortic transplantation study. Circ Res 1982;51:587.

44. Mizuno K, Satomura K, Miyamoto A, et al. Angioscopic evaluation of coronary-artery thrombi in acute coronary syndrome. N Engl J Med 1992; 326:287.

45. Jang IK, Gold HK. Angioscopic evaluation of coronary artery thrombi in acute coronary syndromes. N Engl J Med 1992;327:206.

46. Jang IK, Gold HK, Ziskind AA, et al. Differential sensitivity of erythrocyte-rich and platelet-rich arterial thrombi to lysis with recombinant tissue-type plasminogen activator: a possible explanation for resistance to coronary thrombolysis. Circulation 1989;79:920.

47. Badimon L, Badimon JJ, Turitto VT, et al. Platelet thrombus formation on collagen type I: a model of deep vessel injury: influence of blood rheology, von Willebrand factor, and blood coagulation. Circulation 1988;78:1431.

48. Lassila R, Badimon JJ, Vallabhajosula S, Badimon L: Dynamic monitoring of platelet deposition on severely damaged vessel wall in flowing blood: effects of different stenosis on thrombus growth. Arteriosclerosis 1990;10:306.

49. Badimon L, Badimon JJ. Mechanism of arterial thrombosis in nonparallel streamlines: platelet thrombi grow at the apex of stenotic severely injured vessel wall. Experimental study in the pig model. J Clin Invest 1989;84:1134.

50. Grignani G, Soffiantino F, Zucchella M, et al. Platelet activation by emotional stress in patients with coronary artery disease. Circulation 1991;83: II-128.

51. Yeung AC, Vekshtein VI, Krantz DS, et al. The effect of atherosclerosis on the vasomotor response of coronary arteries to mental stress. N Engl J Med 1991;325:1551.

52. Muller JE, Stone PH, Turi ZG, et al. Circadian variation in the frequency of onset of acute myocardial infarction. N Engl J Med 1985;313:1315.

53. Tofler GH, Brezinski D, Schafer AI, et al. Concurrent morning increase in platelet aggregability and the risk of myocardial infarction and sudden cardiac death. N Engl J Med 1987;316:1514.

54. Fuster V, Chesebro JH, Frye RL, Elveback LR. Platelet survival and the development of coronary artery disease in the young adult: effects of cigarette smoking, strong family history and medical therapy. Circulation 1981;63:546.

55. Badimon JJ, Badimon L, Turitto VT, Fuster V. Platelet deposition at high shear rates is enhanced by high plasma cholesterol levels: in vivo study in the rabbit model. Arteriolscler Thromb 1991;11: 395.

56. Rosengren A, Wilhelmsen L, Eriksson E, et al. Lipoprotein (a) and coronary heart disease: a prospective case-control study in a general population sample of middle-aged men. Br Med J 1990;301: 1248.

57. Hajjar KA, Gavish D, Breslow JL, Nachman RL. Lipoprotein (a) modulation of endothelial surface fibrinolysis and its potential role in atherosclerosis. Nature 1989;339:303.

58. Wilhelmsen L, Svardsudd K, Korsan-Bengtsen K, et al. Fibrinogen as a risk factor for stroke and myocardial infarction. N Engl J Med 1984;311:501.

59. Rosengren A, Wilhelmsen L, Welin L, et al. Social influences and cardiovascular risk factors as determinants of plasma fibrinogen concentration in a general population sample of middle aged men. Br Med J 1990;300:634.

3

THE FIBRINOLYTIC SYSTEM: NORMAL PHYSIOLOGY AND PATHOPHYSIOLOGY

Charles W. Francis

The fibrinolytic system plays a central role in hemostasis, functioning to regulate the extent of fibrin formation and to remove fibrin deposits when they are no longer needed. Like the coagulation system, it is carefully regulated to provide local activation without causing unwanted systemic effects. It differs, however, from the coagulation system in its slower and more prolonged duration of action, which allows formation of a stable hemostatic plug before it is degraded and removed. The fibrinolytic system is controlled through the coordinated interaction of activators, zymogens, and inhibitors (Fig. 3-1) whose properties localize and enhance activity at sites of fibrin deposition.

PLASMINOGEN ACTIVATORS

Plasminogen activators are enzymes that initiate fibrinolysis by converting the zymogen plasminogen to the fibrinolytic enzyme plasmin. Two types of plasminogen activators have been described, including tissue-type plasminogen activator (t-PA) and urokinase-like plasminogen activator (u-PA), and these differ in structural, immunologic, and functional properties (Table 3-1 and Fig. 3-2). Despite these differences, both types of plasminogen activators are serine proteases that have high specific activity in converting plasminogen to plasmin through cleavage of a single peptide bond. Endothelial cells are the principal physiologic source of t-PA,[1-3] but t-PA also has been isolated from other tissues and malignant cell lines.[4-6] Synthesized as a single-chain molecule of 530 amino acid residues,[7] t-PA can be converted to a two-chain form by kallikrein or plasmic cleavage of a single peptide bond,[8-10] and this conversion to the two-chain form increases binding affinity for fibrin.[11] Tissue-type plasminogen activators bind and express greater enzymatic activity in the presence of fibrin,[9,12-14] properties that localize and enhance fibrinolytic potential at sites of fibrin formation. The fibrin affinity of t-PA derives from the kringle structures, which are homologous to those in plasminogen,[7,15] and also from the "finger" domain, which is similar to the fibrin-binding regions of fibronectin.[7,16] Single-chain u-PA has structural similarities to t-PA, but it contains only

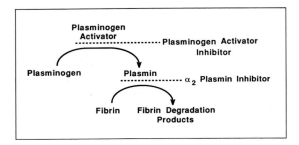

FIGURE 3-1. Schematic diagram of the fibrinolytic system showing the interaction of activators and inhibitors (dotted lines).

a single kringle and lacks the finger domain[17-20] (see Fig. 3-2). Although single-chain u-PA has little enzymatic activity[21] and does not bind avidly to fibrin, it does have fibrin-specific thrombolytic activity, which is possibly due to the ability of fibrin to prevent its inactivation by plasma inhibitors.[22] An alternative explanation for its fibrin specificity proposes that single-chain u-PA has greater affinity for fibrin-bound plasminogen than for circulating plasma plasminogen.[21,23] Either plasmin or kallikrein efficiently converts single-chain u-PA to the two-chain form,[24,25] which can be degraded proteolytically from M_r 54,000 to 33,000.[26,27] The two-chain forms of u-PA are less fibrin-specific than single-chain u-PA but have greater enzymatic

activity.[20,24] The proteolytic inhibitor plasminogen activator inhibitor 1 inhibits both two-chain forms of u-PA but does not inhibit single-chain u-PA.[28,29]

Several plasminogen activators have been developed or are under evaluation for use in treatment. Urokinase for therapeutic use has been purified from human urine and from the culture medium of human embryonic kidney cells. Several preparations are available that contain variable proportions of the larger- and smaller-molecular-weight forms of two-chain u-PA, and these do not differ significantly in their therapeutic effect or changes in blood coagulation.[30] Urokinase also has been cloned recently and expressed in vitro[31] and is under clinical study. Streptokinase is purified for therapeutic use from cultures of β-hemolytic streptococci but has been cloned recently and expressed in vitro,[32] raising the possibility that a more purified preparation with reduced pyrogenic and allergic properties can be produced for therapeutic use. By itself, streptokinase has no enzymatic activity, but it forms an equimolar complex with plasminogen, and the complex functions as a plasminogen activator.[33] Since both streptokinase and urokinase have low fibrin affinity, systemic plasminemia and proteolytic degradation of plasma fibrinogen and other proteins occur during therapeutic adminis-

TABLE 3-1. Molecular Components of the Fibrinolytic System

Molecule	Molecular Weight	Plasma Concentration	Plasma Half-Life	Properties
Plasminogen	88,000	200 μg/ml	2.2 days	Binds to fibrin through lysine binding sites; converted to plasmin by activators
Plasmin	88,000	0	0.1 s	Serine proteinase that cleaves fibrin
Tissue-plasminogen activator	68,000	2 ng/ml	5 min	Binds to fibrin and has greater activity in presence of fibrin; single-chain form rapidly converted to two-chain molecule by plasmin
Single-chain urokinase plasminogen activator	54,000	4 ng/ml	Stable	Little enzymatic activity; converted to two-chain form by plasmin or kallikrein
Two-chain urokinase plasminogen activator	54,000 33,000	0	10 min	Normally present in urine; larger form converted to smaller by plasmin
Streptokinase	48,000	0	30 min	Inactive until complexed with plasminogen
α2-Plasmin inhibitor	70,000	70 μg/ml	3 days	Rapidly inactivates plasmin; factor XIIIa cross-links to fibrin
Plasminogen activator inhibitor 1	52,000	30 ng/ml	—	Inactivates t-PA and two-chain u-PA; circulates in complex with vitronectin; binds to fibrin

tration. A chemically modified streptokinase derivative, acylated plasminogen:streptokinase activator complex, has been synthesized for therapeutic use and contains an unstable blocking group at its active site. This molecule is enzymatically inactive until deacylation of the active site occurs, either in the blood or after attachment to fibrin.[34] These properties give it a relatively long half-life, which results in a sustained fibrinolytic effect after bolus administration.[35,36]

The need for fibrinolytic agents with improved pharmacologic properties has provided the stimulus for development of newer activators.

Biotechnology techniques have been applied successfully in the synthesis of both t-PA and single-chain u-PA. A number of genetically engineered mutants of t-PA have been produced with modifications to either slow clearance from the circulation[37] or prevent inactivation by inhibitors,[38] and study of these mutants has contributed significantly to understanding the biochemistry of fibrinolysis.[39] Other innovative approaches have linked t-PA with monoclonal antibodies specific for fibrin[40] or platelets[41] to further restrict its action to sites of fibrin deposition and to reduce systemic effects. Other naturally occurring activa-

FIGURE 3-2. Schematic representation of the domainal structures of plasminogen, tissue plasminogen activator, and single-chain u-PA. Intact plasminogen has an N-terminal glutamic acid and is called Glu-plasminogen to distinguish it from partially degraded forms with different N-terminal amino acids. Plasminogen activators cleave the Arg_{560}-Val peptide bond that demarcates the heavy and light chains of plasmin. Plasmin attacks other plasminogen molecules at several points, most important at Lys_{76}-Lys_{77}, to liberate an activation peptide from the amino-terminal portion of the heavy chain, leaving Lys-plasminogen. The heavy chain consists mostly of five repeat kringle structures, the first four of which contain a single high-affinity and several low-affinity lysine binding sites for substrate proteins. The serine active site of plasmin (H, histidine; D, asparatic acid; S, serine) is located on the light chain and represents the major site of interaction with α_2-antiplasmin, but antiplasmin also can interact with the lysine binding sites. Tissue-plasminogen activator contains a finger domain similar to those present on fibronectin and a fibrin binding site on its second kringle, which provides fibrin specificity for this protein. Single-chain u-PA is very similar in structure to t-PA except for the presence of the finger domain and the presence of one instead of two kringle structures.

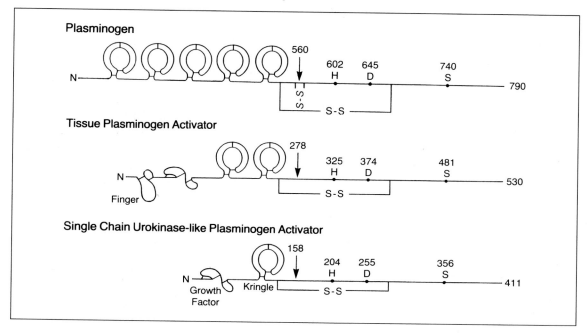

tors with unique properties also have been identified, including staphylokinase from *Staphylococcus aureus*[42,43] and vampire bat plasminogen activator, which is very highly fibrin specific.[44] The potential therapeutic application of these activators is being explored in both in vitro animal and clinical studies.

CONVERSION OF PLASMINOGEN TO PLASMIN

All plasminogen activators share the ability to form plasmin from the inactive plasma zymogen plasminogen, which circulates in plasma at a concentration of approximately 2.4 μM (see Table 3-1). Figure 3-2 illustrates the location of disulfide bonds and functional domains for fibrin binding, plasmin activation, and protease activity. Plasminogen activators hydrolyze the Arg_{560}-Val bond, converting plasminogen to the two-chain molecule plasmin.[45,46] The heavy-chain structures termed *kringles* contain the lysine binding sites that contribute to fibrin binding.[47] The fibrinolytic inhibitory activity of the lysine analogue epsilon aminocaproic acid (EACA) is due to its ability to compete with plasminogen for binding to these lysine binding sites.[48] The activity of the principal physiologic plasmin inhibitor (α_2-plasmin inhibitor) is also mediated in part by its capacity to block fibrin attachment of plasminogen through the lysine binding sites.[49,50]

Plasmic cleavage near the amino terminus liberates a peptide of approximately 70 residues and converts Glu-plasminogen to the smaller Lys-plasminogen, which has increased fibrin affinity and specific activity.[51–55] Therefore, under physiologic conditions, plasminogen may be converted to plasmin through two pathways. In one, intact Glu-plasminogen can be converted directly by plasminogen activators to Glu-plasmin,[56] and plasmin can then cleave Glu-plasminogen to the Lys-form. In the second pathway, Lys-plasminogen can be produced initially by cleavage of the activation peptide, followed rapidly by activation to Lys-plasmin.[57] All forms of plasmin are endopeptidases which hydrolyze susceptible arginine and lysine bonds in fibrin, fibrinogen, and other proteins as well as most synthetic substrates susceptible to trypsin.

FIBRINOLYTIC INHIBITORS

The principal physiologic inhibitor of plasmin is α_2-antiplasmin, which is present in both platelets and plasma[58,59] (see Table 3-1). The very short half-life of plasmin in plasma is due to its rapid reaction with antiplasmin, which results in formation of a stable complex and irreversibly inhibits the enzyme.[50,60,61] When plasmin is bound to fibrin, it is inactivated more slowly than free plasmin[50] because the lysine binding sites that contribute to interaction with the inhibitor are already bound to fibrin and therefore inaccessible. α_2-Antiplasmin also can be cross-linked to fibrin by the action of factor XIIIa,[62] and this contributes to the increased resistance to lysis of cross-linked fibrin clots.[63,64] Other protease inhibitors are less important in regulating fibrinolysis, although α_2-macroglobulin may play a limited physiologic role, particularly if the capacity of α_2-plasmin inhibitor is exceeded.

The principal inhibitor of plasminogen activators is plasminogen activator inhibitor 1 (PAI-1) a 52,000-Da glycoprotein present in platelets,[65] endothelial cells,[66,67] and endothelial cell matrix,[68,69] as well as in plasma at a higher physiologic concentration than that of plasminogen activators (see Table 3-1). Amino acid sequences of both PAI-1 and α_2-antiplasmin have been determined, and they demonstrate homology with other members of the serpin family.[70,71] PAI-1 in plasma is protected from inactivation by circulating in complex with vitronectin.[72,73] PAI-1 binds specifically to fibrin, where it retains activity in inhibiting plasminogen activator,[74] and PAI-1 is also found in the extracellular matrix, where it may inhibit local proteolysis.[68,69] PAI-1 inhibits single-chain t-PA, two-chain t-PA, and two-chain u-PA but has no affinity for single-chain u-PA.[28,29] Plasminogen activator inhibitor 2 (PAI-2) is distinct from PAI-1 and appears in increasing concentration in plasma in the third trimester of pregnancy,[75] but it is otherwise not found in normal plasma. Its role in regulation of fibrinolysis is uncertain.

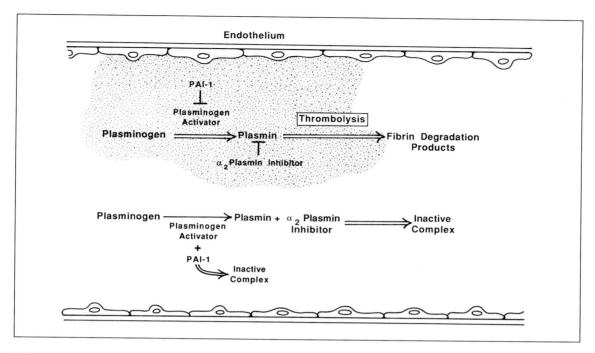

FIGURE 3-3. Molecular interactions of physiologic thrombolysis resulting in local activation and systemic inhibition. Properties of the thrombus promote conversion of plasminogen to plasmin and limit the action of inhibitors, resulting in efficient plasmin generation on the fibrin substrates. Plasmin formation in the blood is inhibited by the action of PAI-1, and free plasmin is efficiently inhibited by α₂-antiplasmin to prevent a systemic proteolytic state that could degrade plasma proteins, especially fibrinogen.

REGULATION OF FIBRINOLYSIS

The coordinated regulation required to achieve efficient, localized activation of fibrinolysis without systemic affects is achieved by complex interactions among blood, thrombus, and endothelial cells (Fig. 3-3). Fibrin formation itself provides an important stimulus for activation of fibrinolysis and also contributes to the regulatory mechanisms (Table 3-2). Approximately 4% of plasma plasminogen binds to fibrin during clotting, and it is incorporated throughout the thrombus,[76,77] with specific binding mediated through sites on the kringle domains (see Fig. 3-2). This makes plasminogen available on the fibrin fibers, where it can be activated efficiently by plasminogen activators. The binding of t-PA to fibrin and the increased enzymatic activity of fibrin-bound t-PA and single-chain u-PA further contribute to rapid conversion of fibrin-bound plasminogen to plas-

min.[9,12–14,21,23] Fibrin-bound plasmin is relatively resistant to inhibition by α₂-antiplasmin,[50] and this property allows degradation of the fibrin matrix to proceed while systemic effects are pre-

TABLE 3-2. Properties of Fibrin
that Regulate Fibrinolysis

Promote fibrinolysis
- Plasminogen binding
- t-PA binding
- Enhancement of t-PA activity
- u-PA binding
- Exposure of new lysine binding sites during fibrinolysis
- Protection of bound plasmin from antiplasmin
- Stimulation of t-PA release from endothelial cells
- Inhibition of PAI-1 release from endothelial cells

Inhibit fibrinolysis
- PAI-1 binding
- Antiplasmin binding and crosslinking
- α-Chain cross-linking

vented. The initial plasmic degradation of fibrin accelerates further fibrinolysis in a positive-feedback mechanism by creating additional sites for plasminogen binding.[78,79] Plasmin action also converts Glu- to Lys-plasminogen, thereby increasing fibrin binding and enzymatic activity.[51–55] Plasmin action also converts single-chain t-PA to the two-chain form, which has greater fibrin affinity.[11] Fibrin also may promote activation of fibrinolysis by inhibiting the secretion of PAI-1 from endothelial cells.[80]

Specific fibrin properties also prevent premature clot dissolution. PAI-1 binds specifically to fibrin, and fibrin-bound PAI-1 can inhibit both t-PA and two-chain u-PA.[74] Factor XIIIa covalently cross-links α_2-plasmin inhibitor to fibrin in roughly equimolar amounts to that of bound plasminogen[62,64] and factor XIIIa mediates cross-linking of α chains into large polymers which increase resistance to plasmic degradation.[81,82] Thrombi containing large amounts of platelets may be relatively resistant to degradation because platelets contain both PAI-1 and antiplasmin and also provide factor XIII required for cross-linking of α_2-antiplasmin and fibrin α chain.

Clot size and blood flow are also determinants of fibrinolytic rate. Large thrombi have a relatively small surface of adjacent endothelium, and this may provide inadequate plasminogen activator for rapid dissolution. In contrast, the high ratio of endothelial cells to fibrin in small hemostatic plugs or microvascular thrombi in conditions such as disseminated intravascular coagulation can support rapid lysis to maintain vascular patency. The speed of delivery of activator and rate of transport into the thrombus are also determinants of fibrinolytic rate which are particularly important in the setting of fibrinolytic therapy when rapid clot dissolution of large thrombi is the goal. In vitro studies demonstrate that the speed of fibrinolysis is related to the rate of transport of activator into the thrombus.[83] Clinical observations also indicate that reperfusion occurs more rapidly if activator can be injected directly into a thrombus rather than infused into the blood proximally,[84,85] providing further evidence for the importance of transport in fibrinolytic therapy.

Endothelial cells also play a critical role in

TABLE 3-3. Effects of Endothelial Cells on Fibrinolysis

- Binding of plasminogen
- Binding of u-PA and t-PA
- Accelerated conversion of bound plasminogen to plasmin
- Rapid conversion of bound Glu- to Lys-plasminogen
- Synthesis of t-PA
- Synthesis of PAI-1
- Protection of bound plasmin and t-PA from antiplasmin and PAI-1

regulation of the fibrinolytic system[86] (Table 3-3). Endothelial cells have specific binding sites for plasminogen and for plasminogen activators,[87–90] and binding accelerates plasmin formation because endothelial cell-bound Glu-plasminogen is rapidly converted to the more active Lys-plasminogen[91] and because the binding of both activators and plasminogen to the cell surface accelerates cleavage to plasmin.[88] Also, t-PA and plasmin bound to the surfaces of endothelial cells are relatively protected from inhibition by their plasma inhibitors.[90] This cell-surface assembly of fibrinolytic proteins that localizes and enhances fibrinolysis at the interface of blood and vessel wall may play an important role in maintaining vascular patency and also contribute to the nonthrombogenic properties of endothelial cells. Endothelial cells play an additional role in regulation of fibrinolysis through synthesis of plasminogen activators and of PAI-1. Endothelial cell synthesis of PAI-1 and of t-PA is regulated by a variety of agents, including growth factors and inflammatory cytokines,[92–96] and these effects could be important in the pathogenesis of thrombotic events associated with inflammation.

Other plasma protein systems also modulate fibrinolysis and may contribute to dysregulation and hemostatic abnormalities. Lipoprotein (a) [Lp(a)] has extensive structural homology with plasminogen, and it can compete with plasminogen for binding to its endothelial cell receptor.[97,98] This property could contribute to the increased risk of atherosclerosis associated with elevated plasma concentrations of Lp(a) by decreasing endothelial cell surface fibrinolytic activity. The protein C system is also involved in regulation of fibrinolysis, since activated protein C can inactivate PAI-1,[99] thereby accelerating clot lysis.

Thrombospondin and histidine-rich glycoprotein interact with plasminogen through lysine binding sites, and these proteins may play an additional role in limiting local fibrinolysis.[100–102]

PLASMIC DEGRADATION OF FIBRINOGEN AND FIBRIN

The pattern of plasmic degradation of fibrinogen and of fibrin is determined by the location and accessibility of bonds susceptible to cleavage by plasmin. The six polypeptide chains of fibrin are arranged in a trinodular form with a central domain joining the two halves of the molecules at their amino-terminal ends (Fig. 3-4). The central domain is connected by α-helical regions to lateral domains containing the carboxyl-terminal portions of all polypeptide chains and from which a long extension of the α chain protrudes. The initial sites of plasmin action are in the Aα chain appendage and generate the fragment X derivatives, the smallest of which has an M_r of 250,000. Following this, the α-helical regions joining the central and lateral domains are cleaved asymmetrically to yield fragment D and fragment Y. Fragment Y is then cleaved into a second fragment D and fragment E, which represents the central domain of the original fibrinogen molecule.[103]

Plasmic degradation of fibrin is similar to that of fibrinogen, with the principal differences resulting from factor XIIIa–mediated covalent cross-linking. Plasmic degradation of non-cross-linked fibrin produces essentially the same degradation products as from fibrinogen except that Bβ15–42 rather than Bβ1–42 is produced by degradation of the amino terminus of the Bβ chain. Degradation of cross-linked fibrin differs in two ways. First, degradation is slower because of the extensive cross-linking of α chains, which increases proteolytic resistance. Second, the degradation products have a distinctive structure primarily because the covalent and noncovalent bonds that hold the terminal domains together remain in soluble derivatives. The initial cleavages degrade the cross-linked α-chain polymer and the connecting α-helical regions at the same sites that are attacked in fibrinogen and non-cross-linked

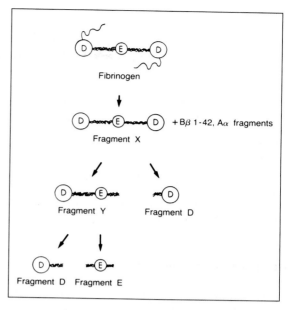

FIGURE 3-4. *Asymmetrical degradation of fibrinogen by plasmin. The principal structures are the three globular domains from which degradation products D and E derive, the α-helical coils that connect them, and the long Aα-chain extensions from each of the terminal (fragment D) domain regions. Fragment X consists of all three domainal regions but lacks the Aα-chain extensions and the Bβ1–42 peptide derived from the N terminus of the Bβ chain. Fragment Y consists of a central E domain with either of the terminal (fragment D) domains connected by the coiled coil. Fragment Y is degraded further to a second fragment D and fragment E by cleavage of the remaining coiled coil.*

fibrin[104] (Fig. 3-5). The largest degradation products consist of domains linked longitudinally by γ-chain cross-links and laterally by noncovalent bonds to the complementary chain of the two-stranded protofibril. The smallest unique degradation product of cross-linked fibrin is fragment DD, which consists of two fragment D domains joined by cross-linking between γ chains.[105] DD may retain noncovalent bonding to fragment E, thereby forming a DD/E complex.[106] Larger complexes consisting of combinations of longer portions of each chain of the protofibril can be degraded progressively by plasmin into smaller complexes,[107] but plasma proteolytic inhibitors may limit such degradation in vitro.

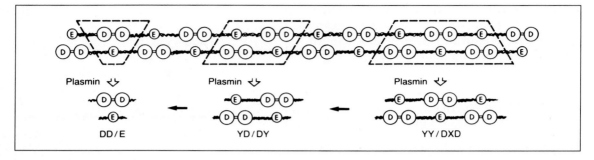

FIGURE 3-5. *Plasmic degradation products of cross-linked fibrin. Plasmic degradation of a two-stranded protofibril results in several noncovalently bound complexes, the smallest of which is DD/E. Each complex consists of fragments derived from each strand of the protofibril attached noncovalently to complementary regions.*

PATHOLOGIC FIBRINOLYSIS

Coagulation and fibrinolysis are carefully coordinated physiologically to provide for prompt control of bleeding followed by resolution and restoration of normal tissue function and structure. Disordered regulation of either the coagulation or fibrinolytic systems can lead to abnormal hemostasis and either bleeding or thrombosis. Hypofunction of the fibrinolytic system can result from either deficient activation or excessive inhibition and ultimately lead to thrombosis (Fig. 3-6). Conversely, bleeding may result from overactive fibrinolysis due to either excessive stimulation or defective inhibition. Congenital disorders of fibrinolysis that cause thrombosis or bleeding are rare, but elucidation of the molecular mechanisms involved has contributed significantly to the understanding of both normal and pathologic fibrinolysis. Acquired fibrinolytic disorders are more frequent but often occur in the setting of systemic diseases that also can affect the coagulation system and platelet function, and this makes it difficult to dissect the contribution of abnormal fibrinolysis to the overall hemostatic disorder. The most common causes of abnormalities in fibrinolysis result from therapeutic administration of plasminogen activators or antifibrinolytic agents, and the clinical results confirm the importance of maintaining the delicate balance between clot formation and dissolution. Thus successful fibrinolytic therapy that dissolves an occluding coronary thrombus and results in reperfusion of ischemic myocardium also may cause troublesome bleeding at the site of arteriotomy or even fatal intracranial hemorrhage. Conversely, antifibrinolytic therapy given to control hemorrhage may similarly tip the balance and predispose to deep vein thrombosis or exacerbate underlying disseminated intravascular coagulation.

FIGURE 3-6. *The hemostatic balance between coagulation and fibrinolysis. Abnormal regulation can lead to either thrombosis or bleeding.*

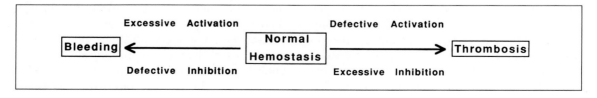

HYPERFIBRINOLYSIS AND BLEEDING

Excessive fibrinolytic activation can cause premature dissolution of hemostatic plugs and result in a bleeding disorder. A congenital disorder due to increased circulating levels of plasminogen activator has been described[108,109] that caused hemorrhagic symptoms, including fatal intracranial hemorrhage. The patients had increased plasma t-PA levels, shortened clot lysis times, and low plasma fibrinogen concentrations, and treatment with fibrinolytic inhibitors resulted in improvement in laboratory parameters. A novel transgenic mouse model of hyperfibrinolytic bleeding due to increased circulating plasminogen activator also has been developed.[110] Increased hepatic expression of u-PA resulted in very high plasma u-PA concentrations and hypofibrinogenemia. Spontaneous and fatal neonatal hemorrhage developed in some mice, but survivors without bleeding were able to transmit the hyperfibrinolytic phenotype to their offspring. This model may permit detailed studies of the pathophysiology of hyperfibrinolysis and the development of potential therapeutic interventions. Hyperfibrinolysis due to congenital deficiency of the plasmin inhibitor α_2-antiplasmin has been described as an autosomal recessive condition resulting in a bleeding disorder.[111–113] The homozygous deficiency of α_2-antiplasmin resulted in nearly undetectable plasma levels and a severe lifelong bleeding disorder, including hemarthrosis and delayed bleeding after trauma or surgery. Systemic fibrinolysis was not present, as indicated by a normal plasma fibrinogen concentration, suggesting that the bleeding was due to premature lysis of hemostatic plugs and not the result of systemic plasminemia. Individuals with heterozygous α_2-antiplasmin deficiency may be either asymptomatic or exhibit a mild bleeding tendency.[114] Antiplasmin deficiency due to synthesis of a dysfunctional molecule with a mutation near the reactive site also has been reported to result in a bleeding disorder.[115] Also, a bleeding disorder due to a dysfunctional PAI-1 molecule with reduced t-PA inhibitory capacity has been described in a patient with a lifelong history of bleeding.[116] Systemic plasminemia was not pres-

ent, and bleeding was treated successfully with EACA. A bleeding disorder due to complete deficiency of PAI-1 as a result of a frame-shift mutation also has been described.[117]

Hyperfibrinolysis may contribute to bleeding in a number of acquired conditions in which excessive amounts of plasminogen activator are released into the blood and exceed the capacity of inhibitors. Excessive release of plasminogen activator may occur with hypotension, surgical trauma, or heat stroke, and tumors such as prostatic carcinoma also may release activator and result in "primary hyperfibrinogenolysis." The hemostatic abnormalities of severe liver disease are complex, but accelerated fibrinolysis may occur and occasionally represent the primary coagulation abnormality, contributing to significant bleeding. Elevated levels of plasminogen activator[118,119] and decreased α_2-plasmin inhibitor[120] may contribute to the heightened fibrinolysis in liver disease. Fibrinolytic hemorrhage may be a particularly important problem during orthotopic liver transplantation, especially during the anhepatic phase of surgery.[121,122] The fibrinolytic activation seen in disseminated intravascular coagulation is usually a secondary response to the presence of microvascular thrombi, and it serves an important function in maintaining vascular patency, but excessive fibrinolysis may contribute to bleeding. For example, in acute promyelocytic leukemia, the leukemic cells can release both t-PA and u-PA, and elevated levels of activators have been found in leukemic patients with accelerated fibrinolysis.[123,124] In such patients with low α_2-plasmin inhibitor levels, treatment with EACA in combination with heparin has led to clinical improvement in bleeding.[125]

HYPOFIBRINOLYSIS AND THROMBOSIS

Hypofunction of the fibrinolytic system alters the hemostatic balance and can lead to thrombosis by inhibiting clot dissolution while clot formation occurs unimpeded. The contribution of defective fibrinolysis to thrombotic disease has been difficult to evaluate because available plasma screening tests are generally less sensitive to decreased than to increased activity and because thrombosis is frequent in the population and often involves a component of primary vascular wall pathology. However, several specific congenital defects in the plasma fibrinolytic system clearly have been associated with thrombosis, including those due to abnormalities of fibrin and of plasminogen. Several cases of variant plasminogens with decreased activity in patients with thrombotic disease have been described.[126–130] However, the pathobiologic importance of the abnormal plasminogen to thrombosis is unclear, and a review of published studies[131] suggests that the relative risk of thrombosis is no higher in individuals who are plasminogen deficient than in those who are not.

Dysfibrinogenemia has been associated with thrombosis in some families, although many cases are asymptomatic and others are associated with bleeding. Several specific abnormalities in the interaction of t-PA, plasminogen, or plasmin with abnormal fibrinogens may explain the thrombotic tendency in some families. For example, fibrinogen Chapel Hill III was identified in a patient with venous thrombosis and exhibits increased resistance to plasmic degradation.[132] Defective thrombolysis also may account for recurrent venous thrombosis and pulmonary embolism in patients with fibrinogen Dussard.[133] Fibrinogen New York I was identified in a family with a thrombotic tendency associated with abnormal fibrinolysis and defective potentiation of plasminogen activation by t-PA.[134] Characterization of the fibrinogen demonstrated a deletion of residues 9 to 72 of the Bβ chain corresponding to exon 2 of the fibrinogen gene and provided evidence for involvement of this sequence in interaction with t-PA.[135] Familial thrombotic disease also has been associated with defective fibrinolytic response to stimulation by either venous occlusion or infusion of DDAVP.[136–138] An improved understanding of these provocative cases awaits further characterization of abnormalities in t-PA and PAI-1 synthesis, release, and endothelial cell binding.

There have been numerous reports of abnormalities of fibrinolysis in patients with sporadic, nonhereditary venous or arterial thrombotic disease. Overall, these reports demonstrate defective fibrinolytic activation in approximately one-third of patients with a history of deep vein thrombosis,[139–141] but further studies will be required to determine whether these abnormalities are causal or the results of the venous thromboembolic disease. A thrombotic predisposition also could result from excessive inhibition of fibrinolysis. This is demonstrated most clearly in a transgenic mouse model in which PAI-1 synthesis is greatly increased, resulting in high plasma levels.[142] In the newborn period, thrombosis in peripheral vessels results in ischemic necrosis of the tails and feet in some animals. Elevated PAI-1 levels have been observed in a small proportion of young patients with otherwise unexplained deep vein thrombosis, and a familial pattern of elevated PAI-1 levels was found in two patients.[143]

Surgical trauma results in a postoperative reduction in fibrinolytic activity related in part to an increase in PAI-1,[144,145] and this could contribute to the increased postoperative risk of venous thrombosis. Pregnancy results in a marked decrease in plasma fibrinolytic activity related to increases in PAI-1 and especially PAI-2, which is produced by the placenta.[146] These changes may contribute to the increased thrombotic risk in pregnancy, and the even greater elevations in PAI-1 in preeclamptic patients can be related to the severity of placental thrombosis.[147] Impaired fibrinolysis, as reflected by decreased fibrinolytic activity after venous occlusion,[148] and elevated PAI-1 levels[149,150] have been related to the pathobiology of coronary artery disease. Elevated PAI-1 has been identified as a risk factor for reinfarction,[151] but the etiologic importance of abnormal fibrinolysis in the development of coronary artery disease will require further population-based prospective studies.

References

1. Booyse FM, Scheinbuks J, Radek J, et al. Immunological identification and comparison of plasminogen activator forms in cultured normal human endothelial cells and smooth muscle cells. Thromb Res 1981;24:495.
2. Goldsmith GH, Ziats NP, Robertson AL. Studies

on plasminogen activator and other proteases in subcultured human vascular cells. Exp Mol Pathol 1981;35:257.

3. Levin EG, Loskutoff DJ. Cultured bovine endothelial cells produce both urokinase and tissue-type plasminogen activators. J Cell Biol 1982;94:631.

4. Cole ER, Bachmann F. Purification and properties of a plasminogen activator from pig heart. J Biol Chem 1977;252:3729.

5. Rijken DC, Wijngaards G, Zaal DeJong M, Welbergen J. Purification and partial characterization of plasminogen activator from human uterine tissue. Biochem Biophys Acta 1079;580:140.

6. Rijken DC, Collen D. Purification and characterization of the plasminogen activator secreted by human melanoma cells in culture. J Biol Chem 1981;256:7035.

7. Pennica D, Holmes WE, Kohn WJ, et al. Cloning and expression of human tissue-type plasminogen activator cDNA in E. coli. Nature 1983;301:214.

8. Ichinose A, Kisiel W, Fukikawa K. Proteolytic activation of tissue plasminogen activator by plasmin and tissue enzymes. FEBS Lett 1984;175:412.

9. Rijken DC, Hoylaerts M, Collen D. Fibrinolytic properties of one-chain human extrinsic (tissue-type) plasminogen activator. J Biol Chem 1982; 257:2920.

10. Ranby M, Bergsdorf N, Nilsson T. Enzymatic properties of the one- and two-chain form of tissue plasminogen activator. Thromb Res 1982;27:175.

11. Husain SS, Hasan AAK, Budzynski AZ. Differences between binding of one-chain and two-chain tissue plasminogen activators to non-cross-linked and cross-linked clots. Blood 1989;74:999.

12. Camiolo SM, Thorsen S, Astrup T. Fibrinogenolysis and fibrinolysis with tissue plasminogen activator, urokinase, streptokinase-activated human globulin, and plasmin. Proc Soc Biol Med 1971; 138:277.

13. Ranby M. Studies on the kinetics of plasminogen activation by tissue plasminogen activator. Biochim Biophys Acta 1982;704:461.

14. Hoylaerts M, Rijken DC, Lijnen HR, Collen D. Kinetics of the activation of plasminogen by human tissue plasminogen activator: role of fibrin. J Biol Chem 1982;257:2912.

15. Sottrup-Jensen L, Claeys H, Zajdel M, et al. The primary structure of human plasminogen: isolation of two lysine-binding fragments and one "mini"-plasminogen (MW, 38,000) by elastase-catalyzed specific limited proteolysis. In: Davidson JF, Rowan RM, Samama MM, Desnoyers PC, eds. vol 3. New York: Raven Press, 1978: 191.

16. Banyai L, Varadi A, Patthy L. Common evolutionary origin of the fibrin-binding structures of fibronectin and tissue-type plasminogen activator. FEBS Lett 1983;163:37.

17. Günzler WA, Steffens GJ, Otting F. The primary structure of high molecular mass urokinase from human urine: the complete amino acid sequence of the A chain. Hoppe Seylers Z Physiol Chem 1982;363:1155.

18. Steffens GJ, Günzler WA, Otting F, et al. The complete amino acid sequence of low molecular mass urokinase from human urine. Hoppe Seylers Z Physiol Chem 1982;363:1043.

19. Verde P, Stoppelli MP, Galeffi P, et al. Identification and primary sequence of an unspliced human urokinase poly(A)$^+$ RNA. Proc Natl Acad Sci USA 1984;81:4727.

20. Zamarron C, Lijnen HR, Van Hoef B, Collen D. Biological and thrombolytic properties of proenzyme and active forms of urokinase: I. Fibrinolytic and fibrinogenolytic properties in human plasma in vitro of urokinases obtained from human urine or by recombinant DNA technology. Thromb Haemost 1984;52:19.

21. Pannell R, Gurewich V: Pro-urokinase. A study of its stability in plasma and of a mechanism for its selective fibrinolytic effect. Blood 1986;67:1215.

22. Lijnen HR, Zamarron C, Blaber M, et al. Activation of plasminogen by prourokinase: I. Mechanism. J Biol Chem 1986;261:1253.

23. Lijnen HR, Van Hoef B, DeCock F, Collen D. The mechanism of plasminogen activation and fibrin dissolution by single chain urokinase-type plasminogen activator in a plasma milieu in vitro. Blood 1989;73:1846.

24. Gurewich V, Pannell R, Louie S, et al. Effective and fibrin-specific clot lysis by a zymogen precursor form of urokinase (pro-urokinase): a study in vitro and in two animal species. J Clin Invest 1984;73:1731.

25. Ichinose A, Fujikawa K, Suyama I. The activation of prourokinase by plasma kallikrein and its inactivation by thrombin. J Biol Chem 1986;261:3486.

26. White WF, Barlow GH, Mozen MM. The isolation and characterization of plasminogen activators (urokinase) from human urine. Biochemistry 1966;5:2160.

27. Barlow GH, Francis CW, Marder VJ. On the conversion of high-molecular-weight urokinase to the low molecular weight form by plasmin. Thromb Res 1981;23:541.

28. Stump DC, Thienpont M, Collen D. Purification and characterization of a novel inhibitor of urokinase from human urine: quantitation and preliminary characterization in plasma. J Biol Chem 1986;261:12759.

29. Kruithof EKO, Tran-Thang CH, Backmann F. The fast-acting inhibitor of tissue-type plasminogen activator in plasma is also the primary plasma inhibitor of urokinase. Thromb Haemost 1986; 55:65.

30. Marder VJ, Donahoe JF, Bell WR, et al. Changes in the plasma fibrinolytic system during urokinase therapy: comparison of tissue culture urokinase with urinary source urokinase in patients with pulmonary embolism. J Lab Clin Med 1978;92: 721.

31. Winkler ME, Blaber M, Bennett GL, et al. Purification and characterization of recombinant urokinase from E. coli. Biotechnology 1985;3:923.

32. Malke H, Ferretti JJ. Streptokinase: cloning, expression, and excretion by Escherichia coli. Proc Natl Acad Sci USA 1984;81:3557.

33. Wohl RC, Summaria L, Arzadon L, Robbins DC. Steady state kinetics of activation of human and bovine plasminogens by streptokinase and its equimolar complexes with various activated forms of human plasminogen. J Biol Chem 1978;253: 1402.

34. Smith RAG, Dupe RJ, English PD, et al. Fibrinolysis with acylenzymes: a new approach to thrombolytic therapy. Nature 1981;290:505.

35. Staniforth DH, Smith RAG, Hibbs M. Streptokinase and anisoylated streptokinase plasminogen complex: their action on haemostasis in human volunteers. Eur J Clin Pharmacol 1983;24:751.

36. Marder VJ, Rothbard RL, Fitzpatrick PG, Francis CW. Rapid lysis of coronary artery thrombi by a (2–4 minute) bolus intravenous injection of APSAC (anisoylated plasminogen:streptokinase activator). Ann Intern Med 1986;104:304.

37. Ahern TJ, Morris GE, Barone KM, et al. Site-directed mutagenesis in human tissue-plasminogen activator: distinguishing sites in the amino-terminal region required for full fibrinolytic activity and rapid cleavance from the circulation. J Biol Chem 1990;265:1.

38. Madison EL, Goldsmith EJ, Gerard RD, et al. Serpin-resistant mutants of human tissue-type plasminogen activator. Nature 1989;339:721.

39. Pannekoek H, deVries C, van Zonneveld A-J. Mutants of human tissue-type plasminogen activator (t-PA): structural aspects and functional properties. Fibrinolysis 1988;2:123.

40. Bode C, Runge MS, Branscomb EE, et al. Antibody-directed fibrinolysis: an antibody specific for both fibrin and tissue plasminogen activator. J Biol Chem 1989;264:944.

41. Dewerchin M, Lijnen HR, Stassen JM, et al. Effect of chemical conjugation of recombinant single-chain urokinase-type plasminogen activator with monoclonal antiplatelet antibodies on platelet aggregation and on plasma clot lysis in vitro and in vivo. Blood 1991;78:1005.

42. Matsuo O, Okada K, Fukao H, et al. Thrombolytic properties of staphylokinase. Blood 1990;76:925.

43. Lijnen HR, Van Hoef B, DeCock F, et al. On the mechanism of fibrin-specific plasminogen activation by staphylokinase. J Biol Chem 1991;266: 11826.

44. Gardell SJ, Hare TR, Bergum PW, et al. Vampire bat salivary plasminogen activator is quiescent in human plasma in the absence of fibrin unlike human tissue plasminogen activator. Blood 1990; 76:2560.

45. Robbins KC, Summaria L, Hsieh B, Shah R. The peptide chains of human plasmin: mechanism of activation of human plasminogen to plasmin. J Biol Chem 1967;242:2333.

46. Summaria L, Hsieh B, Robbins KC. The specific mechanism of activation of human plasminogen to plasmin. J Biol Chem 1967;242:4279.

47. Markus G. DePasquale JL, Wissler FC. Quantitative determination of the binding of epsilon-aminocaproic acid to native plasminogen. J Biol Chem 1978;253:727.

48. Thorsen S. Differences in the binding to fibrin of native plasminogen and plasminogen modified by proteolytic degradation. Influence of ξ-amino carboxylic acids. Biochim Biophys Acta 1975; 393:55.

49. Moroi M, Aoki N. Inhibition of plasminogen binding to fibrin by α_2-plasmin inhibitor. Thromb Res 1977;10:581.

50. Wiman B, Collen D. On the kinetics of the reaction between human antiplasmin and plasmin. Eur J Biochem 1978;84:573.

51. Walther PJ, Steinmann HM, Hill RL, McKee PA. Activation of human plasminogen by urokinase: partial characterization of a preactivation peptide. J Biol Chem 1974;249:1173.

52. Wallen P, Wiman B. Characterization of different molecular forms of human plasminogen. Biochim Biophys Acta 1972;257:122.

53. Summaria L, Arzadon L, Bernabe P, et al. Characterization of the NH$_2$-terminal glutamic acid and NH$_2$-terminal lysine forms of human plasminogen isolated by affinity chromatography and isoelectric focusing methods. J Biol Chem 1973;248: 2984.

54. Lucas MA, Fretto LJ, McKee PA. The binding of human plasminogen to fibrin and fibrinogen. J Biol Chem 1983;258:4249.

55. Lijnen HR. Zamarron C, Collen D. Characterization of the high-affinity interaction between human plasminogen and prourokinase. Eur J Biochem 1985;150:141.

56. Summaria L, Arzadon L, Bernabe P, Robbins KC. The activation of plasminogen to plasmin by urokinase in the presence of plasmin inhibitor trasylol: the preparation of plasmin with the same NH$_2$-terminal heavy (A) chain sequence as the parent zymogen. J Biol Chem 1975;250:3988.

57. Violand BN, Castellino FJ. Mechanisms of the urokinase catalyzed activation of human plasminogen. J Biol Chem 1976;251:3906.

58. Collen D. Identification and some properties of a new fast-reacting plasmin inhibitor in human plasma. Eur J Biochem 1976;69:209.

59. Plow EF, Collen D. The presence and release of α_2-antiplasmin from human platelets. Blood 1981; 58:1069.

60. Christensen U, Clemmensen I. Kinetic properties of the primary inhibitor of plasmin from human plasma. Biochem J 1977;163:389.

61. Wiman B, Collen D. On the mechanism of the reaction between human α_2-antiplasmin and plasmin. J Biol Chem 1979;254:9291.

62. Sakata Y, Aoki N. Cross-linking of α_2-plasmin inhibitor to fibrin by fibrin-stabilizing factor. J Clin Invest 1980;65:290.

63. Gaffney PJ, Whitaker AN. Fibrin crosslinks and lysis rates. Thromb Res 1979;14:85.

64. Sakata Y, Aoki N. Significance of cross-linking of α_2-plasmin inhibitor to fibrin in inhibition of fibrinolysis and in hemostasis. J Clin Invest 1982; 69:536.

65. Erickson LA, Ginsberg MH, Loskutoff DJ. Detection and partial characterization of an inhibitor of plasminogen activator in human platelets. J Clin Invest 1984;74:1465.

66. Loskutoff DJ, Edgington TS. An inhibitor of plasminogen activator in rabbit endothelial cells. J Biol Chem 1981;256:4142.

67. van Mourik JA, Lawrence DA, Loskutoff DJ. Purification of an inhibitor of plasminogen activator (antiactivator) synthesized by endothelial cells. J Biol Chem 1984;259:14914.

68. Levin EG, Santell L. Association of plasminogen activator inhibitor (PAI-1) with the growth substratum and membrane of human endothelial cells. J Cell Biol 1987;105:2543.

69. Mimuro J, Schleef RR, Luskutoff DJ. Extracellular matrix of cultured bovine aortic endothelial cells contains functionally active type I plasminogen activator inhibitor. Blood 1987;70:721.

70. Holmes WE, Nelles L, Lijnen HR, Collen D. Primary structure of human α_2-antiplasmin, a serine protease inhibitor (serpin). J Biol Chem 1987;262: 1659.

71. Ginsburg D, Zeheb R, Yang AY, et al. cDNA cloning of human plasminogen activator-inhibitor from endothelial cells. J Clin Invest 1986;78:1673.

72. Declerck PJ, De Mol M, Alessi M-C, et al. Purification and characterization of a plasminogen activator inhibitor 1 binding protein form human plasma: identification as a multimeric form of S protein (vitronectin). J Biol Chem 1988;263: 15454.

73. Mimuro J, Loskutoff DJ. Purification of a protein from bovine plasma that binds to type 1 plasminogen activator inhibitor and prevents its interaction with extracellular matrix. J Biol Chem 1989; 264:936.

74. Wagner OF, de Vries C, Hohmann C, et al. Interaction between plasminogen activator inhibitor type 1 (PAI-1) bound to fibrin and either tissue-type plasminogen activator (t-PA) or urokinase-type plasminogen activator (u-PA): binding of t-PA/PAI-1 complexes to fibrin mediated by both the finger and the kringle-1 domain of t-PA. J Clin Invest 1989;84:647.

75. Lecander I, Astedt B. Isolation of a new specific plasminogen activator inhibitor from pregnancy plasma. Br J Haematol 1986;62:221.

76. Rakoczi I, Wiman B, Collen D. On the biologic significance of the specific interaction between fibrin, plasminogen and antiplasmin. Biochim Biophys Acta 1978;540:295.

77. Sakata Y, Mimuro J, Aoki N. Differential binding of plasminogen to crosslinked and non-crosslinked fibrins: its significance in hemostatic defect in factor XIII deficiency. Blood 1984;63:1393.

78. Suenson E, Lützen O, Thorsen S. Initial plasmin-degradation of fibrin as the basis of a positive feedback mechanism in fibrinolysis. Eur J Biochem 1984;140:513.

79. Harpel PC, Chang T-S, Verderber E. Tissue plasminogen activator and urokinase mediate the binding of Gly-plasminogen to plasma fibrin I: evidence for new binding sites in plasmin-degraded fibrin I. J Biol Chem 1985;260:4432.

80. Fukao H, Ueshima S, Tanaka N, et al. Suppression of plasminogen activator inhibitor 1 release by fibrin from human umbilical vein endothelial cells. Thromb Res 1990; (suppl 10):11.

81. Francis CW, Marder VJ. Rapid formation of large molecular weight α-polymers in cross-linked fibrin induced by high factor XIII concentrations. J Clin Invest 1987;80:1459.

82. Francis CW, Marder VJ. Increased resistance to plasmic degradation of fibrin with highly cross-linked α-polymer chains formed at high factor XIII concentrations. Blood 1988;70:1361.

83. Blinc A, Planinsic G, Keber D, et al. Dependence of blood clot lysis on the mode of transport of urokinase into the clot: a magnetic resonance study in vitro. Thromb Haemost 1991;65:549.

84. Bookstein JJ, Salinger E. Accelerated thrombolysis: in vitro evaluation of agents and methods of administration. Invest Radiol 1985;20:731.

85. Fraschini G, Jadeja J, Lawson M, et al. Local infusion of urokinase for the lysis of thrombosis associated with permanent central venous catheters in cancer patients. J Clin Oncol 1987;5:672.

86. Nachman RL. Thrombosis and atherogenesis: molecular connections. Blood 1992;79:1897.

87. Bauer PI, Machovich R, Büki KG, et al. Interaction of plasmin with endothelial cells. Biochem J 1984; 218:119.

88. Hajjar KA, Hamel NM, Harpel PC, Nachman RL. Binding of tissue plasminogen activator to cul-

tured human endothelial cells. J Clin Invest 1987;
80:1712.

89. Miles LA, Levin EG, Plescia J, et al. Plasminogen
receptors, urokinase receptors, and their modulation on human endothelial cells. Blood 1988;72:
628.

90. Hajjar K, Harpel P, Jaffe E, Nachman R. Binding of
plasminogen to cultured human endothelial cells.
J Biol Chem 1986;261:11656.

91. Hajjar KA, Nachman RL. Endothelial cell-mediated conversion of Glu-plasminogen to Lys-plasminogen: further evidence for assembly of the fibrinolytic system on the endothelial cell surface.
J Clin Invest 1988;82:1769.

92. Bevilacqua MP, Schleef RR, Gimbrone MA Jr,
Loskutoff DJ. Regulation of the fibrinolytic system
of cultured human vascular endothelium by interleukin 1. J Clin Invest 1986;78:587.

93. Emeis JJ, Kooistra T. Interleukin 1 and lipopoly-
saccharide induce an inhibitor of tissue-type plasminogen activator in vivo and in cultured endothelial cells. J Exp Med 1986;163:1260.

94. Schleef RR, Bevilacqua MP, Sawdey M, et al. Cytokine activation of vascular endothelium: effects
on tissue-type plasminogen activator and type 1
plasminogen activator inhibitor. J Biol Chem 1988;
263:5797.

95. Saksela O, Moscatelli D, Rifkin DB. The opposing
effects of basic fibroblast growth factor and transforming growth factor beta on the regulation of
plasminogen activator activity in capillary endothelial cells. J Cell Biol 1987;105:957.

96. Hopkins WE, Fujii S, Sobel BE. Synergistic induction of plasminogen activator inhibitor type-1 in
HEP G2 cells by thrombin and transforming
growth factor-β. Blood 1992;79:75.

97. Hajjar KA, Gavish D, Breslow JL, Nachman RL.
Lipoprotein (a) modulation of endothelial cell surface fibrinolysis and its potential role in atherosclerosis. Nature 1989;339:303.

98. Miles LA, Fless GM, Levin EG, et al. A potential
basis for the thrombotic risks associated with
lipoprotein (a). Nature 1989;339:301.

99. Sakata Y, Loskutoff DJ, Gladson CL, et al. Mechanism of protein C–dependent clot lysis: role of
plasminogen activator inhibitor. Blood 1986;68:
1218.

100. Silverstein RL, Leung LLK, Harpel PC, Nachman
RL. Complex formation of platelet thrombospondin with plasminogen: modulation of activation by tissue activator. J Clin Invest 1984;74:
1625.

101. Lijnen HR, Hoylaerts M, Collen D. Isolation and
characterization of a human plasma protein with
affinity for the lysine binding sites in plasminogen.
J Biol Chem 1980;255:10214.

102. Ichinose A, Mimuro J, Koide T, Aoki N. Histidine-

rich glycoprotein and α_2-plasmin inhibitor in inhibition of plasminogen binding to fibrin. Thromb
Res 1984;33:401.

103. Marder VJ, Budzynski AZ. The structure of the fi-
brinogen degradation products. In: Spaet T ed.
Progress in Hemostasis and Thrombosis. New
York: Grune and Stratton, 1974:141.

104. Francis CW, Marder VJ. A molecular model of
plasmic degradation of crosslinked fibrin. Semin
Thromb Hemost 1982;8:25.

105. Pizzo SV, Taylor LM Jr, Schwartz ML, et al. Subunit structure of fragment D from fibrinogen and
cross-linked fibrin. J Biol Chem 1973;248:4584.

106. Gaffney PJ, Lane DA, Kakkar VV, Brasher M.
Characterisation of a soluble D-dimer-E complex
in crosslinked fibrin digests. Thromb Res 1975;
7:89.

107. Francis CW, Marder VJ, Barlow GH. Plasmic
degradation of crosslinked fibrin: characterization
of new macromolecular soluble complexes and
a model of their structure. J Clin Invest 1980;
66:1033.

108. Booth NA, Bennett B, Wijngaards G, Grieve JHK.
A new life-long hemorrhagic disorder due to excess plasminogen activator. Blood 1983;61:267.

109. Aznar J, Estellés A, Vila V, et al. Inherited fibrinolytic disorder due to an enhanced plasminogen
activator level. Thromb Haemost 1984;52:196.

110. Heckel JL, Sandgren EP, Degen JL, et al. Neonatal
bleeding in transgenic mice expressing urokinase-
type plasminogen activator. Cell 1990;62:447.

111. Koie E, Kamiya T, Ogata K, Takamatsu J. α_2-
Plasmin-inhibitor deficiency (Miyasato disease).
Lancet 1978;2:1334.

112. Aoki N, Saito H, Kamiya T, et al. Congenital deficiency of α_2-plasmin inhibitor associated with severe hemorrhagic tendency. J Clin Invest 1979;63:
877.

113. Saito H. α_2-Plasmin inhibitor and its deficiency
states. J Lab Clin Med 1988;112:671.

114. Leebeek FWG, Stibbe J, Knot EAR, et al. Mild
haemostatic problems associated with congenital heterozygous alpha-2-antiplasmin deficiency.
Thromb Haemost 1988;59:96.

115. Kluft C, Nieuwenhuis HK, Rijken DC, et al.
Alpha-2-antiplasmin Enschede: a dysfunctional
alpha-2-antiplasmin molecule, associated with an
autosomal recessive hemorrhagic disorder. J Clin
Invest 1987;80:1391.

116. Schleef RR, Higgins DL, Pillemer E, Levitt LJ.
Bleeding diathesis due to decreased functional ac-
tivity of type 1 plasminogen activator inhibitor.
J Clin Invest 1989;83:1747.

117. Fay WP, Shapiro AD, Shih JL, et al. Brief report:
complete deficiency of plasminogen-activator
inhibitor type 1 due to a frame-shift mutation.
N Engl J Med 1992;327:1729.

118. Booth NA, Anderson JA, Bennett B. Plasminogen activators in alcoholic cirrhosis: demonstration of increased tissue type and urokinase type activator. J Clin Pathol 1984;37:772.

119. Hersch SL, Kunelis T, Francis RB Jr. The pathogenesis of accelerated fibrinolysis in liver cirrhosis: a critical role for tissue plasminogen activator inhibitor. Blood 1987;69:1315.

120. Aoki N, Yamanaka T. The alpha-2 plasmin inhibitor levels in liver disease. Clin Chim Acta 1978;84:99.

121. Bohmig HJ. The coagulation disorder of orthotopic hepatic transplantation. Semin Thromb Hemost 1977;4:57.

122. Dzik WH, Arkin CF, Jenkins RL, Stump DC. Fibrinolysis during liver transplantation in humans: role of tissue-type plasminogen activator. Blood 1988;71:1090.

123. Francis RB Jr, Seyfert U. Tissue plasminogen activator antigen and activity in disseminated intravascular coagulation: clinico-pathologic correlations. J Lab Clin Med 1987;110:541.

124. Bennett B, Booth NA, Cross A, Dawson AA. The bleeding disorder in acute promyelocytic leukaemia: fibrinolysis due to u-PA rather than defibrination. Br J Haematol 1989;71:511.

125. Schwartz BS, Williams EC, Conlan MG, Mosher DF. Epsilon-aminocaproic acid in the treatment of patients with acute promyelocytic leukemia and acquired alpha-2 plasmin inhibitor deficiency. An Intern Med 1986;105:873.

126. Aoki NB, Moroi M, Sakata Y, et al. Abnormal plasminogen: a hereditary molecular abnormality found in a patient with recurrent thrombosis. J Clin Invest 1978;61:1186.

127. Miyata T, Iwanaga S, Sakata Y, et al. Plasminogens Tochigi II and Nagoya: two additional molecular defects with Ala-600 → Thr replacement found in plasmin light chain variants. J Biochem 1984;96:277.

128. Wohl RC, Summaria L, Robbins KC. Physiological activation of the human fibrinolytic system: isolation and characterization of human plasminogen variants: Chicago I and Chicago II. J Biol Chem 1979;254:9063.

129. Scharrer IM, Wohl RC, Hach V, et al. Investigation of a congenital abnormal plasminogen, Frankfurt I, and its relationship to thrombosis. Thromb Haemost 1986;55:396.

130. Liu Y, Lyons RM, McDonagh J. Plasminogen San Antonio: an abnormal plasminogen with a more cathodic migration, decreased activation and associated thrombosis. Thromb Haemost 1988;59:49.

131. Prins MH, Hirsh J. A critical review of the evidence supporting a relationship between impaired fibrinolysis and venous thromboembolism. Arch Intern Med 1991;151:1721.

132. Carrell N, Gabriel DA, Blatt PM, et al. Hereditary dysfibrinogenemia in a patient with thrombotic disease. Blood 1983;62:439.

133. Soria J, Soria C, Caen JP. A new type of congenital dysfibrinogenaemia with defective fibrin lysis—Dusard syndrome: possible relation to thrombosis. Br J Haematol 1983;53:575.

134. Al-Mondhiry HAB, Bilezikian SB, Nossel HL. Fibrinogen "New York"—An abnormal fibrinogen associated with thromboembolism: functional evaluation. Blood 1975;45:607.

135. Liu CY, Koehn JA, Morgan FJ. Characterization of fibrinogen New York 1: a dysfunctional fibrinogen with a deletion of Bβ (9–72) corresponding exactly to exon 2 of the gene. J Biol Chem 1985;260:4390.

136. Johansson L, Hedner U, Nilsson IM. A family with thromboembolic disease associated with deficient fibrinolytic activity in vessel wall. Acta Med Scand 1978;203:477.

137. Jorgensen M, Mortensen JZ, Madsen AG, et al. A family with reduced plasminogen activator activity in blood associated with recurrent venous thrombosis. Scand J Haematol 1982;217:1982.

138. Stead NW, Bauer KA, Kinney TR, et al. Venous thrombosis in a family with defective release of vascular plasminogen activator and elevated plasma factor VIII/von Willebrand's factor. Am J Med 1983;74:33.

139. Nguyen G, Horellou MH, Kruithof EKO, et al. Residual plasminogen activator inhibitor activity after venous stasis as a criterion for hypofibrinolysis: a study in 83 patients with confirmed deep vein thrombosis. Blood 1988;72:601.

140. Petäjä J. Fibrinolytic response to venous occlusion for 10 and 20 minutes in healthy subjects and in patients with deep vein thrombosis. Thromb Res 1989;56:251.

141. Korninger C, Lechner K, Niessner H, et al. Impaired fibrinolytic capacity predisposes for recurrence of venous thrombosis. Thromb Haemost 1984;52:127.

142. Erickson LA, Fici GJ, Lund JE, et al. Development of venous occlusions in mice transgenic for the plasminogen activator inhibitor-1 gene. Nature 1990;346:74.

143. Engesser L, Brommer EJP, Kluft C, Briet E. Elevated plasminogen activator inhibitor (PAI), a cause of thrombophilia—A study in 203 patients with familial or sporadic venous thrombophilia. Thromb Haemost 1989;62:673.

144. Clayton JK, Anderson JA, McNicol GP. Preoperative prediction of postoperative deep vein thrombosis. Br Med J 1976;2:910.

145. Rakoczi I, Chamone D, Collen D, Verstraete M. Prediction of postoperative leg-vein thrombosis in gynaecological patients. Lancet 1978;1:509.

146. Kawano T, Morimoto K, Uemura Y. Urokinase inhibitor in human placenta. Nature 1968;217:253.

147. Estellés A, Gilabert J, Aznar J, et al. Changes in the plasma levels of type 1 and type 2 plasminogen activator inhibitors in normal pregnancy and in patients with severe pre-eclampsia. Blood 1989; 74:1332.

148. Francis RB Jr, Kawanishi D, Baruch T, et al. Impaired fibrinolysis in coronary artery disease. Am Heart J 1988;115:776.

149. Olofsson BO, Dahlén G, Nilsson TK. Evidence for increased levels of plasminogen activator inhibitor and tissue plasminogen activator in plasma of patients with angiographically verified coronary artery disease. Eur Heart J 1989;10:77.

150. Hamsten A, Wiman B, DeFaire U, Blombäck M. Increased plasma levels of a rapid inhibitor of tissue plasminogen activator in young survivors of myocardial infarction. N Engl J Med 1985;313: 1557.

151. Hamsten A, Walldius G, Szamosi A, et al. Plasminogen activator inhibitor in plasma: risk factor for recurrent myocardial infarction. Lancet 1987; 2:3.

Anthony J. Comerota (Ed.). *Thrombolytic Therapy for Peripheral Vascular Disease.* Copyright © 1995 J. B. Lippincott Company.

4

THE PLASMINOGEN-PLASMIN ENZYME SYSTEM

Kenneth C. Robbins

The generation of plasmin (Pln) in plasma is regulated by (1) plasminogen (Plg), the zymogen precursor of Pln, (2) Plg activators, urokinase-type (scu-PA and tcu-PA) and tissue-type (sct-PA and tct-PA), synthesized and released from the liver and vascular endothelium into the circulation, (3) protein inhibitors that inactivate Pln, α_2-Pln inhibitor (α_2PI), and α_2-macroglobulin (α_2M), and the Plg activator inhibitors (PAI-1 and PAI-2), and (4) the fibrin-thrombus[1-4] (Fig. 4-1). Other factors that modulate activation of the system are histidine-rich glycoprotein (HRG), which interferes with the binding of Plg to fibrin, and C1-inhibitor, which inactivates kallikrein, generated in a second activator pathway involving prekallikrein, factor (f) XII, and high-molecular-weight kininogen. α_2M is a scavenger protease inhibitor that intervenes only when α_2PI is markedly decreased, e.g., during thrombolytic therapy and in patients with α_2PI deficiencies. The activators, u-PA and t-PA, are serine proteases formed from native proactivators by specific limited proteolysis, either in the circulation or at the surface of the cells secreting these activators. Activation of Plg can occur in the fluid phase surrounding the thrombus, at the thrombus surface, involving both the fibrin clot, the platelet membrane, and circulating white cells (e.g., the monocyte), and at the surface of the vascular endothelial cell. The components of this system, Plg, Plg activators (scu-PA, tcu-PA, sct-PA, and tct-PA), α_2PI, and PAI-1, when assembled at cell surfaces (e.g., endothelial cells and monocytes), are involved in the regulation of the Plg-Pln system.[5]

PLASMINOGEN

Plasminogen Levels in Plasma

Plg is found in human plasma in a concentration of about 12.7 ± 1.8 mg/dl, or about 1.4 μM (functional and antigen)[6] (Robbins and Kozlowski, unpublished results). Plg is determined functionally by adding an excess of streptokinase (SK) to form the equimolar Plg.SK complex with an active site, titrating this active site with a chromogenic substrate (e.g., Kabi S2251) by either initial rate

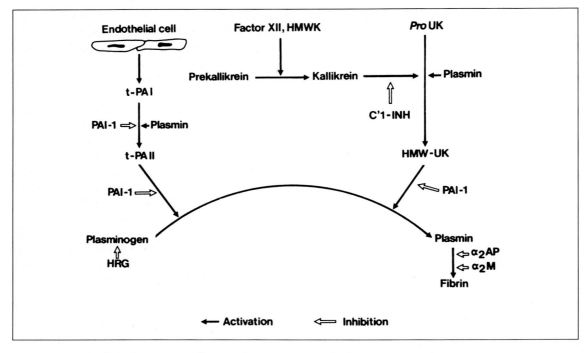

FIGURE 4-1. *The fibrinolytic system of human plasma. t-PA I, single-chain tissue-type plasminogen activator, also called sct-PA; t-PA II, two-chain t-PA (tct-PA); PAI-I, plasminogen activator inhibitor 1 (endothelial type); HMWK, high-molecular-weight kininogen; Pro UK, pro-urokinase, also called single-chain urinary-type PA (scu-PA); HMW-UK, high-molecular-weight urokinase, also called two-chain u-PA (tcu-PA); C'1-INH, C1-inhibitor; α_2AP, alpha$_2$-antiplasmin; α_2M, alpha$_2$-macroglobulin. (Reprinted with permission from Bachman F. In Verstraete M, Vermylen J, Lijnen R, Arnout J, eds. Thrombosis and haemostasis. Leuven: Leuven University Press, 1987:227.)*

(kinetic:net absorbance change/min) or endpoint assays (in IU),[6,7] and converting to milligrams of protein using a specific activity of 28 IU/mg protein for pure Plg. Plg antigen is determined by immunochemical methods: radioimmunoassay, rocket immunoelectrophoresis, radial immunodiffusion, nephelometry, and ELISA; different types of antibody preparations were used in the different methods. The functional and antigen methods require suitable Plg/Pln reference preparations and well-characterized antibody preparations; each method may give different plasma Plg levels and ranges. Plg determined functionally by initial rate assays[7] and immunochemically by either rocket immunoelectrophoresis (Laurell) or radioimmunoassays[8] gave a range of 17 to 24

mg/dl. Plg determined functionally by endpoint assays and immunochemically by either radial immunodiffusion, nephelometry, or ELISA methods gave a range of 9 to 16 mg/dl.[6] Plg levels in females are somewhat higher than in males. In full-term newborns, the Plg functional/antigen levels are about 50% of adult levels[8,9]; Plg levels are lower in premature infants and aborted fetuses (Robbins and Kozlowski, unpublished results).

Synthesis

Plg is found in all mammalian species; it is synthesized primarily in the liver, e.g., human,[10] monkey, and rat. Full-length human Plg clones (cDNA and genomic) have been isolated from a genomic library.[11,12] Recombinant Plg and mutants have been expressed in mammalian cells lines,[13,14] in insect cells,[15] and in *E. coli*.[14]

Characterization of Purified Plasminogens

Affinity chromatography methods with L-lysine–substituted Sepharose are commonly used for the isolation of native Plg from plasma.[16] Purified Plgs can be characterized by various methods: (1) determination of specific proteolytic activities, (2) Pln generation rates, (3) rates of generation of the active site in the Plg.SK equimolar complex, (4) kinetic parameters of Plg activation, (5) SDS-PAGE, (6) formation, conversion, and degradation of the equimolar Plg.SK complexes as studied in PAGE and SDS-PAGE, (7) isoelectric focusing, (8) electrophoretic mobilities, and (9) fibrin clot lysis.[7,17] Molecular defects in the Plg molecule can be determined by both amino acid sequence and nucleotide sequence analyses of both the cellular genomic DNA and RNA.

Structure and Properties

Human Plg is a single-chain glycoprotein with a molecular weight (M_r) of about 92,000, containing 791 amino acid residues and about 2% carbohydrate.[1,3,4] The primary structure of human Plg has been established by amino acid and DNA sequence analysis[11,12] (Fig. 4-2). The M_r calculated from sequence data is 88,320. The molecule has 24 disulfide bridges, no free sulfhydryl groups, and 5 triple-loop, three-disulfide-bridge regions of sequence homology called *kringles*. These five kringles (K-1, K-2, K-3, K-4, and K-5) in the NH_2-terminal domain, or heavy (A) chain region (Glu 1–Arg 561), each with an M_r of about 10,000, exhibit a high degree of sequence homology with similar domains in prothrombin (two), u-PA (one), t-PA (two), lipoprotein (a) (up to 38:37-K4 and 1-K5), and hepatocyte growth factor (four). The kringle regions exist as independent, autonomous domains. The COOH-terminal domain, the light (B) chain region (Val 562–Asn 791), containing the active center or catalytic site, is homologous with the amino acid sequence of the pancreatic serine proteases; this region contains the active site triad, amino acid residues His 603, Asp 646, and Ser 740. Native Plg (Glu 1–Plg) is activated by all Plg activators to native Pln (Glu 1–Pln) by cleavage of the Arg 561–Val peptide bond. The two-chain Pln molecule has the NH_2-terminal heavy (A) chain (M_r of about 62,000), and the COOH-terminal light (B) chain (M_r of about 26,000) connected by two disulfide bridges. Glu 1–Plg is converted by limited Pln digestion to degraded forms, Met 69–Plg and Lys 78–Plg. An elastase-degraded form of Plg designated mini-Plg, Val 443–Plg, and a plasmin-degraded form designated micro-Plg, Lys 531–Plg, have been described. Native Plg can be separated into two affinity chromatography forms, 1 and 2, by L-lysine–substituted Sepharose chromatography. Form 1 contains two oligosaccharide chains, a complex glucosamine containing carbohydrate on Asn 288, and a smaller trisaccharide unit on Thr 345, whereas form 2 contains only the Thr 345 oligosaccharide unit. Native Plg has 10 to 13 isoelectric forms, with isoelectric points between pH 6.2 and 6.6; the degraded Lys 78–Plg form has more alkaline isoelectric forms, between 6.8 and 8.5. The Plg extinction coefficient is 17.0. The biologic half-life ($t_{1/2}$) of native Plg is 2.2 days.

PLASMINOGEN ACTIVATORS

Plasma Plg activators activate circulating plasma Plg to Pln.[1,2,4,19] The physiologic Plg activators are u-PA, and t-PA, both direct activators. SK and staphylokinase (STK) are bacterial proteins that are indirect activators, combining with Plg to form equimolar complexes, which are now direct activators. These Plg activators are serine proteases that have the ability to cleave a single, specific Arg 561–Val peptide bond in Plg, a single-chain molecule, to form Pln, a two-chain molecule.[1] Pln, a serine protease with trypsin-like specificity, has the property of degrading biologically active plasma proteins, particularly the coagulation and complement proteins.

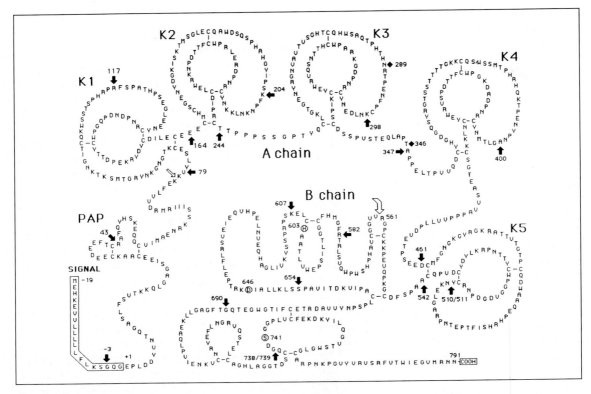

FIGURE 4-2. Amino acid sequence for human plasminogen and the location of the 18 introns in the gene coding for plasminogen. The positions of the introns (A–R) are indicated by solid arrows at or between specific amino acids. The amino acid residues are numbered starting with the amino-terminal glutamic acid residue as number 1 and ending with residue 791. The signal peptide (PAP) is generated primarily by the cleavage between Lys 77 and Lys 78 (shown with an open straight arrow) by plasmin. The conversion of plasminogen to plasmin occurs by the cleavage between Arg 561 and Val 562 (shown by an open curved arrow). K1–K5 refers to kringles 1–5 in the A chain, while the active site His, Asp, and Ser residues in the B chain are circled. Carbohydrate attachment sites (Asn 289, Thr 346) are shown by diamonds. (Reprinted with permission from Petersen TE, et al. Characterization of the gene for human plasminogen, a key proenzyme in the fibrinolytic system. J Biol Chem 1990;265:6101.)

Urokinase

Pro-u-PA (scu-PA), the zymogen precursor of u-PA, is found in endothelial, kidney, and malignant cells and most mammalian tissues and is released from these cells as a virtually inactive proenzyme.[2,19] It is converted to the active enzyme, tcu-PA, by plasmin by limited proteolysis. The zymogen is a single-chain protein without an active center and with negligible Plg activator activity. It is converted to the fully enzymatically active two-chain u-PA, a serine protease. Pro-u-PA and u-PA (HMW-u-PA) have identical molecular weights of about 54,000; a low-molecular-weight, partially degraded form of u-PA (LMW-u-PA), M_r of about 32,000, has been found in urine and tissue culture systems and is derived from the HMW form. On a molar basis, the two u-PA forms have similar specific activities. A scu-PA form with an M_r of 32,000 has been reported; it resembles the M_r 54,000 form and is similar to the M_r 32,000 tcu-PA form. Chimeric (hybrid) u-PA activators have been prepared with both scu-PA and tcu-PA linked to the Pln heavy (A) chain or to a fibrin-specific antibody fragment. The complete primary amino acid and cDNA sequences of pro-u-PA have been determined, and the cDNA gene has been expressed in *Escherichia coli* and in mammalian cells. The human urokinase gene structure has been elucidated and assigned to chromosome 10. Several types of cells, both normal and transformed, have been found to possess specific receptor sites for pro-u-PA and u-PA.

Tissue Plasminogen Activator

t-PA has been found in many mammalian tissues, including endothelial and malignant (transformed) cells.[2,19] A single-chain inactive enzyme, zymogen form, has not been found. It is released into the circulation following exercise and venous occlusion as a single-chain active enzyme (sct-PA) and is easily converted by plasmin to a two-chain active enzyme (tct-PA). Both sct-PA and tct-PA are serine proteases and have identical molecular weights of about 68,000, with similar specific activities. Both t-PAs bind to fibrin, and their Plg activator activities are markedly potentiated in the presence of fibrin. The complete primary amino acid and cDNA sequences of t-PA have been determined, and the cDNA gene has been expressed in *E. coli* and mammalian cells. The human t-PA gene structure has been elucidated and assigned to chromosome 8. Specific receptors have been identified in both normal and transformed, cells.

Streptokinase

SK, M_r of about 50,000, forms an equimolar irreversible activator complex with Plg and Pln (Plg.SK/Pln.SK) with a serine protease active center.[1,2,19] It is species-specific, forming equimolar activator complexes only with human, cat, and dog Plgs. The human Plg.SK/Pln.SK complexes are called *preformed activators*. The complete primary amino acid and cDNA sequences have been determined, and the SK gene has been elucidated.

Staphylokinase

STK, M_r of about 16,500, forms an equimolar irreversible activator complex with Plg (Plg.STK) with a serine protease active center.[20] The gene coding for STK has been cloned. The nucleotide sequence of the STK gene and the deduced amino acid sequence are not related to those of SK.

Catalytic Efficiencies/Assays: International Units

An important property of all Plg activator species is their catalytic efficiency (by kinetic analysis, second-order rate constants) in the activation of native Plg.[21] SK and its complexes with Plg and the Pln-derived COOH-terminal B chain have the highest catalytic efficiencies. Fibrin and fibrin fragments greatly influence the catalytic efficiency of t-PA but minimally influence the catalytic efficiencies of either u-PA or SK. Casein enhances Plg activation by both u-PA and t-PA.

Plasminogen activators, when used as thrombolytic agents, are assayed for theoretical fibrinolytic potency by methods in which the response is dependent only on the concentration of activator.[22] The pharmaceutical industry currently uses a tube fibrin clot lysis assay with a 5- to 6-point parallel line, log lysis time–log activator dose method, where the sample is simultaneously compared against a WHO international reference preparation, and a house standard. The activator assay response is dependent on the Plg substrate concentration, the Plg form, Glu 1- or Lys 78-, and the fibrinogen milieu, plasma or purified fibrinogen. Similar parallel curves are obtained with u-PA, both HMW and LMW preparations, and with different SK and Plg.SK forms, permitting a comparison between u-PA and SK preparations. However, since the t-PA curve is not parallel to the u-PA and SK curves, it is not possible to compare t-PA with other activators. One international unit (IU) is the amount of each WHO international reference preparation, u-PA or SK, which will lyse a clot containing Glu 1–Plg under standard conditions in 10 minutes. Both the current u-PA (HMW) and SK reference preparations are highly purified products; the 10-minute lysis IU will probably change, since the u-PA HMW and LMW forms will not give the same potency values and the second generation of Plg.SK products will require their own specific reference preparations. The amount of WHO international reference preparation of t-PA that will lyse a clot in 10 minutes is about 15 IU. The t-PA IU is based on a longer lysis time and cannot be compared with the u-PA and SK IUs. The specific activities of highly purified two-chain HMW-u-PA, two-chain LMW-u-PA, SK, and t-PA (single-chain and two-chain) are about 100,000, 200,000, 100,000, and about 600,000 to 1,000,000 IU/mg protein, respectively. Some commercial single-chain u-PA preparations have enzymatic activity, about 2 to 5% of tcu-PA. The IU is an in vitro assessment and is needed for labeled potency for each thrombolytic agent; the dose used in patients is not related to clinical efficacy, since each plasminogen activator has a different mechanism of plasminogen activation in the fibrin-thrombus.

Plasminogen Activator Inhibitors

The activity of the physiologic Plg activators (u-PA and t-PA) is controlled in plasma by specific inhibitors.[2,19,23] These inhibitors play an important role in regulating u-PA– and t-PA–dependent fibrinolysis in vivo; they prevent premature fibrinolysis at the adhesion site of clots on the endothelial cell during wound healing, and they prevent and modulate the destruction of vascular walls. Impairment of fibrinolysis may be due to deficient synthesis and/or release of PAI-1 from the vascular wall.

PAI-1

The specific, rapid reacting inhibitor of u-PA and t-PA, with an M_r of about 52,000, is found in plasma, platelets, endothelial cells, fibroblasts, smooth muscle cells, hepatocytes, and malignant cells. In normal human plasma, it is the primary inhibitor of u-PA and t-PA, forming irreversible 1:1 stoichiometric complexes. The platelet releases a latent form. The PAI-1 activity of plasma is associated with a binding protein, vitronectin,

in a complex which stabilizes PAI-1 in the plasma. PAI-1 is a member of the serpin family of protease inhibitor proteins. The complete primary amino acid and cDNA sequences of PAI-1 have been determined, and the cDNA has been expressed in E. coli and mammalian cells. The PAI-1 gene structure has been elucidated and assigned to chromosome 7.

PAI-2

The placental-type inhibitor of u-PA and t-PA, found in pregnancy plasma, is also found in other cells and tissues and in malignant cells. There are two forms of this inhibitor, an HMW form with an M_r of about 70,000 and an LMW form with an M_r of about 47,000. These two react with both u-PA and t-PA to form 1:1 complexes; the u-PA complexes are irreversible, whereas the t-PA complexes are much weaker complexes, particularly the sct-PA–PAI-2 complex. PAI-2 inhibits u-PA about 10 times better than tct-PA and is a poor inhibitor of sct-PA. In contrast to PAI-1, PAI-2 is a stable inhibitor. The reaction rate of PAI-2 is at least one order of magnitude slower than that of PAI-1. The complete primary amino acid and cDNA sequences of PAI-2 have been determined. It is also a member of the serpin family of protease inhibitor proteins.

PAI-3

The plasma heparin–dependent activated protein C inhibitor was found to be similar to the heparin-dependent u-PA inhibitor PAI-3, which is also found in human urine. It is a much less effective inhibitor than either PAI-1 or PAI-2. However, the plasma concentration of PAI-3 is at least two orders of magnitude higher than that of PAI-1, and it is also an inhibitor of both u-PA and t-PA.

Interactions of Plasminogen and Plasminogen Activators with Fibrin (Fibrin-Thrombus)

Since formation of plasmin at the surface of and in the fibrin-thrombus is the critical event in clot dissolution, it is important to consider the interactions of the various components of the fibrinolytic system at the fibrin surface. Native Glu 1–Plg contains specific lysine binding sites (LBS), both strong and weak, located in the kringle regions of the NH$_2$-terminal heavy (A) chain of the molecule. Compounds such as 6-aminohexanoic acid (EACA) bind to these structures, inhibit activation of Plg, and inhibit the functional activity of Pln. They inhibit the fibrinolytic activity of Pln both in vitro and in vivo. These LBSs regulate the interaction of the native Glu 1–Plg and also degraded Lys 78–Plg molecules, with fibrin(ogen), α_2PI, HRG, and thrombospondin, to endothelial cells and platelets. Platelets have the potential to enhance fibrinolysis by localizing Plg in a thrombus.

Plg binding sites are hidden in fibrin(ogen), uncovered by proteolysis (plasmic degradation), and found in fragments D and E. Removal of the NH$_2$-terminal Glu 1–Lys 77 peptide(s) from Glu 1–Plg to give Lys 78–Plg causes a marked increase in fibrin binding. The Glu 1–Lys 78 domain inhibits the binding of native Plg to cross-linked fibrin. Plg binding to fibrin is inhibited by α_2PI, which is cross-linked to fibrin by activated fXIII. Plg activators mediate the binding of Glu 1–Plg to fibrin. Thrombospondin and t-PA form trimolecular complexes with native Plg and HRG. Native Plg is also activated on the platelet surface.

The binding of Plg activators to fibrin also depends on the kringle structures of the activators. Plg/Pln.SK binding also depends on the Plg/Pln kringle structures; other Pln.SK derivatives without kringle domains do not bind. The binding of t-PA to fibrin depends on one of its two kringle structures (NH$_2$-terminal domain) and the fibronectin and finger domains. Single-chain t-PA appears to bind more efficiently to fibrin than tct-PA. With the u-PA species, the single-kringle domain in the NH$_2$ terminus does not bind avidly to fibrin. Single-chain u-PA, without an active center (no titratable active sites) does not bind to fibrin. However, a scu-PA isolated from a transformed cell culture medium has been reported with fibrin-binding properties; this u-PA has 54% titratable active sites, indicating the possibility of a different three-dimensional structure. Hybrids of t-PA and u-PA serine protease domains

(COOH-terminal regions) with the Pln NH$_2$-terminal domain containing the kringle regions bind well to fibrin.

MECHANISM OF ACTIVATION OF PLASMINOGEN

Sreptokinase

In Purified Systems

SK is an indirect activator that forms with native Plg an equimolar irreversible Plg/Pln.SK activator complex.[24] The Glu 1–Plg.SK complex converts to the final Glu 1–Pln.SK complex in which SK is extensively degraded; all intermediate complex forms are also activator species. SK also forms activator complexes with Plg-derived domains, such as partially degraded Lys 78–Plg and Lys 78–Pln, Val 443–Plg and Val 443–Pln, and Val 562–Pln [light (B) chain]. These activator complexes are preformed Plg activators, and all are serine proteases. Acyl derivatives of Plg/Pln.SK have been prepared using inverse acylating agents in which enzyme activity is regenerated by hydrolysis.[25] All the SK activator species will generate Pln from Plg.

In Plasma Milieu

The addition of SK to human plasma or the intravenous infusion of a clinical dose of SK into a human subject with a fibrin-thrombus will produce a plasma fibrinolytic state. In the plasma milieu, antibodies to SK may be found that could prevent SK from forming Plg.SK complexes if present in high concentrations. However, since large amounts of SK are infused, the circulating antibodies play a minor role in preventing the formation of a fibrinolytic state. Also, there are no apparent plasma inhibitors to any of the Plg/Pln.SK activator complexes; these complexes are not inhibited by α_2PI. However, Pln.SK, once formed, can react with α_2M, with SK dissociating from the Pln.SK–α_2M complex; the importance of this reaction during thrombolytic therapy has not been established.[26] The SK activator species in plasma will activate Plg to Pln. Lipoprotein (a) inhibits SK-mediated activation of Plg by competing with Plg for SK; it inhibits the binding of native Plg to fibrin.

In the Fibrin-Thrombus

The dissolution of fibrin in the fibrin-thrombus depends on a number of factors. During thrombolytic therapy, in a patient with a myocardial infarct, a bolus dose of SK of approximately 15 mg, or 1,500,000 IU, or an equivalent dose of anisoylated Lys 78–Plg.SK would be infused in a relatively short period of time. SK does not bind to fibrin. With SK, the Plg/Plg.SK activator complexes will form rapidly; with anisoylated Lys 78-Plg.SK, the activator complex will form after deacylation over a period of several hours. The resulting SK.Pln activator complexes will rapidly activate circulating Plg to Pln, which will be complexed to the α_2PI and inactivated. In the fibrin-thrombus, circulating Plg "bathing" the thrombus, together with fibrin-bound Plg, is rapidly activated to Pln, which will then be complexed to both circulating and fibrin-bound α_2PI. Free Pln in both the plasma milieu and the fibrin-thrombus will degrade fibrinogen and dissolve fibrin, respectively, and could convert the small amount of bound Glu 1–Plg to the degraded Lys 78–Plg form, which is more readily activated. Pln will cleave susceptible peptide bonds in the fibrin, making available more binding sites for the native Plg. The fibrin-bound native Plg appears to have a Lys 78–Plg conformation and is more readily activatable. Also, the catalytic efficiency of the Pln.SK activator species is enhanced about 1.4-fold in the presence of fibrin. The important factors in clot lysis of the fibrin-thrombus by the SK activator species are (1) some binding of native Plg to intact fibrin and then increased binding to partially degraded fibrin, (2) conversion of fibrin-bound native Plg to the degraded Lys 78–Plg form, (3) the binding of the Plg/Pln.SK activator species to fibrin, (4) the removal of Pln by both circulating and fibrin-bound α_2PI, and (5) the possible dissociation of Pln.SK by circulating α_2M, liberating free SK. The plasma milieu could contain SK antibodies that inhibit some SK and Pln.SK. During thrombolytic therapy, large amounts of fibrinogen and fibrin degradation products are present. Finally, the biologic half-life of these activator species plays an important role in the duration of the thrombolytic effect.

Staphylokinase

In Purified Systems

STK is an indirect activator similar to SK that forms an equimolar irreversible Plg.STK activator complex.[20] Its reaction with Pln has not been studied; however, one can assume that a complex forms with the enzyme. The complexes are serine proteases and will activate Plg to Pln.

In Plasma Milieu

The addition of STK to human plasma produces a fibrinolytic state. In the absence of fibrin, the active site of the Plg.STK complex, when formed, will be rapidly neutralized by α_2PI; however, the active site of the Plg.SK complex is not neutralized. The affinity of the Plg.STK complex for Plg is about 10-fold lower than that of the Plg.SK complex, thus preventing Plg activation in plasma. It was found that 50% activation of Plg and 50% fibrin degradation in human plasma in vitro requires 180-fold (molar basis) more STK than SK.

In the Fibrin-Thrombus

STK, like SK, does not bind to fibrin, but fibrin stimulates the initial rate of Plg activation by STK, about four-fold. The initial rate of Plg activation by Plg.STK is about fourfold lower than Plg.SK activation of Plg. Plg.STK is rapidly neutralized in plasma by α_2PI, but not at the fibrin surface. In the presence of fibrin, some of the lysine binding sites of the Plg.STK complex are occupied, and therefore, inhibition by α_2PI is impaired, thus allowing for efficient Plg activation. STK is more fibrin-specific than SK. The thrombolytic efficiency of STK in human plasma, compared with SK and t-PA, showed that the relative molar potency of STK is about two times more effective than SK but about half that of t-PA.

Prourokinase and Urokinase

In Purified Systems

Normally, scu-PA has little or no intrinsic enzymatic activity, indicating a potential active site that will not activate Plg.[1,2,19] However, an active scu-PA has been prepared with 54% active sites from a transformed cell line with a specific activity of about 64,000 IU/mg protein. It probably has a different three-dimensional structure, where the active center is in a different structural position and available for activation of Plg. The scu-PA zymogen can be converted to the fully active tcu-PA form by either plasmin or trypsin-like enzymes by cleaving the Lys 158–Ile peptide bond. The two-chain HMW-u-PA can be converted to the LMW-u-PA form by limited proteolysis by cleaving the Lys 135–Lys peptide bond. On a molar basis, the HMW- and LMW-u-PA forms have similar specific activities and similar thrombolytic properties. All active u-PA forms, both HMW and LMW and two-chain forms, are serine proteases and will convert Plg to the two-chain Lys 78–Pln form, however, with different catalytic efficiencies.

In Plasma Milieu

The addition of tcu-PA to plasma or the intravenous infusion of a clinical dose of tcu-PA into a human subject with a fibrin-thrombus will produce a plasma fibrinolytic state. Single-chain u-PA will produce a plasma fibrinolytic state only if the preparation has about 1 to 2% of the potential enzymatic activity of tcu-PA; Pln will be generated that will convert the single-chain form to the two-chain fully active form. PAI-1 plays a major role in regulating the concentration of u-PA in plasma. Single-chain u-PA may be completely bound to Plg in the circulation under normal physiologic conditions and could provide a possible explanation for the fibrin specificity of this activator. Plg activation by the intrinsic activity of scu-PA can be stimulated exclusively by fibrin fragment E-2; this structural segment is unavailable in intact fibrin.

In the Fibrin-Thrombus

Since neither scu-PA nor tcu-PA (HMW or LMW forms) binds to the fibrin-thrombus, the dissolution of fibrin is primarily due to both the generation of circulating plasma Pln "bathing" the fibrin-thrombus and thrombus-bound Pln. Glu 1–Plg, bound to both native fibrin and degraded-fibrin, will be activated by u-PA to generate additional Pln at the thrombus surface. Also, scu-PA

can be activated at the fibrin surface by fibrin-bound Pln to yield the two-chain active form. There is a small enhancing effect of fibrin on the catalytic efficiency of activation of Plg by the active u-PA species. Single-chain u-PA is considered to be a fibrin-selective activator, like t-PA, since it does not produce a plasma fibrinolytic state.

Tissue Plasminogen Activator

In Purified Systems
Single-chain t-PA can be converted by Pln to the two-chain form by cleavage of the Arg 275–Ile peptide bond; both forms are serine proteases.[2,19] Single-chain t-PA does not appear to be a zymogen. Fibrin enhances the catalytic efficiency of sct-PA with native Glu 1–Plg from about 10- to 2000-fold depending on the assay method used.

In Plasma Milieu
The addition of sct-PA or tct-PA to human plasma or the intravenous infusion of a clinical dose of either form into a human subject with a fibrin-thrombus should not produce a plasma fibrinolytic state unless it is given in a bolus dose. The two-chain form, which appears to be the more active form, may produce a plasma fibrinolytic state, particularly at higher doses. PAI-1 will regulate the concentration of t-PA in the plasma.

In the Fibrin-Thrombus
Since both the sct-PA and tct-PA forms bind to fibrin, the activation of fibrin-bound and soluble native Plg at the surface of the fibrin-thrombus is greatly enhanced. Once fibrin degradation takes place, additional native Plg molecules will be bound to new fibrin binding sites. The configuration of bound native Plg may be changed to that of the Lys 78–Plg form by surface-bound Pln. The Glu 1– to Lys 78–Plg conversion takes place during t-PA–mediated lysis of plasma clots. Also, Lys 78–Plg is converted more rapidly than native Glu 1–Plg to Pln by all Plg activators. The binding and enhanced activity of t-PA in the fibrin-thrombus also can be enhanced by thrombospondin and proteoglycans. t-PA is probably the most fibrin-selective plasminogen activator.

KINETICS OF PLASMINOGEN ACTIVATION

Mathematical models for studying Plg activation kinetics have recently been developed.[21] The derived equations can accommodate both the u-PA and SK activators, with the Glu 1–Plg, Lys 78–Plg, and Val 443–Plg substrate species. The zymogen-to-enzyme conversion obeys Michaelis-Menten kinetics. The data obtained fit the established molecular mechanism of conversion of Glu 1–Plg through Glu 1–Pln to Lys 78–Pln but not through the Lys 78–Plg intermediate. The steady-state kinetic parameters of plasminogen activation are the catalytic rate constants (k_{Plg}), or turnover members, and the apparent Michaelis constants (K_{Plg}). The K_{Plg} is the concentration of substrate at which the initial rate of formation of product(s) is equal to half the maximum velocity. The second-order rate constant, k_{Plg}/K_{Plg}, reflects the catalytic efficiency and substrate specificity of the activator species.

With SK and lysyl substrates, the lowest second-order rate constants (the lowest activator efficiencies) were with either Glu 1– or Lys 78–Plg.SK or Lys 78–Pln.SK activating Glu 1–Plg; these activators have the lowest k_{Plg}, approximately 9 min^{-1}. Higher, intermediate second-order rate constants were found with the smaller-molecular-weight activator species, namely, the Val 562–Pln.SK (B.SK) and Val 443–Pln.SK complexes activating Glu 1–Plg; these activator species have a k_{Plg} of approximately 26 min^{-1}. The highest catalytic efficiencies were found with the various SK complexes activating Lys 78–Plg rather than Glu 1–Plg; these activator species have a k_{Plg} of approximately 50 min^{-1}. It has been suggested that the "Glu" NH$_2$ terminus of the substrate affects the number of binding subsites in the Plg/Pln.SK activator active site. The K_{Plg} of activation varies between 0.1 and 0.2 μM for both the Glu 1– and the Lys 78–Plg substrates. Fibrinogen, fragment D, soluble fibrin, and fibrin fragments enhanced the rates of activation of Plg by the SK complexes.

With u-PA, the activation kinetic parameters, with lysyl substrates, depend somewhat on the type of activator used, either the HMW or LMW species. The K_{Plg} varies from approximately 1 to 2 μM for both the Glu 1– and Lys 78–Plg substrates, with both HMW-u-PA and LMW-u-PA and the functionally active chain derived from HMW-u-PA; these values are 10-fold higher than those found for SK with the same zymogen substrates. The k_{Plg} values for HMW-u-PA and LMW-u-PA are similar to one another, approximately 50 min^{-1} on both the same and the two different zymogen substrates. These constants are similar to the constants obtained with SK, with the highest catalytic efficiencies for the Lys 78–Plg substrate. The differences in the activation parameters of both the Glu 1– and the Lys 78–Plg substrates by either u-PA or SK are dependent on the specific characteristics of the activator preparation and the zymogen substrate used. The steady-state kinetic parameters for the Val 443–Plg substrate were more similar to those for the Lys 78–Plg substrate than to those for the Glu 1–Plg substrate with both SK and u-PA. The data on kinetics of activation of Glu 1–Plg and Lys 78–Plg with u-PA show that the second-order rate constants or catalytic efficiencies are identical, indicating that u-PA does not activate Lys 78–Plg faster than Glu 1–Plg, as has been postulated in the literature with nonkinetic data. The catalytic efficiency of u-PA with Glu 1–Plg is increased from 2- to 10-fold in the presence of cyanogen bromide–degraded fibrinogen. A monoclonal antibody to kringle 4 accelerates the activation of Glu 1–Plg with u-PA, increasing the catalytic efficiency about 5-fold.

The K_{Plg} values of activators such as trypsin and STK with the Glu 1–Plg substrate were 2 and 0.1 μM, respectively, with k_{Plg} values of 0.3 and 0.1 min^{-1}, respectively. In these kinetic systems, Pln, kallikrein, and thrombin did not have measurable activator activity; the k_{Plg} of activation for these enzymes would have to be above 10 μM and the k_{Plg} of activation under 0.1 min^{-1}. Hageman factor, kallikrein, and factor XIa have at least 10^4 times lower second-order rate constants for Plg activation in solution than do either u-PA or SK. Thus, to invoke substrate and activator specificities for this class of Plg activators, one has to propose different physiologic conditions and possibly even a different mechanism of Plg activation (e.g., surface activation).

The kinetic parameters of Plg activation of five native mammalian species (cat, dog, bovine, rabbit, and horse) with u-PA, human Glu 1–Plg.SK, and Val 562–Pln.SK, when compared with human Plg, revealed great differences in the tertiary structures of the various Plg scissle bonds.[27] The k_{Plg} values varied by as much as 100-fold, while differences in the K_{Plg} values were relatively small. The second-order rate constants varied by as much as 1400-fold. The results of this study confirm the activation mechanism previously postulated, namely, that rapid equilibrium rather than steady-state conditions prevail and that k_2 (acylation) is the catalytic rate constant and the rate-determining step, while K_s is a true dissociation constant. Calculations of the free energy of interaction of the Plg activation reactions indicate three to five subsite binding interactions for u-PA and four to six binding interactions for SK for the activation catalytic event. Val 562–Pln.SK is more like u-PA than SK as an activator in activating nonhuman Plg species; it is a preformed activator and does not have to form an activator complex as SK does.

The kinetic parameters of Plg activation by t-PA are influenced greatly by fibrin; in the presence of fibrin, t-PA has an increased affinity for the Plg substrate, as shown in a decreased K_{Plg}. In the presence of fibrin(ogen) (e.g., fibrin monomer, fibrin films, CNBr-degraded fibrinogen), the K_{Plg} for Glu 1–Plg activation drops from approximately 65 to approximately 0.16 µM, with a slight increase in k_{Plg} from approximately 2 to 4 min^{-1}. The catalytic efficiencies or second-order rate constants (k_{Plg}/K_{Plg}) increase from approximately 5 to approximately 32 µM^{-1} min^{-1}, a 6-fold increase. Single-chain, two-chain, and recombinant t-PA show similar results. The reported kinetic data are variable and depend primarily on the fibrin(ogen) cofactor. The proposed mechanism of activation of Plg by t-PA involves the binding (strong) of t-PA to fibrin and the binding (weak) of native Glu 1–Plg to fibrin, resulting in plasmin generation at the fibrin surface.

Fibrinogen and its plasmic cleavage products also affect the kinetics of activation parameters of u-PA. The second-order rate constants (k_{Plg}/K_{Plg}) of activation of Glu 1–Plg with HMW-u-PA increase approximately 4-fold in the presence of fibrinogen, or fragment D, and increase approximately 2-fold in the presence of fragment E; these proteins do not affect the second-order rate constants of u-PA activation of Lys 78–Plg. Glu 1–Plg can bind to the fragment D region of fibrinogen/fibrin through its low-affinity binding sites, and when lysine binds to these sites, the activation to Glu 1–Plg is accelerated. The conversion of Glu 1–Plg to Lys 78–Plg by Lys 78–Pln is enhanced by interaction with the fibrinogen domains. Also, the binding of Lys 78–Plg to the fragment E region, which occurs through the high-affinity binding site (kringle 1 region), must localize Pln on the substrate as well as protect Pln from inhibitors and autolytic degradation.

Isolated components of the extracellular matrix (ECM) also affect the kinetics of activation parameters of t-PA with native Glu 1–Plg and degraded Lys 78–Plg (form 2).[28] Several of the ECM protein components studied stimulated the activation of both Plgs. With Glu 1–Plg, the catalytic efficiencies of activation (k_{Plg}/K_{Plg}) increased due to a decrease in K_{Plg} and an increase in k_{Plg}: CNBr-degraded fibrinogen, 10-fold; collagen IV, 21-fold; gelatin IV, 55-fold; and laminin, 5-fold. With Lys 78–Plg, the K_{Plg} changes were small, but the k_{Plg} changes were relatively large: CNBr-degraded fibrinogen, 7-fold; collagen III, 9-fold; collagen IV, 5-fold; collagen V, 9-fold, fibronectin, 6-fold; and laminin, 8-fold. However, amidolytic activity of t-PA was enhanced 12-fold by ECM proteins. Actin (muscle, spleen, and platelet) accelerates Pln generation from native Glu 1–Plg by t-PA; the k_{Plg}/K_{Plg} increases several-fold due to a decrease in K_{Plg}.[29] Actin has been found to bind to the kringle domains of Pln, inhibiting its enzymatic activity.

Lipoprotein (a) [Lp(a)] inhibits native Glu 1–Plg activation by SK, u-PA, and t-PA.[30] Sequencing of cloned human Lp(a) cDNA showed that it is very similar to human Plg.[31] With SK, Lp(a) inhibits Plg activation by competitive and uncompetitive inhibition. Lp(a) competes with Pg for SK and forms a stable complex with SK. Lp(a) does not inhibit Plg activation by the Pln-SK preformed activator complex. The Plg.SK, with an active site (virgin enzyme, single-chain Pln) is a possible target for Lp(a) uncompetitive inhibition. The competitive inhibition constant is 45 nM and the uncompetitive inhibition constant is 140 nM, corresponding to physiologic and pathophysiologic Lp(a) concentrations, respectively. The activity of Plg.SK was unaffected by heparin, whether or not fibrin was present. With u-PA, Lp(a) is a competitive inhibitor of native Plg activation with an inhibition constant of 20 nM. The glycosaminoglycans heparin, and heparan stimulate the rate of u-PA activation of native Plg by increasing k_{Plg} by 5.3-fold and 3.5-fold, respectively, but not K_{Plg}.[30] They may enhance the rate of Plg activation through an interaction with the catalytic domain of u-PA with dissociation constants of approximately 30 nM. Fibrin potentiates the activity of heparin on u-PA. Lp(a) inhibits heparin and heparan stimulation of Pln formation. Lp(a) is a competitive inhibitor of t-PA–mediated Plg activation with an inhibition constant of 30 nM. Heparin and heparan enhance native Plg conversion to Pln by t-PA; they increase the k_{Plg} by 25-fold and 3.5-fold, respectively, but not the K_{Plg}.[30] They stimulate t-PA activity by interacting with the finger domain of t-PA, with association constants of 1000 and 200 nM, respectively. The stimulation of t-PA activity by fibrin is attenuated by heparin. Lp(a) is a competitive inhibitor of t-PA–mediated Plg activation with an inhibition constant of 30 nM.

PLASMIN

Pln, a serine protease with trypsin-like specificity, is formed when Plg is activated by various types of physiologic and pathologic activators, e.g., u-PA (pro-u-PA), t-PA, and SK.[1,32] Although its basic physiologic function in the circulation is probably to digest fibrin clots and thrombi, this enzyme also can convert other plasma zymogens by specific limited proteolysis to active enzymes. Also, increased activation of the fibrinolytic system in some diseases can result in free Pln in the circulation, resulting in extensive degradation of many of the components of the blood coagulation, kinin generation, and complement systems. This process is controlled by circulating Pln inhibitors, particularly α_2PI. The active center of Pln is found in the COOH-terminal light (B) chain portion of the enzyme (Val 562–Pln). In purified systems, Glu 1–Pln (M_r of about 92,000) can be prepared by activating Glu 1–Plg with u-PA in the presence of Pln inhibitors such as Trayslol (aprotinin), leupeptin, α_1-antitrypsin, antithrombin III (ATIII) (plus heparin), and α_2PI. In the absence of inhibitors, Glu 1–Plg is always activated to Lys 78–Pln (M_r of about 83,000). Similarly, partially degraded Lys 78–Plg can be activated to Lys 78–Pln, and substantially degraded Val 443–Plg is activated to Val 443–Pln (M_r of about 38,000). The physiologic Pln form is probably Glu 1–Pln. The selective reduction of the two interchain disulfide bonds connecting the heavy (A) chain and light (B) chain components of Lys 78–Pln gives a functionally active Val 562 light (B) chain that can be readily separated from the Lys 78 heavy (A) chain by affinity chromatography on L-lysine–substituted Sepharose. The Val 562 light (B) chain has the same enzymatic characteristics as the other Pln forms and is the smallest of the enzyme forms. The Lys 78 heavy (A) chain portion of the enzyme contains the ω-aminocarboxylic acid and fibrin binding sites. Lys 78–Plg$_a$, the virgin enzyme with an active site (single-chain Pln), has the same enzymatic properties as Lys 78–Pln.[33] The Arg 561–Val peptide bond of the single-chain plasmin can be cleaved by both u-PA and Plg.SK to yield the two-chain Lys 78–Pln.

The Glu 1, the Lys 78, and the Val 443 forms of Pln are two-chain monomers connected by two interchain disulfide bonds, Cys 548–Cys 666 and Cys 558–Cys 465. The COOH-terminal chain of the enzyme is the Val 562 light (B) chain (Val 562–Asn 791) and contains a single DFP-sensitive serine residue and a single TLCK (L-1-chloro-3-tosylamido-7-amino-heptanone)–sensitive histidine residue. This chain has a molecular weight of about 26,000 and is homologous in primary structure to the pancreatic serine proteases. It contains four intrachain disulfide bonds: Cys 588–Cys 604, Cys 680–Cys 747, Cys 710–Cys 726, and Cys 737–Cys 765. The interchain Cys 558–Cys 566 disulfide loop contains the essential Arg 561–Val activation-site peptide bond. The amino acid residues His 603, Asp 646, and Ser 741 in the Val 562 light (B) chain portion of the zymogen form the catalytic site. The functionally active human Pln-derived Val 562 light (B) chain has been prepared in both the carboxymethyl and sulfhydryl forms. The SK binding site is located on the Val 561 light (B) chain. The NH_2-terminal chains of the enzymes are the heavy (A) chains; these chains can be either Glu 1–Arg 561 (M_r of about 63,000), or Lys 78–Arg 561 (M_r of about 58,000), or Val 441–Arg 561 (M_r of about 12,000). The ω-aminocarboxylic acid and fibrin binding-sites are located on the Glu 1 and Lys 77 chains but not on the Val 442 chain; they are located on the kringle 1 to 4 regions with none on the kringle 5 region. The fibrin binding sites are physiologically important since the Glu 1– and Lys 77–Plns and the Lys 77 heavy (A) chain bind to both fibrinogen-Sepharose and fibrin-Sepharose. There are 16 disulfide bonds in the Lys 77 heavy (A) chain, three each per kringle region and one connecting the kringle 2 and 3 regions. There are two disulfide bonds in the Glu 1–Lys 77 NH_2 terminus. One of the two carbohydrate moieties is found in the kringle 3 region and the other between the kringle 3 and 4 regions. The Glu 1– and Lys 77–Plgs and the Lys 77 heavy (A) chain also contain specific p-aminobenzamidine binding sites that are found only in the kringle 5 region. Functionally active sulfhydryl forms of the Val 562 light (B) chain and the Val 562–light (B) chain.SK complex have been prepared and recombined with a sulfhydryl form of the Lys 77 heavy (A) chain to form native recombinant Pln and native recombinant Pln.SK complex. A covalent hybrid Plg activator (M_r of about 92,000) has been prepared from the sulfhydryl form of the Lys 77 heavy (A) chain and the sulfhydryl form of the Ile 159 heavy (B) chain of u-PA. The plasminogen activator activity of the covalent hybrid was stimulated in the presence of soluble fibrin, about five-fold over u-PA, and this hybrid could be adsorbed to a fibrin clot. Its specific fibrinolytic activity was increased fourfold over u-PA in a clot lysis assay. A similar covalent hybrid (M_r of about 92,000) has been prepared from the sulfhydryl form of the Ile 279 light (B) chain of t-PA. The Plg activator activity with fibrin was about 40% of the parent t-PA. In a clot lysis assay, the hybrid has the same fibrinolytic activity as the parent t-PA.

The Pln-derived light (B) chain (residues 562–791) and the pancreatic serine proteases are found on the same branch of the evolutionary tree, whereas the clotting enzymes thrombin and activated factor X are on a second branch. All these enzymes cleave with varying restrictions after either arginine or lysine residues, except for chymotrypsin and elastase, which cleave instead after certain hydrophobic residues. These latter two enzymes share a critical amino acid substitution at position 189 (in chymotrypsinogen) which is associated with this change in specificity. The preparation of stable Pln solutions has been described. The Pln form generated in an activation mixture depends on the Plg form used, the activator, the molar ratio of zymogen to activator, the presence and concentration of stabilizers (e.g., glycerol, lysine, EACA), the pH and temperature, and the presence or absence of a reversible inhibitor (e.g., leupeptin). The Lys 78–Pln form in 25% to 50% glycerol is probably the major form currently being used and can be prepared from either the highly purified native Glu 1 or partially degraded Lys 78 zymogens. Human Lys 78–Pln reference preparations have been prepared and standardized in international units (IU).

Pln cleaves proteins and peptides at arginyl and lysyl peptide bonds and basic amino acid esters and amides. The enzyme has a preference for lysyl peptide bonds in proteins (e.g., fibrinogen and fibrin) and ester substrates. Functional assay methods have been described for the zymogen (after activation) and the enzyme with the use of protein substrates, synthetic esters, chromogenic substrates, and fluorescent substrates. Guanidinobenzoates and nitroanilides have been used to determine the enzyme concentration in solution by active-site titration methods and to determine active-site formation in the zymogen during the interaction of stoichiometric amounts of Plg and SK. Specific functional assays have been developed with the use of Trasylol and α_2PI to determine enzyme concentration; these inhibitors bind irreversibly to the Pln active center in all enzyme species to form irreversible mole:mole enzyme-enzyme inhibitor complexes. Methods have been described for determining the molar concentration of both zymogen and enzyme in solution through the use of the specificity of their interactions with SK, which form stoichiometric complexes. Also, the equimolar Plg.SK and Pln.SK complexes have Plg activator activity that can be measured quantitatively with either highly purified human or bovine or porcine Plg as substrates. Radioimmunoassays and immunochemical methods have been used to measure Plg levels in plasma. Quantitative clot lysis assays also have been developed.

The specific proteolytic activities of highly purified Lys 77–Pln (>95% active sites), Val 443–Pln (>95% active sites), and Val 562 light (B) chain (about 35% active sites) on a casein substrate are approximately 30, 60, and 3 IU/mg protein, respectively. The formation of the Val 561–light (B) chain.SK complex from the individual pure components increases the titratable active sites to greater than 85%, indicating that the Val 562 light (B) chain is not in a well-organized three-dimensional structure; it apparently requires the two interchain disulfide bonds together with a small part of the Lys 77 heavy (A) chain (maximum of Val 442–Arg 561) to stabilize the active center. The Val 562–light (B) chain.SK complex, whether prepared from individual components or from the Glu 1– or Lys 77–Plg.SK complex, has similar human Plg activator and bovine Plg activator activities and the same specific proteolytic activity as the Val 562 light (B) chain component of the complex.

Steady-state kinetic parameters, the apparent Michaelis constant (K_m), and the catalytic rate constant (k_{cat}), have been used to describe the catalytic reaction between enzyme and substrate. These parameters have been determined for various types of Plns on a variety of synthetic substrates at different pHs and temperatures. The K_m varies from 10 to 1000 μM, and the k_{cat} varies from 1 to 75 s^{-1}, with second-order rate constants (k_{cat}/K_m) of approximately 0.1 $\mu M^{-1}s^{-1}$. These summary data also include the amidase parameters of different Pln.SK species. The Val 562 light (B) chain has a K_m value of 1260 μM and a k_{cat} value of 14.5 s^{-1}, with a k_{cat}/K_m value of approximately 0.01 $\mu M^{-1}s^{-1}$. With tripeptidyl-p-nitroanilide substrates, subsite amino acids greatly influence the catalytic efficiency (k_{cat}/K_m) of the enzyme. ω-aminocarboxylic acids both enhance and inhibit Pln activity; they increase both the K_m values (inhibition) and the k_{cat} values (enhancement). Specific antibodies to Plg (Pln) inhibit both activation of Plg and Pln activity.

PLASMA PLASMIN INHIBITORS

Human plasma contains inhibitors that regulate the activity of proteolytic enzymes generated during the activation of the fibrinolytic, clotting, complement, and kinin-generating systems.[1,34] These protease inhibitors react at different rates with generated Pln and depend on the concentration and type of Plg activator used and the concentration of Plg in the system. α_2PI (concentration of about 1 μM) is the most specific Pln inhibitor and has the strongest affinity for Pln, giving inactive, irreversible Pln.Pln inhibitor complexes. α_2M (concentration of about 3 μM) binds Pln after α_2PI is depleted. It is a slow-binding Pln inhibitor. The Pln-α_2M complexes are active and are rapidly removed from the circulation. It has been postulated that α_2M is a "trap" for endopeptidases. The other plasma protease inhibitors, α_1AT (concentration of about 37 μM), ATIII (concentration of about 5 μM), and C1 inhibitor (concentration of about 2 μM), are effective Pln inhibitors in purified systems. Pln activity also may be regulated by fibrinogen, inhibited via its LBS. Actin, a cellular protein found in micromolar concentrations in plasma, was found to be a noncompetitive inhibitor of Pln; covalent complexes were not found. Thrombospondin, another cellular protein found in normal and transformed cells, appears to be a slow tight-binding stoichiometric inhibitor of Pln.[34] Kringle domains of Plg are involved in these processes.

α_2PI is a single-chain glycoprotein with a carbohydrate content of 13 to 14% with two disulfide bridges and a molecular weight of about 58,000.[35] Its concentration in plasma is about 1 μM, corresponding to 7 mg/dl. DNA and protein sequencing revealed that it contains 452 amino acids and 4 Asn-linked glycosylation sites. α_2PI in normal plasma is heterogeneous and consists of functionally active and inactive proteins. Complete activation of the Plg present in normal plasma converts only 70% of the α_2PI antigen into a complex with Pln; 30% of the inhibitor-related antigen appears to be functionally inactive. Human plasma also contains two forms of the inhibitor that differ in their binding to Plg. The form that does not bind remains an active Pln inhibitor but reacts much more slowly with Pln. This form lacks a 26-residue peptide from the COOH-terminal end of α_2PI. This peptide inhibits the interaction of α_2PI with Pln, suggesting that it contains the Pln (Plg) binding site. The weak-binding form is converted from the strong-binding form in the circulation.

α_2PI has three functional sites: (1) the Pln (Plg) binding site, (2) the reactive site, and (3) the cross-linking site. It has a strong affinity for Pln (Plg) and preferentially binds to the LBSs or fibrin binding sites on the Pln (Plg) molecule. α_2PI competitively inhibits the binding of Plg to fibrin. The naturally occurring fibrinolytic process is the result of fibrin-associated Plg activation and depends on the amount of both Plg and Plg activator bound to fibrin. Therefore, inhibition of Plg binding to fibrin by α_2PI results in retardation of the initiation of the fibrinolytic process. The Pln (Plg) binding site in α_2PI is located in its COOH-terminal region at Lys 436 and Lys 452. This binding site plays an important role in the inhibition of Pln. α_2PI rapidly forms a reversible complex with Pln through noncovalent binding between the LBS in Pln and the Pln (Plg) binding site of α_2PI. This step in the reaction can be competitively inhibited by Plg fragments containing the LBS or by EACA, which binds to the LBS. The partially degraded form of α_2PI, without the Pln (Plg) binding site, reacts less readily with Pln, indicating a significant contribution of the Pln (Plg) binding site to the efficient inhibition of Pln. In the second step, a covalent bond is formed between the active-site serine of Pln and the reactive site of α_2PI resulting in the loss of Pln proteolytic activity. The reactive site of α_2PI is located at Arg 364.

Another important function of α_2PI is its cross-linking to fibrin. When blood clots, part of the α_2PI present in plasma is rapidly cross-linked to the fibrin α chain by activated fXIII. While clot retraction is progressively taking place, the fibrin-bound α_2PI becomes condensed in the clot and contributes to the resistance of the clot against lysis. Fibrin-fibrin cross-linking is only of minor importance in endowing the clot with resistance to lysis. The α_2PI cross-linking site is located at the second amino acid from the NH$_2$ terminus, Gln. The residue in the fibrin(ogen) molecule where the Gln residue of α_2PI cross-links is Lys 303 of the Aα chain. No other serine protease inhibitor has a fXIIIa–catalyzed cross-linking site under physiologic conditions. When homologous amino acid sequences of α_2PI and the other members of the serine protease inhibitor family (serpins), e.g., ATIII, α_1AT, and PAI-1, are aligned, α_2PI extends 50 to 52 amino acids beyond the COOH-terminal ends of the other members of the serpin family. This extra COOH-terminal end that is specific for α_2PI contains the Pln (Plg) binding site. Although the cross-linking reaction proceeds rapidly, the maximum level of cross-linking is limited to only 20 to 25% of the αPI present in plasma before clotting. Most of the α_2PI cross-linked to the α chain of fibrin is in the form of the α-chain monomer–α_2PI complex, which is gradually transformed into the α-chain polymer–α_2PI complex as polymerization proceeds. Another plasma protein, fibronectin, is also cross-linked to the fibrin α chain by activated fXIII when blood coagulation takes place. However, these two proteins, α_2PI and fibronectin, are independently cross-linked to fibrin without affecting the cross-linking of the other. Although the amount of αPI cross-linked to fibrin is low, it is significant in the inhibition of clot lysis. However, the inhibitor effect of free α_2PI on clot lysis is limited. The absence of cross-linking of α_2PI to fibrin, in addition to an increased affinity of non-crossed-linked fibrin for Pln (Plg), may contribute to the instability of hemostatic plugs in fXIII deficiency by increasing the susceptibility of fibrin clots to the naturally occurring fibrinolytic process. The congenital deficiency of α_2PI results in a lifelong severe hemorrhagic tendency due to the premature degradation of hemostatic plugs by the physiologically occurring fibrinolytic process.

ABNORMAL PLASMINOGENS: DYSPLASMINOGENEMIAS

Inherited disorders of the Pln-dependent fibrinolytic system can result in thromboembolic disease.[17,36,37] Congenital deficiencies of Plg in patients with normal hemostatic parameters associated with impaired fibrinolysis may be a risk factor in coronary artery disease and cerebral infarction. Abnormal Plg may be regarded as a predisposing factor but not the causative factor in the development of thrombophilia. Patients with Plg deficiencies, hypoplasminogenemias, and dysplasminogenemias with normal hemostatic parameters and with a history of thromboembolism are rare. Plg deficiencies associated with thrombosis with familial involvement have been described in about 20 families.

Two types of familial Plg deficiencies have been described—the hypoplasminogenemias and the dysplasminogenemias. The true hypoplasminogenemias, congenital Plg deficiencies, have lower antigen levels with a plasma functional-to-antigen ratio of about 1:1 with Plg levels below 70% of normal. The dysplasminogenemias, with abnormalities in the Plg molecule, have a reduced functional activity with a plasma functional-to-antigen ratio of from about 0.9:1 to 0.2:1 with normal plasma Plg antigen levels.

CHARACTERIZATION OF VARIANT PLASMINOGENS

Yields and Specific Activities

The characterization of the dysfunctional Plg and the determination of the molecular defect require highly purified proteins. The isolation of Plg from normal and variant plasmas using the classical L-lysine–substituted Sepharose method gives yields of about 10 to 14 mg/dl, with specific activities (after activation) of about 28 IU/mg protein for normal plasmas that will vary from about 10 to 20 IU/mg protein for the variant plasmas depending on the plasma functional-to-antigen ratio. With the hypoplasminogenemias, where there is a parallel decrease in the functional and antigen levels, the Plg yields will be lower and will depend

on the plasma levels, but the specific activities of the isolated Plgs also will vary from 28 IU/mg protein (normal) to 15 to 20 IU/mg protein (abnormal); the lower specific activities indicate dysfunctional/abnormal proteins. With true heterozygotes, the specific activities will be about 50% of the normal value, indicating that 50% of the molecules are normal. With the isolated, highly purified Plgs, yields and specific activities are important parameters for characterizing these proteins.

Plasmin Generation

Another important parameter for defining an abnormal protein is its ability to generate Pln. Pln generation has proven to be useful in identifying a number of dysfunctional proteins, e.g., Chicago I, II, and III, Frankfurt I and II, and Maywood I; all these abnormal proteins have low plasmin generation rates. The methods used to study Pln generation from normal and abnormal Plgs are (1) measuring initial velocities (rates) of Plg activation at either a fixed concentration of Plg with varying concentrations of two or three activators or varying concentrations of Plg with a fixed concentration of two or three activators using specific Pln substrates and (2) measuring Plg activation by two-stages: activation for a fixed time with a fixed concentration of Plg and activator and followed by the addition of a specific Pln substrate (endpoint assay). These comparative Pln generation methods differ significantly from the kinetic methods, where substantially higher concentrations of Plg, 10- to 100-fold, are being used with similar concentrations of activator.

Generation of Active Sites in the Equimolar Plasminogen-Streptokinase Complexes

Human Plg reacts with SK to form a stoichiometric 1:1 complex that is a specific Plg activator. SK's only known function is to form an equimolar complex with human Plg, as well as with several other mammalian Plgs, which are then converted into Plg activators. After formation of the complex, the inactive zymogen is rapidly transformed by SK into a molecule with an active site without any apparent peptide bond cleavages in either protein. Following this initial event, a series of transformations involving limited specific peptide bond cleavages takes place in both proteins. The Plg.SK complex with intact SK and with an active site is functionally the "virgin" activator with the highest specific activity. SK undergoes progressive intramolecular degradation in the complex to large protein fragments of molecular weights from about 44,000 to 26,000 and a smaller peptide with a molecular weight of about 10,000 without any apparent loss of protein/peptide material from the complex. The native Glu 1–Plg converts to Glu 1–Pln by intramolecular cleavage of the Arg 561–Val peptide bond and then to Lys 78–Pln in the complex by cleavage of the Lys 77–78 peptide bond. The final activator complex is the Lys 78–Pln.SK form.

The rate of active site generation in the Pln.SK complex varies with abnormal Plgs. Variant Plgs can easily be identified by the slow formation of this active site, which means slower generation of the activator complex. The measurement of plasma Plg with excess SK depends on the rate of generation of the active site in the complex; both initial rate and two-stage (endpoint) assays will quickly show the presence of abnormal Plg.SK complexes with normal and all abnormal Plgs. SK forms complexes with both normal and abnormal Plgs. Heterozygote Plgs with 50% inert molecules will form the complexes without generation of an active site in the defective molecules.

Amidase Parameters/Kinetics of Plasminogen Activation Parameters

The functional defect in the variant Plgs is in the potential active center of the zymogen. When approximately equal amounts of normal and abnormal molecules are found in the patient's plasma, the abnormal molecules have no potential to generate Pln (e.g., heterozygotes Tochigi I and Frankfurt I) due to an inert active center. The normal molecules will generate Pln and will generally have normal amidase and kinetics of activation parameters. All plasminogen activators will con-

vert Plg to Pln by cleavage of a single specific peptide bond, Arg 561–Val, in the zymogen to generate the active site. A molecular defect in the active site will produce an inert enzyme.

A mathematical model for studying Plg activation has been developed to accommodate all activator species. The amidase parameters of the enzymes, different Pln and activator species, Plg.SK complexes, u-PA, and t-PA, vary with second-order rate constants from 0.01 to 0.30 $\mu mol^{-1}s^{-1}$. The kinetics of Plg activation parameters for the activator species with normal Plgs also vary, with second-order rate constants from about 28 to 170 $\mu mol^{-1}min^{-1}$. CNBr-degraded fibrinogen will enhance the activation about 1.3-fold for the Plg.SK and u-PA species and about 12-fold for the t-PA species; this enhancement will vary from 10- to 2000-fold, depending on the assay methodology used.

Patients have been described with variant Plgs with plasma functional levels from 26% (Maywood I), to 41% (Chicago I), to 80% (Chicago III), to 88% (Chicago II), with normal antigen levels and kinetic defects. The interpretation of the kinetic data with these variant Plgs is possible only in terms of a homogeneous population of molecules, because 85 to 100% active sites can be generated in these molecules (patients are homozygotes). These variants are all catalytically less efficient than normal molecules, but the kinetics of the Plg activation parameters of the variants with different activators gave lower second-order rate constants and were different from one another. The kinetics of activation defects were in the binding properties of the activators to the variants, deviation from Michaelis-Menten activation kinetics, K_{Plg}, and in the active sites formed in the Plg moiety of the zymogen.SK complexes, with impaired cleavage of the Arg 561–Val scissile board, k_{Plg}. The u-PA kinetics of Plg activation data with the variants I and II point to an activation mechanism identical to that proposed for SK, namely, the formation of a Plg.u-PA complex analogous to the Plg.SK complex. FTN Plg was found to have lower second-order rate constants with t-PA compared with adult Plg due to an increased K_{Plg} and to a decreased k_{Plg}, indicating a dysfunctional molecule.

Equimolar Plasminogen-Streptokinase Complexes

The binding of SK to Plg, the rate of formation of the equimolar Plg.SK complex, and the generation of the active site in the complex are properties that reflect the fundamental integrity of the native Plg molecule—its three-dimensional, two-dimensional, and primary structures, particularly the COOH-terminal domain that contains the SK binding sites. All Plg variants, both zymogens and inert proteins, bind SK. Normal Plg.SK complexes form zymogen.SK complexes with an active site that then converts to the Pln.SK complexes; all these complexes are Plg activators. In the complex, the zymogen-to-enzyme conversion results in the cleavage of the Arg 561–Val peptide bond and a secondary bond cleavage of the Lys 77–Lys peptide bound; these are the typical Glu 1– to Lys 78–zymogen and –enzyme conversions. SK, in the complex with an active site, undergoes a series of intramolecular bond cleavages to give large and small fragments, all bound to the zymogen. There is little loss in mass or activator activity during these conversions; maximum Plg activator activity remains in the complexes.

The formation, conversion, and degradation of the Plg.SK complexes can be followed in PAGE and SDS-PAGE systems. The PAGE gels permit, with time, the visualization of the various complexes and fragments. Also, scanning of these gels will permit one to estimate and quantitate the concentrations of the various components in the mixtures. With normal Plg, the zymogen.SK and enzyme.SK complexes are readily identified, both before and after reduction. Many variant Plgs form complexes with SK that do not readily convert to Pln.SK. Different types of complexes form: (1) two types of Plg.SK complexes, I (abnormal) and II (normal), are found, and both convert to Pln.SK; also, complex I converts to complex II; (2) two Pln.SK complexes, I and II, are found; also, complex I converts to complex II; and (c) a major degraded Plg/Pln.SK complex is formed instantaneously on mixing the components. Not only do the patients show these different types of complexes, but family members, with no history of thrombophilia, also show similar complexes.

These usual complexes also may permit us to characterize variant plasminogen types by PAGE methods.

Plasminogen Polymorphism: Isoelectric Forms

Plg polymorphism has been described using isoelectric focusing techniques with plasma in PAGE systems; the plasma Plg forms can be detected by immunofixation and zymographic methods. Plg is coded by an autosomal gene with two common alleles, Plg A and Plg B. These common alleles, A and B, are found in all investigated races, but with different allele frequencies (from 0.98 for A in mongoloids to 0.69 for A in caucasoids); they are fairly constant within each race. Rare alleles, in all races, have a frequency of about 0.01 to 0.03; these rare alleles are found in patients with variant proteins. A nomenclature for Plg polymorphism has been proposed (Fig. 4-3). A nonfunctional Plg variant, Tochigi I, was detected in a Japanese population with a gene frequency of 0.018; this abnormal variant was not detected in an American white population, suggesting the very rare occurrence of this variant in the white population.

Isoelectric focusing of purified Plg in PAGE and in columns using both normal and several variant Plgs (e.g., Chicago I, II, and III) gave about 10 to 12 normal isoelectric forms, with isoelectric points from pH 5.64 to pH 7.05. Major forms were found at pH values 5.72, 5.97, 6.20, 6.30, and 6.37,.and each of these major forms can be isolated when column isoelectric focusing systems are used. The Tochigi I heterozygote is a mixture of some 10 to 12 normal isoelectric forms with a similar number of abnormal forms in "doublets." The Frankfurt I heterozygote gave an isoelectric form pattern with fewer bands than normal Plg, including several missing anodic bands and with quantitatively more negatively charged bands. The position of each of the variant Plg bands along the pH gradient was not identical to the position of any of the normal Plg bands. Electrophoresis and crossed immunoelectrophoresis showed that Frankfurt I was more negatively charged than normal Plg.

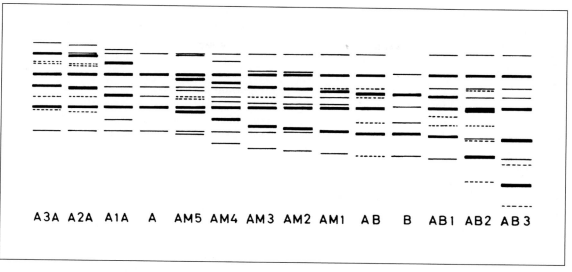

FIGURE 4-3. Schematic representation of plasminogen phenotypes with recognized variants, a proposed nomenclature. (Reprinted with permission from Skoda V, et al. Proposal for the nomenclature of human plasminogen polymorphism. Vox Sanguinis 1986;51:244.)

Charge Mutation: Electrophoretic Mobility

Charge mutations of variant Plgs have been described (e.g., Frankfurt I and San Antonio). Frankfurt I gave a more negative charge when compared with normal Plg in electrophoresis, in crossed immunoelectrophoresis, and in isoelectric focusing. However, with San Antonio, a more positive charge was found, with an extra band, in the more anodic isozyme range and without a corresponding normal band.

Molecular Defect

The primary structure of human Plg has been established by amino acid and DNA sequence analysis (see Fig. 4-2). The full-length cDNA is 2.7 kilobases. The organization and structure of the gene coding for Plg have been determined; the gene spans about 52.5 kilobases of DNA with 19 exons, interrupted by 18 introns. They code for the domains of the molecule involved in (1) fibrin binding (the five kringle structures are coded by two exons), (2) activator cleavage of the Arg 561–Val peptide bond, and (c) catalysis (the potential active center of the enzyme). The Plg gene was mapped to the long arm of chromosome 6 at bands q26–q27. The Plg gene is closely related to the lipoprotein (a) gene.

DNAs from 11 individuals from 3 unrelated Japanese families were analyzed for gene abnormalities. Five individuals from two families were found to have a substitution of Ala 601 to Thr 601 in the active center region in exon 15 (type I abnormality). This substitution is close to His 603, Asp 645, and Ser 741 in the active site. Three members of a third family were found to have a Val 355 to Phe 355 substitution in the kringle 4 region in exon 6 (type II abnormality). These two mutations have been found only in Japanese families, where both heterozygotes and homozygotes have been identified. These mutations have not been found in either American or European families, where other abnormal Plgs have been identified with active center defects.

Classification of Abnormal Plasminogens

An attempt has been made to classify the well-characterized abnormal Plgs. Because the variants do not have the same properties, it is necessary to establish a classification in which similar proteins are grouped together. Those variants with an active center defect that are heterozytes (50% normal Plg molecules and 50% abnormal Plg molecules) can be grouped into one class; they are Tochigi I and II, Nagoya I and II, Kagoshima, Paris I, Tokyo, Frankfurt I, II, and III, and San Antonio and Cleveland. Frankfurt I and San Antonio also have a charge mutation. In this class, the functionally abnormal molecules do not form an active enzyme on activation with Plg activators; the Tochigi I homozygote has 94% abnormal molecules, and the Kagoshima homozygote has 92% abnormal molecules. Those variants with an active center defect and with kinetic defects are classified as homozygotes and are grouped into another class; they are Chicago I, II, and III and Maywood I. In this class, the abnormal molecules form active enzyme, and greater than 85% active sites are formed in the equimolar Plg.SK complex. Frankfurt II and Cleveland are hypoplasminogen-emias with an active center defect, and Cleveland also has a kinetic defect.

The abnormal Plgs can be subdivided into two types: type 1a, b, and c dysplasminogenemias and type 2a and c dysplasminogenemias. The type 1a dysplasminogenemias, with an active center defect, are Tochigi I and II, Nagoya I and II, Kagoshima, Paris I, Tokyo, and Frankfurt III. The type 1b dysplasminogenemias, with an active center defect and a charge mutation, are Frankfurt I and San Antonio. The type 1c dysplasminogenemias, with active center and kinetic defects, are Chicago I, II, and III and Maywood I. The type 2a dysplasminogenemia, with an active center defect, is Frankfurt I, a hypoplasminogenemia. The type 2c dysplasminogenemia, with active center and kinetic defects, is Cleveland, a hypoplasminogenemia. The classification is found in Table 4-1. This classification will change when complete information on the molecular defect of each variant Plg is available.

TABLE 4-1. Classification of Abnormal Plasminogens: Dysplasminogenemias

		Plasma		
		Functional Level,* % of Normal	Antigen Level[†]	Reference[‡]
Type 1: Dysplasminogenemia				
a. Active center defect	Heterozygotes[§]			
Tochigi I		46	N	(38)
Tochigi II		45	N	(39)
Nagoya		19	N	(39, 40)
Nagoya II		55	N	(40)
Kagoshima		44	N	(40)
Paris I		28	N	(41)
Tokyo		20	N	(42)
b. Active center defect and charge mutation	Heterozygotes			
Frankfurt I		48	N	(43)
San Antonio		44	N	(44)
c. Active center and kinetic defects	Homozygotes[¶]			
Chicago I		41	N	(45)
Chicago II		88	N	(45)
Chicago III		80	N	(46)
Maywood I		26	N	(47)
Type 2: Dysplasminogenemia: Hypoplasminogenemia				
a. Active center defect	Heterozygotes			
Frankfurt II		62	66	(48)
c. Active center and kinetic defects	Heterozygotes			
Cleveland		40	64	(49)

*Functional % of normal value, not % of normal range values.
[†]N, normal, range 70–130%, varies in different laboratories.
[‡]See reference list.
[§]Heterozygotes—normal and abnormal plasminogen molecules, mainly 50% each; Togichi I has homozygote niece—6% normal and 94% abnormal molecules; the abnormal molecules do not form active enzyme.
[¶]Homozygotes—homogeneous population of abnormal plasminogen molecules, with greater than 85% forming active molecules.

Thrombophilia and Dysplasminogenemaia

Many patients with thrombophilia have been found to have abnormal variant Plgs. These patients will have both normal and low-normal Plg antigen levels, with lower than normal functional levels. In these patients, the functional-to-antigen ratio is always less than 1:1. Patients have been found with a congenital Plg deficiency, about 65% antigen level, with a functional-to-antigen ratio of about 1:1 and with an abnormal Plg (see Table 4-1). There are many reports of patients with congenital Plg deficiencies, hypoplasminogenemias, where the hemostatic parameters are normal; however, no studies were performed to determine if these patients also have abnormal proteins and dysplasminogenemias. The methodologies described in this review can easily identify those patients with variant Plgs. The identification depends on the ability of a laboratory to quantitatively determine Plg functional and antigen levels and to characterize the isolated Plg by the methods described above.

The factors involved in the precipitation of the thrombotic event in those patients with abnormal Plgs are not known. One usually does not find a history of thromboembolic disease in family members. It is possible that there is a defective assembly of Plg, Plg activators, and inhibitors on the fibrin-thrombus in addition to slow activation of Plg and defective clot lysis. Also, defective assembly on the endothelial cell surface is possible due to poor binding of Plg to surface Plg receptors, preventing the generation of Pln. It should be possible to develop in vitro models to study the assembly of the fibrinolytic components on cell and thrombus surfaces in order to study the role of abnormal variant Plgs in clot dissolution.

PLASMINOGEN RECEPTORS

Assembly of Fibrinolytic System Components of Fibrin-Thrombus and Cell Surfaces

The components of the fibrinolytic system assemble on the surface of the fibrin-thrombus and on cell surfaces, generating Pln.[50–53] The fibrin surface and many cell surfaces regulate fibrinolysis in the vascular system. The fibrin surface assembles Plg, Plg activators, and Plg inhibitors, regulating clot dissolution. Once formed on the fibrin surface, Pln begins the process of fibrin degradation, including the generating of new binding sites (COOH-terminal residues) for native Plg, the conversion of native Plg to the degraded Lys 78–Plg form, which activates at more rapid rates than native Glu 1–Plg to Lys 78–Pln. The fibrin surface protects bound Pln from inactivation by α_2PI.

A striking analogy exists between the role of cells and fibrin surfaces on the binding of the fibrinolytic system components in the regulation of Plg activation and generation of Pln (Fig. 4-4). The similarities include (1) the presence of specific binding sites for Plg and Plg activator, (2) the enhanced efficiency of Plg activation, (3) a role for COOH-terminal lysines in mediating Plg and Pln binding, and (4) the protection of bound Pln from α_2PI on both surfaces.

Interaction of Plasminogen with Cells/Receptors-Binding Proteins

Many cell types express receptors for Plg[54–56] and Plg activators (e.g., u-PA).[57–59] Pro-u-PA and u-PA bind to cells, and the conversion of the single-chain proenzyme to the two-chain enzyme occurs on the cell surface. The colocalization of u-PA and/or t-PA and Plg allows Pln formation to proceed, and the activation is catalytically more favorable on the cell surface than in solution. Pln is retained by cell surfaces, perhaps with higher affinity than Plg, and cell-bound Pln is protected from inactivation by α_2PI. As a consequence of these interactions, the cells are able to harness Pln activity. In addition to its capacity to degrade fibrin, Pln has broad substrate recognition, allowing it to cleave a variety of molecules on cell surfaces and within the pericellular environment, e.g., degradation of matrix constituents and activation of various zymogens.[50, 51] Assembly of the Plg system arms the cell surface with a proteinase that is capable of contributing broadly not only to normal cellular functions but also to pathophysiologic processes, including cancer cell invasion and metastasis.

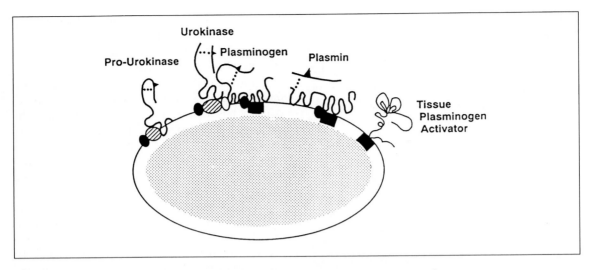

FIGURE 4-4. *Assembly of the fibrinolytic system on cell surfaces. Cells can express specific receptors for the plasminogen activators, tissue-type plasminogen activator and urokinase-type plasminogen activator, and for plasminogen. As a consequence of colocalization of activators and zymogen, plasminogen is converted to plasmin, and plasmin is retained on the cell surface. Cell-bound plasmin may convert single-chain u-PA to its two-chain form, which, in turn, propagates plasmin formation. By virtue of its broad substrate recognition, cell-bound plasmin may be used to execute a variety of cellular functions. (Reprinted with permission from Plow EF, Felez J, Miles LA. Cellular regulation of fibrinolysis. Thromb Haemost 1991;66:33.)*

Many cells types have been shown to bind native Plg in a time-dependent specific and saturable manner.[50,51] Peripheral blood cells (with the exception of erythrocytes), endothelial cells, hepatocytes, monocytoid cells, lymphoid cells, and fibroblasts bind Plg with high capacity, from 0.37 to 49×10^5 sites per cell for white cells and from 141 to 310×10^5 sites per cell for the other cells, with a K_d of approximately 1 μM (0.3 to 2.8 μM) for all the cells studied, with approximately half the Plg binding sites on the cells, exposed to a 1.1 to 1.5 μM plasma concentration of Plg, occupied. Plg receptors are present at extremely high densities on cells. The number of Plg binding sites can exceed 10^7 sites per cell, and both adherent (fibroblasts, hepatocytes, and endothelial) cells and nonadherent (monocytoid and lymphoid) cells can express such high numbers of receptors. Plg binding to all cells types is inhibited by lysine and lysine analogues, indicating a common mechanism of ligand recognition. The LBSs of Plg are involved in the binding interactions. The existence of two cellular recognition sites within Plg could create a heterogeneity in the orientation of the molecule on the cell surface.[60] It is generally accepted that Plg and Pln can bind to the same sites but that Pln interacts with at least a subset of these sites with higher affinity; differences in affinity range from 2- to 50-fold. Glu 1–Plg appears to have a lower binding affinity than Lys 78–Plg. FTN Plg differs from adult Plg in carbohydrate composition, kinetics of activation second-order rate constants (with t-PA), and decreased binding to cellular receptors.[61]

It has not been established that a single cell membrane component serves exclusively as a Plg receptor. Both nonprotein and protein constituents have been implicated in Plg binding. Gangliosides have been identified as candidate receptors.[59] They inhibit Plg binding, they bind to cell membranes and enhance Plg binding, and Plg binds directly to gangliosides. This interaction is inhibited by lysine analogues. Peptides with COOH-terminal lysyl residues inhibit Plg binding to cells. The COOH-terminal 19 amino acids of α_2PI is a potent inhibitor. The alpha isoform of enolase (M_r of about 54,000) which has a COOH-terminal lysine residue binds to Plg with high affinity; it is present in extracts of the U937 monocytoid cells and was found to be localized on the cell surface.[56] An α-enolase–related protein is expressed on the cell surface and can function as a Plg receptor. Synovial fibroblasts have receptors for both Plg and SK. PMA stimulation of monocytes and monocytoid cells increases their expression of Plg binding sites. The nonadherent populations bound Plg with a 5- to 17-fold higher affinity. The capacity of cells to modulate their receptors for fibrinolytic components provides a means for regulating cell surface and pericellular proteolysis. Extracellular matrix basement-membrane type IV collagen has a specific binding site for Plg.[62]

Plasminogen Activation at the Surface of Normal and Malignant Cells

Plg and Plg activators assemble on the surface of both normal (e.g., endothelial cells and monocytes) and malignant cells and generate Pln. Plg receptors on these cells localize this zymogen within a defined microenvironment. Coexpression of u-PA receptors on these cells is critical for the generation of Pln. Plg activation is enhanced when the zymogen is bound to the cell surface; binding of Plg to the cell surface may change its conformation, rendering it more readily activatable. Also, activation of cell-bound native Plg is enhanced by its conversion to degraded Lys 78–Plg, a more readily activable form. This conversion may be via a membrane-bound serine protease or by means of Pln. Pln bound to the receptor appears to be protected from inactivation by α_2PI. Pln-α_2PI complexes apparently form on cell surfaces or are bound to cell surfaces. Surface-bound Plg activators may be protected from the specific physiologic activator inhibitors. The enhancement of the catalytic efficiency of Plg activation by cell surfaces (e.g., endothelial cells and monocytes) is an important regulatory mechanism for in situ fibrinolysis. Surface-bound Pln on transformed cells (e.g., U937 monocytoid cells,

HT 1080 fibrosarcoma cells, and melanoma Mel Juso cells) is an essential component of the proteolytic cascade for Plg activation during invasiveness of malignant cells, namely, pericellular proteolysis. Plg and Pln receptors have been identified in human malignant cells; bound Pln retains its enzymatic activity. These receptors can be solubilized by detergents; the solubilized receptors also bind both Plg and Pln.[54–56,63]

References

1. Robbins KC. The plasminogen-plasmin system. In: Colman RW, Hirsh J, Marder VJ, Salzman EW, eds. Hemostasis and thrombosis: basic principals and clinical practice. 2nd ed. Philadelphia: JB Lippincott, 1987:340.
2. Bachmann F. Fibrinolysis. In: Verstraete M, Vermylen J, Lijnen R, Arnout J, eds. Thrombosis and haemostasis. Leuven: International Society on Thrombosis and Haemostasis and Leuven University Press, 1987:227.
3. Nilsson TK, Wallen PB. The fibrinolytic system: biochemistry and assay methods. In: Nilsson TK, Boman K, Jansson JH. eds. Clinical aspects of fibrinolysis. Stockholm: Almqvist and Wiksell International, 1991:9.
4. Henkin J, Marcotte P, Yang H. The plasminogen-plasmin system. Prog Cardiovas Dis 1991;34:135.
5. Plow EF, Felez J, Miles LA. Cellular regulation of fibrinolysis. Thromb Haemost 1991;66:32.
6. Friberger P. Chromogenic peptide substrates: their use for the assay of factors in the fibrinolytic and plasma kallikrein-kinin systems. Scand J Clin Lab Invest 1982;42(suppl 162):49.
7. Wohl RC, Sinio L, Robbins KC. Methods for studying fibrinolytic pathway components in human plasma. Thromb Res 1982;27:523.
8. Rabiner SF, Goldfine, Hart A, et al. Radioimmunoassay of human plasminogen and plasmin. J Lab Clin Med 1969;74:265.
9. Estelles A, Aznar J, Gilabert J, et al. Dysfunctional plasminogen in a full-term newborn. Pediatr Res 1980;14:1180.
10. Raum D, Marcus D, Alper CA, et al. Synthesis of human plasminogen by the liver. Science 1980; 208:1036.
11. Forsgren M, Raden B, Israelsson M, et al. Molecular cloning and characterization of a full-length cDNA clone of human plasminogen. FEBS Lett 1987;213:254.
12. Petersen TE, Martzen MR, Ichinose A, et al. Characterization of a gene for human plasminogen, a

key proenzyme in the fibrinolytic system. J Biol Chem 1990;265:6101.

13. Busby SJ, Mulvihill E, Rao D, et al. Express of recombinant human plasminogen in mammalian cells is augmented by suppression of plasmin activity. J Biol Chem 1991;266:15286.

14. Gonzalez-Gronow M, Grenett HE, Fuller GM, et al. The role of carbohydrate in the functon of human plasminogen: comparison of the protein obtained from molecular cloning and expression in *Escherichia coli* and COS cells. Biochim Biophys Acta 1990;1039:269.

15. Whitefleet-Smith J, Rosen E, McLinden J, et al. Expression of human plasminogen cDNA in a Baculovirus vector-infected insect cell system. Arch Biochem Biophys 1989;271:390.

16. Robbins KC, Summaria L. Plasminogen and plasmin. Methods Enzymol 1976;45:257.

17. Robbins KC. Dysplasminogenemias. Prog Cardiovas Dis 1992;34:295.

18. Sottrup-Jensen L, Claeys H, Zajdel M, et al. The primary structure of human plasminogen: isolation of two lysine-binding fragments and one "mini" plasminogen (MW, 38,000) by elastase-catalyzed specific limited proteolysis. Prog Chem Fibrinol Thrombol 1978;3:191.

19. Bachmann F. Plasminogen activators. In: Colman RW, Hirsh J, Marder VJ, Salzman EW, eds. Hemostasis and thrombosis: basic principals and clinical practice. 2nd ed. Philadelphia: JB Lippincott 1987: 318.

20. Lijnen HR, Van Hoef B, DeCook F, et al. On the mechanism of fibrin-specific plasminogen activation by staphylokinase. J Biol Chem 1991;266: 11826.

21. Wohl RC, Summaria L, Robbins KC. Kinetics of activation of human plasminogen by different activator species at pH 7.4 and 37°C. J Biol Chem 1980;255:2005.

22. Robbins KC, Barlow GH, Nguyen G, et al. Comparison of plasminogen activators. Semin Thromb Hemost 1987;13:131.

23. Kruithof EKO. Plasminogen activator inhibitors-a review. Enzyme 1988;40:113.

24. Robbins KC, Markus G. The interaction of human plasminogen with streptokinase. In: Gaffney PJ, Balkuv-Ulutin, eds. Fibrinolysis: current fundamental and clinical concepts. London: Academic Press, 1978:61.

25. Fears R. Development of anisoylated plasminogen-streptokinase activator complex from acyl enzyme concept. Semin Thromb Hemost 1989;15: 129.

26. Rajagopalan S, Gonias SL, Pizzo SV. The temperature-dependent reaction between α_2-macroglobulin and streptokinase-plasmin (ogen) complex. J Biol Chem 1987;262:3660.

27. Wohl RC, Sinio L, Summaria L, et al. Comparative activation kinetics of mammalian plasminogens. Biochim Biophys Acta 1983;745:20.

28. Stack S, Gonzalez-Gronow M, Pizzo SV. Regulation of plasminogen activation by components of the extracellular matrix. Biochemistry 1990;29: 4966.

29. Lind SE, Smith CJ. Actin accelerates plasmin generation by tissue plasminogen activator. J Biol Chem 1991;266:17673.

30. Edelberg JM, Pizzo SV. Lipoprotein (a): the link between impaired fibrinolysis and atherosclerosis. Fibrinolysis 1991;5:135.

31. McLean JW, Tomlinson JE, Kuang W-J, et al. cDNA sequence of human apolipoprotein (a) is homologous to plasminogen. Nature 1987;330: 132.

32. Robbins KC. Plasmin. In: Markwardt F, ed. Fibrinolytics and antifibrinoolytics. Berlin: Springer-Verlag, 1978:317.

33. Summaria L, Wohl RC, Boreisha IG, et al. A virgin enzyme derived from human plasminogen: specific cleavage of the arginyl-560–valyl peptide bond in the disopropoxyphosphinyl virgin enzyme by plasminogen activators. Biochemistry 1982;21:2056.

34. Harpel PC. Blood proteolytic enzyme inhibitors: their role in modulating blood coagulation and fibrinolytic enzyme pathways. In: Colman RW, Hirsh J, Marder VJ, Salzman EW, eds. Hemostasis and thrombosis: basic principles and clinical practice. 2d ed. Philadelphia: JB Lippincott, 1987:219.

35. Aoki N. Alpha$_2$ plasmin inhibitor. In: Tanaka K, ed. Recent advances in thrombosis and fibrinolysis. Tokyo: Academic Press, 1991:91.

36. Dolan G, Preston FE. Familial plasminogen deficiency and thromboembolism. Fibrinolysis 1988; 2(suppl 2):26.

37. Conard J, Horellou MH, Samama M. Incidence of thromboembolism in association with congenital disorders in coagulation and fibrinolysis. Acta Chir Scand 1988;(suppl 543):15.

38. Aoki N, Moroi M, Sakata Y, et al. Abnormal plasminogen: a hereditary molecular abnormality found in a patient with recurrent thrombosis. J Clin Invest 1978;61:1186.

39. Miyata T, Iwanaga S, Sakata Y, et al. Plasminogen Tochigi II and Nagoya: two additional molecular defects with Ala 600 to Thr replacement found in plasmin light chain variants. J Biochem 1984;96: 277.

40. Ichinose A, Espling ES, Takamatsu J, et al. Two types of abnormal genes for plasminogen in families with a predisposition for thrombosis. Proc Natl Acad Sci USA 1991;88:115.

41. Soria J, Soria G, Bertrand O, et al. Plasminogen Paris I: congenital abnormal plasminogen and its

incidence in thrombosis. Thromb Res 1983;32: 229.

42. Kazama M, Tahara C, Suzaki Z, et al: Abnormal plasminogen, a case of recurrent thrombosis. Thromb Res 1981;21:517.

43. Scharrer IM, Wohl RC, Robbins KC, et al. Investigation of a congenital abnormal plasminogen, Frankfurt I, and its relationship to thrombosis. Thromb Haemostas 1986;55:396.

44. Liu Y, Lyons RM, McDonagh J. Plasminogen San Antonio: an abnormal plasminogen with a more cathodic migration, decreased activation and associated thrombosis. Thromb Haemost 1988;59:49.

45. Wohl RC, Summaria L, Robbins KC. Physiological activation of the human fibrinolytic system: isolation and characterization of human plasminogen variants, Chicago I and II. J Biol Chem 1979;254: 9063.

46. Wohl RC, Summaria L, Robbins KC, et al. Human plasminogen variant Chicago III. Thromb Haemost 1982;48:146.

47. Robbins KC, Boreisha IG, Godwin JE. Abnormal plasminogen Maywood I. Thromb Haemost 1991; 66:575.

48. Robbins KC, Boreisha IG, Hach-Wunderle V, et al. Congenital plasminogen deficiency with an abnormal plasminogen: Frankfurt II, dysplasminogen-emia-hypoplasminogenemia. Fibrinolysis 1991;5: 145.

49. Furlan AJ, Lucas FV, Wohl RC, et al. Stroke in a young adult with familial plasminogen disorder. Stroke 1991;22:1598.

50. Miles LA, Plow EF. Plasminogen receptors: ubiquitous sites for cellular regulation of fibrinolysis. Fibrinolysis 1988;2:61.

51. Plow EF, Miles LA. Plasminogen receptors in the mediation of pericellular proteolysis. Different Develop 1990;32:293.

52. Vassalli J-D, Sappino A-P, Belin D. The plasminogen activator/plasmin system. J Clin Invest 1991; 88:1067.

53. Pollanen J, Stephens RW, Vaheri A. Directed plasminogen activation at the surface of normal and malignant cells. Adv Cancer Res 1991;57:273.

54. Felez J, Miles LA, Plescia J, et al. Regulation of plasminogen receptor expression on human monocytes and monocytoid cell lines. J Cell Biol 1990; 111:1673.

55. Hajjar KA: The endothelial cell tissue plasminogen activator receptor: specific interaction with plasminogen. J Biol Chem 1991;266:21962.

56. Miles LA, Dahlberg CM, Plescia J, et al. Role of cell-surface lysines in plasminogen binding to cells. Biochemistry 1991;30:1682.

57. Blasi F, Vassalli J-D, Dano K: Urokinase-type plasminogen activator: proenzyme, receptor and inhibitors. J Cell Biol 1987;104:801.

58. Manchanda N, Schwartz BS. Single chain urokinase: augmentation of enzymatic activity upon binding to monocytes. J Biol Chem 1991;266: 14580.

59. Haddoch RC, Spell ML, Baker III CD, et al. Urokinase binding and receptor indentification in cultured endothelial cells. J Biol Chem 1991;266: 21466.

60. Gonzalez-Gronow M, Edelberg JM, Pizzo SV. Further characterization of cellular plasminogen binding site: evidence that plasminogen 2 and lipoprotein a compete for the same site. Biochemistry 1989;28:2374.

61. Edelberg JM, Enghild JJ, Pizzo SV, et al. Neonatal plasminogen displays altered cell surface binding and activation kinetics: correlation with increased glycosylation of the protein. J Clin Invest 1990; 86:107.

62. Stack MS, Moser TL, Pizzo SV. Binding of human plasminogen to basement membrane (type IV) collagen. Biochem J 1992;284:103.

63. Burtin P, Fondaneche MC. Solubilization of the plasmin receptor from human carcinoma cells. Biochem Biophys Res Commun 1990;170:748.

5

THE HISTORY AND DEVELOPMENT OF THROMBOLYTIC THERAPY

Sol Sherry

Anticoagulants that can prevent blood clotting have been available for physician use for 50 years, but there wasn't a medical way to dissolve a blood clot until the development of thrombolytic therapy.

Now that thrombolytic therapy has become established as an important modality in the treatment of various thromboembolic disorders, it is timely to describe its origin and development. The story is an interesting one that spans more than half a century: It began with a serendipitous observation made over 50 years ago, first applied to patients over 40 years ago, followed by a landmark study some 30 years ago, and where patience, perseverance, and a continuum of sound clinical investigation were ultimately successful in overcoming the impediments and skepticism that delayed its acceptance.

Thrombolytic therapy as it is practiced today involves the activation of the body's own mechanism for dissolving fibrin. Consequently, in tracing the development of fibrinolytic therapy, it is appropriate to consider what we knew about fibrinolysis before the advent of thrombolytic therapy.

SPONTANEOUS FIBRINOLYSIS OF CLOTTED BLOOD

The knowledge that human blood contains fibrinolytic activity is very old. Denis, and then Zimmerman, in the first half of the nineteenth century observed that the fibrin of human blood obtained from wet cupping dissolved in 12 to 24 hours.[1] Dastre, in the late nineteenth century, noted that the fibrin yield of dog blood decreased with the rate and magnitude of the phlebotomy.[2] Although his observations may have been a result of hemodilution, Dastre postulated that the decreased yield was caused by actual destruction or lysis of the fibrin and defined the phenomenon as "fibrinolysis." Nolf, one of the great pioneers in the concepts of blood coagulation, believed that the coagulation process was a proteolytic one and that fibrinolysis of blood clots simply represented a continuation of the process by which clotting originally took place.[3]*

Interest in the spontaneous fibrinolysis of human blood clots was reawakened by Yudin in the Soviet Union.[4] He demonstrated the possibility of utilizing cadaver blood without anticoagulants for transfusion purposes. Yudin used blood from fresh corpses, selecting donors who were the victims of accidental or sudden death rather than those who died from a chronic illness. Following phlebotomy, the blood clotted, but it subsequently reliquefied in several hours and remained in a fluid state thereafter. The fairly rapid activation of fibrinolytic activity in some patients with severe shocking episodes is now well recognized and may account for the usually reported low incidence of coronary thrombi in some patients dying suddenly and for the accelerated spontaneous resolution of coronary thrombi in patients with an acute transmural myocardial infarction.

Tissue Fibrinolysis

In their pioneering tissue culture studies, Fleisher and Loeb[5] observed that cells growing in plasma clots led to the clot's liquefaction; this suggested a source for the initiation of fibrinolysis. Though their observation was not pursued for many years, it ultimately provided a major stimulus for the important studies on tissue fibrinolysis and its mechanisms.

Proteolytic Activity in Blood

Information concerning fibrinolysis also related to observations on a powerful proteolytic enzyme in serum with many similarities to trypsin. In 1889, Denys and Marbaix[6] found that a thermolabile proteolytic substance developed in serum

*The action of thrombin and other coagulation enzymes as proteolytic enzymes is now firmly established. It is also well known that the processes involved in clotting, while they may be interrelated with those of fibrinolysis, are distinct from each other. Nevertheless, it is to Nolf's credit that he introduced the view that fibrinolysis was caused by a proteolytic enzyme in plasma.

previously treated with chloroform. Deleżene and Pozerski,[7,8] some years later, demonstrated that chloroform treatment of serum removed the inhibition to proteolytic enzymes and was followed by the appearance of an active enzyme in the serum. In 1911, Opie et al.[9] demonstrated that the proteolytic enzyme that appeared in serum following chloroform treatment had many of the characteristics of trypsin (pH optima and ability to digest casein and gelatin). It is of interest that Tagnon et al.[10] reported in 1942 that the globulin fraction of chloroform-treated serum was strongly fibrinolytic.

Streptococcal Fibrinolysis

Our understanding of this subject received its major impetus in 1933 when Tillett and Garner,[11] at the Johns Hopkins Medical School, where Tillett was an associate professor of medicine and head of the Department of Medicine's Biological Division, reported that filtrates of broth cultures of certain strains of hemolytic streptococci contained a substance capable of inciting the rapid fibrinolysis of human plasma clots. This substance was termed *streptococcal fibrinolysin,* and serendipity played a great role in its discovery.

Tillett (Fig. 5-1) had observed that hemolytic streptococci were clumped or agglutinated by normal plasma but not by normal serum, suggesting that this clumping was mediated by fibrinogen.[12] (Interestingly, fibrinogen's ability to clump certain bacteria subsequently served as the basis for the staphylococcal clumping test for quantitating the amount of fibrinogen/fibrin degradation products in serum.[13] In this regard, it is noteworthy that fibrinogen has the capacity to bridge the cell membranes of several types of opposing cells, including its importance in platelet aggregation and red blood cell clumping.) Tillett reasoned that if this clumping of hemolytic streptococci was due to a reaction between fibrinogen and streptococci, the addition of a heavy inoculum of a streptococcal culture to oxalated human plasma would bind up all the fibrinogen so that clotting would not occur upon recalcification. However, he was disappointed when clotting oc-

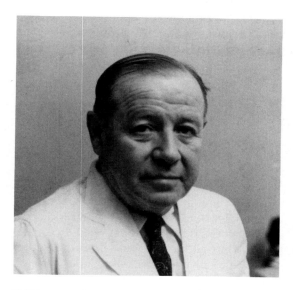

FIGURE 5-1. Photograph of William S Tillett, discoverer of streptococcal fibrinolysin, later renamed streptokinase.

curred upon recalcification just as rapidly as in the control test tube. However, upon leaving the laboratory, he left the tubes in the incubator. When he returned several hours later and was about to discard the tubes, he noticed that the tube to which the streptococcal culture had been added was now liquid, but not so for the control. This puzzled him, since he was sure the plasma mixture had clotted upon recalcification. When he repeated the experiment, the plasma clotted and then after a number of minutes suddenly liquefied. Tillett immediately suspected that this was an important observation.

To facilitate the study of this substance, Tillett teamed up with a young Ph.D. biochemist, Garner, who undertook a fellowship in the Department of Medicine, and they began a much more extensive investigation of this fibrin dissolving phenomenon. In a series of studies, they demonstrated that the streptococcal fibrinolysin probably was a protein present in the broth culture filtrate of the culture medium and presumably a highly selective enzyme specific only for human fibrin and that the digestion of fibrin was a limited hydrolytic process with the slow release of amino nitrogen.[14,15] Interestingly, they also indicated that after a period of time, incubation of their human fibrinogen preparation with the fibrinolysin rendered the fibrinogen incoagulable. Since little was made of this latter observation, they based the specificity of the streptococcal fibrinolysin for fibrin on the evidence that the former did not degrade casein or gelatin, as did trypsin; was distinct in characteristics from the proteolytic enzyme that could be released from disrupted streptococcal cells; only human but not rabbit fibrin could be dissolved readily by the fibrinolysin; and the lysis of human fibrin was accomplished with relatively little release of amino nitrogen. Nevertheless, in light of their various observations,[14,15] including the effects on his human fibrinogen preparation, I suspect that had Garner continued with his studies, he would have recognized that fibrinolysis as induced by the streptococcal protein was a two-step reaction and involved the action of a nonspecific proteolytic enzyme.[16-19]

After Garner left Johns Hopkins to join the faculty in the Department of Chemistry at the University of Michigan, where his research took an entirely different direction, Tillett continued tenaciously to pursue his original observation. However, based on his bacteriologic research training at the Rockefeller Institute under Avery, with emphasis on the biologic effects of bacterial infections, he concentrated on characterizing the streptococcal strains that did and did not elaborate a fibrinolysin, studied a variety of other bacterial strains in search of a similar type of substance, demonstrated the appearance of a specific antifibrinolysin in the sera of patients recovering from hemolytic streptococcal infections, and showed that the production of a fibrinolysin had little to do with the virulence of the organism or the course or complications associated with a streptococcal infection.[20-22] He believed that the biologic purpose of the streptococcal fibrinolysin was to provide the streptococcus with a soluble form of nutrient from any fibrin that had been deposited in and around a hemolytic streptococcal infection. Nevertheless, it is difficult to conceive that this streptococcal protein has little to do with the ability of this organism to spread rapidly through tissues.

In 1941, Milstone, also working as a fellow in Tillett's laboratory, but now at New York University School of Medicine where Tillett had become chief of medicine and head of the Third Medical Division at Bellevue Hospital, demonstrated that clots made with highly purified human fibrinogen and thrombin were not lysed by streptococcal fibrinolysin. However, if a small amount of a euglobulin from human serum was added to the mixture, rapid lysis of the clot resulted. The serum euglobulin could be readily isolated in a partially purified form by isoelectric precipitation at pH 5.2. Milstone named this substance *plasma lysing factor* and believed that it interacted with streptococcal fibrinolysin to form an active lysing system.[23]

From 1943 to 1945, Christensen, a microbiologist at New York University, and Kaplan, an immunologist then working in the Respiratory Diseases Commission Laboratory at Fort Bragg, independently demonstrated that the plasma lysing factor described by Milstone was in reality an inactive precursor of a proteolytic enzyme capable of readily degrading insoluble fibrin into soluble fragments and that this precursor enzyme could be rapidly activated by streptococcal fibrinolysin.[24–28] Because the streptococcal product was an activator rather than a fibrinolysin, Christensen suggested that it be renamed *streptokinase*.

INTEGRATED CONCEPT OF THE FIBRINOLYTIC ENZYME SYSTEM

Thus the stage was set for Christensen, on the basis of his extensive and classic study, to point out that the phenomenon of fibrinolysis was due to the same proteolytic enzyme that had been observed in chloroform-treated serum, that this existed in the natural state as an inactive precursor, and that it could be rapidly activated by streptokinase. Thus all the previous observations were unified into one integrated concept, as shown in Figure 5-2. Christensen's view, which was fundamental to all subsequent research, is summarized in Figure 5-3. The naturally occurring precursor of the proteolytic (and fibrinolytic) enzyme of plasma was referred to as *plasminogen* so as to denote its source of origin. However, the term *profibrinolysin* remained a favorite among many "coagulationists" for many years. In the presence of

FIGURE 5-2. *Four independent sources of information that ultimately were explained by the presence of a fibrinolytic and proteolytic enzyme in human blood.*

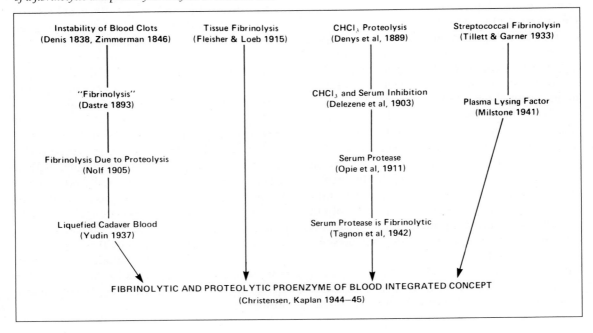

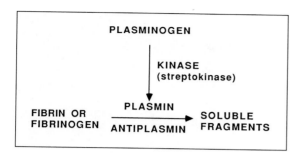

FIGURE 5-3. Original concept of Christensen of the fibrinolytic and proteolytic enzyme of blood and its action.

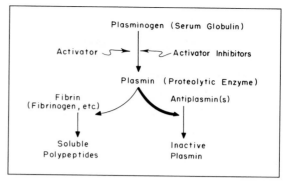

FIGURE 5-4. Original simplified and generalized overview of the components of the fibrinolytic and proteolytic enzyme system of blood with its various checks and balances.

an activator or kinase, this plasma globulin was rapidly converted to an active proteolytic enzyme termed *plasmin* to denote its source of origin.

Although plasmin digested fibrin into several soluble incoagulable fragments, its action was not restricted to fibrin. It proved to be a proteolytic enzyme resembling trypsin in its pH optima and the types of amino acid linkages it split.[27–29] For this reason, the terminology *plasminogen* and *plasmin* proved preferable and was in keeping with the terminology of *trypsinogen* and *trypsin*.

Christensen also noted that like all biologically active proteolytic enzyme systems with their checks and balances, plasma contains considerable antiplasmin activity. A simplified and generalized overview of the components of the human fibrinolytic enzyme system at that time is shown schematically in Figure 5-4.

Subsequently, the development of knowledge concerning the fibrinolytic enzyme system stemmed primarily from two major sources: (1) investigation of the biochemical and physiologic aspects of fibrinolysis and (2) the use of fibrinolytic agents for therapeutic purposes.

Early Studies on the Physiologic Role of Fibrinolysis

Studies on the physiologic role of this newly discovered fibrinolytic enzyme system were led by Astrup, Permin, Mullertz, and others at the Carlsberg Institute in Copenhagen and by Macfarlane and Biggs at Oxford. Astrup (Fig. 5-5) and his associates developed a simple assay system, the fibrin plate method (Fig. 5-6), which when un-

heated served as a measure of activator activity and when heated so as to destroy the plasminogen present served as a measure of plasmin activity. Astrup's interest was in the native mechanisms for fibrinolytic activity and in identifying the tissue sources of plasminogen activators. In effect, the studies of Astrup and his associates laid the groundwork for subsequent studies on tissue

FIGURE 5-5. Photograph of Tage Astrup, a pioneer in fibrinolysis research whose investigational team was involved in the initial discovery of both tissue plasminogen activator and urokinase.

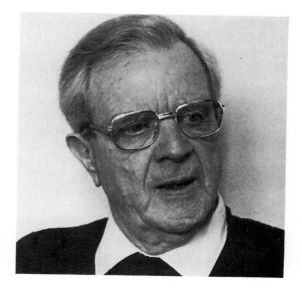

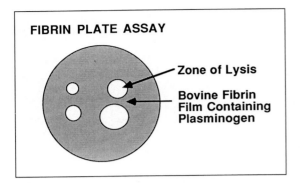

FIGURE 5-6. Schematic of the fibrin plate method originally developed by Astrup and collaborators for demonstrating the presence of plasminogen activators and/or
plasmin in tissue and body fluids.

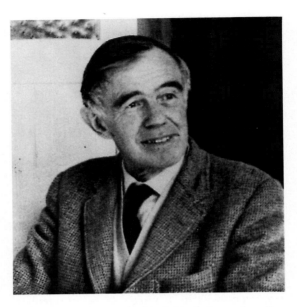

FIGURE 5-7. Photograph of R. G. Macfarlane, whose Oxford group pioneered the early studies of the physiology of
fibrinolytic activity in humans.

plasminogen activator and their sites of concentration as well as potential for release in human
organs. Macfarlane, professor of pathology at the
Radcliffe Infirmary (Fig. 5-7), then a world leader
in coagulation research, and his chief associate,
Biggs, provided a series of interesting observations on the dynamics of the fibrinolytic enzyme
system in response to stressful stimuli, e.g., intense physical activity and surgery and its con-
templation. This stimulated other pioneers in fibrinolysis research, such as Von Kaulla, Ferguson,
my group in the United States, Fantl in Australia,
and Kwaan and McFadzean in Hong Kong, to begin to investigate the native mechanisms involved
in regulating fibrinolytic activity under a variety
of situations. As a result of these studies carried
out in the late 1940s and 1950s, it became apparent that the fibrinolytic enzyme system was as
dynamic as the coagulation system in human biology (like the former, its action was usually localized) and that fibrin would now have to be
considered in terms of the interplay or balance between two opposing reactions, fibrin formation
and fibrin resolution.

EARLY THERAPEUTIC STUDIES

Simultaneously with early developments on the
physiology of the native fibrinolytic enzyme system, there was the desire to manipulate this sys-

tem for therapeutic purposes, initially to activate
it for fibrinolysis and later to inhibit it for improving hemostasis. A potent activator of this enzyme
system was a partially purified preparation of
streptokinase which Christensen made available
to Tillett and me for clinical investigation. Beginning in 1946, we began to pursue the goal of fibrinolysis and clot dissolution.

It was my privilege to work with Tillett for
5 years (1946–1951) and, at his request, to undertake the initial clinical investigation and application of fibrin and clot dissolving therapy in human beings. This was a rewarding experience for
me, not only to be involved in starting a new field
of therapy but to be associated with a man of the
caliber of Tillett, whose discovery provided the
impetus to the development of thrombolytic therapy and the key to unraveling a hitherto little
recognized human fibrinolytic enzyme system.
Tillett (1892–1974) was born and raised in North
Carolina, where at the University of North Carolina he excelled as a student and gained fame as
an All-American quarterback on their football
team. After graduating from the Johns Hopkins

University Medical School in 1917, he spent 2 years in France during World War I and then returned to Baltimore for clinical training. The period 1922–1930, i.e., before returning to Hopkins as an associate professor of medicine, proved to be the most formative years of his career. These were spent at the Rockefeller Institute under the tutelage of several of the outstanding infectious disease investigators of that period (Thomas Rivers, Rufus Cole, and most important, the biologically oriented and brilliant Oswald Avery). Under Avery's influence, Tillett developed a strong biologic interest centered primarily around the pneumococcus, which he referred to as a "regal organism not dependent on the production of extracellular toxins, but still capable of producing a devastating illness," and the hemolytic streptococcus, which he described as having "no fat or gristle, just metabolic machinery."

Tillett, in his approach to science, was not concerned with minutiae nor particularly impressed with statistics; he was primarily interested in opening up new areas of investigation. Perhaps some understanding of the man and what he believed to be important in medial research may be seen in his remarks at the 1957 dedication of the newly constructed laboratories at Bellevue Hospital that were to bear his name. In his remarks, Tillett stated that he hoped one of the laboratories would have only benches for sitting and thinking and a single plant growing in the center of the room. He though this could be one of the most important of the Tillett laboratories, i.e., a place for investigators to reflect both on the wonders of nature and whether their approach to medical research had biologic significance.

Tillett's approach to science also was reflected in his enjoyment of what he called "dinosaur egg experiments." When I questioned him as to its meaning, he gave the following explanation: Once there was an American paleontologist who had just returned from the Gobi Desert with the major find of a lifetime of work—two dinosaur eggs. Upon his return to the United States, he gave one to the Smithsonian Institution and kept the other for himself. A businessman, noting a small newspaper item about this event, asked the professor whether he would sell his egg and urged

him to think the matter over. The professor gave it some thought and, considering the meagerness of his pension, decided that for a million dollars he would part with it. Thereupon the businessman quickly wrote out a check. A reporter, after confirming the sale, said to the businessman, "That was an enormous price to pay for that egg. You don't really think it will hatch, do you?" To which the businessman, with a twinkle in his eye and a shake of his index finger, quickly retorted, "Ah! But what if it does?"

Tillett's own investigational career balanced "dinosaur egg experiments" with the more conventional techniques of research. When he made an observation that he believed was worthy of further study, he was tenacious in following it up. Under the influence of Avery, he had become very interested in acute-phase reactants—new or increased amounts of reactive substances which appeared in the circulation after an inflammatory event—following a pneumococcal or streptococcal infection. While at the Rockefeller Institute, he and Thomas Francis, Jr., described the appearance of a protein present in the acute-phase sera of pneumonia patients but not in the sera of convalescent individuals which precipitated the "C fraction" carbohydrate present in all strains of pneumococci. This precipitin reaction was later found to occur in the acute phase of a wide variety of diseases of diverse etiology in which there was an acute inflammatory reaction. Assay of this "C-reactive protein" (CRP), like the erythrocyte sedimentation rate (ESR), became a very useful clinical test for determining the presence of acute inflammation. Subsequently, it was also shown that C-reactive protein was capable of triggering the alternative pathway of complement activation. It was this type of background training and interest that led to Tillett's discovery of streptococcal fibrinolysin, as described previously.

When Christensen made available "purified" preparations of streptokinase[30] for clinical investigation, Tillett decided to bypass animal studies, since streptokinase was not a very effective activator of animal plasminogens. In mid-1946, Tillett had asked me to join him in the clinical evaluation of streptokinase and to be responsible for the

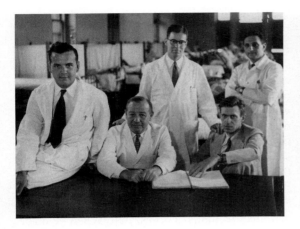

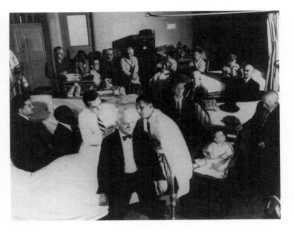

FIGURE 5-8. Pioneering team involved in the original clinical investigation of fibrinolytic therapy. Photograph taken in 1950; Tillett is seated in the center, Christensen is on his right, and George Hazlehurst, a research fellow working with me, is on his left. Standing on the left is Alan Johnson, who initiated studies on the ability of Christensen's streptokinase preparation to dissolve clots induced in rabbit ear veins. I am on his right and was responsible for the clinical and laboratory observations in the patient studies. A ward of Bellevue Hospital in New York City is in the background.

FIGURE 5-9. Group of patients successfully treated for a wide variety of conditions with Christensen's streptokinase preparation, which contained other streptococcal enzymes. Hazlehurst (left) and Sherry (right) are shown examining the remnants of a chronic neck infection in one of the patients.

laboratory and patient studies.* As has been recounted previously,[31,32] we chose hemothorax and empyema cases to initiate the investigation because serial radiographs would allow us to observe the effects, and samples of fluid could be removed for analysis. While the ultimate goal would be to evaluate its usefulness intravascularly, this would have to wait until less toxic preparations were made available (Christensen's preparation proved to be only 10% pure, and its intrapleural administration was associated frequently with significant pyrogenic reactions), and at the time, angiography and venography were

not available to determine the effects. Documentation of the ability of the streptokinase preparation when administered intrapleurally to lyse clotted blood and fibrin in the chest appeared in 1949[33] and was followed shortly by a series of reports on the application of this type of therapy in the management of hemothorax[34] and postpneumonic and chronic empyemas.[35,36] Our team at that time is shown in Figures 5-8 and 5-9.

Laboratory studies revealed that the streptokinase preparation also contained a variety of other streptococcal enzymes which, like streptokinase, were released into the culture medium and purified along with streptokinase.[37] These included a deoxyribonuclease, ribonuclease, hyaluronidase,* and various nucleotidases, nucleosidases, deaminases, and phosphatases.[33,38,39] Since the deoxyribonuclease was able to depolymerize rapidly the thick viscous strands of deoxyribonucleoprotein that accumulated in purulent exu-

---

*At the time, I was finishing a residency in internal medicine on the 3rd (NYU) Medical Division at Bellevue Hospital, where Tillett was the chief. However, what attracted me to him was that I had a considerable experience in research as a medical student, as a fellow in metabolism and endocrinology following graduation from medical school (NYU) before beginning my internship and residency training, and in typhus control during World War II, where I served in the European Theater of Operations as a flight surgeon with a B26 Bomb Group.

*Interestingly, the streptokinase preparation originally prepared by Christensen and later by Lederle Laboratories as streptokinase-streptodornase was the most potent deoxyribonuclease available at the time (personal communication from Arthur Kornberg), as was the hyaluronidase in it (personal communication from Karl Meyer).

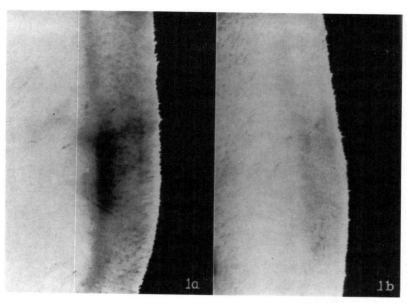

FIGURE 5-10. *Lysis of blood clots induced in rabbit ear vein by systemic infusion of streptokinase. The clot was induced by local injection of sodium morrhuate. On right, patency of vessel has been restored following the intravenous infusion of Christensen's streptokinase preparation. (Used with permission from Johnson AJ, Tillett WS: Lysis in rabbits of intravascular blood clots by the streptococcal fibrinolytic system [streptokinase]. J Exp Med 1952;95:449.)*

dates from the chromosomal material of dead, degenerating granulocytes and other inflammatory cells,[40] the preparation not only dissolved fibrin but facilitated the drainage of purulent exudates. Accordingly, the preparation also was used to effect an enzymatic debridement by direct application to a variety of dirty and infected areas.[41]

THROMBOLYTIC THERAPY

However, the major interest in the development of the clot-lysing ability of streptokinase was its potential for the treatment of acute thrombotic disorders, especially acute coronary thrombosis. At the time, *coronary thrombosis* was a term used synonymously with *acute myocardial infarction,* a common medical problem with a $\geq 30\%$ in-hospital mortality rate. The reason for this interest was that several well-known pathologists in the 1930s[42,43] and again in the 1960s and 1970s[44–46] had pointed out that the most common cause of a

myocardial infarction was a thrombus superimposed on the cracked surface of an atheromatous plaque.* However, the streptokinase preparations elicited severe febrile reactions when administered intravenously or injected into closed spaces. Though these preparations were not suitable for intravenous therapy, Lederle Laboratories initiated a program to develop preparations that would be acceptable for intravenous therapy, and in 1952, Johnson and Tillett[47] reported that experimental thrombi in rabbit ear veins could be lysed by the intravenous administration of streptokinase into a peripheral vessel (Fig. 5-10).

---

*Interestingly, as pointed out later in this chapter, the 1960s and 1970s were a period during which cardiologists no longer accepted coronary thrombosis as the causative mechanism in acute myocardial infarction on the basis of mistaken reasoning, i.e., the failure of anticoagulants to reduce mortality significantly. They believed the sustained ischemic event was due to spasm in the presence of underlying arteriosclerotic stenosis.

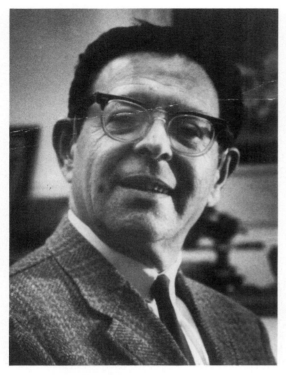

FIGURE 5-11. Photograph of Daniel Kline, a pioneer in plasminogen purification.

Studies on Plasminogen Activator for Thrombolysis

Shortly thereafter, Daniel Kline (Fig. 5-11), then at Yale University, developed a technique that allowed for purification of human plasminogen.[48] Because human plasmin could now be prepared in vitro by the addition of streptokinase, it was possible to consider human plasmin, rather than streptokinase, for thrombolysis. However, in vitro studies on clot lysis[49] indicated that the rate of fibrinolysis and its selectivity as a process were dependent on the presence of both a plasminogen activator and plasminogen, but not on plasmin alone.

The late 1950s proved to be a most productive period in the development of thrombolytic therapy. I was fortunate to be joined in St. Louis, where I had set up my own laboratory, by two outstanding investigators, Anthony Fletcher and Norma Alkjaersig (Fig. 5-12). First, we attacked the problem of whether it would be best to use a plasminogen activator or the fibrinolytic enzyme plasmin. A variety of observations, both in vitro and in vivo,[50–52] led us to conclude that plasminogen activators would be more successful as thrombolytic agents than would the proteolytic enzyme plasmin. This view was based mostly on the demonstration that the primary and most sensitive mechanism for thrombolysis was the penetration of an activator into a thrombus, with activation of the plasminogen that bound to fibrin during clotting.[52] However, we knew that the intravenous infusion of a plasminogen activator such as streptokinase would result in two different actions (Fig. 5-13). Diffusion of streptokinase into a thrombus would result in clot lysis, but the agent also would activate plasminogen in the systemic circulation, producing fibrinogenolysis and an impaired hemostatic mechanism.

FIGURE 5-12. Senior members of the team of investigators in St. Louis responsible for establishing the basis for the use of plasminogen activators as the most desirable agents for thrombolytic therapy and the introduction of streptokinase and, later, urokinase for the treatment of a wide variety of thromboembolic disorders including acute myocardial infarction. Shown from left to right are the late Anthony P. Fletcher, his wife, Norma Alkjaersig, and Sol Sherry.

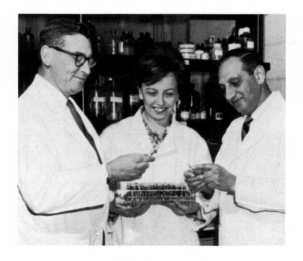

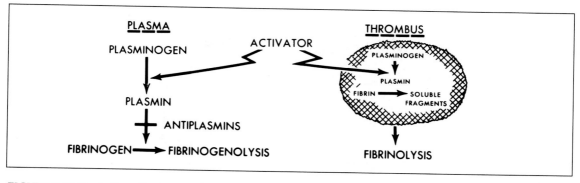

FIGURE 5-13. *Dual effect of intravenously administered streptokinase.*

Studies on Streptokinase for Thrombolysis

In the meantime, Lederle Laboratories had been successful in developing purified preparations of streptokinase that were well tolerated by patients and, in the absence of trauma or invasive procedures, with few bleeding complications. In 1957, we reported[53] on a rational approach to thrombolysis with streptokinase. It involved a loading dose and a sustaining infusion sufficient to increase the clot-dissolving activity of plasma several hundred-fold and maintain a streptokinase concentration in plasma of about 10 μg/ml (Fig. 5-14, *top panel*). This resulted in a short-lived proteolytic state because, once the plasma plasminogen was exhausted, fibrinogen levels began to rise even though the streptokinase infusion was being maintained (Fig. 5-14, *second panel*). However, the clot-dissolving activity of the plasma was sustained as long as streptokinase was being infused (Fig. 5-14, *third panel*). The therapy resulted in a prolongation of the prothrombin time (resulting from fibrinogenolysis) and the appearance of breakdown products (Fig. 5-14, *bottom panel*).

Johnson, who had remained in New York, demonstrated that a similar system was effective in dissolving experimental thrombi in human volunteers. An intravenous infusion into the opposite arm resulted, in most cases, in lysis of the clot and reestablishment of the patency of the vessel[54] (Fig. 5-15).

First Studies on Acute Myocardial Infarction

The interest of our group, however, was to evaluate this regimen for clinical purposes, and in 1958, we reported the first study of intravenously administered streptokinase in patients with various acute thrombotic and embolic disorders, including myocardial infarction. The stated objective, for the latter, then, as now, was that "the rapid resolution of a coronary thrombus by enzymatic means could result in reduction of the final area of muscle infarction, reduction of the degree of electrical instability present during the early critical phase of infarction, and prevent the appearance of or lyse mural thrombi,"[55] similar to current objectives. However, ours was primarily a pilot study to determine how well the patient and the heart would tolerate a 30-hour infusion of streptokinase.

Not only were we encouraged by the lack of complications we observed, but patients treated within the first 14 hours after symptom onset had a very low in-hospital mortality rate (Table 5-1), whereas patients treated anywhere from 20 to 72 hours after symptom onset had a mortality rate similar to that of untreated patients. We also were the first to describe (Fig. 5-16) the early peaking of serum transaminase in streptokinase-treated patients, that is, at an average of 14 hours rather than the 24 hours, as observed in untreated patients.

The details of these studies, which provided

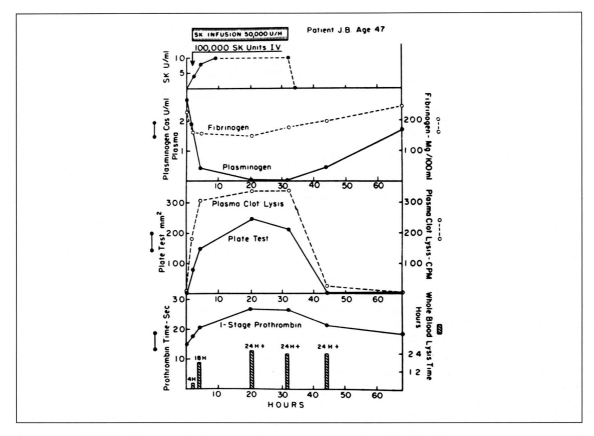

FIGURE 5-14. Serial biochemical determinations in a patient during a 30-hour infusion of streptokinase (SK) administered intravenously. See text for details. (Used with permission from Fletcher AP,
Alkjaersig N, Sherry S: The maintenance of a sustained thrombolytic state in man: I. Induction and
effects. J Clin Invest 1959;38:1096.)

the basis for the use of plasminogen activators as thrombolytic agents, as well as the pharmacologic and clinical observations on intravenous therapy with streptokinase, were published in 1959[55–57] and attracted wide attention.[58] As a result, a number of fellows who went on to become leaders in thrombosis research joined our research group. These included Edward Genton, Nils Bang, Fedor Bachmann (who in 1964, while in our laboratory, was responsible for the first major purification of tissue plasminogen activator from pig heart[59]), Robert Colman, Jack Hirsh, Heinz Joist, Zbigniew Latallo, George McNicol, Michael Mosesson, Josef Vermylen, and Per Wallen. These fellows added much knowledge to the subject of fibrinolysis and

helped in the clinical development of urokinase.[60] The latter was the result of recognition that streptokinase therapy was associated with two problems: (1) antigenicity and occasional allergic reactions and (2) bleeding complications that were assumed, at that time, to be caused by the hemostatic defect (reduced fibrinogen and increased breakdown products) resulting from the action of the plasmin formed in the circulating plasma. Consequently, beginning in 1959, interest in the United States in the further development of thrombolytic therapy began to center on the production of a nonantigenic activator whose action would be more selective for fibrin than fibrinogen; i.e., the ratio of fibrinolysis/fibrinogenolysis

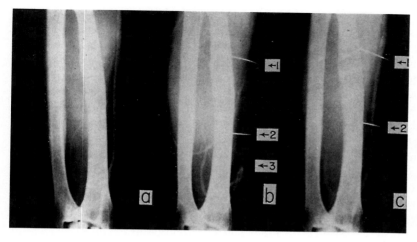

FIGURE 5-15. Radiographic demonstration of the lysis of an experimentally induced clot in a human volunteer. (a) A control venogram before the induction of a clot showing a patent vessel. (b) Venogram taken 24 hours after the induction of a clot by traumatizing the intima of an antecubital vein by a dental burr inserted through a needle. The radiopaque lines at 1 and 2 were made by nichrome wires on the skin surface to define the extent of the clot; the arrow at 3 indicates the distal portion of the clot. (c) Venogram 24 hours after the streptokinase infusion showing complete lysis of the clot without reformation. (Used with permission from Johnson AJ, McCarty WR: The lysis of artificially induced intravascular clots in man by intravenous infusions of streptokinase. J Clin Invest 1959;38:1627.)

would be greater than observed with streptokinase therapy. Hopefully, moderation of the systemic fibrinogenolytic effect would reduce the incidence of bleeding complications.

THE DEVELOPMENT OF UROKINASE

Two pharmaceutical firms, Abbott Laboratories and Sterling-Winthrop, and two investigational groups, those who originally had developed

FIGURE 5-16. Serial serum glutamic oxaloacetic transaminase (SGOT) observations in patients after the onset of an acute myocardial infarction who were treated with a 30-hour intravenous infusion of streptokinase. Note the early peaking of the serum transaminase at 14 hours. (Used with permission from Fletcher AP, Alkjaersig N, Smyrniotis FE, Sherry S: Treatment of patients suffering from early myocardial infarction with massive and prolonged streptokinase therapy. Trans Assoc Am Physicians 1958;71:287.)

TABLE 5-1. Mortality in Patients with Acute Myocardial Infarction Treated with Streptokinase

	Number Treated	Died
Early treatment (6 to 14 h)	15	1
Delayed treatment (20 to 72 h)	9	3

Results of a 30-hour infusion of intravenously administered streptokinase when treatment was begun 6 to 14 h after the onset of symptoms of acute myocardial infarction or when therapy started 20 to 72 hours later.
From Fletcher AP, Alkjaersig N, Smyrniotis FE, Sherry S: Treatment of patients suffering from early myocardial infarction with massive and prolonged streptokinase therapy. Trans Assoc Am Physicians 1958;71: 287.

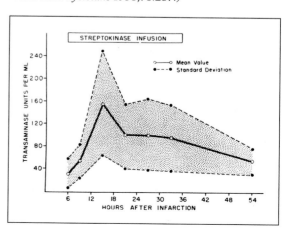

streptokinase for therapeutic thrombolysis, i.e., the St. Louis Group, and Alan Johnson and his group in New York, turned their attention to urokinase, a plasminogen activator that had been shown to be present in human urine independently by Williams,[61] Astrup and Sterndoff,[62] and Sobel et al.,[63] in the early 1950s. By the late 1950s, this activator had been partially purified and characterized by Ploug and Kjeldgaard.[64,65] Besides being a native and presumably nonantigenic activator, in vitro studies also showed that it had a higher fibrinolytic/fibrinogenolytic ratio than did streptokinase,[66] suggesting that it might be safer because it would produce less fibrinogenolysis than streptokinase when administered systemically. The pharmaceutical firms set up pilot plants for the production of urokinase from human urine by collecting large amounts from major military installations (Great Lakes Naval Station and Fort Dix) and transporting the initially treated material to processing plants by large tank trucks (it took the processing of 300 gallons of urine to provide enough material for the treatment of one patient).

In 1963, the further development of urokinase as a thrombolytic agent was aided by James Stengle, chief of the Blood Program within the National Heart and Lung Institute, who involved experts in the academic community by establishing a National Institutes of Health Committee on Thrombolytic Agents (CTA). This committee focused on two aspects of development that it also helped to solve: (1) under the leadership of Anthony Fletcher, the committee defined the minimum requirements for an acceptable therapeutic preparation (in terms of specific activity and freedom from thromboplastic contaminants), and (2) through the efforts of Norma Alkjaersig, Daniel Kline, and Alan Johnson, the committee established a standard unit for urokinase (the CTA unit) which subsequently served as the basis for the international reference unit adopted by the World Health Organization. Thus the development of a urokinase preparation suitable for therapeutic purposes proved to be a remarkable collaborative program among industry, government, and the scientific community. The members of the

scientific community who played a major role in the clinical development of urokinase as a thrombolytic agent are shown in Figure 5-17.

By the midsixties, Abbott Laboratories, whose program was headed by Grant Barlow, and Sterling-Winthrop Pharmaceuticals, whose program was directed by Alex Lesuk, had developed preparations[67,68] that met all the criteria of the Committee on Thrombolytic Agents. Our group in St. Louis then provided the initial pharmacologic, biochemical, and clinical data associated with its use in patients for the treatment of thromboembolic disorders.[60] As anticipated, the urokinase preparations were nonantigenic, and when administered in appropriate dosage intravenously, they induced a level of plasma thrombolytic activity similar to that achieved with streptokinase but associated with a milder hemostatic defect. Furthermore, the inhibitory activity of plasma to urokinase was more uniform in patients as compared with the wide differences previously observed in antistreptokinase antibody levels. Consequently, a fixed-dose schedule based on body weight was introduced for urokinase from the very beginning; this simplified its use.

LYSIS OF PULMONARY THROMBI (UROKINASE AND STREPTOKINASE)

By the 1960s, pulmonary angiography had become an available technique, and this allowed for the demonstration of in vivo clot lysis of pulmonary emboli by urokinase and streptokinase as compared with heparin in National Institutes of Health–sponsored trials.[69-71] These were the first quantitative studies of clot lysis in patients. Figure 5-18 shows the marked hypoperfusion of the right lung resulting from a large embolus in the right main pulmonary artery (*left panel*) and its disappearance within 24 hours with the restoration of lung perfusion after a course of thrombolytic therapy with urokinase (*right panel*). These trials taught us that local factors were more important in determining the success of therapy than were measurable activities in the systemic circulation and that bleeding complications were

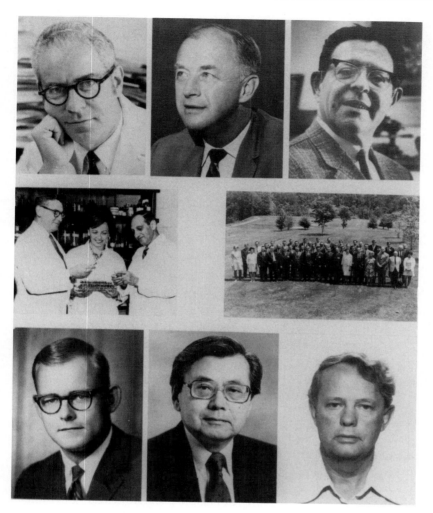

FIGURE 5-17. Besides the pharmaceutical firms (Abbott and Sterling-Winthrop), those members of the scientific community who were prominent in the active development of urokinase for therapeutic purposes included (from top left clockwise). Alan Johnson, of New York University, James M. Stengle, then chief of the Blood Program at the National Heart and Lung Institute, Daniel Kline, of the University of Cincinnati, the various investigators in the Urokinase-Pulmonary Embolism Trial, William Bell, of Johns Hopkins, Arthur Sasahara, of Harvard, Peter Walsh, of the National Heart and Lung Institute, the liaison officer for the Urokinase-Pulmonary Embolism Trial, and the St. Louis group of Fletcher, Alkjaersig, and Sherry, who provided the basis background clinical investigation underlying urokinase's further development.

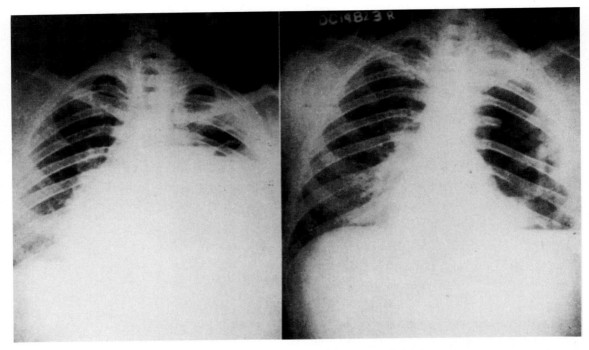

FIGURE 5-18. *Lysis of a large pulmonary embolus in the right main pulmonary artery by 12-hour infusion of urokinase in the Urokinase-Pulmonary Embolism Trial.*[69, 70] (Left panel) *Pulmonary angiogram before treatment.* (Right panel) *Pulmonary angiogram 24 hours later (that is, after treatment).*

related to the lysis of hemostatic plugs at sites of vessel injury and were unrelated to the extent of the hemostatic defect induced in the patient.

SUBSEQUENT DEVELOPMENTS WITH THROMBOLYTIC THERAPY

Although a fixed-dose regimen was introduced initially for urokinase, this was not so for the regimen we developed for streptokinase; originally, streptokinase therapy required a considerable amount of laboratory control to determine the amount of the loading dose and the adjustments made in the sustaining infusion to maintain the desired level of activator activity in plasma. This problem was overcome by Verstraete et al.,[72] who developed a standard-dose therapy based on a loading dose that proved to be effective in overcoming the antistreptokinase resistance of $\geq 90\%$

of patients and a fixed maintenance dose that sustained a fairly intense clot-dissolving state; this simplified therapy enormously.

When Lederle Laboratories ran into difficulties in quality control of streptokinase preparations, the 1960s and thereafter saw the production of streptokinase undertaken by European pharmaceutical firms (Behringwerke in Germany, a subsidiary of Hoechst-Roussel, and Kabi in Sweden). These firms made improvements in quality control and production, and this led to many trials of thrombolytic therapy for the treatment of acute deep vein thrombophlebitis, arterial thrombosis and embolism, and acute myocardial infarction. Table 5-2, which is based on a review by Yusuf et al.,[73] lists 18 trials of streptokinase and 4 of urokinase administered intravenously for the treatment of acute myocardial infarction. These trials were conducted between 1963 to 1979, usually by a 24-hour infusion and most

TABLE 5-2. Randomized Trials of Thrombolytic Therapy in Acute Myocardial Infarction Conducted Between 1959 and 1979 and Utilizing Sustained Intravenous Infusions of Streptokinase or Urokinase

Streptokinase	Urokinase
Fletcher et al. (1959)	Lippschutz et al. (1965)
Dewar et al. (1963)	Gormsen (1973)
Amery et al. (1967)	Brochier et al. (1975)
Heikenheimo et al. (1967)	European Collaborative Group (1975)
European Working Party (1971)	Dioguardi et al. (1971)
Bett et al. (1973)	
Breddin et al. (1973)	
Ness et al. (1974)	
Frank (1975)	
Valere et al. (1975)	
Klein et al. (1976)	
Aber et al. (1976)	
Australian (1977)	
Benda et al. (1977)	
Lasiera et al. (1977)	
Poliwoda et al. (1977)	
Wischitz et al. (1977)	
European Cooperative Study Group (1979)	

Adapted from review by Yusuf S, Collins R, Peto R, et al: Intravenous and intracoronary fibrinolytic therapy in acute myocardial infarction: Overview of results on mortality, reinfarction, and side effects from 33 randomized controlled trials. Eur Heart J 1985;6:556, which also cites references. Year of the report is shown in parentheses.

often within 12 to 24 hours after symptom onset. Though some of these trials were well designed and conducted, e.g., that of the European Cooperative Study Group,[74,75] they were never taken seriously for the following reasons: (1) cardiologists no longer stressed coronary thrombosis as the cause of an acute infarct because of the observations of Roberts, the pathologist at the National Heart and Lung Institute,[76] whose view contrasted with that held by most other leading pathologists on this subject during this period,[44] (2) there were delays in admitting patients into trials because biometricians insisted that randomization be delayed until there was unequivocal proof of an infarct as based on serial electrocardiographic changes and enzyme elevations (by this time the infarction was essentially completed), (3) coronary care units were coming into promi-

nence, and most of the reported studies did not involve such units, (4) bleeding complications became more frequent as the number of invasive procedures increased, and (5) there was no technique available for adequately measuring infarct size or ventricular function. Nevertheless, a retrospective meta-analysis of these trials[73, 77] indicated that overall there was a significant (approximately 20%) reduction in the mortality rate when the therapy, even though delayed, was carried out within the first day of infarction.

Besides these trials with intravenous therapy, efforts at directly infusing a fibrinolytic agent into the coronary arteries of patients suffering from an acute myocardial infarction began with the ingenious approach of Boucek and Murphy[78] in 1960. Subsequently, Chazov et al.[79] described its accomplishment by coronary catheterization in 1976. Local perfusion also became the method of choice for the treatment of peripheral arterial thrombotic and thromboembolic occlusions.

This brings us to the modern era of thrombolytic therapy, spurred in large part by the accomplishments of thrombolytic therapy, especially in acute myocardial infarction but, in addition, in the management of deep vein thrombophlebitis, peripheral arterial thrombotic and thromboembolic occlusions, and pulmonary embolism as well. These accomplishments have spurred the development of a number of new plasminogen activators, including prourokinase,[80] recombinant tissue-type plasminogen activator (rt-PA),[81] and anisoylated plasminogen streptokinase activator complex (APSAC).[82]

Today, after a long developmental period, thrombolytic therapy has become well established as an important therapeutic modality though modifications in techniques of administration, regimens, and adjunctive treatments that continue to evolve.

REFERENCES

1. MacFarlane RG, Biggs R. Fibrinolysis: its mechanism and significance. Blood 1948;3:1167.
2. Dastre A. Fibrinolyse dans le sang. Arch Norm Pathol 1893;5:661.

3. Nolf P. Des modifications de la coagulation du sang chez le chien apres extirpation du fois. Arch Int Physiol Biochim 1905;3:1.

4. Yudin SS. Transfusion of cadaver blood. JAMA 1936;106:997.

5. Fleisher MS, Loeb L. On tissue fibrinolysis. J Biol Chem 1915;21:477.

6. Denys J, De Marbaix H. Les peptonisations provoquees par le chloroforme. Cellule 1889;5:197.

7. Delezenne C, Pozerski E. Action du serum sanguin sur la gelatine en presence du chloroforme. C R Soc Biol (Paris) 1903;55:327.

8. Delezenne C, Pozerski E. Action kinasique du serum sanguin preablement traite par le chloroforme. C R Soc Biol (Paris) 1903;55:693.

9. Opie EL, Barker BI, Dochez AR. Changes in the proteolytic enzymes and antienzymes of the blood serum produced by substances (chloroform and phosphorus) which cause degenerative changes in the liver. J Exp Med 1911;13:162.

10. Tagnon HJ, Davidson CS, Taylor FHL. The coagulation defect in hemophilia: a comparison of the proteolytic activity of chloroform preparations of hemophilic and normal plasma. J Clin Invest 1943;22:127.

11. Tillett WS, Garner RL. The fibrinolytic activity of hemolytic streptococci. J Exp Med 1933;58:485.

12. Tillett WS, Garner RL. The agglutination of hemolytic streptococci by plasma and fibrinogen. Bull Johns Hopkins Hosp 1934;54:145.

13. Hawiger J, et al. Measurement of fibrinogen and fibrin degradation products in serum by staphylococcal clumping test. J Lab Clin Med 1970;75:93.

14. Garner RL, Tillett WS. Biochemical studies on the fibrinolytic activity of hemolytic streptococci: I. Isolation and characterization of fibrinolysin. J Exp Med 1934;60:239.

15. Garner RL, Tillett WS. Biochemical studies on the fibrinolytic activity of hemolytic streptococci: II. Nature of the reaction. J Exp Med 1934;60:255.

16. Mullertz S, Lassen M. An activator system in blood indispensable for formation of plasmin by streptokinase. Proc Soc Exp Biol Med 1953;82:264.

17. Sherry S. The fibrinolytic activity of streptokinase activated human plasmin. J Clin Invest 1954;3:1054.

18. Troll W, Sherry S. The activation of human plasminogen by streptokinase. J Biol Chem 1955;213:881.

19. Davies MC, Englert ME, DeRenzo EC. Interaction of streptokinase and human plasminogen: I. Combining of streptokinase and plasminogen observed in the ultracentrifuge under a variety of experimental conditions. J Biol Chem 1964;239:2651.

20. Tillett WS. The fibrinolytic activity of hemolytic streptococci in relation to the source of strains and to cultural reactions. J Biol Chem 1935;29:111.

21. Tillett WS. The occurrence of antifibrinolytic properties in the blood of patients with acute hemolytic streptococcus infections. J Clin Invest 1935;14:276.

22. Tillett WS. The fibrinolytic activity of hemolytic streptococci. Bacteriol Rev 1938;2:161.

23. Milstone H. A factor in normal human blood which participates in streptococcal fibrinolysis. J Immunol 1941;42:116.

24. Christensen LR. The mechanism of streptococcal fibrinolysis (abstract). J Bacteriol 1944;47:471.

25. Christensen LR. Streptococcal fibrinolysis: a proteolytic reaction due to a serum enzyme activated by streptococcal fibrinolysis. J Gen Physiol 1945;28:363.

26. Christensen LR. The activation of plasminogen by chloroform. J Gen Physiol 1946;30:149.

27. Christensen LR, MacLeod CM. A proteolytic enzyme of serum: characterization, activation, and reaction with inhibitors. J Gen Physiol 1945;28:559.

28. Kaplan MH. Nature and role of the lytic factor in hemolytic streptococcal fibrinolysis. Proc Soc Exp Biol Med 1944;57:40.

29. Troll W, Sherry S, Wachman J. The action of plasmin on synthetic substrates. J Biol Chem 1954;208:85.

30. Christensen LR. Protamine purification of streptokinase and effect of pH and temperature on reversible inactivation. J Gen Physiol 1947;30:465.

31. Sherry S. The origin of thrombolytic therapy. J Am Coll Cardiol 1989;14:1085.

32. Sherry S. Revisiting the development of thrombolytic therapy: an historical perspective. Trans Stud Coll Physicians Phila 1989;11:337.

33. Tillett WS, Sherry S. The effect in patients of streptococcal fibrinolysin (streptokinase) and streptococcal deoxyribonuclease on fibrinous, purulent and sanguineous pleural exudations. J Clin Invest 1949;28:173.

34. Sherry S, Tillett WS, Read CT. The use of streptokinase-streptodornase in the treatment of hemothorax. J Thorac Surg 1950;20:393.

35. Tillett WS, Sherry S, Read CT. The use of streptokinase-streptodornase in the treatment of postpneumonic empyema. J Thorac Surg 1951;21:275.

36. Tillett WS, Sherry S, Read CT. The use of streptokinase-streptodornase in the treatment of chronic empyema. J Thorac Surg 1951;21:325.

37. Sherry S, Goeller JP. The extent of the enzymatic degradation of desoxyribonucleic acid (DNA) in purulent exudates by streptodornase. J Clin Invest 1950;29:1588.

38. Tillett WS, Sherry S, Christensen LR. Streptococcal desoxyribonuclease: significance in lysis of purulent exudates and production by strains of hemolytic streptococci. Proc Soc Exp Biol Med 1948;68:184.

39. Sherry S, Johnson A, Tillett WS. Action of streptococcal desoxyribose nuclease (streptodornase) in vitro and on purulent pleural exudations of patients. J Clin Invest 1949;28:1094.

40. Sherry S, Tillett WS, Christensen LR. Presence and significance of desoxyribose nucleoprotein in the purulent pleural exudates of patients. Proc Soc Exp Biol Med 1948;68:179.

41. Tillett WS, Sherry S, Christensen LR, et al. Streptococcal enzymatic debridement. Ann Surg 1949; 131:12.

42. Leary T. Experimental arteriosclerosis in the rabbit compared with human (coronary) arteriosclerosis. Arch Pathol 1934;17:453.

43. Clark E, Graef I, Chasis H. Thrombosis of the aorta and coronary arteries. Arch Pathol 1936;22:183.

44. Chandler AB, Chapman I, Erhardt L, et al. Coronary thrombosis in myocardial infarction: report of a workshop on the role of coronary thrombosis in the pathogenesis of acute myocardial infarction. Am J Cardiol 1974;34:823.

45. Constantinides P. Plague fissures in human coronary thrombosis. J Atherscler Res 1966;65:1.

46. Friedman den Bovenkamp GJ. The pathogenesis of coronary thrombus. Am J Pathol 1966;48:19.

47. Johnson AJ, Tillett WS. Lysis in rabbits of intravascular blood clots by the streptococcal fibrinolytic system (streptokinase). J Exp Med 1952;95:449.

48. Kline DL. Purification and crystallization of plasminogen (profibrinolysin). J Biol Chem 1953;204:949.

49. Sherry S. Fibrinolytic activity of streptokinase activated human plasmin. J Clin Invest 1954;33:1054.

50. Sherry S, Titchener A, Gottesman L, et al. The enzymatic dissolution of experimental intravascular thrombi in the dog by trypsin, chymotrypsin and plasminogen activators. J Clin Invest 1954;33:1303.

51. Sherry S, Lindemeyer RI, Fletcher AP, Alkjaersig N. Studies on enhanced fibrinolytic activity in man. J Clin Invest 1959;38:810.

52. Alkjaersig N, Fletcher AP, Sherry S. The mechanism of clot dissolution by plasmin. J Clin Invest 1959;38:1086.

53. Sherry S, Fletcher AP, Alkjaersig N, Smyrniotis FE. An approach to intravascular fibrinolysis in man. Trans Assoc Am Physicians 1957;70:288.

54. Johnson AJ, McCarty WR. The lysis of artificially induced intravascular clots in man by intravenous infusions of streptokinase. J Clin Invest 1959; 38:1627.

55. Fletcher AP, Alkjaersig N, Smyrniotis FE, Sherry S. Treatment of patients suffering from early myocardial infarction with massive and prolonged streptokinase therapy. Trans Assoc Am Physicians 1958;71:287.

56. Fletcher AP, Alkjaersig N, Sherry S. The maintenance of a sustained thrombolytic state in man: I. Induction and effects. J Clin Invest 1959;38:1096.

57. Fletcher AP, Sherry S, Alkjaersig N, et al. The maintenance of a sustained thrombolytic state in man: II. Clinical observations on patients with myocardial infarction and other thromboembolic disorders. J Clin Invest 1959;38:1111.

58. Reference 52 noted in Life Sciences, July 23, 1984, as a citation classic; and in Current Contents, February 23, 1987, as one of 50 classics from J Clin Invest.

59. Bachmann F, Alkjaersig N, Fletcher AP, Sherry S. Partial purification and properties of plasminogen activator from pig heart. Biochemistry 1964;3:1578.

60. Fletcher AP, Alkjaersig N, Sherry S, et al. Development of urokinase as a thrombolytic agent: maintenance of a sustained thrombolytic state in man by its intravenous infusion. J Lab Clin Med 1965;654:713.

61. Williams JRB. Fibrinolytic activity of urine. Br J Exp Pathol 1951;32:530–537.

62. Astrup T, Sterndorff I. An activator of plasminogen in normal urine. Proc Soc Exp Biol Med 1952;81:675.

63. Sobel GW, Mohler SR, Jones NW, et al. Urokinase, an activator of profibrinolysin extracted from urine. Am J Physiol 1952;171:768–769.

64. Ploug J, Kjeldgaard NO. Urokinase, an activator of plasminogen from human urine: I. Isolation and properties. Biochim Biophys Acta 1957;24:282–288.

65. Kjeldegaard NO, Ploug J. Urokinase, an activator of plasminogen from human urine: II. Mechanism of plasminogen activation. Biochim Biophys Acta 1957;24:283–289.

66. Sawyer WD, Alkjaersig N, Fletcher AP, Sherry S. Comparison of fibrinolytic and fibrinogenolytic effects of plasminogen activators and proteolytic enzymes in plasma. Thromb Diath Haemorrh 1960;5:149–161.

67. White WF, Barlow GH, Mozen MM. The isolation and characterization of plasminogen activators (urokinase) from human urine. Biochemistry 1966;5:2160–2169.

68. Lesuk A, Terminiello L, Traver JH. Crystalline human urokinase: some properties. Science 1965;147:880.

69. Urokinase-Pulmonary Embolism Trial Study Group. Urokinase-pulmonary embolism trial: phase I results. JAMA 1970;214:2163.

70. Urokinase Pulmonary Embolism Trial. A national cooperative study. Circulation 1973;47(suppl II):II-1.

71. Urokinase-Streptokinase Pulmonary Embolism Trial. Phase II results: a national cooperative trial. JAMA 1974;229:1606.

72. Verstraete M, Tytgat G, Amery A, Vermylen J. Thrombolytic therapy with streptokinase using a standard dosage. Thromb Diath Haemorrh 1966; 16(suppl 21):494.

73. Yusuf S, Collins R, Peto R, et al. Intravenous and intracoronary fibrinolytic therapy in acute myocardial infarction: overview of results on mortality, reinfarction and side effects from 33 randomized controlled trials. Eur Heart J 1985;6:556.

74. European Cooperative Study Group for Streptokinase Treatment in Acute Myocardial Infarction. Streptokinase in acute myocardial infarction. N Engl J Med 1979;301:797.

75. European Cooperative Study Group for Streptokinase in Acute Myocardial Infarction. Extended report of the European cooperative trial. Acta Med Scand 1981;(suppl 648):7.

76. Roberts WR, Buja LM. The frequency and significance of coronary arterial thrombi and other observations in fatal acute myocardial infarction: a study of 107 necropsy patients. Am J Med 1972; 52:425.

77. Stampfer MJ, Goldhaber SZ, Yusuf S, et al. Effects of intravenous streptokinase on acute myocardial infarction: results pooled from randomized trials. N Engl J Med 1982;307:1180.

78. Boucek RJ, Murphy WP Jr. Segmental perfusion of the coronary arteries with fibrinolysin in man following myocardial infarction. Am J Cardiol 1960; 6:525.

79. Chazov EL, Mateeva LS, Mazaev AV, et al. Intracoronary administration of fibrinolysin in acute myocardial infarction. Terr Arkh 1976;48:8.

80. Hussain SS, Gurewich V, Lipinski B. Purification of a new high molecular weight form of urokinase from urine (abstract). Thromb Haemost 1981; 46:11.

81. Rijken DC, Collen D. Purification and characterization of the plasminogen activator secreted by human melanoma cells in tissue culture. J Biol Chem 1981;256:7035.

82. Smith RAG, Dupe RJ, English PD, Green J. Fibrinolysis with acyl enzymes: a new approach to thrombolytic therapy. Nature 1981;290:505.

6

STREPTOKINASE

Ronald N. Rubin

PHYSIOLOGY OF FIBRINOLYSIS

Fibrinolysis is a normal physiologic process in humans whereby insoluble fibrin deposited in intravascular areas during hemostasis or tissue injury is rendered soluble by proteolytic digestion and removed. Fibrinolysis in humans is mediated primarily by the plasminogen-plasmin proteolytic enzyme system. Plasminogen is a native plasma component synthesized in concentrations of 20 mg/dl by hepatocytes.[1]

Plasminogen exists in an inactive zymogen form in the β-globulin portion of plasma in two moieties: a major species of 89,000 Da possessing a glutamic acid N terminal (Glu-plasminogen) and a minor species with a lysine N terminal (Lys-plasminogen).[2] Abnormalities of plasminogen have been found that as a group manifest defective (i.e., absent, slow) activation to plasmin. As one might expect, patients found to have such variant molecules have been associated with thromboembolic diatheses.[3–5] Any of a broad variety of plasminogen activators can effect a cleavage of peptide bonds of the inactive zymogen, yielding the active, proteolytic plasmin, which is a two-chained species connected by a disulfide bond.[6] Plasmin has its greatest affinity (K_m) for fibrin and fibrinogen but manifests nonspecific protease activity that has the capability of digesting many other plasma proteins, including coagulation factors V, VIII, and XII as well as complement and kinin system proteins.[7] Thus, in the presence of plasmin, plasma proteolysis yields a variety of degradation products, many of which are "nonspecific" and only some of which are fibrinogen- or fibrin-specific. Specific fibrinogen degradation products include fragment X, a poorly clottable fibrinogen derivative, and smaller, nonclottable, antithrombotic fragments Y, D, and E.[8,9] Such products will be detected in most of the older fibrinogen/fibrin degradation product assays. The derivatives of plasmin digestion of fibrin are different, since cross-linking usually has occurred, and include the D-dimer piece, which has some specificity for the occurrence of plasmin digestion of cross-linked fibrin and which is now assuming a place in coagulation testing for thrombotic disorders and in patients receiving thrombolytic agents.[10,11]

Plasmin also has naturally occurring inhibitors in plasma to bind and control free plasmin, especially away from the site of thrombus. The major inhibitor is α_2-antiplasmin (α_2AP), which has a plasma concentration of 7 mg/dl and has the capability of converting active plasmin into stable, inert 1:1 stoichiometric complexes with the inhibitor.[12] Just as patients having deficient or defective plasminogen activation due to molecular defects manifest a thrombotic diathesis, rare patients have been found with quantitatively or qualitatively deficient α_2AP function who, as is predictable, manifest excessive plasmin effects with a subsequent clinical bleeding tendency.[13] In situations of marked plasmin activation, α_2-macroglobulin also acts as a secondary plasmin inhibitor[12] (Fig. 6-1).

Activation of plasminogen to plasmin can occur through a variety of pathways. In humans, two mechanisms for endogenous activation exist: intrinsic and extrinsic. The intrinsic activation involves factor XIIa converting prekallikrein to kallikrein, which then serves as a plasminogen activator.[14] Of interest is the direct and early interrelationship of thrombus formation with the fibrinolytic removal pathway that this intrinsic schema demonstrates.

Extrinsic plasmin activation plays the more dominant role in vivo and is mediated by the release of plasminogen activators from endothelial cells. Vascular endothelial cells release plasminogen activators in response to fibrin thrombi, ischemia, or the presence of vasoactive stimuli.[15] Both the extrinsic and intrinsic pathways of plasminogen activation are physiologic mechanisms usually activated by clot formation or inflammation/tissue damage.

Exogenous pathways for plasminogen activation also exist and involve the wide variety of thrombolytic agents now in use. All these involve the administration into the circulation of activators capable of activating plasmin without the mediation of either the intrinsic or extrinsic pathways (Fig. 6-2).

Special considerations come into play at the site of thrombus formation. Unique interactions between plasminogen, plasmin, and an evolving fibrin clot result in some differences from the fibrinogenolysis that occurs in a plasma system. These interactions result in a local enhancement of fibrinolytic activity at the site of thrombus formation. Plasminogen-binding sites that are "covered" in native fibrin or fibrinogen become uncovered during initial proteolysis by plasmin, thus rendering the molecule more readily available to further plasmin and plasminogen binding and subsequent proteolysis.[16] In addition, several of the high-affinity binding sites of plasminogen for fibrin(ogen) are also the binding sites for the previously noted rapid, stoichiometric, irreversible inactivation of plasmin by α_2AP.[17] In plasma, with its abundant α_2AP, plasminogen activation with free plasmin generation is quickly controlled by availability and competition for these binding

FIGURE 6-1. Basic physiology of fibrinolysis.

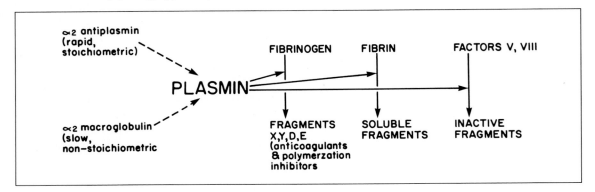

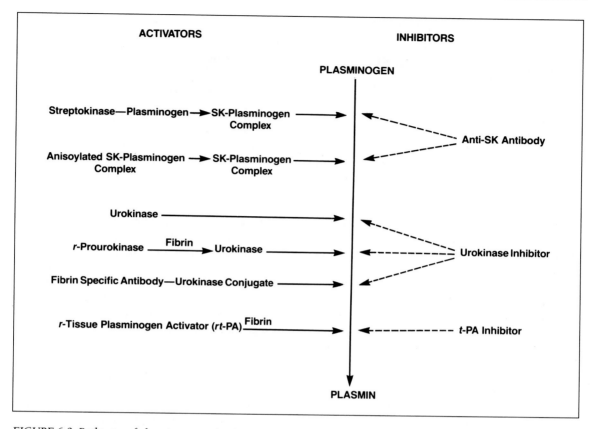

FIGURE 6-2. Pathways of plasminogen activation.

sites by α_2AP. In the region of thrombus formation, however, there is much less competition for these sites. There is a marked excess in availability of fibrin(ogen) binding sites for plasmin rather than α_2AP, so the fibrinolytic reaction can occur in a relatively inhibitor-free environment. The affinity of plasmin for fibrin cannot be overcome by its affinity for α_2AP, and the plasmin formed is present at the site of its action.[18,19] Thus there are differences between the degree and duration of fibrinolysis in the plasma phase compared with the fibrin-bound phase. Events monitored in plasma, such as degree of plasminogen and fibrinogen lowering, alterations in gross plasma clotting times, etc., may not particularly correlate with events occurring in thrombi, either pathologic or physiologic.

STREPTOKINASE

Biochemical Considerations

Streptokinase (SK) is the oldest of the clinically available thrombolytic agents. SK is produced by cultures of Lancefield group C β-hemolytic streptococci and has a molecular weight of around 50,000.[20,21] SK does not cleave plasminogen directly, rather first forming an equimolar stoichiometric 1:1 complex of plasminogen or plasmin with SK. This complex of plasminogen or plasmin is the true activator which can convert plasminogen to plasmin.[21,22] The plasmin(ogen)-SK activators behave as serine proteases.

SK introduced into patients activates both plasma plasminogen and thrombus-bound plasminogen. Most people have experienced streptococcal infection previously and therefore possess antistreptokinase neutralizing antibody in variable titer which is capable of binding to and inactivating SK.[23] This results in a biphasic half-life for SK, a rapid $t_{1/2}$ of about 16 minutes, which represents anti-SK antibody complexing and removal, and then a second slower $t_{1/2}$ of about 90 minutes, which seems to be the true biologic half-life of the protein.[24,25] Although there are no inhibitors of the plasminogen-SK complex in plasma, any active plasmin eluted from the complex can be inactivated by the α_2-antiplasmin inhibitor.[17,18] Thus, in plasma, SK usually will effect a state of hyperplasminemia, the level and duration of which depend on the level of preexisting anti-SK neutralizing antibody present (large "loading doses" infused initially usually are sufficient to neutralize such antibody in most cases), the concentrations of inhibitors α_2AP and less so α_2M, and the rate of clearance of plasmin by the body. The degree and duration of plasma hyperplasminemia thus can be quite variable within a population of patients but in most instances will be most striking in the initial hours of SK administration, with a tapering effect even as SK therapy continues.[26,27] It is during the period of plasma hyperplasminemia that the majority of fibrinogen digestion (with subsequent hypofibrinogenemia) and the digestion of other plasma proteins such as factors V and VIII (with subsequent prolongation of clotting time assays) occur.

Events at the site of fibrin thrombus after SK infusion are somewhat different. Once in the site of fibrin, the plasmin(ogen)-SK complex and eluted plasmin is protected somewhat from α_2AP and α_2M and protected to a significant degree from anti-SK antibody. The fibrin-bound plasminogen is quickly activated to locally active plasmin, which then enhances the fibrinolytic process by (1) converting Glu-plasminogen into more readily activated Lys-plasminogen in the thrombus[11] and (2) starting to digest fibrin, which creates more binding sites for plasminogen. Thus, at the clot site, the SK-complex is relatively free from inhibition, and the initial digestions create biochemical synergism for further, more rapid digestion of fibrin. These characteristics result in a significant degree of localization of the throm-

bolytic process, particularly in the later stages of SK therapy.[17-19,28]

Pharmacologic Considerations and Adverse Reactions

SK is a foreign protein that elicits antigenic responses in patients. Binding, neutralizing antibody to SK can be demonstrated even during the initial phases of treatment and usually reaches peak titers from days 7 to 10. Titers remain elevated for about 3 months and then decline toward baseline by 6 months.[28,29] Baseline titers and the need to overcome them with free SK are the reasons large initial loading doses, such as 250,000 units for venous thrombosis and roughly 1 million units for myocardial infarction, have been used. Higher titers may be expected in patients retreated within 6 to 12 months, and other thrombolytic agents need to be considered in such patients.

In a similar fashion, true allergy to SK can be encountered due to the formation of allergic antibodies. As purification methods have improved, the incidence has continued to decline. I reviewed data of cases treated between 1977 and 1985 and found the incidence of severe allergic reactions (angioedema, periorbital edema, bronchospasm, anaphylaxis) to be roughly 2%. Less severe allergic side effects (rash, urticaria) were reported to occur in up to 9% of cases in early studies.[30] The large myocardial infarction trials, which have studied many thousands of patients, have demonstrated a marked lowering of incidence for both severe and mild allergic reactions to about 1% and <3%, respectively.[31,32] These already low incidence figures can be further improved on with prophylactic measures such as pretreatment with antithistamines or corticosteroids. In my practice spanning more than a decade, such maneuvers have resulted in a total allergic incidence of less than 3%.

Pyrexia also may be encountered, despite SK being nonpyrogenic in standard animal tests. Non-aspirin-containing antipyretics almost always are adequate to address this.

Other nonhemorrhagic side effects encountered with SK therapy include increases in most hepatic enzymes which are dose-dependent.[33] This has been totally reversible after cessation of treatment, and no chronic sequelae or hepatic dysfunction has been seen.[34]

Bleeding

The major toxicity encountered with the use of SK is bleeding. Since almost all thrombolytic-related bleeding can be anticipated and prevented with careful patient selection, a discussion of these aspects is appropriate at this juncture.

Streptokinase can exert an effect on the clotting function of patients in a variety of ways. The therapeutic goal of lytic therapy, which is plasmin digestion of thrombi, can result in bleeding complications. This is so because SK and subsequently generated plasmin cannot differentiate physiologic fibrin thrombi (postoperative wounds, procedure-related trauma) from pathologic fibrin thrombi (deep venous thrombi, thrombi in occluded peripheral arteries). In fact, most bleeding episodes encountered with SK do not result from plasmin-induced derangements of the coagulation cascade but rather from plasmin lysis of hemostatic plugs.[35] This explains the high incidence of hemorrhage in the urokinase-streptokinase pulmonary embolism trials,[36] in which patients had frequent invasive procedures during the study in addition to invasive procedures establishing the diagnosis (pulmonary angiogram) and many patients developed postoperative pulmonary embolism. With time, experience, and more care to patient selection, the incidence of bleeding complications has diminished from 20% to 40% to more current observations of 0.5% to 1.0% for major bleeding and 7% to 11% for minor bleeding, respectively.[31] A representation of modern bleeding incidence figures is shown in Table 6-1 and is all the more remarkable because much larger doses of SK as well as concurrent aspirin and/or heparin were used in many of these studies.[31,32,37] Thus it is now well accepted that much of SK-related (and hemorrhage that of any other lytic agent) can be traced to poor technique—including the treatment of patients who would be expected to bleed as well as the concomitant use of invasive procedures during therapy.[35,38] The

TABLE 6-1. Incidence of Adverse In-Hospital Clinical Events with Streptokinase Derivatives

Event	Incidence (%)
Hemorrhagic stroke	0.5–1.0
Major bleeding—non CNS	0.7–1.0
Other bleeding events	5.1–11.0
Hypotension	4.4
Allergy	2.0–5.0

most effective means to avoid or at least lessen the hemorrhagic problem with SK is to try to prevent it, which has been shown to be possible in most instances by (1) strict, careful patient selection, (2) an established diagnosis, (3) therapy only for those likely to benefit (proper indication, recent "fresh" thrombi or emboli which are much more susceptible to plasmin digestion using thrombolysis, and (4) careful consideration of the contraindications, absolute and relative, as shown in Table 6-2. Once an appropriate decision to use SK has been made, meticulous medical and nursing care with avoidance of invasive procedures and patient manipulation is necessary.

Another source that contributes to bleeding is the proteolytic depletion of other plasma coagulation proteins in addition to fibrinogen. The most strikingly affected proteins are fibrinogen and factors V and VIII.[7] Patients receiving SK, particularly during the early plasma hyperplasminemia phase, uniformly display lowering of these proteins as well as significant prolongation

TABLE 6-2. Contraindications to Streptokinase Therapy

Absolute
  Active internal bleeding
  Recent (within 3–6 months) cerebrovascular accident or
    other intracranial damage (e.g., tumor)
Major Relative Contraindications
  Recent (fewer than 14 days) surgery or closed deep biopsy
  Recent (fewer than 14 days) serious trauma
  Gastrointestinal or genitourinary bleeding
  Uncontrolled hypertension (>110 mmHg diastolic)
Minor Relative Contraindications
  Other bleeding disorders such as thrombocytopenia,
    uremia, or hepatic failure
  Pregnancy
  Age over 75
  Diabetic retinopathy

of in vitro clotting times, specifically the pro-thrombin time (PT), partial thromboplastin time (PTT), and thrombin time (TT).[35,38] Additionally, some fibrinogen degradation products (fragments D, E, and Y) are relatively potent anticoagulants that further exacerbate plasmin-induced coagulopathy.[8,9] Still, these changes, though pronounced in laboratory findings, are not nearly as important in causing bleeding as is the lysis of hemostatic plugs previously discussed. Almost all earlier studies and reviews failed to demonstrate a correlation between the results of classic coagulation tests (fibrinogen level, PTT) and bleeding.[35,38] This observation was further supported by the findings in the TIMI trial and similar SK versus t-PA trials, which found that there was no more bleeding (and, in fact, almost always less) with SK compared with t-PA, despite consistent findings of greater aberrations in the PTT and fibrinogen level with SK preparations.[39,40] These coagulation changes do *not* induce spontaneous bleeding. A preexisting pathology, wound, or other hemostatic plug is required for that. Once bleeding begins, coagulation factor depletion can be expected to worsen the degree and extent of bleeding, and attention to repleting such coagulation function is needed (see blow).

Finally, an SK-related defect in platelet function has been demonstrated and is currently thought to be related to fibrinogen alterations which diminish the ability of fibrinogen to function in its platelet-aggregation role.[40,41] This defect is subtle and seems of uncertain clinical significance, since in recent studies in myocardial infarction and peripheral arterial indications, further antiplatelet therapy in the form of aspirin has been required to maintain vascular patency, and very little excess bleeding has been seen compared with identical SK dosage regimens without aspirin.[31,32,42]

Management of Adverse Reactions

The preceding reactions are amenable to preventive and/or therapeutic measures. There are a variety of empirical regimens to address the side effects of pyrexia and allergy, including one or more of acetaminophen, antihistamines, and short courses of corticosteroids. Appropriate use of such regimens can be expected to bring the overall incidence of all such nonhemorrhagic adverse reactions to <5%.[31,32]

Experience has established the principles of management for bleeding episodes. The most common instances are "nuisance" bleeding and consist of oozing from invasive sites such as vascular punctures. These respond to local pressure and should not be viewed as reasons to stop therapy when the indications are firm.

For more serious free bleeding and bleeding into an inaccessible site, the first maneuver should be discontinuation of SK therapy. Even the second-phase plasma half-life for SK is less than 90 minutes,[24,43] so within 3 to 4 hours very little SK remains in circulation. Usually, an additional measure is to replenish the depleted plasma coagulation factors during this time interval. Since the major plasma proteins being replenished are factors V and VIII and fibrinogen, appropriate sources include fresh-frozen plasma and cryoprecipitates. Investigators have reported that these measures can return hemostatic function to normal in less than 1 hour,[44] which should certainly be adequate in all but the most serious situations. In cases of cerebral bleed, probably the most serious complication encountered with SK, the plasmin inhibitor epsilon-aminocaproic acid (EACA) has been used.[44–46] This and related compounds bind to the lysine binding sites of plasminogen, thereby interfering with the required interaction and binding between plasminogen and fibrin(ogen), and they also inhibit the functional activity of plasmin itself.[19] The effect is very rapid in onset but should be reserved only for the most severe, life-threatening cases. The dosage of EACA is a 5-g loading dose, intravenously, and then 1 g/h.

Laboratory Findings and Monitoring during Streptokinase Therapy

Streptokinase, in its activation of plasminogen to active proteolytic plasmin, effects changes in plasma and at the sites of fibrin deposition, including pathologic thrombi as well as hemostatic plugs. The aim of successful thrombolytic therapy is dissolution of fibrin. It should be clear, therefore, that a certain amount of bleeding, resulting from the lysis of hemostatic plugs, will be a concomitant side effect of all thrombolytic therapy, regardless of indication, agent, and dose. Findings in the large acute myocardial infarction trials in the last decade provide evidence in favor of this assumption. These patients, as a group, are not postoperative, have not spent much prior time in intensive-care settings, and had few, if any, invasive procedures. Their bleeding incidence demonstrates the "core" morbidity of lytic agents and demonstrates a rather consistent 5% to 6% bleeding incidence (specifically 0.5% to 0.6% intracranial hemorrhage) which remains essentially constant regardless of thrombolytic agent used (i.e., streptokinase, tissue plasminogen activator, or acylated streptokinase) and regardless of the degree and extent of changes in the standard laboratory tests used to monitor thrombolytic therapy.[40,47-49] Earlier studies using very small doses of streptokinase for acute arterial thrombi,[50] as well as earlier studies of local infusions of SK for pulmonary embolism,[51] similarly showed little, if any, differences in laboratory findings or bleeding morbidity and provide further credibility to the concept that laboratory monitoring is useful to identify the presence of an active thrombolytic state but far less reliable and useful (if at all) in predicting bleeding complications or effectiveness of treatment.[38,52,53]

A brief review of the previous discussion of the physiology of thrombolysis will indicate what plasma and fibrin changes occur and therefore predict what might be measurable in the clinical laboratory. In the plasma phase, free plasmin, which is routinely encountered in the hyperplasminemic phase of streptokinase therapy, will cleave plasma fibrinogen into its known plasmin degradation fragments X, Y, D, and E. Fragments Y, D, and E are anticoagulants in their own right and prolong the thrombin clotting time.[8,9] They are also routinely detectable in the clinical coagulation laboratory using a variety of assay methods.[54] Thus plasmin effects on the plasma fibrinogen are easily demonstrable by measurements of (1) plasma fibrinogen itself, which usually is markedly lowered, (2) generation of high titers

of fibrinogen degradation products (FDPs), and (3) prolongation of the thrombin clotting time due to hypofibrinogenemia to levels below 1 g/L and the presence of significant titers of FDPs. None of the preceding tests, however, necessarily predicts successful lysis or bleeding complications during streptokinase therapy.

Other changes are also encountered in plasma and relate to the relative nonspecificity of plasmin. Plasmin will proteolyze other proteins, specifically factors V and VIII, and thus also result in prolongation of the prothrombin time and even more so the partial thromboplastin time.[55]

Finally, plasmin activity in plasma is countered in vivo by the two major inhibitors, α_2-antiplasmin and, to a far lesser extent, α_2-macroglobulin. A decrease in α_2-antiplasmin and the presence of plasmin-antiplasmin complexes in plasma constitute indirect but specific evidence of plasmin generation in circulating blood.[56,57] Such measurements are being used by some investigators and may become more preferred in clinical laboratories in the future.[57,58]

Changes induced by plasmin activation specifically at the site of fibrin deposition traditionally have been more difficult to measure. Even now, actual serial contrast study of the vessel involved by the fibrin clot remains the standard procedure for evaluating effectiveness of therapy for essentially all indications.[59-61] Recently, however, the measurement of fibrin digestion products after the cross-linking step has become available. Measurements of the YD fragment and D-dimer fragments have been successful, and D-dimer measurement in particular is becoming available in many clinical coagulation laboratories.[10,62] Although not as specific as earlier believed, their presence can be evidence of active plasmin digestion of clotted fibrin and may be considered as evidence of "successful" thrombolytic treatment.

The proteolytic products of plasmin digestion for fibrinogen and fibrin are shown on Figure 6-3. Laboratory findings expected with streptokinase-induced hyperplasminemia are summarized on Table 6-3.

The following is a reasonable approach to coagulation testing in patients undergoing streptokinase utilizing most of the standard protocols.

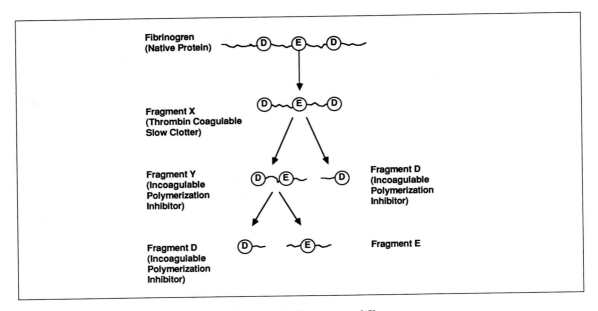

FIGURE 6-3. Proteolytic products of plasmin digestion for fibrinogen and fibrin.

Baseline fibrinogen levels and prothrombin and partial thromboplastin times should be obtained. In North America, anti-SK titers are rarely measured, since standard "loading doses" are designed to effectively overcome any preexisting neutralizing antibody. In patients having received SK within 6 to 12 months, high levels are anticipated, and alternative lytic agents should be chosen. In those rare instances of other patients having high neutralizing antibody titers, a fibrinogen level 1 to 2 hours into therapy points out their resistance

and the need to change to another agent as well. Once therapy is initiated, care to technique of specimen collection is important, since in vitro plasmin activity can have a marked effect on laboratory measurements.[63] Therefore, it is suggested that following blood collection, the plasma should be separated promptly at low temperature (4°C), followed by quick freezing to avoid in vitro formation of plasmin-antiplasmin complexes.[64,65] Also, most investigators suggest that in addition to citrate, collecting tubes contain a proteolytic inhibitor, such as Aprotinin, to slow in vitro fibrinogenolysis.[14] Thrombin times, partial thromboplastin times, fibrinogen levels, and FDP titers have rapid turnaround times in clinical coagulation laboratories and remain the preferred serial monitoring tests. These studies can be performed by any of a variety of commonly available methods with reasonably reliable results. With SK, changes are rapid and should be expected to occur within an hour, certainly within two, and the presence of markedly decreased fibrinogen (to less than 1 g/L), elevated FDPs (to levels above 1000 µg/mL), and prolongation of thrombin times and/or partial thromboplastin times to twice baseline or more provides direct evidence of

TABLE 6-3. Incidence of Adverse In-Hospital Clinical Events with Streptokinase Derivative

Coagulation Parameter	Alteration
Fibrinogen	Marked depletion, often to <0.50 g/L
Thrombin clotting times (e.g., partial thromboplastin time, thrombin time)	Moderate prolongation to >2× control
Fibrinogen degradation products (fragments D, X, Y, E)	Markedly elevated
Fibrin specific degradation products (D-dimers)	Markedly elevated

active plasmin in blood and therefore indirect evidence that plasmin also should be effecting lysis at sites of fibrin thrombi. Other tests, including depletion of plasminogen (to levels 5% to 15% of baseline) and formation of α_2-antiplasmin complexes, correlate with the preceding findings but are complicated to perform and are currently experimental. As noted, the measurement of crosslinked D-dimer is now available and in theory should be a more specific indicator of successful thrombolysis at actual fibrin sites rather than plasma proteolysis. Pre-liminary results have demonstrated correlation of D-dimer concentration in successful lytic treatments of deep vein thrombosis[11] and coronary artery occlusions.[10] Rapid identification of D-dimer fragments using monoclonal antibody techniques[32,62,66] and the increased availability of such tests in clinical coagulation laboratories likely will result in D-dimer being used along with the standard fibrinogen and thrombin-based clotting times as the "standard" serial tests for patients receiving SK.

Laboratory Testing and Bleeding Risk

In most studies, major and lethal bleeding episodes could not be predicted by alterations in laboratory testing. No differences are usually demonstrable between patients suffering major or CNS bleeding compared with patients who do not bleed. Laboratory and patient characteristics that have been suggested to point out a population at increased risk include longer duration of SK therapy[67] and patients undergoing SK therapy for peripheral arterial disease in comparison with myocardial infarction.[56] Presently, however, there is no single or, for that matter, no combination of laboratory testing methods, able to predict bleeding. The bleeding risk is linked to the drug's efficacy. When there is systemic lysis, fresh fibrin thrombi also will undergo proteolysis. If such fresh thrombi are in coronary arteries, pulmonary arteries, deep veins of the legs, or peripheral arteries, lysis is efficacy. If such fresh thrombi are in surgical wounds, areas of invasive diagnostic or therapeutic procedures, or hemostasic plugs in the fragile cerebral vasculature of a poorly controlled hypertensive patient or a patient with diffuse peripheral vascular disease, then lysis is hemorrhagic toxicity.

References

1. Robbins KC. The plasminogen-plasmin enzyme system. In: Colman R, Hirsh J, Marder VJ, Salzman EW, eds. Hemostasis and thrombosis: basic principles and clinical practice. 2nd ed. Philadelphia: JB Lippincott, 1987:340.
2. Wiman B. Biochemistry of the plasminogen to plasmin conversion. In: Gafney P, Balkur-Ulutin S, eds. Fibrinolysis: current fundamental and clinical aspects. London: Academic Press, 1978:46.
3. Aoki N. Genetic abnormalities of the fibrinolytic system. Semin Thromb Hemost 1984;10:42.
4. Lijnen HR, Collen D. Congenital and acquired deficiencies of components of the fibrinolytic system and their relation to bleeding and thrombosis. Fibrinolysis 1989;3:67.
5. Robbins KC. Classification of abnormal plasminogens: dysplasminogenemias. Semin Thromb Hemost 1990;16:217.
6. Wiman B, Walen P. The specific interaction between plasminogen and fibrin: a physiologic role of the lysine binding site in plasminogen. Thromb Res 1977;10:213.
7. Bell WR. Physiology of the fibrinolytic enzyme system. In: Sherry S, Bell WR, Chandler AB, Gurewich V, Mammen E, Marder VJ, Weiss HJ, eds. Thrombosis and thrombolysis. Princeton: Hoechst Medication Press, 1979:25.
8. Marder VJ, Budzynski AZ, James H. High molecular weight derivatives of human fibrinogen produced by plasmin. J Biol Chem 1972;247:4775.
9. Marder VJ, Budzynski AZ. Fibrinogen and its derivatives: hereditary and acquired abnormalities. Schweiz Med Wochenschr 1974;104:1338.
10. Soria J, Soria C, Mirshahi M, Mirshahi M, et al. Specific determination and identification of crosslinked fibrin degradation products in patients under thrombolytic therapy for myocardial infarction. Semin Thromb Hemost 1987;13:223.
11. Brenner B, Francis CW, Kessler C, et al. Noninvasive quantitation of venous clot lysis during fibrinolytic therapy using a D-dimer assay after correction for degradation of soluble fibrin. Circulation 1990;81:1818.
12. Harpel PC. Blood proteolytic enzyme inhibitors: their role in modulating blood coagulation and fibrinolytic enzyme pathways. In: Colman RW, Hirsh J, Marder VJ, Salzman EW, eds. Hemostasis and thrombosis: basic principles and clinical practice. 2nd ed. Philadelphia: JB Lippincott, 1987: 219.

13. Aoki N, Saito H, Kamiya H, et al. Congenital deficiency of α_2-plasmin inhibitor associated with severe hemorrhagic tendency. J Clin Invest 1979; 63:877.

14. Ogston D, Bennett B. Surface mediated reactions in the formation of thrombin, plasmin and kallikrein. Br Med Bull 1978;34:107.

15. Robbins KC, Barlow G, Nguyen G, Samama MM. Comparison of plasminogen activators. Semin Thromb Hemost 1987;13:131.

16. de Serrano VS, Vrano T, Gaffney PJ, Castellano FJ. Influence of various structural domains of fibrinogen and fibrin on the potentiation of plasminogen activation by recombinant tissue plasminogen activator. J Protein Chem 1989;8:61.

17. Christensen U, Clemmensen I. Kinetic properties of the primary inhibitor of plasmin from human plasma. Biochem J 1977;163:389.

18. Alkjaersig N, Fletcher AP, Sherry S. The mechanism of clot dissolution by plasmin. J Clin Invest 1959;38:1086.

19. Robbins KC. Fibrinolytic therapy: biochemical mechanisms. Sem Thromb Hemost 1991;17:1.

20. Davis MC, Englert ME, De Rezo EC. Interaction of streptokinase and human plasminogen observed in the ultra centrifuge under a variety of experimental conditions. J Biol Chem 1964;239:2651.

21. Reddy KN. Streptokinase: biochemistry and clinical applications. Enzyme 1988;40:79.

22. Reddy KN, Markus G. Mechanisms of activation of human plasminogen by streptokinase. J Biol Chem 1972;246:1683.

23. McGrath K, Patterson R. Immunology of streptokinase in human subjects. Clin Exp Immunol 1985;62:421.

24. Fletcher AP, Alkjaersig N, Sherry S. The clearance of heterologous proteins from the circulation of normal and immunized man. J Clin Invest 1959; 37:1306.

25. Scully MF, Strachan C, Kakkar VV. Binding of iodinated proteins to forming and preformed thrombi. Biochem Soc Trans 1973;1:1204.

26. Collen D. On the regulation and control of fibrinolysis. Thromb Haemost 1980;43:77.

27. Collen D. On the regulation and control of fibrinolysis. Thromb Haemost 1981;45:77.

27a. Suenson E, Thorsen S. The course and prerequisite of Lys-plasminogen formation during fibrinolysis. Biochemistry 1988;27:2435.

28. Jostring H, Barth U, Naidu R. Changes of antistreptokinase titer following long-term streptokinase therapy. In: Martin M, Schoop W, Hirsh J, eds. New concepts of streptokinase dosimetry. Vienna: Hans Huber, 1978:110.

29. James DC. Antistreptokinase levels in various hospital groups. Postgrad Med 1973;49:26.

30. Marbet G, Eichlisberger HL, Duckert F, et al. Side effects of thrombolytic therapy with porcine plasmin and low dose streptokinase. Thromb Haemost 1982;48:196.

31. Rubin RN. Choosing a thrombolytic agent in acute myocardial infarction. Pharm Therap 1992;17: 617.

32. ISIS-2 (Second International Study of Infarct Survival) Collaborative Group. Randomized trial of intravenous streptokinase, oral aspirin, both or neither among 17,187 cases of suspected acute myocardial infarction: ISIS-2. Lancet 1988;332: 349.

33. Hurnage D, Keller HE, Nienhaus KH, Wenzel W. On the behavior of serum enzymes during long term treatment with streptokinase. In: Martin M, Schoop W, Hirsh J, eds. New concepts of streptokinase dosimetry. Vienna: Hans Huber, 1978:105.

34. Shepard IT, Rao S, Lawrence IR, et al. Streptokinase and serum enzymes. Br Med J 1976;273:562.

35. Marder V, Sherry S. Thrombolytic therapy: current status. N Engl J Med 1988;318:1512.

36. Urokinase-Streptokinase Embolism Trial. Phase 2 results: a cooperative study. JAMA 1974;229: 1606.

37. The International Study Group. In-hospital mortality and clinical course of 20,891 patients with suspected acute myocardial infarction randomized between alterplase and streptokinase with or without heparin. Lancet 1990;33:71.

38. Bell WR, Meeh AG. Guides for the use of thrombolytic agents. N Engl J Med 1979;301:1266.

39. Sheehan F, Braunwald E, Canner P, et al. The effects of intravenous thrombolytic therapy on left ventricular function: a report on tissue type plasminogen activator and streptokinase from the thrombolysis in myocardial infarction (TIMI phase I) trial. Circulation 1987;75:817.

40. The TIMI Study Group. The thrombolysis in myocardial infarction (TIMI) trial: phase I findings. N Engl J Med 1985;312:932.

41. Brogden RN, Speight TM, Avery GS. Streptokinase: a review of its clinical pharmacology, mechanism of action and therapeutic uses. Drugs 1973;5:357.

42. Verstraete M. Use of thrombolytic agents in noncoronary disorders. Drugs 1989;38:801.

43. Staniforth DH, Smith RA, Hibbs M. Streptokinase and anisoylated streptokinase plasminogen complex-their action on haemostasis in human volunteers. Eur J Clin Pharmacol 1983;24:751.

44. Sherry S, Fletcher AP, Alkjaersig N, et al. ϵ-Amino caproic acid: a potent antifibrinolytic agent. Trans Assoc Am Physicians 1959;72:62.

45. Hull R, Raskob GE. Pulmonary thromboembolism. In: Kelly W, ed. Textbook of internal medicine, 2nd ed. Philadelphia: JB Lippincott, 1992: 1783.

46. Mantia AM, Balint BW, Stulken EH Jr. Does ep-

silon aminocaproic acid limit intraoperative bleeding in patients with greater coagulation derangements after streptokinase thrombolysis? Anaesth Rev 1989;16:41.

47. Rao AK, Pratt C, Berke A, et al. Thrombolysis in myocardial infarction (TIMI) trial phase I: hemorrhagic manifestations and changes in plasma fibrinogen and the fibrinolytic system in patients treated with recombinant tissue plasminogen activator and streptokinase. J Am Coll Cardiol 1988; 2:1.

48. Gruppo Italiano per lo studio della streptochinasi nell'Infarto Miocardico (GISSI). Effectiveness of intravenous thrombolytic treatment in acute myocardial infarction. Lancet 1986;314:1465.

49. Rubin RN. Choosing a thrombolytic agent in acute MI. Drug Ther 1992;17:17.

50. Rubin RN, Comerota AC, Soulen R, et al. Intra-arterial thrombolytic therapy for peripheral arterial disease. Blood 1982;60:221.

51. Sasahara AA, Sharma G. Thrombolytic therapy in the treatment of pulmonary embolism: short and long-term benefits. In: Comerota AJ, ed. Thrombolytic therapy. Philadelphia: Grune & Stratton, 1988:51.

52. Marder V, Soulen R, Atichartakarn V, Budzynski A. Qualitative venographic assessment of deep vein thrombosis in the evaluation of streptokinase and heparin therapy. J Lab Clin Med 1977;89: 1018.

53. Sharma G, Cella G, Parisi A, Sasahara A. Thrombolytic therapy. N Engl J Med 1982;306:1268.

54. Marder VJ. Molecular aspects of fibrin formation and dissolution. Semin Thromb Hemost 1982;8:1.

55. Donaldson VH. Effect of plasmin in vitro on clotting factors in plasma. J Lab Clin Med 1960;56: 644.

56. Conard J, Samama MM. Theoretic and practical considerations on laboratory monitoring of thrombolytic therapy. Semin Thromb Hemost 1987;13: 212.

57. Collen D, Verstraete M. α_2-Antiplasmin consumption and fibrinogen breakdown during thrombolytic therapy. Thromb Res 1979;14:631.

58. Harpel PC. α_2-Plasmin inhibitor and α_2-macroglobulin-plasmin complexes in plasma: quantitation by an enzyme-linked differential antibody immunoabsorbent assay. J Clin Invest 1983;68:46.

59. Comerota AJ. Intra-arterial thrombolytic therapy. In: Comerota AJ, ed. Thrombolytic therapy. Philadelphia: Grune & Stratton, 1988:125.

60. Van Breda A, Robinson JC, Feldman L, et al. Local thrombolysis in the treatment of arterial graft occlusions. J Vasc Surg 1984;1:103.

61. Carabello BA, Spann JF. Thrombolytic therapy in acute myocardial infarction. In: Comerota AJ, ed. Thrombolytic therapy. Philadelphia: Grune & Stratton, 1988:165–189.

62. Soria J, Soria C, Boucheix C, et al. Monoclonal antibodies that react preferentially with fibrinogen degradation products or with fibrin degradation products. Ann NY Acad Sci 1983;408:665.

63. Lurie AA, Gross LF, Rogers WJ. The measurement of fibrinogen by the Dupont Aca and Dade methods in patients receiving streptokinase infusions. Am J Clin Pathol 1985;84:526.

64. Conard J, Samama M. Laboratory control of streptokinase therapy. Thromb Diatherm Haemorrh (Suppl) 1973;56:191.

65. Collen D, Bounameaux H, de Cock F, et al. Analysis of coagulation and fibrinolysis during intravenous infusion of recombinant tissue-type plasminogen activator in patients with acute myocardial infarction. Circulation 1986;73:511.

66. Connagtian DG, Francis CW, Lane DA, Marder VJ. Specific identification of fibrin polymers, fibrinogen degradation of fibrin polymers, fibrinogen degradation products and cross-linked fibrin products in plasma and serum with a new, sensitive technique. Blood 1985;65:589.

67. Van Breda A. Thrombolysis in arterial bypass grafts. Semin Thromb Hemost 1991;17:7.

7

UROKINASE

Marc Verstraete

The fibrinolytic activity of human urine was originally described by Williams[1] and Astrup et al.,[2] and this finding resulted in the name of *urokinase.* This protein also can be isolated from tissue cultures of human embryonic kidney cells.

PHYSICOCHEMICAL PROPERTIES

Urokinase is a trypsin-like enzyme composed of two polypeptide chains (molecular weight 20,000 and 34,000). It may occur in two molecular forms designated S_1 (molecular weight 31,600, 276 amino acids: *low-molecular-weight urokinase*) and S_2 (molecular weight 54,000, 411 amino acids: *high-molecular-weight urokinase*), the former being a proteolytic degradation product of the latter.[3] The high-molecular-weight form is found predominantly in the urinary commercial preparations,[3] and the low-molecular-weight forms are isolated from long-term cultures of human fetal kidney cells collected at 26 to 32 weeks of gestation.[4] Both forms of urokinase have common pharmacologic properties in vivo and do not differ in terms of clinical results.

The complete primary structure of high-molecular-weight urokinase has been elucidated.[5] The light chain contains 158 amino acids, and the heavy chain contains 253. The interchain disulfide bond Cys_{194}-Cys_{222} was shown to be required for the activity of urokinase.[6] The catalytic center is located in the COOH-terminal chain and is composed of Asp_{255}, His_{204}, and Ser_{356}. The NH_2-terminal chain contains a growth-factor domain (residues 9 to 45) and one kringle domain (residues 45 to 134). A low-molecular-weight tcu-PA (M_r 33,000) can be generated with plasmin by hydrolysis of the Lys_{135}-Lys_{136} peptide bond following previous cleavage of the Lys_{158}-Ile_{159} peptide bond.[7]

MECHANISM OF PLASMINOGEN ACTIVATION

Urokinase activates plasminogen directly following Michaelis-Menten kinetics. This double-chain molecule has no specific activity for fibrin and activates fibrin-bound and circulating plasminogen relatively indiscriminately. Extensive plasminogen activation and depletion of α_2-antiplasmin may occur following treatment with urokinase, leading to degradation of several plasma proteins, including fibrinogen, factor V, and factor VIII. The half-life of urokinase is approximately 15 minutes; urokinase is cleared mainly by the liver, with about 3% to 5% being cleared by the kidneys.

Although the S_1 and S_2 forms are equipotent, the high-molecular-weight form preferentially activates Glu-plasminogen circulating in plasma, and the low-molecular-weight form is more directed to Lys-plasminogen.[8] The latter type of plasminogen has specific Lys binding sites, whereby the molecule binds to the fibrin surface and can accumulate on the thrombus.[9] Furthermore, upon minimal digestion of fibrin, additional Lys binding sites are exposed.[10]

INHIBITORS OF UROKINASE

Several inhibitors of plasminogen activators (PAIs) have been described. Plasminogen activator inhibitor 1 (PAI-1) is released by endothelial cells and different neoplastic cell lines and is also found in platelets and plasma.[11-13] PAI type 2 (PAI-2) was first detected in placental extracts and is also released from cell lines and macrophages.[14] These two PAIs are proteins with molecular weights of about 50,000 to 60,000 and differ in immunologic reactivity and several physiologic characteristics.[15] Both belong to the serpin superfamily (serine protease inhibitor family). A third PAI (protease nexin) was found predominantly in the extracellular matrix and inhibits plasminogen activators but also plasmin and thrombin.[16] All three PAI molecules crossreact with tcu-PA but not with scu-PA.

A single bolus of urokinase given intravenously in humans is cleared with a half-life of 14 ± 6 minutes; most of urokinase is degraded to inert metabolites by the liver.[17]

DOSE OF UROKINASE

For over a decade, an initial intravenous dose of 4000 units/kg of body weight over 10 minutes followed by the same maintenance dose per kilogram hourly was recommended for the treatment of acute major pulmonary embolism. A bolus dose in the right atrium of 15,000 units/kg of body weight was recently proposed in this indication; an intravenous infusion of 3 million units of urokinase (1 million units over 10 minutes and 2 million units over the next 110 minutes) is presently being tested.

In the early trials in acute myocardial infarction, intracoronary urokinase (6000 U/min) was given for 90 to 120 minutes.[18] At present, the systemic dose of urokinase is 2 million units given as an intravenous bolus[19] or 1.5 million units given as a bolus, followed by the same dose administered over 90 minutes.[20] Another, more conservative administration scheme recently tested was 1 million units over 15 minutes, followed by 1 million units over less than 3 hours.[21]

ADVERSE EFFECTS OF UROKINASE

Purified urokinase preparations are nonantigenic and nonpyrogenic, and their proper use is most often associated with a milder coagulation defect than that with streptokinase, but with a similar incidence of bleeding to that shown for streptokinase-treated patients. Since the level of inhibitors in plasma is relatively constant, a fixed dosage regimen can readily be used. Rigors and bronchospasm are not expected to occur after administration of a natural human protein; they have been reported, however, although at a low frequency and in patients previously exposed to streptokinase.[22]

REFERENCES

1. Williams JRB. The fibrinolytic activity of urine. Br J Exp Pathol 1951;32:530.
2. Astrup T, Sterndorff I. An activator of plasminogen in normal urine. Proc Soc Exp Biol Med 1952; 81:675.
3. White WF, Barlow GH, Mozen MM. The isolation and characterization of plasminogen activators (urokinase) from human urine. Biochemistry 1966;5:2160.
4. Barlow GH. Urinary and kidney cell plasminogen

activator (urokinase). In: Lorand L, ed. Methods in Enzymology, Vol 45. San Diego, Academic Press, 1976:239.

5. Guenzler WA, Steffens GJ, Oetting F, et al. The primary structure of high-molecular-mass urokinase from human urine: the complete amino acid sequence of the A chain. Hoppe-Seylers Z Physiol Chem 1982;363:1155.

6. Miwa N, Sawada T, Suzuki A. Conformational changes in human urokinase induced by a specific reduction of disulfide bond in Cys_{194}-Cys_{222} associated with exhibition of enzymatic activity. Biochim Biophys Acta 1984;791:1.

7. Steffens GJ, Guenzler WA, Oetting F, et al. The complete amino acid sequence of low molecular mass urokinase from human urine. Hoppe-Seylers Z Physiol Chem 1982;363:1043.

8. Collen D. On the regulation and control of fibrinolysis. Thromb Haemost 1980;43:77.

9. Rákóczi I, Wiman B, Collen D. On the biological significance of the specific interaction between fibrin, plasminogen and antiplasmin. Biochim Biophys Acta 1978;540:295.

10. Harpel PC, Chang TS, Verderber E. Tissue plasminogen activator and urokinase mediate the binding of Glu-plasminogen to plasma fibrin I. J Biol Chem 1985;260:4432.

11. Andreasen PA, Nielsen LS, Kristensen P, et al. Plasminogen activator inhibitor from human fibrosarcoma cells binds urokinase-type plasminogen activator, but not its proenzyme. J Biol Chem 1986;261:7644.

12. Gelehrter TD, Barouski-Miller PA, Coleman PL, Cwikel BJ. Hormonal regulation of plasminogen activator in rat hepatoma cells. Mol Cell Biochem 1983;53/54:11.

13. Loskutoff DJ, van Mourik JA, Erickson LA, Lawrence D. Detection of an unusually stable fibrinolytic inhibitor produced by bovine endothelial cells. Proc Natl Acad Sci USA 1983;80:2956.

14. Astedt B, Lecander T, Brodin T, et al. Purification of specific placental plasminogen activator inhibitor by monoclonal antibody and its complex formation with plasminogen activator. Thromb Haemost 1985;53:122.

15. Hekman CM, Loskutoff DJ. Endothelial cells produce a latent inhibitor of plasminogen activators that can be activated by denaturants. J Biol Chem 1985;260:11581.

16. Scott RW, Bergmann BL, Bajpai A, et al. Protease nexin: properties and a modified purification procedure. J Biol Chem 1985;260:7029.

17. Collen D, De Cock F, Lijnen HR. Biological and thrombolytic properties of proenzyme and active forms of human urokinase: II. Turnover of natural and recombinant urokinase in rabbits and squirrel monkeys. Thromb Haemost 1984;52:24.

18. Cernigliaro C, Sansa M, Campi A, et al. Clinical experience with urokinase in intracoronary thrombolysis. Clin Cardiol 1987;10:222.

19. Mathey DG, Schofer J, Sheehan FH, et al. Intravenous urokinase in acute myocardial infarction. Am J Cardiol 1985;55:878.

20. Neuhaus KL, Tebbe U, Gottwik M, et al. Intravenous recombinant tissue plasminogen activator (rt-PA) and urokinase in acute myocardial infarction: results of the German Activator Urokinase Study (GAUS). J Am Coll Cardiol 1988;12:581.

21. Masini G. Intravenous urokinase in acute myocardial infarction: a critical review of an Italian multicentre experience. Drug Invest 1991;3(5):368.

22. Matsis P, Mann S. Rigors and bronchospasm with urokinase after streptokinase (letter). Lancet 1992;340:1552.

8

RECOMBINANT TISSUE PLASMINOGEN ACTIVATOR

Juergen Froehlich

David L. Stump

IDENTIFICATION / DISCOVERY

Tissue plasminogen activator (t-PA) is a naturally occurring activator of plasminogen that plays an important physiologic role in the regulation of hemostasis and fibrinolysis. In the normal organism, it is produced and released by endothelial cells[1] in response to local stimuli and regulatory mechanisms. The human form of t-PA has been isolated from various sources such as postmortem vascular perfusates,[2,3] postexercise blood,[2] and uterine tissue.[4]

Molecular cloning techniques that became available in the early 1980s were used to clone and express the complementary DNA that encodes human t-PA.[5] Early expression experiments were performed using mRNA derived from cultures of human Bowes melanoma cells which had led to the purification of natural t-PA from the cell culture fluid.[6-8] Subsequently, recombinant t-PA (rt-PA) was produced in sufficient quantities for use in pilot clinical trials. An initial small-scale process using Chinese hamster ovary cells (CHO) in roller bottles resulted in a two-chain form of t-PA. The generation of CHO cells in suspension culture has allowed the large-scale production of alteplase, the predominantly single-chain form of human t-PA. Under the trade name Activase, alteplase was approved in 1987 in the United States for treatment of acute myocardial infarction and in 1990 for treatment of massive pulmonary embolism.

MOLECULAR BIOLOGY

Natural t-PA is a serine protease composed of a single polypeptide chain of 527 amino acids.[5] Its primary structure, illustrated in Figure 8-1, shows sequences of amino acids which are homologous with dominant sequences (domains) of other naturally existing and biologically active proteins.[5,9] The amino-terminal end of t-PA has a total of five domains of four different types: a fibrinonectin-type finger domain of about 44 amino acid residues, a growth factor-type domain of about 40 residues, and two kringle domains of 81 residues each. The carboxy-terminal end of the

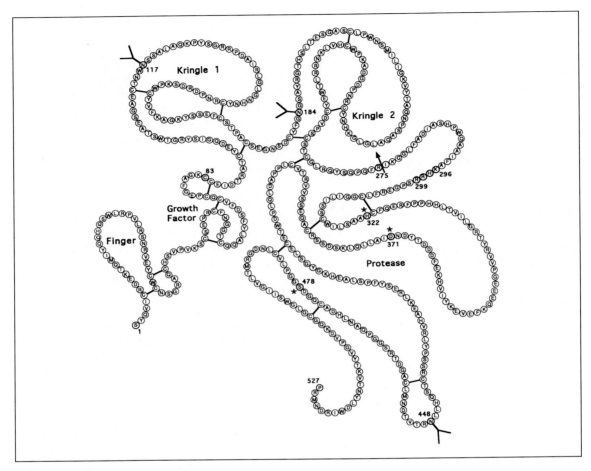

FIGURE 8-1. The primary structure of t-PA. Disulfide bonds are indicated by bars. Sites known to be glycosylated on native t-PA are marked with a Y, and residues related to the catalytic triad are marked with an asterisk. The arrow indicates the plasmin cleavage site.

t-PA molecule has the sequence of a serine protease domain with about 260 residues. Linker regions bring the total to 527 residues for the mature protein.[5] Occasionally, three additional residues (Gly-Ala-Arg) are found at the amino-terminal end, which is generally thought to be the result of incomplete precursor processing without imparting functionality.[10–13]

Cysteine-linked disulfide bonds stabilize the secondary and tertiary structures of t-PA. Mature t-PA contains 35 cysteines that form 17 disulfide bonds, as indicated in Figure 8-1.[5,9] Most of the disulfides are intradomain linkages. The most

likely site for the unpaired disulfide is at position 83, in the growth factor domain.[14] It is not known whether this unpaired disulfide is involved in any specific function of the t-PA molecule.

The human t-PA gene has been localized to chromosome 8.[15–17] It is divided into exons coding separately for the various domains. Thirteen intervening sequences divide the gene into 14 coding regions. The mRNA for t-PA codes for a precursor of 35 additional residues at the amino-terminal end. The first 20 amino acids of the precursor constitute a hydrophobic signal peptide involved in the secretion of t-PA. They are followed by a positively charged decapeptide that may be a processing signal.[5] The signal peptide, propeptide, finger, and growth factor regions are encoded by individual exons, whereas the kringles and the protease domain are encoded by multiple exons.[18]

Plasmin converts t-PA to a two-chain molecule by hydrolysis of the Arg_{275}-Ile_{276} peptide bond[7,19]: the A chain or heavy chain (amino acids 1 to 275, containing the finger, growth factor-type, and both kringle domains) and the B-chain or protease domain (amino acids 276 to 527). A disulfide (Cys_{264}-Cys_{395}) connects both chains with each other. Alteplase represents a mixture of predominantly single-chain t-PA (approximately 80%) and two-chain t-PA.

The molecular weight of t-PA varies from 63,000 to 65,000.[5] This heterogeneity is due to different patterns of glycosylation at four potential N-linked glycosylation sites of the t-PA molecule. Three of these sites, at positions 117, 184, and 448, are known to be glycosylated under certain circumstances.[20,21] Mammalian cells have been found to not glycosylate at the fourth position 218.[11,19,21]

Different glycosylation sites characterize the two types of t-PA.[19,20,22] Type I t-PA is glycosylated at positions 117, 184, and 448, whereas type II is glycosylated only at positions 117 and 448. The carbohydrate at positions 184 and 448 are complex oligosaccharides, position 117 carries a high-mannose oligosaccharide carbohydrate.[19,21,23] Type II t-PA has been shown to have slightly higher specific activity[12] compared with type I t-PA. Alteplase, produced by CHO in suspension culture cells, is an approximately 1:1 mixture of type I and type II t-PA. It contains by weight approximately 7% carbohydrate.

BIOLOGIC CHARACTERIZATION AND STRUCTURE-FUNCTION RELATIONS

Early studies of structure-function relationships used t-PA variant molecules with domain deletions or site-directed modifications. Newer techniques utilizing an algorithm to mutate clustered charged amino acids (Glu, Asp, His, Lys, Arg) to alanine resulted in an increasing number of t-PA variants and new insights into functional groups. The majority of studied variant molecules were reviewed by Higgins and Bennett,[24] Lijnen and Collen,[25] and Bennett et al.[26]

The accepted physiologic role of t-PA is to cleave the Arg_{560}-Val_{561} peptide bond of plasminogen, converting it to plasmin, and thus to initiate or accelerate the process of fibrinolysis. The active site for this enzymatic activity is located in the protease domain of the t-PA molecule with its carboxy-terminal region. Earlier reports suggested that a catalytic triad composed of His_{322}, Asp_{371}, and Ser_{478} is responsible for the enzymatic activity.[5] Recent research using the clustered "charged-to-alanine scan" to obtain mutant variants further associated the Lys-His-Arg-Arg 296–299 region of t-PA with enzymatic activity and regulation of fibrinolysis.[26–30]

In contrast to most serine proteases, the single-chain form of the t-PA molecule has appreciable enzymatic activity. In the absence of fibrin, in vitro assays demonstrate greater activity of the two-chain form. However, in the presence of fibrin, the two forms of t-PA are equally active.[31,32] Fibrinogen accelerated the t-PA activity to about six times the unstimulated value.[26] From the measurement of its affinity to plasminogen, it is known that in plasma very little plasminogen activation occurs with physiologic levels of t-PA. Its Michaelis constant (K_m) of 65 μM is well above the 2 μM concentration of plasminogen in plasma. When t-PA and plasminogen are both bound to the fibrin surface, the conformation of the two molecules then greatly facilitates plasminogen activation.[33] The K_m for the reaction falls to a 0.16 μM, yielding nearly 400-fold more efficient activation of plasminogen than in the absence of fibrin (Fig. 8-2).

It is now known that all domains of t-PA are involved in fibrin binding, especially the finger and the growth factor domains. In contrast to earlier observations, newer studies with a variety of point t-PA mutants suggest that kringle 2 is less involved in fibrin binding than originally expected. A functional lysine binding site on the same kringle 2 does not seem to be required for fibrin binding, fibrin stimulation, or clot lysis.[26] The protease domain of t-PA contains multiple

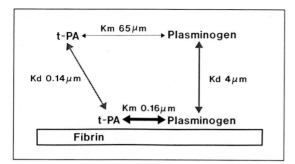

FIGURE 8-2. Mechanism of action of t-PA. In the absence of fibrin, t-PA is efficient only at high concentrations of plasminogen (K_m = 65 μM). When fibrin is present, the efficiency of t-PA increases nearly 400-fold (K_m = 0.16 μM), now capable of activation at well below the concentration (2 μM) of plasminogen in blood. (Used with permission from Stump DC, Collen D: The fibrinolytic system: implications for thrombolytic therapy. In: Acute coronary care in the thrombolytic era. Chicago: Year Book Medical Publishers, 1988.)

sites that mediate the interaction with fibrin and also seems to be related to fibrin-specificity. This is demonstrated by the above-mentioned Lys-His-Arg-Arg 296–299 Ala-Ala-Ala-Ala variant, which has 8- to 10-fold increased fibrin specifity compared with the native t-PA.[26]

ROLE OF t-PA IN PHYSIOLOGY AND PATHOPHYSIOLOGY OF HEMOSTASIS

Physiologic Regulation of t-PA Secretion

t-PA is synthesized and secreted by endothelial cells.[1] Under physiologic conditions, t-PA antigen levels in human plasma at rest range between 3.4 and 6.6 μg/L, measured by immunoradiometric assay[34] or by enzyme-linked immunosorbent assay.[35] After venous occlusion,[35] and after acute exercise,[37,38] t-PA levels are known to increase in normal subjects. A variety of agents, such as thrombin, dexamethasone, histamine, butyrate, interleukin-1, epinephrine, and arginine vasopressin, were shown to stimulate secreted t-PA antigen levels or to induce t-PA mRNA expression in vitro. Gonadotropin may play a role in the regulation of t-PA activity to induce ovulation.

Inhibition/Regulation of t-PA Activity

Like other serine proteases, t-PA can be irreversibly inhibited by general inhibitors such as diisopropylfluorophosphate[4,22] and by some selective inhibitors containing arginine, such as Phe-Pro-Arg-chloromethylketone.[39–41] The peptide inhibitor aprotinin, which does inhibit plasmin and urokinase, is ineffective against t-PA. In plasma, several higher-molecular-weight inhibitors react with and inhibit the t-PA molecule. Relatively slow and physiologically less important plasma inhibitors are α_2-antiplasmin, C1-esterase inhibitor,[22] and α_2-macroglobulin.[41] The protease nexin and the placenta-derived plasminogen activator inhibitor 2 (PAI-2) demonstrate moderate rates of inhibition.[42]

A relatively fast-acting physiologic inhibitor is thought to be the serpin-related protein plasminogen activator inhibitor 1 (PAI-1) reviewed elsewhere.[43,44] It is present in plasma, endothelial cells, and platelets. t-PA cleaves PAI-1 at the Arg_{346}-Met_{347} peptide bond and forms a stable t-PA/PAI-1 complex. It is interesting to note that this cleavage site bears little resemblance with the site at which plasminogen is cleaved by t-PA. In the t-PA molecule, the specific amino acids Lys_{296}-His-Arg-Arg-Ser-Pro-Gly_{302} and Arg_{304} have been identified to be responsible for the interaction with PAI-1.[30,45] Recent results with the Lys-His-Arg-Arg 296–299 Ala-Ala-Ala-Ala variant of t-PA support this finding, since this molecule exerts a 10-fold resistance to PAI-1 compared with native t-PA.[28,29]

The level of plasma PAI-1 appears to be responsible for the regulation of the fibrinolytic process through the t-PA/PAI-1 interaction. The physiologic concentrations of PAI-1 in plasma are less than 20 ng/mL[46,47] and would not be high enough to interfere significantly with physiologic t-PA levels or the supraphysiologic levels achieved during t-PA therapy. Administration of t-PA to healthy subjects by infusion resulted in an immediate formation of t-PA/PAI-1 complex with levels of free PAI-1 returning to normal (5 ng/ml) over the subsequent 24 h.[48] Some of the previously mentioned t-PA stimulating agents (thrombin, dexamethasone) as well as others, such as endotoxin, are also known to stimulate PAI-1 antigen levels, resulting in a regulatory effect on local fibrinolytic activity.

Pathophysiology of t-PA Regulation

In certain pathologic conditions, such as acute myocardial infarction[49] and others,[44,50–52] PAI-1 can be markedly increased, leading to a predisposition for thrombotic occlusions. Similar changes resulting in a reduction of the plasma fibrinolytic activity were seen in patients with arterial occlusive disease.[53,54] The important role of PAI-1 in the regulation of fibrinolytic activity is further evidenced by recent findings of a decrease in PAI-1 levels and consequently increased fibrinolytic activity after acute arterial and venous occlusions[55] as well as exercise programs in normal subjects and patients with coronary artery disease.[56,57] Whether PAI-1 interactions with t-PA may contribute to the appearance of thrombotic reocclusion after successful reperfusion[58] remains to be established.

Excessive Fibrinolysis

Certain inherited or acquired bleeding disorders may be related to deficiencies of PAI-1 or α_2-antiplasmin or excess circulating t-PA or may occur in patients with acute leukemia or amyloidosis. The recent development of orthotopic liver transplantation in patients with severe hepatic failure has led to the observation of cases with profound intraoperative bleeding in part due to compromised clearance of circulating t-PA during the procedure.[59]

PHARMACOLOGY

Animal Models

For an overview of animal models, see Collen et al.[60] and Gold et al.[61] A number of animal models in different species, such as rabbits, rats, dogs, and baboons, have been performed to investigate the fibrinolytic characteristics of t-PA. Experimental thrombotic or embolic occlusions in arterial and venous locations were induced by various techniques. In summary, the fibrinolytic activity of t-PA did not depend on the type of vasculature (arterial or venous) or the mode of administration. t-PA administration did not result in the magnitude of fibrinogen breakdown observed with streptokinase and urokinase. The extent of fibrinolysis by t-PA was mainly dependent on the administered dose and much less dependent on the age of the thrombotic. Increasing doses of t-PA shortened time to reperfusion. Local delivery close to or into thrombus/embolic occlusions improved the fibrinolytic efficacy with reduced doses of t-PA necessary for clot lysis as compared with intravenous infusion.

In a rabbit jugular vein thrombosis model, t-PA activity was found to be sustained for more than 1 h beyond its time of clearance from the circulation. In contrast, the thrombolytic effect of streptokinase closely paralleled its activity in the circulation.[62,63] High doses of intravenous t-PA given over a short period of time (15 min) resulted in improved thrombolysis compared with longer (4 h) infusion of similar or higher total t-PA doses.[63] Other investigators confirmed the improved thrombolytic activity using a strategy of either single or multiple boluses. In particular, speed of thrombolysis seems to be increased with bolus regimens.[64,65]

Clinical Pharmacology

Elaborate details of the pharmacokinetics of t-PA in normal volunteers and acute myocardial infarction (AMI) patients can be reviewed in the articles by Baughman[66] and Tanswell et al.[67] Recent pharmacokinetic studies using extensive data sets have best described the kinetic characteristics of t-PA by a three-compartment model with a dominating central and two peripheral compartments. In normal volunteers having received different doses of intravenous t-PA infusions, no major difference was found between t-PA antigen and t-PA activity levels. The approximate values for the initial volume of distribution between 3 and 4 L and the steady-state volume of distribution between 9 and 12 L indicate that t-PA is confined to the plasma and well-perfused tissues. t-PA is cleared from the plasma with a half-life of approximately 4 minutes. The terminal half-life, mainly representing the clearance from tissue, was found to be in the range of 30 to 40 minutes. Area-under-the-curve measurements demonstrated that mainly the plasma compartment with its short half-life contributes to the elimination of t-PA. No major difference was found in the pharmacokinetic characteristics between the single-chain form and the two-chain form of t-PA.

t-PA is primarily eliminated by specific uptake and degradation by the liver[68–70] involving parenchymal cells, endothelial cells, and Kupffer cells.[71] Two types of receptors seem to be responsible for t-PA binding and uptake. A specific t-PA receptor on parenchymal cells accounts for about 55% of liver uptake. Mannose receptors on endothelial cells contribute 40%. Kupffer cells contribute to a much lesser degree (6%) to the elimination process.[70,72]

Experimental studies have shown that the removal of t-PA from the blood depends significantly on its oligosaccharide structure.[73–75] Periodate oxidation of the carbohydrate residues with destruction of the terminal residues at the high-mannose oligosaccharide at position Asn_{117} and the complex oligosaccharides at positions 184 and 448 resulted in a decrease in t-PA clearance in rabbits of approximately threefold. The same reduction in clearance was seen with the more specific endo-β-N-acetylglucosaminidase H removal of the high-mannose asparagine-linked oligosaccharides.[73] Another t-PA variant molecule was created using directed mutagenesis to generate a new consensus carbohydrate attachment at position 103 in the first kringle domain of t-PA. This modification resulted in a 5.8-fold reduction in clearance in rats and a 13.3-fold reduction in clearance in rabbits as compared with native t-PA.[28] Mutagenesis to alter the asparagine at position 117 to glutamine resulted in a molecule with similarly reduced clearance. These studies indicate that the high-mannose carbohydrate of Asn_{117} is a minor contributor to carbohydrate-mediated t-PA clearance.

ANTIGENICITY

Since recombinant t-PA is identical to the naturally occurring human tissue plasminogen activator, its immunogenic potential is expected to be very low. A study of serum samples from 1686 patients enrolled in several clinical trials for acute myocardial infarction, deep venous thrombus, peripheral arterial occlusion, and unstable angina measured t-PA antibodies. Alteplase was given in various doses (60–150 mg) and treatment regimens (1–24 h). Three patients (0.18%) were identified with positive titers within 7 to 32 days of treatment.[76] Reexaminations at 12 to 440 days were negative. No correlation could be found with dose, dosing regimen, or clinical diagnosis, and no clinical sequelae related to the appearance of antibodies in these patients were observed.

SYNERGY / POTENTIATION OF THROMBOLYSIS

Heparin is currently being used in conjunction with t-PA administration to inhibit thrombin activation, which was found to be promoted by t-PA–induced fibrinolysis,[77–79] and to prevent rethrombosis of successfully lysed occlusions. Conflicting experimental data exist on the interaction between heparin and t-PA when given concomitantly. Some reports have suggested that heparin may compromise the fibrinolytic activity of t-PA,[80–82] whereas other experiments could either not demonstrate negative interactions[83,84] or even reported enhancement of pharmacologic effect.[85–87] Newer anticoagulants (e.g., hirudin or hirulog) have been demonstrated experimentally to enhance the fibrinolytic activity of t-PA and sustain reperfusion.[84,88–90] New generations of antiplatelet agents (e.g., combined thromboxane synthetase and thromboxane receptor inhibitors and inhibitors of the platelet IIb-IIIa receptor, also have shown promising experimental results toward enhancement of the fibrinolytic activity of t-PA.[88,91–93] Prostaglandin accelerated fibrinolysis with t-PA in a rabbit jugular vein thrombosis model[94] but did not sustain coronary blood flow in a dog model.[95] Whether these experimental effects of new agents may translate into clinical benefit remains to be established by large-scale clinical trials, some of which are currently underway.

CLINICAL STUDIES CONFIRMATIVE OF BIOLOGIC CHARACTERISTICS

In a trial giving different doses of t-PA and streptokinase to AMI patients, the sustained action of t-PA could be demonstrated. Cross-linked fibrin degradation products (XL-FDPs) and fibrinopeptides were measured at several time points. All patients given t-PA exhibited higher elevations of XL-FDPs than those given streptokinase. This difference was particularly striking 7 h or more after thrombolysis. The levels of fibrinopeptides were significantly higher after t-PA compared with streptokinase beginning 3 h after treatment. These results are consistent with a greater fibrinolytic response to t-PA as well as prolonged fibrinolytic activity.[96] In several other studies, analyses of fibrinogen levels before and after fibrinolysis in AMI patients were performed. Because of the supraphysiologically high doses and plasma levels of t-PA in these studies, systemic plasminogen activation was to be expected. However, the decrease in fibrinogen after initiation of fibrinolysis with t-PA was significantly less pronounced as compared with streptokinase[97–99] or anisoylated plasminogen activator complex (APSAC).[100] Similar changes were seen for plasminogen and α_2-antiplasmin levels.

In the TAMI-3 study, the concomitant use of IV heparin did result in similar patency rates measured 2 h after initiation of t-PA treatment in AMI patients as compared with deferred IV heparin administration starting immediately after termination of t-PA infusion.[101] Two AMI studies performed in the United States demonstrated significantly higher patency rates 19 to 72 h after 100 mg t-PA given over 3 h was administered with IV heparin as compared with aspirin only[102] or when no IV heparin was administered.[103] A European study resulted in higher patency rates 48 to 120 h after t-PA and aspirin administration with IV heparin as compared with placebo.[104]

The TIMI-1 study in AMI patients demonstrated significantly higher patency rates (62% versus 31%) 90 minutes after administration of 80 mg t-PA given over a period of 3 h as compared with the standard streptokinase regimen of 1.5 million units given over 90 minutes.[105] Heparin was administered concomitantly with either fibrinolytic agent. Subsequently, a dose regimen administering 100 mg over 3 h (10-mg bolus, 50 mg over 60 min and 40 mg over 120 min) was developed, yielding patency rates of 70% to 77% at 90 minutes.[106,107] A front-loaded dose regimen of t-PA, with more than 50% of the total dose of 100 mg given in the first 30 minutes, demonstrated improved 90-minute patency rates of 81% to 91% as compared with the conventional 100 mg over 3 h regimen.[100,107–109] Similar patency results were achieved administering a double-bolus regimen of two 50-mg boluses given 30 minutes apart.[110]

In patients with peripheral arterial occlusion, local intraarterial infusion of t-PA using different doses, catheters, and catheter placement techniques resulted in reperfusion rates of 50% to 90%.[111–114] In these studies, the observed alterations in hemostatic parameters were less pronounced as those seen in AMI trials.

The recently reported results of the GUSTO study in 41,000 AMI patients demonstrated higher patency rates along with reduced mortality in a group receiving a front-loaded t-PA dosing regimen and concomitant IV heparin as compared with streptokinase with either subcutaneous (SC) or IV heparin.[109] Furthermore, the significant differences in allergic reactions (1.6% versus 5.7% and 5.8%) and anaphylaxis (0.2% versus 0.7% and 0.6%) between the front-loaded t-PA arm and both the SC and IV streptokinase arms confirm the very low immunogenic potential of t-PA.

Currently, mutant human t-PA molecules and nonhuman variants are being investigated to further improve the fibrinolytic characteristics and enable improved thrombolytic dosing regimens.

REFERENCES

1. Levine EG, Loskutoff DJ. Cultured bovine endothelial cells produce both urokinase and tissue-

type plasminogen activators. J Cell Biol 1982;94:631.

2. Aoki N. Preparation of plasminogen activator from vascular trees of human cadavers: its comparison with urokinase. J Biochem 1974;75:731.

3. Allen RA, Pepper DS. Isolation and properties of human vascular plasminogen activator. Thromb Haemost 1981;45:43.

4. Rijken DC, Wijngaards G, Zaal-de Jong M, Welbergen J. Purification and partial characterization of plasminogen activator from human uterine tissue. Biochim Biophys Acta 1979;580:140.

5. Pennica D, Holmes WE, Kohr WJ, et al. Cloning and expression of human tissue-type plasminogen activator cDNA in E. coli. Nature 1983;301:214.

6. Collen D, Rijken DC, Van Damme J, Billiau A. Purification of human tissue-type plasminogen activator in centigram quantities from human melanoma cell culture fluid and its conditioning for use in vivo. Thromb Haemost 1982;48:294.

7. Wallen P, Pohl G, Bergsdorf N, et al. Purification and characterisation of a melanoma cell plasminogen activator. Eur J Biochem 1983;132:681.

8. Kruithof EKO, Schleuning WD, Bachmann F. Human tissue-type plasminogen activator: production in continuous serum-free cell culture and rapid purification. Biochem J 1985;226:631.

9. Bányai L, Váradi A, Patthy L. Common evolutionary origin of the fibrin-binding structures of fibronectin and tissue-type plasminogen activator. FEBS Lett 1983;163:37.

10. Jörnvall H, Pohl G, Bergsdorf N, Wallen P. Differential proteolysis and evidence for a residue exchange in tissue plasminogen activator suggest possible association between two types of protein microheterogeneity. FEBS Lett 1983;156:47.

11. Vehar GA, Kohr WJ, Bennett WF, et al. Characterization studies on human melanoma cell tissue plasminogen activator. Biotechnology 1984;2:1051.

12. Einarsson M, Brandt J, Kaplan L. Large-scale purification of human tissue-type plasminogen activator using monoclonal antibodies. Biochim Biophys Acta 1985;830:1.

13. Rickles RJ, Darrow AL, Strickland S. Molecular cloning of complementary DNA to mouse tissue plasminogen activator mRNA and its expression during F9 teratocarcinoma cell differentiation. J Biol Chem 1988;263:1563.

14. Sehl LC, Nguyen HV, Arcila P, et al. A comparison of the properties of C83A and C84A mutants of tissue-type plasminogen activator (t-PA): evidence indicating that C83 is unpaired (abstract). Thromb Haemost 1993;69:577.

15. Rajput B, Degen SF, Reich E, et al. Chromosomal locations of human tissue plasminogen activator and urokinase genes. Science 1985;230:672.

16. Verheijen JH, Visse R, Wijnen JT, et al. Assignment of the human tissue-type plasminogen activator gene (PLAT) to chromosome 8. Hum Genet 1986;72:153.

17. Yang-Feng TL, Opdenakker G, Volckaert G, Francke U. Human tissue-type plasminogen activator gene located near chromosomal breakpoint in myeloproliferative disorder. Am J Hum Genet 1986;39:79.

18. Ny T, Elgh F, Lund B. The structure of the human tissue-type plasminogen activator gene: correlation of intron and exon structural domains. Proc Natl Acad Sci USA 1984;81:5355.

19. Vehar GA, Spellman MW, Keyt BA, et al. Characterization studies of human tissue-type plasminogen activator produced by recombinant DNA technology. Cold Spring Harbor Symp Quant Biol 1986;51:551.

20. Bennett WF. Two forms of tissue-type plasminogen activator differ at a single, specific glycosylation site (abstract). Thromb Hemost 1983;50:106.

21. Pohl G, Källström M, Bergsdorf N, et al. Tissue plasminogen activator: peptide analyses confirm an indirectly derived amino acid sequence, identify the active site serine residue, establish glycosylation sites, and localize variant differences. Biochemistry 1984;23:3701.

22. Rånby M, Bergsdorf N, Wallén P. Isolation of two variants of native one-chain tissue plasminogen activator. FEBS Lett 1982;146:289.

23. Pohl G, Kenne L, Nilsson B, Einarsson M. Isolation and characterization of three different carbohydrate chains from melanoma tissue plasminogen activator. Eur J Biochem 1987;170:69.

24. Higgins DL, Bennett WF. Tissue plasminogen activator: the biochemistry and pharmacology of variants produced by mutagenesis. Annu Rev Pharmacol Toxicol 1990;30:91.

25. Lijnen HR, Collen D. Strategies for the improvement of thrombolytic agents. Thromb Haemost 1991;66:88.

26. Bennett WF, Paoni NF, Keyt BA, et al. High resolution analysis of functional determinants on human tissue-type plasminogen activator. J Biol Chem 1991;266:5191.

27. Paoni NF, Refino CJ, Brady K, et al. Involvement of residues 296–299 in the enzymatic activity of tissue-type plasminogen activator. Protein Eng 1992;5:259.

28. Paoni NF, Keyt BA, Refino CJ, et al. A slow clearing, fibrin-specific, PAI-1 resistant variant of t-PA (T103N, KHRR 296–299 AAAA). Thromb Haemost 1993;70:307.

29. Refino CJ, Paoni NF, Keyt BA, et al. A variant of t-PA (T103N, KHRR 296–299 AAAA) that, by bolus, has increased potency and decreased sys-

temic activation of plasminogen. Thromb Haemost 1993;70:313.

30. Madison EL, Goldsmith EJ, Gerard RD, et al. Amino acid residues that affect interaction of tissue-type plasminogen activator with plasminogen activator inhibitor 1. Proc Natl Acad Sci USA 1990;87:3530.

31. Tate KM, Higgins DL, Holmes WE, et al. Functional role of proteolytic cleavage at arginine-275 of human tissue plasminogen activator as assessed by site-directed mutagenesis. Biochemistry 1987; 26:338.

32. Lijnen HR, Van Hoef B, De Cock F, Collen D. Effect of fibrin-like stimulators on the activation of plasminogen by tissue-type plasminogen activator (t-PA): studies with active site mutagenized plasminogen and plasmin resistant t-PA. Thromb Haemost 1990;64:61.

33. Hoylaerts M, Rijken DC, Lijnen HR, Collen D. Kinetics of the activation of plasminogen by human tissue plasminogen activator: role of fibrin. J Biol Chem 1982;257:2912.

34. Rijken DC, Juhan-Vague I, De Cock F, Collen D. Measurement of human tissue-type plasminogen activator by a two-site immunoradiometric assay. J Lab Clin Med 1983;101:274.

35. Holvoet P, Cleemput H, Collen D. Assay of human tissue-type plasminogen activator (t-PA) with an enzyme-linked immunosorbent assay (ELISA) based on three murine monoclonal antibodies to t-PA. Thromb Haemost 1985;54:684.

36. Holvoet P, Boes J, Collen D. Measurement of free, one-chain tissue-type plasminogen activator in human plasma with an enzyme-linked immunosorbent assay based on an active site-specific murine monoclonal antibody. Blood 1987;69:284.

37. Booth NA, Walker E, Maughan R, Bennett B. Plasminogen activator in normal subjects after exercise and venous occlusion: t-PA circulates as complexes with C1-inhibitor and PAI-1. Blood 1987; 69:1600.

38. Beisiegel B, Treese N, Hafner G, et al. Increase in endogenous fibrinolysis and platelet activity during exercise in young volunteers. Agents Actions 1992;37(suppl):183.

39. Lijnen HR, Uytterhoeven M, Collen D. Inhibition of trypsin-like serine proteinases by tripeptide arginyl and lysyl chloromethylketones. Thromb Res 1984;34:431.

40. Green GDJ. The inactivation of one- and two-chain forms of tissue plasminogen activator by a series of peptidyl chloromethyl ketones. Thromb Res 1986;44:175.

41. Higgins DL, Lamb MC. Incorporation of a fluorescent probe into the active sites of one- and two-chain tissue-type plasminogen activator. Arch Biochem Biophys 1986;249:418.

42. Korninger C, Collen D. Neutralization of human extrinsic (tissue-type) plasminogen activator in plasma: no evidence for a specific inhibitor. Thromb Haemost 1981;46:662.

43. Kruithof EO. Plasminogen activator inhibitors—a review. Enzyme 1988;40:113.

44. Dawson S, Henney A. The status of PAI-1 as a risk factor for arterial and thrombotic disease: a review. Atherosclerosis 1992;95:105.

45. Sambrook J, Hanahan D, Rodgers L, Gething MJ. Expression of human tissue-type plasminogen activator from lytic viral vectors and in established cell lines. Mol Biol Med 1986;3:459.

46. Takada Y, Takada A. Measurements of the concentration of free plasminogen activator inhibitor (PAI-1) and its complex with tissue plasminogen activator in human plasma. Thromb Res 1988; (suppl 8):15.

47. Kluft C, Jie AH, Rijken DC, Verheijen JH. Daytime fluctuations in blood of tissue-type plasminogen activator (t-PA) and its fast-acting inhibitor (PAI-1). Thromb Haemost 1988;59:329.

48. Takada A, Hou P, Mori T, Takada Y. Changes in various parameters of fibrinolysis in persons infused with tissue plasminogen activator: special reference to plasminogen activator inhibitor. Thromb Res 1988;(suppl 8):23.

49. Almer L, Öhlin H. Elevated levels of the rapid inhibitor of plasminogen activator (t-PAI) in acute myocardial infarction. Thromb Res 1987;47: 335.

50. Hersch SL, Kunelis T, Francis RBR. The pathogenesis of accelerated fibrinolysis in liver cirrhosis: a critical role for tissue plasminogen activator inhibitor. Blood 1987;69:1315.

51. Neerstrand H, Hedner U, Lutzen O, et al. The influence of surgery on plasminogen activator inhibitor (abstract). Thromb Haemost 1987;58:557.

52. Kruithof EKO, Gudinchet A, Bachmann F. Plasminogen activator inhibitor 1 and plasminogen activator inhibitor 2 in various disease states. Thromb Haemost 1988;59:7.

53. Earnshaw JJ, Westby JC, Hopkinson BR, Makin GS. Resting plasma fibrinolytic activity and fibrinolytic potential in peripheral vascular disease. J Cardiovasc Surg 1988;29:300.

54. Hartl D, Tiso E, Anderle K, et al. Reduced fibrinolytic potential in patients with arterial occlusive disease (AOD) in comparison with normal subjects. Haemostasis 1988;18(Suppl 1):93.

55. Schneiderman J, Adar R, Savion N. Changes in plasmatic tissue-type plasminogen activator and plasminogen activator inhibitor activity during acute arterial occlusion associated with severe ischemia. Thromb Res 1991;62:401.

56. Estelles A, Aznar J, Tormo G, et al. Influence of a rehabilitation sports program on the fibrinolytic

activity of patients after myocardial infarction. Thromb Res 1989;55:203.

57. Chandler WL, Levy WC, Veith RC, Stratton JR. A kinetic model of the circulatory regulation of tissue plasminogen activator during exercise, epinephrine infusion, and endurance training. Blood 1993;81:3293.

58. Verstraete M, Collen D. Thrombolytic agents. In: Fuster V, Verstraete M, eds. Thrombosis in cardiovascular disorders. Philadelphia: WB Saunders, 1992:175.

59. Stump DC, Taylor FB, Nesheim ME, et al. Pathologic fibrinolysis as a cause of clinical bleeding. Semin Thromb Hemost 1990;16:260.

60. Collen D, Lijnen HR, Todd PA, Goa KL. Tissue-type plasminogen activator: a review of its pharmacology and therapeutic use as a thrombolytic agent. Drugs 1989;38:346.

61. Gold HK, Yasuda T, Jang IK, et al. Animal models for arterial thrombolysis and prevention of reocclusion. Circulation 1991;83:iv.

62. Agnelli G, Buchanan MR, Fernandez F, et al. Sustained thrombolysis with DNA-recombinant tissue type plasminogen activator in rabbits. Blood 1985;66:399.

63. Agnelli G, Buchanan MR, Fernandez F, Hirsh J. Thrombolytic and hemorrhagic effects of tissue type plasminogen activator: influence of dosage regimens in rabbits. Thromb Res 1985;40:769.

64. Cercek B, Lew AS, Yano J, et al. Thrombolytic effect of recombinant tissue-type plasminogen activator administered as a bolus (abstract). Clin Res 1987;35:370a.

65. Eisert WG, Müller TH. Bolus treatment regimen of TPA expedites rate of lysis in vivo without increasing risk of bleeding (abstract). Blood 1987;70 (suppl 1):370a.

66. Baughman RA. Pharmacokinetics of tissue plasminogen activator. In: Sobel BE, Collen D, Grossbard EB, eds. Tissue plasminogen activator in thrombolytic therapy. New York: Marcel Dekker, 1987:41.

67. Tanswell P, Seifried E, Krause J. Pharmacokinetics of human tissue-type plasminogen activator. In: Reidenberg, ed. The clinical pharmacology of biotechnology products. Amsterdam: Excerpta Medica, 1991:103.

68. Korninger C, Collen D. Studies on the specific fibrinolytic effect of human extrinsic (tissue-type) plasminogen activator in human blood and in various animal species in vitro. Thromb Haemost 1981;46:561.

69. Fuchs HE, Berger H, Pizzo SV. Catabolism of human tissue plasminogen activator in mice. Blood 1985;65:539.

70. Krause J, Seydel W, Heinzel G, Tanswell P. Different receptors mediate the hepatic catabolism of tissue-type plasminogen activator and urokinase. Biochem J 1990;267:647.

71. Rijken DC, Otter M, Kuiper J, van Berkel TJC. Receptor mediated endocytosis of tissue-type plasminogen activator (t-PA) by liver cells. Thromb Res 1990;(suppl 10):63.

72. Kuiper J, Otter M, Rijken DC, van Berkel TJC. Characterization of the interaction in vivo of tissue-type plasminogen activator with liver cells. J Biol Chem 1988;263:18220.

73. Hotchkiss A, Refino CJ, Leonard CK, et al. The influence of carbohydrate structure on the clearance of recombinant tissue-type plasminogen activator. Thromb Haemost 1988;60:255.

74. Lucore CL, Fry ETA, Nachowiak DA, Sobel BE. Biochemical determinants of clearance of tissue-type plasminogen activator from the circulation. Circulation 1988;77:906.

75. Ord JM, Owensby DA, Billadello JJ, Sobel BE. Determinants of clearance of tissue-type plasminogen activator and their pharmacologic implications. Fibrinolysis 1990;4:203.

76. Reed BR, Chen AB, Tanswell P, et al. Low incidence of antibodies to recombinant human tissue-type plasminogen activator in treated patients. Thromb Haemost 1990;64:276.

77. Eisenberg PR, Sherman L, Rich M, et al. Importance of continued activation of thrombin reflected by fibrinopeptide A to the efficacy of thrombolysis. J Am Coll Cardiol 1986;7:1255.

78. Owen J, Friedman KD, Grossman BA, et al. Thrombolytic therapy with tissue-plasminogen activator or streptokinase induces transient thrombin activity. Blood 1988;72:616.

79. Rapold HJ, Kuemmerli H, Weiss M, et al. Monitoring of fibrin generation during thrombolytic therapy of acute myocardial infarction with recombinant tissue-type plasminogen activator. Circulation 1989;79:980.

80. Andrade-Gordon P, Strickland S. Interaction of heparin with plasminogen activators and plasminogen: effects on the activation of plasminogen. Biochemistry 1986;25:4033.

81. Paques EP, Stohr HA, Heimburger N. Study on the mechanism of action of heparin and related substances on the fibrinolytic system: relationship between plasminogen activators and heparin. Thromb Res 1986;42:797.

82. Görög P, Ridler CD, Kovacs IB. Heparin inhibits spontaneous thrombolysis and the thrombolytic effect of both streptokinase and tissue-type plasminogen activator: an in vitro study of the dislodgement of platelet-rich thrombi formed from native blood. J Int Med 1990;227:125.

83. Fry ETA, Sobel BE. Lack of interference by heparin with thrombolysis or binding of tissue-type

plasminogen activator to thrombi. Blood 1988;71: 1347.

84. Mirshahi M, Soria J, Soria C, et al. Evaluation of the inhibition by heparin and hirudin of coagulation activation during r-tPA–induced thrombolysis. Blood 1989;74:1025.

85. Cercek B, Lew AS, Hod H, et al. Enhancement of thrombolysis with tissue-type plasminogen activator by pretreatment with heparin. Circulation 1986;74:583.

86. Tomora T, Uchida Y, Nakamura F, et al. Enhancement of arterial thrombolysis with native tissue-type plasminogen activator by pretreatment with heparin or batroxobin: an angioscopic study. Am Heart J 1989;117:275.

87. Rapold HJ, Lu HR, Wu Z, et al. Requirement of heparin for arterial and venous thrombolysis with recombinant tissue-type plasminogen activator. Blood 1991;77:1020.

88. Yao SK, Ober JC, Ferguson JJ, et al. Combination of inhibition of thrombin and blockade of thromboxane A_2 synthetase and receptors enhances thrombolysis and delays reocclusion in canine coronary arteries. Circulation 1992;86:1993.

89. Klement P, Borm A, Hirsh J, et al. The effect of thrombin inhibitors on tissue plasminogen activator induced thrombolysis in a rat model. Thromb Haemost 1992;68:64.

90. Agnelli G, Pascucci C, Cosmi B, Nenci GG. Effects of hirudin and heparin on the binding of new fibrin to the thrombus in t-PA treated rabbits. Thromb Haemost 1991;66:592.

91. Gold HK, Coller BS, Ysauda T, et al. Rapid and sustained coronary artery recanalization with combined bolus injection of recombinant tissue-type plasminogen activator and monoclonal antiplatelet GPIIb/IIIa antibody in a canine preparation. Circulation 1988;77:670.

92. Fitzgerald DJ, Wright F, FitzGerald GA. Increased thromboxane biosynthesis during coronary thrombolysis: evidence that platelet activation and thromboxane A_2 modulate the response to tissue-type plasminogen activator in vivo. Circ Res 1989; 65:83.

93. Golino P, Rosolowsky M, Yao SK, et al. Endogenous prostaglandin endoperoxides and prostacyclin modulate the thrombolytic activity of tissue plasminogen activator: effects of simultaneous inhibition of thromboxane A_2 synthase and blockade of thromboxane A_2/prostaglandin H_2 receptors in a canine model of coronary thrombosis. J Clin Invest 1990;86:1095.

94. Vaughan DE, Plavin SR, Schafer AI, Loscalzo J. Prostaglandin E_1 markedly accelerates thrombolysis by tissue plasminogen activator. Blood 1989; 73:1213.

95. Nichols WW, Nicolini FA, Khan S, et al. Failure of prostacyclin analogue iloprost to sustain coronary blood flow after recombinant tissue-type plasminogen-induced thrombolysis in dogs. Am Heart J 1993;126:285.

96. Eisenberg PR, Sherman LA, Tiefenbrunn AJ, et al. Sustained fibrinolysis after administration of t-PA despite its short half-life in the circulation. Thromb Haemost 1987;57:35.

97. Collen D, Bounameaux H, De Cock F, et al. Analysis of coagulation and fibrinolysis during intravenous infusion of recombinant human tissue-type plasminogen activator in patients with acute myocardial infarction. Circulation 1986;73: 511.

98. Rao KA, Pratt C, Berke A, et al. Thrombolysis in myocardial infarction (TIMI) trial—phase 1: hemorrhagic manifestations and changes in plasma fibrinogen and the fibrinolytic system in patients treated with recombinant tissue plasminogen activator and streptokinase. J Am Coll Cardiol 1988;11:1.

99. Magnani B, Plasminogen Activator Italian Multicenter Study (PAIMS) Group. Comparison of intravenous recombinant single-chain human tissue-type plasminogen activator (rt-PA) with intravenous streptokinase in acute myocardial infarction. J Am Coll Cardiol 1989;13:19.

100. Neuhaus KL, Von Essen R, Tebbe U, et al. Improved thrombolysis in acute myocardial infarction with front-loaded administration of alteplase: results of the rt-PA–APSAC patency study (TAPS). J Am Coll Cardiol 1992;19:885.

101. Topol EJ, George BS, Kereiakes DJ, et al. A randomized, controlled trial of intravenous tissue plasminogen activator and early intravenous heparin in acute myocardial infarction. Circulation 1989;79:281.

102. Hsia J, Hamilton WP, Kleiman N, et al., for the Heparin-Aspirin Reperfusion Trial (HART) investigators. A comparison between heparin and low-dose aspirin as adjunctive therapy with tissue plasminogen activator for acute myocardial infarction. N Engl J Med 1990;323:1433.

103. Bleich SD, Nichols TC, Schumacher RR, et al. Effect of heparin on coronary arterial patency after thrombolysis with tissue plasminogen activator in acute myocardial infarction. Am J Cardiol 1990; 66:1412.

104. de Bono DP, Simoons ML, Tijssen J, et al. Effect of early intravenous heparin on coronary patency, infarct size, and bleeding complications after alteplase thrombolysis: results of a randomised double blind European Cooperative Study Group trial. Br Heart J 1992;67:122.

105. Chesebro JH, Knatterud G, Roberts R, et al. Thrombolysis in myocardial infarction (TIMI) trial, phase 1: a comparison between intravenous

tissue plasminogen activator and intravenous streptokinase. Circulation 1987;76:142.

106. Verstraete M, Bernard R, Bory M, et al. Randomised trial of intravenous recombinant tissue-type plasminogen activator versus intravenous streptokinase in acute myocardial infarction. Lancet 1985;1:842.

107. Carney RJ, Murphy GA, Brandt TR, et al. Randomized angiographic trial of recombinant tissue-type plasminogen activator (alteplase) in myocardial infarction. J Am Coll Cardiol 1992;20:17.

108. Neuhaus KL, Feuerer W, Jeep-Tebbe S, et al. Improved thrombolysis with a modified dose regimen of recombinant tissue-type plasminogen activator. J Am Coll Cardiol 1989;14:1566.

109. The GUSTO Angiographic Investigators. An angiographic study within the global randomized trial of aggressive versus standard thrombolytic strategies in patients with acute myocardial infarction. N Engl J Med 1993;329:1615.

110. Purvis JA, Trouton TG, Roberts MJD, et al. Effectiveness of double bolus alteplase in the treatment of acute myocardial infarction. Am J Cardiol 1991;68:1570.

111. Graor RA, Risius B, Lucas FV, et al. Thrombolysis with recombinant human tissue-type plasminogen activator in patients with peripheral artery and bypass graft occlusions. Circulation 1986;74 (suppl 1):1.

112. Verstraete M, Hess H, Mahler F, et al. Femoropopliteal artery thrombolysis with intra-arterial infusion of recombinant tissue-type plasminogen activator—report of a pilot trial. Eur J Vasc Surg 1988;2:155.

113. Meyerovitz MF, Goldhaber SZ, Reagan K, et al. Recombinant tissue-type plasminogen activator versus urokinase in peripheral arterial and graft occlusions: a randomized trial. Radiology 1990; 175:75.

114. The STILE Investigators. Results of a prospective randomized trial evaluating surgery versus thrombolysis for ischemia of the lower extremity: the "STILE" trial. Ann Surg, in press.

9

ANISOYLATED PLASMINOGEN-STREPTOKINASE ACTIVATOR COMPLEX

Jeffrey L. Anderson

The past decade has witnessed the development and widespread application of the plasminogen activators in clinical medicine for the treatment of thrombotic and thromboembolic vascular disease.[1,2] These agents have been subgrouped into those which are systemically active (non-fibrin-selective), including streptokinase, urokinase, and anistreplase, and those which are relatively fibrin-selective [tissue plasminogen activator (t-PA) and prourokinase]. Their initial introduction into clinical medicine was for the treatment of pulmonary embolism (streptokinase, urokinase) and deep vein thrombosis. Subsequently, intense interest in development and application of these agents for acute myocardial infarction has occurred.[2,3] Clinical trial data have firmly established that timely therapy can reduce infarct size and improve functional outcome and survival.[4] This success in treating myocardial infarction has in turn renewed interest in the application of thrombolytic agents to other vascular disease processes, including cerebrovascular and peripheral vascular thromboembolic disease.

This chapter will focus on the development and clinical application of the systemically active plasminogen activator *anistreplase,* common name *anisoylated plasminogen-streptokinase activator complex* (APSAC) (marketed as Eminase-R, Smith-Kline Beecham, Philadelphia, PA).[5,6] It should be noted that the development of anistreplase has focused on its application for acute myocardial infarction (AMI), rather than for peripheral vascular disease, pulmonary embolism, etc. However, APSAC's ease of administration and long duration of activity suggest promise for these as yet largely unexplored clinical applications.

HISTORY

Anistreplase was synthesized in the late 1970s by chemists at Beecham Laboratories (London, United Kingdom) to improve on the perceived disadvantages of streptokinase.[7] The molecule was "custom designed" to allow for (1) simpler administration, (2) a longer plasma half-life, and (3) enhanced fibrin (thrombus) affinity and fibrinolytic efficiency.[8] Modification of streptokinase was accomplished by acylation, and the anisoy-lated compound, patented in 1979, was selected for further development. Preclinical and clinical studies followed shortly thereafter, leading to approval of anistreplase for clinical application in AMI in several countries, including the United States (1989).

CHEMISTRY AND PHARMACOLOGY

APSAC is an equimolar complex of streptokinase and *para*-anisoylated human Lys-plasminogen possessing a molecular weight of 131,000.[7] In the synthesis of APSAC, native human Glu-plasminogen is modified by removal of a small N-terminal peptide, yielding Lys-plasminogen. Lys-plasminogen is then further modified by acylation of the serine residue at the center of the active site, temporarily masking its activity. This protected form of Lys-plasminogen is then combined with streptokinase in 1:1 molar ratio to form anistreplase (Fig. 9-1), a proenzyme, which is stable in lyophilized form for at least 1 year at 5°C.

When APSAC is placed in aqueous solution or plasma, deacylation occurs by a simple ester hydrolysis reaction that follows pseudo-first-order kinetics in a temperature-dependent fashion.[7-9] *p*-Anisic acid and free Lys-plasminogen streptokinase activator complex are released. Deacylation (activation) also occurs with fibrin-bound APSAC at rates equal to those in free plasma, generating the potent fibrinolytic enzyme plasmin. Biologic activity of APSAC is expressed in specific units (1 mg = 1 unit). The clinically used dosage for AMI of 30 units contains 1.1 million units of streptokinase.

Preclinical and early clinical evaluations suggested that the pharmacologic objectives of the chemical synthesis of APSAC were largely achieved[9] (Table 9-1). First, anistreplase could be given as a single bolus (over ≤5 min) without causing the hypotension that prevents the rapid administration of streptokinase. Second, substantial lengthening of the plasma half-life of total fibrinolytic activity (to 90 to 105 min) as compared with the parent drug streptokinase (averaging 20 to 30 min) was shown. Third, enhanced fibrin (thrombus) affinity was demonstrated for the Lys-plasminogen–containing compound compared with activators using the native Glu-plasminogen. Improved enzymatic efficiency compared with streptokinase was demonstrated.

FIGURE 9-1. *Schematic representation of the structure of anistreplase (APSAC, Eminase-R).* (Courtesy of H. Ferres, SmithKline Beecham Laboratories, U.K.)

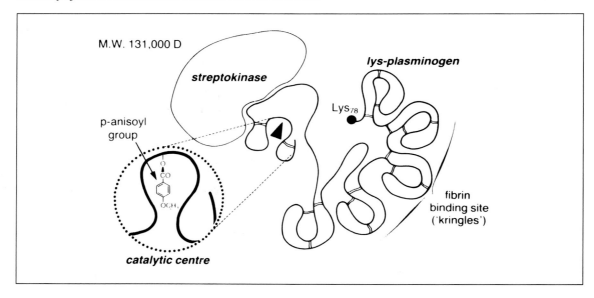

TABLE 9-1. Objectives in the Synthesis of Anistreplase

Pharmacologic Objectives
   Simplified administration regimen
   Long half-life of plasma activity
   Enhanced affinity for fibrin
Clinical Expectations
   Increased ease and efficiency in patient management
   Improved early thrombolytic efficiency
   Prolonged action associated with reduced risk of
      rethrombosis
   Improved patient outcome

In these preclinical studies, APSAC was found to be stable in plasma; its streptokinase moiety did not dissociate or exchange with non-acylated plasminogen in plasma,[10] and acylation rendered the plasminogen-streptokinase activator complex less susceptible to autoproteolytic degradation.[11]

Acylation of plasminogen was shown to cause dramatic gains in persistence rates of total potential fibrinolytic activity (i.e., activity resulting from both acylated and nonacylated forms) in several animal species (guinea pigs, rabbits, dogs) from about 2 to 45 to 90 min.[9,11,12] In human plasma, in vitro and in vivo studies showed that APSAC achieved a half-life of fibrinolytic activity of 90 to 120 min, compared with 20 to 30 min for streptokinase[9,13–19](Fig. 9-2). The half-life of de-acylation was shown to be the rate-limiting step in clearance and hence was similar to the half-life for fibrinolytic activity.[9,17] These in vitro and in vivo studies also indicated that acylation was successful in protecting APSAC against plasma inhibitors of activator activity, autodegradation, and rapid hepatic clearance.

Lys-plasminogen (contained in APSAC) was shown to be taken up more rapidly into pre-formed human clots than native Glu-plasminogen (a component of the streptokinase activator complex).[19] In other experiments, the fibrin binding capacity of APSAC (accumulation rate into clot) was shown to be on the relative order of APSAC = rt-PA > Lys-plasminogen > urokinase, indicating that additional fibrin affinity was conferred on Lys-plasminogen by the formation of the acylated stabilized activator complex.[20] The clot-retentive ability of APSAC exceeded that of streptokinase and urokinase in in vitro studies.[9]

FIGURE 9-2. Stability of APSAC (8×10^{-8} M, triangles) and streptokinase (SK) plasmin(ogen) (8×10^{-8} M, squares) in human plasma in vitro (mean ± SE) for three experiments. (From Standing, Fears, and Ferres: Fibrinolysis 1988;2:157–163, with permission.)

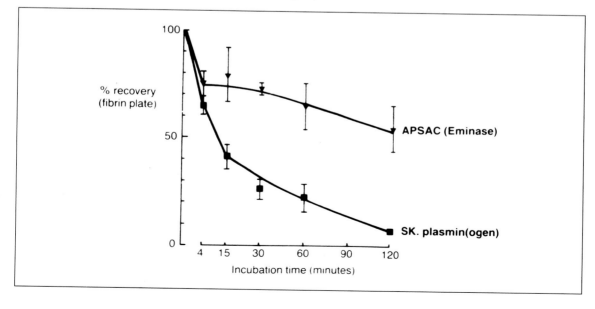

Superior thrombolytic efficiency of APSAC was demonstrated in a guinea pig in vivo pulmonary embolism model, in which the dose-response curve was shifted substantially up and to the left of that for streptokinase-plasmin (APSAC 15 times more potent) when both agents were given as a bolus.[9] In a canine model, bolus doses of anistreplase did not cause the profound transient hypotension caused by equivalent bolus doses of streptokinase[21] (Fig. 9-3).

In summary, APSAC, given in inactive form as a single injection, can circulate without initially causing systemic effects, find and bind to fibrin-containing clot with high affinity, and be activated efficiently and in a semiselective fashion at the site of the clot. In the doses given clinically, additional, systemic fibrinolytic activity is generated which promotes ongoing fibrinolysis and reduces the risk of reocclusion. Thus the synthesis of APSAC resulted in an agent which was more easily administered and had improved thrombolytic efficiency compared with streptokinase, as demonstrated in several animal species and human beings.

Results of Clinical Trials

Applications in Acute Myocardial Infarction

General Considerations

The development of thrombolytic agents for AMI began with feasibility studies (generally, uncontrolled or historically controlled observations) and was followed by controlled trials to assess three primary endpoints: (1) establishment of coronary artery reperfusion and patency, (2) reduction in infarct size and improvement in left ventricular function, and (3) reduction in AMI-associated mortality, both short and long term. Simultaneous assessments of safety also were made, the primary safety concern being bleeding. Controlled comparisons were made initially with placebo or nonthrombolytic (standard) therapies; subsequent comparisons used active thrombolytic therapy controls.

Initial and Feasibility Trials

Kasper et al.[22] showed that anistreplase had similar efficacy to streptokinase when administered by

FIGURE 9-3. *Blood pressure response to bolus injections of anistreplase (Eminase) or streptokinase (SK)-plasmin(ogen)(Plg) and plasma plasmin/kallikrein flux in dogs. (From Green J, Dupe RJ, Smith RAG, et al. Comparison of hypotensive effects of streptokinase [human]–plasmin activator complex and BRL 26921 [anisoylated streptokinase-plasminogen activator complex] in the dog after high dose bolus administration. Thromb Res 1984;36:2936, with permission.)*

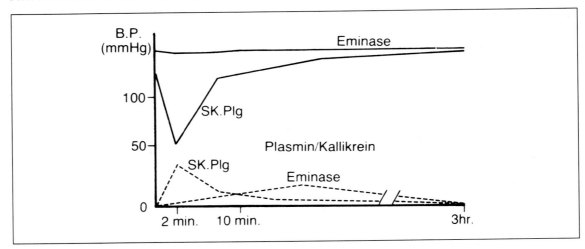

the intracoronary route. However, the unique features of anistreplase favor intravenous administration as the optimal route of application. Most subsequent clinical trials have thus used the intravenous route of administration. Initial tolerance and feasibility studies used a variety of doses and study designs, most focusing on coronary reperfusion or patency rates as study endpoints.[23,24] A pooled analysis ($n = 160$ patients) indicated a dose-response relationship.[24,25] Response rates were inadequate (21% perfusion) at doses causing little systemic fibrinogenolysis (5 to 10 units), intermediate (49% overall response) at doses of 15 to 20 units, and optimal (70% average perfusion response) at doses of 25 to 30 units. The vast majority of patients in subsequent trials have received an anistreplase dose of 30 units.

Controlled Trials of APSAC versus Placebo and Nonthrombolytic Therapies

REPERFUSION

The potential of anistreplase for achieving rapid reperfusion was evaluated by Timmis et al.[26] in a double-blind, placebo-controlled design. Coronary occlusion was documented by pretreatment angiography, performed an average of 3.4 h (range 2.1 to 6.0 h) after the onset of symptoms. At the primary 90-min posttreatment angiographic endpoint, reperfusion had occurred in 9 (56%) of 16 patients given APSAC but in only 1 (8%) of 13 patients given placebo ($p < 0.01$).

LEFT VENTRICULAR FUNCTION

The potential of anistreplase to reduce infarct size and improve left ventricular function was investigated in a French multicenter study.[27] The study was designed as a double-blind, parallel comparison of APSAC (30 units/5 min) versus heparin (5000-IU bolus) in 231 patients with AMI and symptoms of less than 5 h duration. Therapy in both groups included heparin, reintroduced 4 h after initial therapy. Left ventricular ejection fraction (EF), measured during the first week following therapy using contrast ventriculography, favored anistreplase by 6 percentage points (53% versus 47%; $p < 0.01$). Ejection fraction was higher after anistreplase in both the ante-

rior and inferior infarct groups. Associated infarct-related coronary artery patency was found in 77% of anistreplase versus 36% of heparin patients ($p < 0.01$). Infarct size was assessed during the third week following AMI using thallium single-photon-emission computed tomography (SPECT). Infarct size was reduced 33% in the anterior AMI group and 16% in the inferior AMI group by APSAC in comparison with heparin therapy alone (Fig. 9-4). The difference in radionuclide EF, measured during the third week, averaged 4 percentage points in favor of APSAC and was significant for the anterior infarct group (6 percentage point differential). A significant inverse relationship was found between tomographically determined infarct size and radionuclide EF.

In a separate German study,[28] anistreplase therapy was associated with a substantial reduction in mortality, although EF did not differ in the two groups. Variability in EF benefits with therapy also has been observed in studies with streptokinase and rt-PA.[29]

MORTALITY

Early trials with anistreplase were too small to individually assess mortality effects. However, pool-

FIGURE 9-4. *Infarct size reduction by APSAC versus heparin in anterior and inferior AMI patients measured by thallium scintigraphy (single-photon-emission computed tomography technique) during week 3. (Data from Bassand et al. JACC 1989;13:988.)*

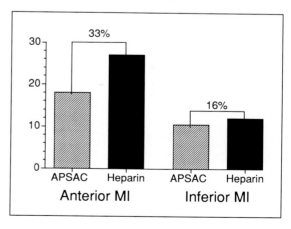

ing the early controlled trials in an overview strongly suggested a mortality benefit.[24] In these studies, 708 patients received nonthrombolytic treatment and 1386 received anistreplase. Early mortality (in-hospital or within 1 month) was 6.1% in the anistreplase group, compared with 12.3% after standard therapy ($p < 0.001$). This potential for survival benefit was subsequently tested in the prospective Anistreplase Intervention Mortality Study (AIMS).[30, 31]

AIMS (Anistreplase Interventional Mortality Study) was a double-blind, multicenter United Kingdom trial that randomized AMI patients presenting within 6 h of symptom onset to anistreplase or placebo, along with heparin, subsequent warfarin, and other standard therapy (i.e., timolol).[30] Mortality outcome, the primary endpoint, was assessed at 1 month and 1 year. AIMS was stopped early by the Safety Monitoring Board before completion of the intended recruitment of 2000 patients because of a substantial mortality difference in favor of thrombolytic therapy. In the final report of 1258 patients[31](Fig. 9-5), mortality at 30 days was 6.4% (40 of 624) in the anistreplase group versus 12.1% (77 of 634) in the placebo group, an odds reduction in mortality of 51% (confidence interval 26% to 67%; $p = 0.006$). Survival benefit was maintained over the next 11 months, with an additional 29 in the anistreplase group and 36 in the placebo group dying. Overall mortality at 1 year was thus 11.1% (69 of 624)

after anistreplase and 17.8% (113 of 634) after placebo, a 43% odds reduction (confidence interval 21% to 59%; $p = 0.0007$).

SAFETY ASSESSMENTS FROM CONTROLLED TRIALS

Possible Allergic Events. As a compound containing the bacterial protein streptokinase, anistreplase is potentially antigenic and allergenic. Although minor allergic-type reactions have been reported in 5% to 10% of patients receiving streptokinase or APSAC, anaphylaxis has been rare (4 of 624, or 0.6%, in AIMS after APSAC, 0 after placebo).[31] Other allergy (early urticaria/rash/asthma) was infrequently recorded in AIMS and was not significantly greater after APSAC.[31]

Hypotension. Streptokinase activates both the plasminogen-plasmin and prekallikrein-kallikrein-bradykinin systems, generating potent vasodilator activity; hypotension thus restricts the rapid administration of streptokinase.[21] In AIMS,[31] blood pressure fall after APSAC was greater than after placebo, but the differences were modest (<5 to 10 mmHg average); falls to <100 mmHg occurred in 25% of treated versus 18% of control patients; falls to <80 mmHg occurred in 4% versus 3%.

Bleeding/Stroke. Using the placebo-controlled database for AIMS,[31] the risk of serious bleeding in patients not undergoing routine interventions (angiography, angioplasty) after APSAC administration can be assessed. Any hemorrhagic event was reported in 14% of APSAC patients versus 4% of placebo patients (a 10 percentage point absolute difference). However, most of these events were benign and most commonly puncture site–related. Transfusions were given to <1% in each group. Two anistreplase versus one placebo patient suffered a proven intracranial hemorrhage; the total (including undefined) stroke rates were 1.3% versus 0.6%.

In-Hospital Reinfarction. A differential rate of reinfarction is expected after thrombolytic reperfusion, but the difference in AIMS for reinfarction was small and not statistically significant comparing anistreplase-treated patients (6.1%) with placebo-treated patients (4.7%)(absolute difference 1.4%; $p = 0.3$).[31]

FIGURE 9-5. Survival curves up to 1 year after myocardial infarction in patients receiving anistreplase (Eminase) or placebo. (From the AIMS Trial Study Group. Lancet 1990;335:427, with permission.)

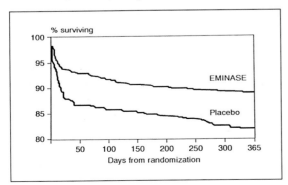

Other Events. In general, major cardiovascular complications of AMI (including shock, cardiac arrest, and ventricular fibrillation) were less frequent with anistreplase than placebo, whereas ventricular arrhythmias and bradycardia (arrhythmias potentially related to reperfusion) were more common after treatment with anistreplase.[31]

Comparisons of Anistreplase with Active Therapies

EFFICACY COMPARISONS

Patency. Comparisons of early (90-min) patency have suggested that APSAC is superior or equivalent to streptokinase (direct comparisons), equivalent to standard-regimen t-PA (indirect comparisons), and lower than front-loaded t-PA. Comparisons of late ($\geq$1 day) patency suggest a greater rate, approximately equivalent to the late patency rate for streptokinase and similar to one exceeding that for t-PA.

Initial trials required angiographic demonstration of occlusion prior to entry (reperfusion design) and used *intracoronary* streptokinase as the comparator regimen, then the "gold standard." In these studies, intravenous APSAC was as effective as intracoronary streptokinase (and more convenient) when administered to patients within 4 h of symptom onset (60% to 65% reperfusion success at 90 min).[32,33] As noted earlier with streptokinase, anistreplase showed time dependence in its reperfusion rate, with patients presenting later after the onset of symptoms (>4 to 6 h) achieving lower rates of reperfusion success by 90 minutes than those presenting earlier (33% versus 60%).[32]

Subsequent studies used *intravenous* (IV) streptokinase as the comparator regimen. In an open design multicenter French study,[34] 116 patients with AMI and symptoms of <6 h duration were randomized to therapy with either anistreplase (30 units/2 to 5 min) or streptokinase (1.5 million units/60 min) and treated at a mean of 2.8 h after symptom onset. Posttreatment angiography, performed after about 90 minutes (range 22 to 330 min), demonstrated an overall patency (grade 2/3 flow) rate of 70% (38 of 54 patients) in the anistreplase group versus 51% (27 of 53 patients) in the streptokinase group ($p < 0.05$).

These reperfusion rates compared quite closely with those observed earlier in the European Cooperative Study comparison of recombinant rt-PA versus IV streptokinase (patency rates of 70% versus 55%, respectively),[35] suggesting relative equivalence in efficacy between anistreplase and standard-dose regimens of rt-PA.

A Scottish study[36] randomized 128 patients with AMI of duration of 6 h or less (median 3 to 4 h) to anistreplase or streptokinase and determined angiographic early and late patency. No difference in patency was observed at 90 minutes (55% versus 53%) or 24 h (81% versus 87%) between the anistreplase and streptokinase groups.

In a much larger U.S. multicenter comparative trial,[37] 370 patients were entered and treated within 4 h of symptom onset (mean 2.6 h). Early coronary patency was determined at a mean of 140 minutes. The combined grade 2 and 3 perfusion rate was large and equal after both drugs (72% and 73%), but the achievement of grade 3 (complete) perfusion was greater after anistreplase (60%) than streptokinase (53%), and residual coronary stenosis was slightly less in patent arteries early after anistreplase (mean stenosis diameter 74%) than streptokinase (77%; $p = 0.02$).

The German t-PA–Anistreplase Patency Study (TAPS)[38] randomized 421 patients with AMI to either a front-loaded regimen of rt-PA (65 mg/30 min, 35 mg/subsequent 60 min) or to APSAC (30 units). Coronary angiography at 90 min revealed a patent infarct-related artery in 84% of rt-PA patients ($n = 199$) versus 70% of APSAC patients ($n = 202$)($p < 0.001$). However, reocclusion was greater after rt-PA, despite heparin, and the 1- to 2-day patency determination favored APSAC (93% versus 85% patency; $p < 0.03$).

A more valid comparison of 1-day patency between APSAC and t-PA (standard-regimen) was obtained in the TEAM-3 study ($n = 325$ patients), in which results were not confounded by early angiography or interventions.[39] In TEAM-3, 1-day coronary patency rates were large and similar in both groups (APSAC = 89%, rt-PA = 86%). Both regimens were supplemented by IV heparin, begun during the t-PA infusion and continued through the time of the patency determination.

Late patency at an average of 5 ± 2 days also

was compared among 169 patients in a French randomized study of APSAC versus rt-PA (standard dose) and found to be comparable (72% in the APSAC group, 76% in the rt-PA group; p = NS).[40]

A patency profile overview is shown in Figure 9-6 for APSAC, streptokinase, t-PA (standard regimen), and placebo or heparin.

Comparative Reocclusion Rates. Documented coronary reocclusion and/or reinfarction have occurred with low rates after anistreplase, comparable with those after SK and lower than those after t-PA, in controlled comparative trials. Reocclusion assessment is complicated by the requirement for a second angiographic study and is confounded by interventions such as angioplasty and surgery. Information on reocclusion within 1 to 3 days after initially successful anistreplase therapy was available for 289 patients evaluated in several clinical studies;[6] reocclusion was documented in only 9 (3.1%). In six trials, intravenous streptokinase was used as the comparator agent. Among 181 patients given IV streptokinase, reocclusion was noted in 8 (4.4%; p = NS versus anistreplase). In the largest single comparative study (TEAM-2), reocclusion within 1 to 2 days was

found in 1 of 96 patients given anistreplase and 2 of 94 given streptokinase plus heparin.[37] In a comparison with front-loaded t-PA, reocclusion within 1 to 2 days occurred in 10.3% (18 of 174) given rt-PA, despite IV heparin, versus 2.5% (4 of 163) given APSAC (p = 0.003).[38] The reocclusion risk after APSAC also was lower when restricting analysis to patients without additional interventions [9.4% (15 of 159) after t-PA versus 0% (0 of 130) after APSAC; p = 0.0003].[38] Reocclusion thereafter to the 2- to 3-week angiogram was similar in the two groups.

In contrast to angiographic reocclusion rates, clinically detected reinfarction rates were actually slightly less after t-PA (2.9%) than after APSAC (3.5%) or streptokinase (3.5%) in the ISIS-3 study,[41] suggesting that very early reocclusions after rt-PA may not have been detected as events distinct from the initial infarction.

Ejection Fraction/Infarct Size. Functional outcome after anistreplase versus rt-PA has been compared in two studies. In a French study of 183 patients treated at a mean of 2.9 h after symptom onset, ejection fractions were found to average 50% after APSAC and 52% after rt-PA at the 5 ± 2-day angiographic study and 47% versus 48% at

FIGURE 9-6. *Comparative patency profiles of anistreplase, streptokinase, t-PA, and placebo (or heparin). (Reprinted from JL Anderson. Am J Cardiol 1991;67:14E, with permission.)*

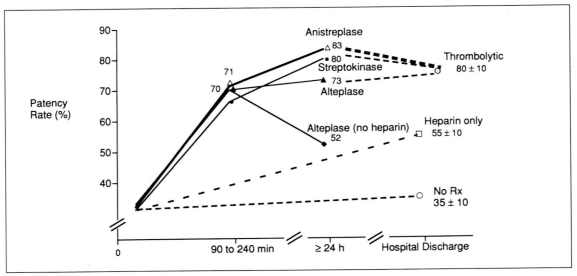

the 18 ± 5-day convalescent radionuclide study.[40] The 1 to 2 percentage point intergroup differences and the parallel differences in regional wall motion and infarct size were not significant. In a larger U.S. comparative trial in 325 patients treated at a mean of 2.6 h after symptom onset, ejection fraction at predischarge study averaged 51.3% after APSAC versus 54.3% after rt-PA ($p <$ 0.05), and at the 1-month convalescent study, 50.2% versus 54.8%, respectively ($p <$ 0.01).[39] Functional and volumetric analyses suggested that differences by treatment were explained primarily by differences in infarct zone function and end-systolic volumes. Other outcome measures, including exercise augmentation in ejection fraction, cardiac enzyme release, and clinical morbidity, were similar in the two groups.

Comparative Mortality Results. The Third International Study of Infarct Survival (ISIS-3) performed a randomized, double-blind comparison of anistreplase, streptokinase, and t-PA, plus aspirin with or without heparin, among 41,299 cases of suspected AMI.[41] No significant difference in mortality was seen among groups after 35 days (APSAC = 10.5%, SK = 10.6%, t-PA = 10.3%) and after 6 months (13.7%, 14.0%, 14.1%, respectively).

SAFETY OUTCOME
IN COMPARATIVE STUDIES

Allergy. In the large three-way comparative study (ISIS-3)[41] allergic reactions were recorded slightly more commonly after APSAC (5.1%) than after streptokinase (3.6%) and more frequently than after t-PA (0.8%)(both comparisons significant). However, only 10% of allergic reactions (0.5% incidence) caused persistent symptoms. In the other (smaller) comparative trials,[37–40] allergy was reported after APSAC in 5% ± 3% of patients and differed from the comparative agent in only 1 study.[38]

Hypotension. Compared with the standard, slow (1-h) infusion of streptokinase, rapid injection of anistreplase (over 2 to 5 min) was associated with an additional modest reduction in blood pressure averaging 4 to 5 mmHg at 5 to 10 min.[37] The incidence of clinical hypotension did not differ between treatments. In the U.S. multicenter

comparison of APSAC and t-PA,[39] maximal measured differences in blood pressure occurred at 10 min after starting therapy, when pressures averaged 106/69 mmHg in the APSAC group versus 125/79 mmHg in the t-PA group ($p <$ 0.01). The increment in reported cases of transient clinical hypotension at any time during hospitalization was 14%, comparing APSAC with t-PA, in one study[39] and −2% in another.[40] In the large ISIS-3 study,[41] hypotension was reported with a similar incidence after APSAC (12.5%) and streptokinase (11.8%) but more frequently than after t-PA (7.1%). In all these reports, hypotensive events after APSAC and streptokinase were generally transient and readily managed.

Bleeding Comparisons. In the ISIS-3 comparative study,[41] noncerebral bleeding events were reported in 5.4% of APSAC patients, 4.5% of streptokinase patients, and 5.2% of t-PA patients. Only about one-fifth of these bleeding events required transfusions, which were given with equal frequency in the three groups. Compared with streptokinase, there was a slight excess of total stroke with APSAC (1.3% versus 1.0%); the small excess could be attributed to definite or probable cerebral hemorrhage (0.55% versus 0.24% incidence). The largest rate of total stroke (1.4%) and cerebral hemorrhage (0.66%) occurred in the t-PA group. Bleeding rates after APSAC and comparator drug(s) were equivalent in the smaller randomized trials of APSAC versus SK[37] and APSAC compared with rt-PA.[40] In two trials of APSAC versus t-PA in which initial heparin was given in association with APSAC (to match that required for t-PA), the bleeding rate was somewhat greater after APSAC.[38,39]

Overview of Efficacy/Safety
of Anistreplase for AMI (Table 9-2)
PATENCY

A literature review culled 15 studies in 859 patients in which early patency (at 90 to 240 mins) was assessed.[42] Overall early patency rate was 71%. Seventeen studies including 1093 patients were found in which late (plateau) patency rates were determined at ≥1 day after therapy.[42] Late patency rate was 83%. A similar review was performed for studies using standard-dose alteplase

TABLE 9-2. Summary of Efficacy/Safety of Anistreplase for AMI

Usual IV dose	30 units (30 mg), injected over 5 min
Patency success	At 90 min: 70%[†]
	At 1–21 days: 80–85%[†]
Myocardial salvage/improved function (therapy in <4 h)	
Increase in ejection fraction	4–6%[‡]
Decrease in infarct size	16–33%[‡]
Mortality reduction (therapy in <6 h)	
Odds reduction	51% at 30 d[§]
	43% at 1 y[§]
Absolute reduction (Lives saved/ 100 pts treated)	5.7% at 1 y[§]
	6.7 at 1 y[§]
Hemorrhagic risk:	
Noncerebral bleeding events*	5.4%[¶]
Events requiring transfusion*	1.0%[¶]
Probable cerebral hemorrhage	0.55%[¶]
Allergic-type reactions	
Any	5.1%[¶]
Severe (persistent symptoms)	0.5%[¶]
Hypotensive risk (associated with AMI or therapy)	
Anytime	12.5%[¶]
Requiring therapy	7%[¶]

*Higher rates of bleeding (10–20% events) and transfusion (2–3%) have been reported from studies using IV heparin, invasive procedures, or more stringent definitions for (mild) hemorrhagic events.
[†]Ref. 42.
[‡]Ref. 27.
[§]Ref. 31.
[¶]Ref. 41.

and streptokinase. The early patency rate for anistreplase (71%) was similar to that for alteplase (70%) and greater than that for streptokinase (65%). The late patency rate for anistreplase (83%) was similar to that for streptokinase (80%) and greater than that for alteplase given with or without heparin (73%). Additional observations (noted above) suggest that rates of reperfusion with APSAC, as with other systemically active agents, are greater when anistreplase is given earlier (within 4 h) after the onset of symptoms than when treatment is delayed. Front-loaded regimens of rt-PA appear to achieve patency earlier than after anistreplase,[38] but late patency rates are similar or less (despite heparin) due to an increased reocclusion risk after rt-PA.[38]

The influence of pretreatment antistreptokinase antibody on efficacy of intravenous anistreplase and streptokinase was evaluated in a TEAM-2 comparison.[43] Within the population defined by this study (which precluded previous receipt of streptokinase or anistreplase), pretreatment antistreptokinase immunoglobin G was not a significant determinant of efficacy response. However, very high titers of antistreptokinase antibody are known to occur after treatment with anistreplase and streptokinase and may persist for 1 to 2 years or longer. Because these very high titers may be of clinical relevance, it has been suggested that retreatment with these agents be avoided within the window of 5 days to at least 2 years after initial therapy.

REOCCLUSION POTENTIAL

Angiographic coronary artery reocclusion was assessed in an open multicenter study in 156 patients (Anistreplase Reocclusion Multicenter Study, ARMS)[44] and found to be 4% within the first 24 h after treatment. Similarly, in an overview of other patency studies (see above), angiographic reocclusion within 1 to 3 days was low (averaging 3.1%).[6] As documented by serial angiographic studies, the rate of ongoing reperfusion exceeds that of reocclusion within the first 1 to 2 days. Late reocclusion/reinfarction rates are approximately similar for the three thrombolytic agents[41] and relate more to ancillary therapies and individual patient characteristics.

EJECTION FRACTION/ FUNCTIONAL OUTCOME

The advantage of early-administered (within 3 to 4 h) APSAC, compared with nonthrombolytic/ heparin control therapy, has been demonstrated (i.e., a 6 percentage point advantage)[27] and is similar to that established for early treatment with streptokinase and rt-PA.[4] Direct comparisons with t-PA have suggested either equivalent[40] or slightly smaller convalescent EF benefits after early-administered anistreplase.[39] In the latter, however, ejection fraction augmentation with exercise and functional class were equivalent to those after rt-PA.[39]

MORTALITY

The survival benefits of anistreplase have been clearly established. The AIMS trial[30,31] confirmed results of a pooled analysis of earlier studies,[24,25] demonstrating an absolute reduction of 6 lives per 100 patients treated at 30 days, with the advantage being maintained at 1 year. Proportionate reductions in mortality were observed in low-, medium-, and high-risk patients, but the greatest absolute differences were in high-risk patients (15 percentage point reduction) compared with medium- (4 point change) and low- (3 point change) risk patients selected by classic clinical and ECG criteria of AMI.[31] Although indirect comparisons suggested potentially greater survival benefits after APSAC than SK or t-PA, the ISIS-3 study[41] showed that under similar study conditions, survival benefits are comparable among agents. Some questions still remain, however, about the comparative outcomes of patients treated well outside of the median time range in ISIS-3, that is, at ≤ 1 to 2 h or at ≥ 6 to 8 h after the onset of symptoms.

OVERVIEW OF SAFETY

To the adverse event summaries presented above from the large AIMS and ISIS-3 experiences,[31,41] a summary of the entire clinical trials database (prior to ISIS-3) can be added based on 5275 patients treated with anistreplase.[24,25] Overall, hemorrhagic events were reported in 14.6% of patients and most commonly consisted of hemorrhage or hematoma at puncture sites (5.7% of patients). Hemorrhagic events were severe in only 1.6%. Not surprisingly, the incidence of hemorrhagic events was higher in studies incorporating invasive (angiographic) rather than noninvasive techniques (22% versus 13%), the difference being accounted for by puncture-site hemorrhages. The overall incidence of cerebrovascular accidents, occurring at any time after anistreplase, was 0.99% versus 0.80% after nonthrombolytic therapy. An excess of events after anistreplase was noted within the first 1 to 7 days, after which slightly fewer events than after nonthrombolytic therapy occurred. Etiology of stroke was reported as definitely or possibly hemorrhagic in 0.57% and 0.34%, respectively; these rates after APSAC are comparable with those observed in the ISIS-3 study.[41] The impact on severe hemorrhagic events of adding aspirin to anistreplase was assessed by a retrospective review. No difference was noted in any severe event (3.3% versus 3.9%) or in the rate of stroke [hemorrhagic or unknown etiology (0.88% versus 0.86%)] comparing patients in whom aspirin was given versus not given.[25]

As noted above, the incidence of possible allergic reactions after APSAC has averaged about 5% $\pm$ 3%. In contrast, the incidence of anaphylactoid reactions has been very low, 0.2% overall after anistreplase (11 of 5275 patients), similar to the 0.3% incidence found in patients treated in parallel with streptokinase (1 of 327).[24,25]

Role of Concomitant Therapy in AMI

ASPIRIN

Early studies evaluated APSAC in the absence of concomitant aspirin therapy.[30–33,37] After the ISIS-2 report,[45] trials of anistreplase incorporated initial and daily aspirin.[38–40] No direct, controlled assessment of the impact of aspirin on outcome after anistreplase therapy has been made, although the impact of aspirin is believed to be similar to that noted after streptokinase.[45] As noted earlier, a retrospective review of hemorrhagic events suggests that aspirin may be administered safely as concomitant therapy with anistreplase without significantly increasing hemorrhagic events.

HEPARIN

The heparin regimens given with APSAC have varied. In the majority of studies, heparin has been administered intravenously beginning as an infusion (e.g., 1000 units/h) at 4 to 6 h after anistreplase, the time when systemic thrombolytic effects begin to resolve, and adjusted so as to maintain PTT at $1\frac{1}{2}$ to 2 times the upper limits of normal for 1 to 7 days. These studies suggested an acceptable hemorrhagic risk with this regimen. In some more recent studies,[38–40] more aggressive heparin regimens (begun immediately or within 1 h of APSAC and given with concurrent aspirin) have been used, mimicking regimens recommended for t-PA. In these studies, the risk of bleeding after APSAC has been greater than in older studies and somewhat greater than with regimens using the shorter-acting rt-PA.[38,39] The question of added benefit versus risk of heparin, given in addition to aspirin, has thus been raised. In the large ISIS-3 trial,[41] no benefit of concomitant subcutaneous heparin on the mortality outcome after APSAC was noted whether heparin was (10.5% mortality) or was not given (10.6% mortality). Hemorrhagic events tended to be somewhat more common with subcutaneous heparin and were substantially more frequent in patients given intravenous heparin (out-of-protocol, nonrandomized comparison experience). A recent randomized comparison (Duke University) of heparin versus no heparin (added to aspirin) after APSAC also suggested an excess rate of hemorrhage in the absence of a clear outcome advantage.[46] Thus current data do not support a role for routine intravenous or subcutaneous heparin when aspirin is given with APSAC. The long-acting thrombolytic and systemic anticoagulant effects of APSAC, together with the antiplatelet effects of aspirin, generally appear to achieve an optimal benefit/risk ratio.

BETA BLOCKADE
Beta-blocker therapy (timolol), begun before hospital discharge and continued chronically, was well tolerated after APSAC in the AIMS mortality trial and was associated with an excellent long-term outcome.[31] Beta-blocker therapy also has been used routinely both acutely and chronically, as clinically indicated, in most other trials of APSAC. Thus beta-blocker and other standard concomitant therapies (nitroglycerin, oxygen, etc.) commonly used in myocardial infarction appear to be appropriate.

WARFARIN
In the AIMS study,[31] completed before the ISIS-2 evaluation of aspirin,[45] long-term anticoagulation was achieved with warfarin. Chronic warfarin and beta-blocker therapy preserved at 1 year the initial advantages of early APSAC observed in AIMS at 1 month. In patients at high risk for reocclusion, including those intolerant of chronic aspirin therapy, warfarin may continue to be viewed as a therapeutic option.

ADJUNCTIVE ANGIOPLASTY/SURGERY
The SWIFT (Should We Intervene Following Thrombolysis?) trial study group evaluated the hypothesis that early elective angiography with a view to coronary angioplasty or bypass grafting of a stenosed infarct-related vessel would improve outcome in AMI patients treated by thrombolysis with anistreplase.[47] Twenty-one district hospitals and regional cardiac centers in Great Britain and Ireland participated, enrolling 800 of 993 qualifying patients presenting with AMI up to 3 h after symptom onset. After treatment with anistreplase, randomization to intervention or no intervention was performed. Of 397 patients randomized to early angiography, 43% underwent angioplasty, and an additional 15% underwent coronary grafting (58% intervention rate). At the 1-year endpoint, mortality (5.8% versus 5.0%) and rates of reinfarction (15.1% versus 12.9%) were similar in the intervention and conservative-care groups. No significant differences in rates of angina or rest pain were observed, and left ventricular ejection fraction at 3 and 12 months was the same in both groups. The study concluded that for most patients given thrombolytic therapy for AMI, a strategy of angiography and intervention is appropriate only when required for clinical indications. These results and conclusions are similar for those obtained in t-PA trials.[48–51]

Combination Thrombolysis
Given that a front-loaded regimen of t-PA (a "fibrin-selective agent") appears to achieve reperfusion most rapidly among agents[38] but has a high reocclusion rate,[38] and given that the long-acting thrombolytic and antithrombotic effects of anistreplase are associated with optimal late patency rates[38,42] and a very low reocclusion risk,[6] the suggestion had been made that a combination of anistreplase with t-PA might result in an optimal overall reperfusion profile. It also had been hoped that somewhat reduced dosages of each agent, when combined, would result in a favorable safety profile. The Fourth Thrombolysis In Myocardial Infarction (TIMI-4) trial tested this hypothesis. Endpoints included serial assessments of angiographic patency, left ventricular functional outcome, and overall morbidity. Preliminary results did not suggest an added benefit of the combination regimen, however.[51a]

Prehospital Thrombolysis
Because the benefits of thrombolytic therapy are time-dependent, strategies to reduce the "symp-

tom to needle time," "door to needle time," and "symptom to reperfusion time" are being evaluated. It is known that the average time delay to thrombolytic therapy from hospital admission is about 60 to 90 min. A rapid checklist protocol for inclusion or exclusion was tested in one hospital in an effort to target 15 min as an optimal "door to needle time."[52] Among 39 consecutive patients treated with APSAC, a median in-hospital delay to treatment of only 13 min was achieved.[52]

Another approach to further shortening the delay between onset of pain and treatment is to give treatment at home. The European Myocardial Infarction Project (EMIP) demonstrated the feasibility of such an approach, administered by a trained medic team, first in a pilot study[53] and has now compared its impact with that of in-hospital therapy in a full study. Results were recently reported.[54] Although initially projected to evaluate 10,000 patients, funding issues required that the study be truncated to 5454 patients. Compared with in-hospital therapy, those randomized to in-field therapy were treated with a time savings of 56 min (i.e., therapy at a mean of about 2 h after onset of symptoms for prehospital compared with 3 h for the in-hospital group). Prehospital therapy was associated with reductions in cardiac mortality averaging 17% ($p < 0.05$) and total mortality averaging 13% ($p = 0.1$). A strong association was noted between benefit and reductions in time delays to therapy. Further analysis of the EMIP data may allow the question to be answered, do the benefits of in-field therapy outweigh the strategic and cost difficulties? The preliminary analysis already indicates the potential for earlier therapy to provide an additional increment of benefit and suggests the need for more efficient treatment strategies, beginning with reductions in emergency department and hospital delays.

APPLICATION OF ANISTREPLASE IN UNSTABLE ANGINA

Unstable angina is believed to be associated with intracoronary pathology resembling that in acute myocardial infarction, that is, endothelial injury with superimposed thrombus formation. However, the benefits of thrombolytic therapy have not been demonstrated in those with either a clinical history of unstable angina or its most frequent associated electrocardiographic finding, ST-segment depression.[45,55,56] To study this problem, a multicenter Dutch group entered 159 patients into a double-blind, placebo-controlled trial.[57] Patients without previous AMI with a typical history of unstable angina and ECG abnormalities suggestive of ischemia were included. Baseline angiography was performed and medication (double-blind) with either anistreplase or placebo was given. Repeat angiography at 12 to 28 h demonstrated a significant decrease in diameter stenosis in the anistreplase group compared with the placebo group (11% versus 3%; $p = 0.008$). This difference was accounted for by reopening of occluded vessels in a subgroup of patients in the thrombolytic group. However, no overall improvement in clinical outcome in the thrombolytic therapy group was demonstrated, and bleeding complications were more frequent in those receiving thrombolytic therapy (21 versus 7; $p = 0.001$). On the basis of these data, thrombolytic therapy is not recommended in patients diagnosed as having unstable angina. These results are similar to accumulating results in these patient groups treated with streptokinase or t-PA and indicate that unless demonstrated otherwise in specific patient subgroups, standard, nonthrombolytic therapy continues to be indicated in unstable angina.

APPLICATION OF ANISTREPLASE IN PULMONARY EMBOLISM

Because of its ease of administration, long duration of activity, and theoretical advantages compared with streptokinase, APSAC is an appealing drug to consider for treatment of massive pulmonary embolism. To date, no controlled studies have been performed with APSAC in pulmonary embolism. However, case reports indicate the feasibility and potential benefit of anistreplase in this condition. Schalij et al.[58] recently reported their experience in treating two patients with clinically massive pulmonary embolism of recent onset (confirmed by lung perfusion scans) with APSAC (30-unit injection) followed by systemic heparinization for 7 days. Both patients were reported to show considerable improvement following APSAC. Follow-up perfusion scans made after 2 days revealed marked reduction of perfusion defects.[58] In another report, Santo et al.[59] described the clinical case of a patient suffering from massive pulmonary embolism with circulatory shock who was treated successfully with a single bolus of APSAC (30 units). APSAC was viewed as a safe and effective therapy.[59] On the basis of its theoretical advantages and these favorable initial case reports, further evaluation of anistreplase for massive pulmonary embolism seems appropriate.

APPLICATION OF ANISTREPLASE IN ARTERIAL THROMBOSIS, DEEP VEIN THROMBOSIS, AND OTHER CONDITIONS

Although clinical trials have focused on the application of anistreplase for AMI, its ease of administration and long-acting systemic lytic and antithrombotic effects suggest that it may be an excellent candidate agent for use in peripheral vascular (venous and arterial) thromboembolic disease, including disease with large clot burdens. In these conditions, it would be anticipated that its efficacy may be greater than that of streptokinase, with similar tolerance and with greater ease of administration. No controlled studies have been performed for these conditions, but they should be encouraged for the future.

SUMMARY / PERSPECTIVES

Anistreplase is an efficient thrombolytic agent which is most easily administered and requires the least ancillary therapy support (aspirin alone) among the approved agents for treatment of coronary thrombosis. Controlled trial data are so far are lacking for use of APSAC in pulmonary embolism, but case reports indicate it to have therapeutic potential. Similarly, clinical experience is not yet available for its application in peripheral thromboembolic disease, although from a theo-

retical standpoint it would appear to be a promising agent. A summary of its benefits and risks in AMI may be useful to its applications in other areas. For patients treated within 4 to 6 h of symptom onset, a coronary patency rate of about 70% is achieved within 90 min and a rate of about 85% within 1 day. With timely therapy (within 2 to 3 h of symptom onset), improvement in left ventricular function (averaging 6%) and reduction in infarct size (averaging 15% to 30%) are achieved. In patients selected by classic ECG criteria, a reduction in the odds of mortality of 50% may be achieved (survival benefit of 6 patients per 100 patients treated) that persists long term (≥ 1 year). In a three-drug comparison, mortality outcome was similar among all thrombolytic agents begun simultaneously. The ease of APSAC lends itself to earlier (timelier) administration than the other agents, however, and the potential for further reductions in cardiovascular mortality by very early APSAC therapy (17% additional reduction in cardiovascular mortality for at-home versus in-hospital therapy) has been demonstrated. The primary risks of anistreplase are allergy (similar to those of streptokinase) and hemorrhage (most important, as with other agents, cerebral hemorrhage, 0.5% risk). Minor allergy is seen occasionally (about 5% of cases) but rarely is problematic, and severe allergy (i.e., anaphylaxis) has been extremely rare (0.2%). It appears to be wise to avoid anistreplase reuse or its first use in patients previously given streptokinase, at least within the window of 5 days to 2 years. The bleeding risks after anistreplase can be reduced by avoiding concomitant IV heparin, which appears to be unnecessary as a routine when aspirin is given as concomitant therapy. The risk of cerebral hemorrhage after APSAC is somewhat greater than after streptokinase (consistent with its greater thrombolytic efficiency) but less than that of rt-PA. The excess risk of cerebral hemorrhage with APSAC (0.2% excess in the absence of heparin, 0.5% with heparin) appears to be related to age, suggesting that its use in patients over about 70 years of age be selective, that heparin be omitted, that smaller doses of APSAC in older patients be considered, or that streptokinase be substituted in these patients.

INDICATIONS / CONTRAINDICATIONS (TABLE 9-3)

Anistreplase is indicated for use in management of acute myocardial infarction, including lysis of obstructing coronary thrombi, reduction in infarct size, improvement in ventricular function following AMI, and reduction in AMI-associated mortality. Treatment should be initiated as soon as possible after the onset of symptoms.

Contraindications to anistreplase are similar to those for other lytic agents and involve primar-ily the risks of increased bleeding noted in the following situations: active internal bleeding, history of cerebrovascular accident, recent (within 2 months) intracranial or intraspinal surgery or trauma, intracranial neoplastic or arterial-venous malformation or aneurysm, known bleeding diathesis, and severe, uncontrolled hypertension. Additional relative contraindications exist that should be considered in overall risk/benefit profiling.

TABLE 9-3. Anistreplase: Indications and Applications

Approved indication	Acute myocardial infarction
Usual dose	30 units (30 mg), injected IV over 5 min
Potential (investigational) applications:	1. Pulmonary embolism 2. Other arterial thromboses or thromboemboli 3. Venous thrombosis

Recommended concomitant therapy	Aspirin initially and qd (162–325 mg)
	Heparin
	  With aspirin—not routinely indicated (ISIS-3)
	  Without aspirin—may infuse at 1000 U/h (or to keep PTT at 1½–2 × control), starting after 4–6 h (AIMS). May begin an infusion (e.g., 1000 U/h) without a bolus, starting after 4–6 h[27, 33] and continue for 1–7 days. Adjust to keep PTT at 1½ to 2 times control (i.e., about 60–90 s).
	Other standard therapies—as indicated in postthrombolysis patients

Contraindications	1. Surgery or major trauma in <10 days 2. Internal bleeding (e.g., bleeding ulcer) in <6 mos 3. Known bleeding diathesis 4. History of cerebrovascular accident 5. Severe, uncontrolled hypertension 6. Known intracranial neoplasm or aneurysm 7. Recent (<2 mos) neurosurgical procedure

DOSE / ADMINISTRATION / COST

Anistreplase is marketed in vials of lyophilized powder containing 30 units (30 mg) of drug at a pharmacy cost of about $1700 per vial. APSAC is reconstituted by dissolving the contents of a vial with 5 ml of sterile water or saline, and the solution is administered by intravenous injection over 2 to 5 min. Although anistreplase can be given by intraarterial (intracoronary) infusion, APSAC was designed and approved specifically for intravenous therapy.

REFERENCES

1. Sherry S. Fibrinolysis thrombosis, and hemostasis: concepts, perspectives, and clinical applications. Philadelphia: Lea & Febiger, 1992.
2. Marder VJ, Sherry S. Thrombolytic therapy: current status. N Engl J Med 1988;318:1512.
3. Laffel GL, Braunwald E. Thrombolytic therapy: a new strategy for the treatment of acute myocardial infarction. N Engl J Med 1984;311:710.
4. Yusuf S, Sleight P, Held P, McMahon S. Routine medical management of acute myocardial infarction: lessons from overviews of recent randomized controlled trials. Circulation 1990;82(suppl II): II–117.
5. Anderson JL. Anisoylated plasminogen-streptokinase activator complex. In: Messerli FH, ed. Cardiovascular drug therapy. Philadelphia: WB Saunders, 1990:1496.
6. Anderson JL. Review of anistreplase (APSAC) for acute myocardial infarction. In: Modern management of acute myocardial infarction in the community hospital. New York: Marcel Dekker, 1991: 149.
7. Smith RAG, Dupe RJ, English PD, Green J. Fibri-

nolysis with acyl-enzymes: a new approach to thrombolytic therapy. Nature 1981;290:505.

8. Fears R. Development of anisoylated plasminogen-streptokinase activator complex from the acyl enzyme concept. Semin Thromb Hemost 1989;15: 129.

9. Ferres H. Pre-clinical pharmacological evaluation of Eminase (APSAC). Drugs 1987;33(suppl 3):33.

10. Smith RAG. Non-exchange of streptokinase from anisoylated plasminogen streptokinase activator complex and other acylated streptokinase-plasminogen complexes. Drugs 1987;33(suppl 3):75.

11. Nunn B, Esmail A, Fears R, et al. Pharmacokinetic properties of anisoylated plasminogen streptokinase activator complex and other thrombolytic agents in animals and in humans. Drugs 1987; 33(suppl 3):88.

12. Standring R, Fears R, Ferres H. The protective effect of acylation on the stability of APSAC (Eminase) in human plasma. Fibrinolysis 1988;2:157.

13. Been M, de Bono DP, Muir Al, et al. Clinical effects and kinetic properties of intravenous APSAC—anisoylated plasminogen-streptokinase activator complex (BRL 26921)—in acute myocardial infarction. Int J Cardiol 1986;11:53.

14. Doenecke P, Schwerdt H, Hellsten P, et al. Bolus injection of anisoylated plasminogen-streptokinase activator complex (BRL 26921): a new approach to intravenous thrombolytic treatment of acute myocardial infarction. Klin Wochenschr 1986;64:682.

15. Mentzer RL, Budzynski AZ, Sherry S. High-dose, brief-duration intravenous infusion of streptokinase in acute myocardial infarction: description of effects in circulation. Am J Cardiol 1986;57:1220.

16. Fears R, Ferres H, Standring R. The protective effect of acylation of the stability of anisoylated plasminogen streptokinase activator complex in human plasma. Drugs 1987;33(suppl 3):57.

17. Ferres H, Hibbs M, Smith RAG. Deacylation studies in vitro on anisoylated plasminogen streptokinase activator complex. Drugs 1987;33(suppl 3):80.

18. Fears R, Ferres H, Glasgow E, et al. Comparison of fibrinolytic and aminolytic methods for the measurement of streptokinase pharmacokinetics with acute myocardial infarction. Fibrinolysis 1989;3: 175.

19. Fears R, Ferres H, Standring R. Pharmacological comparison of anisoylated Lys-plasminogen streptokinase activator complex with its Glu-plasminogen variant and streptokinase–Glu-plasminogen: binding to human fibrin and plasma clots. Fibrinolysis 1989;3:93.

20. Fears R, Standring R, Ferres H. Evidence for a continuing accumulation of APSAC (anisoylated plasminogen streptokinase activator complex) by human clots: comparison with the binding of other plasminogen activators and plasminogen. Fibrinolysis 1987;1:215.

21. Green J, Dupe RJ, Smith RAG, et al. Comparison of the hypotensive effects of streptokinase (human)–plasmin activator complex and BRL 26921 (anisoylated streptokinase-plasminogen activator complex) in the dog after high dose bolus administration. Thromb Res 1984;36:2936.

22. Kasper W, Erbel R, Meinertz T, et al. Intracoronary thrombolysis with an acylated streptokinase plasminogen activator (BRL 26921) in patients with acute myocardial infarction. J Am Coll Cardiol 1984;4:357.

23. Marder VJ, Rothbard RL, Fitzpatrick PG, Francis CW. Rapid lysis of coronary artery thrombi with anisoylated plasminogen-streptokinase activator complex: treatment by bolus intravenous injection. Ann Intern Med 1986;104:304.

24. Johnson ES, Cregeen RJ. An interim report of the efficacy and safety of anisoylated plasminogen streptokinase activator complex (APSAC). Drugs 1987;33(suppl 3):298.

25. Cregeen R. Report to the US FDA Advisory Committee, Bureau of Biologies. Anistreplase review meeting, Bethesda, MD, Oct 31, 1989.

26. Timmis AD, Griffin B, Crick JCP, Sowton E. APSAC in acute myocardial infarction: a placebo-controlled arteriographic coronary recanalization study. J Am Coll Cardiol 1987;10:205.

27. Bassand J-P, Machecourt J, Cassagnes J, et al, for the APSIM Study Investigators. Multicenter trial of intravenous anisoylated plasminogen streptokinase activator complex (APSAC) in acute myocardial infarction: effects on infarct size and left ventricular function. J Am Coll Cardiol 1989;13:988.

28. Meinertz T, Kasper W, Schumacher M, et al. The German multicenter trial of anisoylated plasminogen streptokinase activator complex versus heparin for acute myocardial infarction. Am J Cardiol 1988;62:347.

29. Califf RM, Harrelson-Woodlief L, Topol EJ. Left ventricular ejection fraction may not be useful as an end point of thrombolytic therapy comparative trials. Circulation 1990;82:1847.

30. AIMS Trial Study Group. Effect of intravenous APSAC on mortality after acute myocardial infarction: preliminary report of a placebo-controlled clinical trial. Lancet 1988;1:545.

31. AIMS Trial Study Group. Long-term effects of intravenous anistreplase in acute myocardial infarction: final report of the AIMS study. Lancet 1990; 335:427.

32. Anderson JL, Rothbard RL, Hackworthy RA, et al, for the APSAC Multicenter Investigators. Multi-

center reperfusion trial of intravenous anisoylated plasminogen streptokinase activator complex (APSAC) in acute myocardial infarction: controlled comparison with intracoronary streptokinase. J Am Coll Cardiol 1988;11:1153.

33. Bonnier HJRM, Visser RF, Klomp HD, Hoffman HMJL, and the Dutch Invasive Reperfusion Study Group. Comparison of intravenous anisoylated plasminogen streptokinase activator complex and intracoronary streptokinase in acute myocardial infarction. Am J Cardiol 1988;62:25.

34. Pacouret G, Charbonnier B, Curien ND, et al. Invasive reperfusion study: II. Multicenter European randomized trial of anistreplase vs streptokinase in acute myocardial infarction. Eur Heart J 1991; 12:179.

35. Verstraete M, Bernard R, Bory M, et al. Randomized trial of intravenous recombinant tissue-type plasminogen activator versus intravenous streptokinase in acute myocardial infarction. Lancet 1985;1:842.

36. Hogg KJ, Gemmill JD, Burns JMA, et al. Angiographic patency study of anistreplase versus streptokinase in acute myocardial infarction. Lancet 1990;335:254.

37. Anderson JL, Sorensen SG, Moreno FL, et al, and the TEAM-2 Investigators. Multicenter patency trial of intravenous anistreplase compared with streptokinase in acute myocardial infarction. Circulation 1991;83:126.

38. Neuhaus K-L, Von Essen R, Tebbe U, et al. Improved thrombolysis in acute myocardial infarction with front-loaded administration of alteplase: results of the rt-PA–APSAC patency study (TAPS). J Am Coll Cardiol 1992;19:885.

39. Anderson JL, Becker LC, Sorensen SG, et al, for the TEAM-3 Investigators. Anistreplase versus alteplase in acute myocardial infarction: comparative effects on left ventricular function, morbidity and 1-day coronary artery patency. J Am Coll Cardiol 1992;20:753.

40. Bassand JP, Cassagnes J, Machecourt J, et al. Comparative effects of APSAC and rt-PA on infarct size and left ventricular function in acute myocardial infarction. Circulation 1991;84:1107.

41. ISIS-3 Collaborative Group. ISIS-3: a randomized comparison of streptokinase vs tissue plasminogen activator vs anistreplase and of aspirin plus heparin vs aspirin alone among 41,299 cases of suspected acute myocardial infarction. Lancet 1992;339:753.

42. Anderson JL. Consideration of patency as an end point of thrombolytic therapy. Am J Cardiol 1991; 67:11E.

43. Fears R, Hearn J, Standring R, et al. Lack of influence of pretreatment antistreptokinase antibody on efficacy in a multicenter patency comparison of intravenous streptokinase and anistreplase in acute myocardial infarction. Am Heart J 1992; 124(2):305.

44. Relik-van Wely L, Visser RF, van der Pol JM, et al. Angiographically assessed coronary arterial patency and reocclusion in patients with acute myocardial infarction treated with anistreplase: results of the anistreplase reocclusion multicenter study (ARMS). Am J Cardiol 1991;68:296.

45. ISIS-2 Collaborative Group. Randomized trial of intravenous streptokinase, oral aspirin, both, or neither among 17,187 cases of suspected acute myocardial infarction: ISIS-2. Lancet 1988;2:349.

46. O'Connor CM, Meese R, Carney R, et al. for the DUCCS 1 Investigators. A randomized trial of intravenous heparin in conjunction with anistreplase in acute myocardial infarction. J Am Coll Cardiol 1994;23:11.

47. SWIFT Trial Study Group. SWIFT trial of delayed elective intervention vs conservative treatment after thrombolysis with anistreplase in acute myocardial infarction. Br Med J 1991;302:555.

48. Topol EJ, Califf RM, George BS, et al. A randomized trial of immediate versus delayed elective angioplasty after intravenous tissue plasminogen activator in acute myocardial infarction. N Engl J Med 1987;317:581.

49. Simoons ML, Betriu A, Col J, et al. Thrombolysis with tissue plasminogen activator in acute myocardial infarction: no additive benefit from immediate coronary angioplasty. Lancet 1988;1:197.

50. The TIMI Research Group. Immediate vs delayed catheterization and angioplasty following thrombolytic therapy for acute myocardial infarction: TIMI-IIA results. JAMA 1988;260:2849.

51. The TIMI Study Group. Comparison of invasive and conservative strategies after treatment with intravenous tissue plasminogen activator in acute myocardial infarction: results of the thrombolysis in myocardial infarction (TIMI) phase II trial. N Engl J Med 1989;320:618.

51a. Cannon CP, McCabe CH, Dives DJ, et al. for the TIMI-4 Investigators. Clinical benefit of front-loaded t-PA over combination thrombolytic therapy or APSK for acute MI. Circulation 1993; 88:I-291.

52. MacCallum AG, Stafford PJ, Jones C, et al. Reduction in hospital time to thrombolytic therapy by audit of policy guidelines. Eur Heart J 1990; 11(suppl F):48.

53. Castaigne AD, Herv'e C, Duval-Moulin AM, et al. Pre-hospital thrombolysis, is it useful? Eur Heart J 1990;11(suppl F):43.

54. The European Myocardial Infarction Project Group. Prehospital thrombolytic therapy in pa-

tients with suspected acute myocardial infarction. N Engl J Med 1993;329:383.

55. Topol EJ, Nicklas JM, Kander NH, et al. Coronary revascularization after intravenous tissue plasminogen activator for unstable angina pectoris: results of a randomized double-blind, placebo-controlled trial. Am J Cardiol 1988;62:368.

56. Williams DO, Topol EJ, Califf RM, et al. Intravenous recombinant tissue-type plasminogen activator in patients with unstable angina pectoris: results of a placebo-controlled, randomized trial. Circulation 1990;82:376.

57. Bar FW, Verheugt FW, Col J, et al. Thrombolysis in patients with unstable angina improves the an-giographic but not the clinical outcome: results of UNASEM, a multicenter, randomized, placebo-controlled, clinical trial with anistreplase. Circulation 1992;86:(1):131.

58. Schalij MJ, van de Meeberg PC, Marsman JW, Maingay D. Pulmonary embolism treated with a single dose of anisoylated Lys-plasminogen streptokinase activator complex and systemic heparinization: a report of two cases. Neth J Med 1992;40 (1–2):69.

59. Santo ME, da Silva G, Pimenta A. Pulmonary embolism: a propos of a case treated with APSAC. Rev Port Cardiol 1991;10:339.

10

PROUROKINASE: A NEW CLOT-SELECTIVE THROMBOLYTIC AGENT

John C. Sobolski

Arthur A. Sasahara

Patrick A. Marcotte

Jack Henkin

Victor Gurewich

Prourokinase (pro-UK) is the zymogen form of urokinase (UK) and has alternatively been named *single-chain urokinase-type plasminogen activator* (scu-PA) (Fig. 10-1); it is now produced by recombinant DNA technology[1] in the United States and Europe, while it is produced from kidney cell cultures in Japan. It has a molecular weight of about 50,000, and the protein consists of 411 amino acids and has a N-terminal domain with homology to the growth factor domain of other proteins, followed by a kringle domain, homologous to domains on plasminogen, tissue plasminogen activator, and other proteins involved in coagulation.[2,3] However, the kringle domain of UK, or its zymogen, does not contain a lysine binding site, and it does not confer fibrin binding properties to the enzyme.[4] The zymogen or pro-enzyme property of pro-UK is of special pharmacologic importance and identifies pro-UK as different from other plasminogen activators. It is the only activator which is inert in plasma and does not form inhibitor complexes.[5]

ACTIVATION OF PLASMINOGEN BY PRO-UK

In the presence of a fibrin clot, pro-UK becomes active and induces plasminogen activation. However, the fibrin-dependent mechanisms by which pro-UK induces plasminogen activation, unlike tissue plasminogen activator (t-PA), are independent of fibrin binding.[6] At the pH of circulating blood, little binding to fibrin appears to take place, but nevertheless, pro-UK has been shown in vitro and in vivo to be at least as fibrin-specific as t-PA.[7,8]

The mechanism for this fibrin specificity appears to be related to several factors: the pro-enzyme property of pro-UK, the conformational change of plasminogen when it binds to fibrin, and the plasma inhibitors which help to confine the proteolytic activity to the clot surface.[5]

Pro-UK is readily activated by plasmin to the two-chain form of UK, with a resultant increase of at least 500-fold in its plasminogen-activating activity[9,10] (Fig. 10-2). Therefore, pro-UK and plasminogen are mutually activated, and this provides

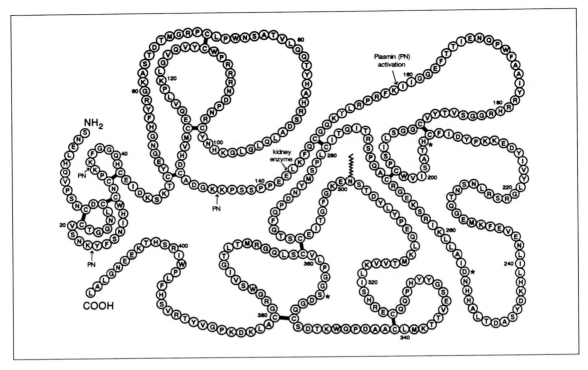

FIGURE 10-1. *Amino acid sequence of single-chain prourokinase, cloned and expressed in mouse hybridoma cell line.*

a positive feedback which greatly amplifies plasmin generation on the clot surface.[11-13] Since pro-UK has only a low intrinsic activity (less than 0.2% of the rate of u-PA), the active principle of pro-UK is UK.[14,15] However, unlike UK, pro-UK reaches the clot intact without being partially quenched by the formation of inhibitor complexes and without inducing nonspecific plasminogen activation.

FIBRIN SPECIFICITY OF THROMBOLYSIS

Clinical thrombolysis with streptokinase (SK), UK, anisoylated plasminogen-streptokinase activator complex (APSAC), or t-PA, in contrast to physiologic fibrinolysis, is invariably accompanied by systemic plasmin generation that may compromise the safety and efficacy of therapy. These potential adverse effects are related to the multiple substrates of plasmin. Plasmin is an en-

zyme that has broad activity, inducing a number of proteolytic reactions: degradation of certain clotting factors (I, V, VIII, and vWF), proteolysis of certain constituents of platelets and basement membrane, and activation of the complement system through activation of C1, C3, and C5. The most important clinical consequence of plasminemia is compromised hemostasis because of degradation of clotting factors and the generation of fibrinogen degradation products which may interfere with platelet aggregation and fibrin polymerization and may increase vascular permeability. However, the generation of fibrinogen degradation products may be viewed as advantageous by reducing the risk of rethrombosis. Plasmin, paradoxically, also induces platelet aggregation and the platelet release reaction and may therefore contribute to a prothrombotic state.[16]

Plasmin generation also results in a major depletion of the circulating substrate for fibrinolysis, plasminogen. It was shown years ago that re-

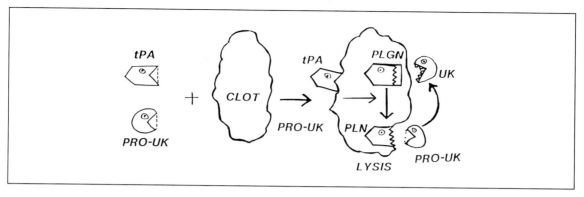

FIGURE 10-2. *Graphic depiction of a collision between pro-UK and a "protected" plasmin within the clot (PLN), converting single-chain pro-UK to two-chain urokinase. t-PA, in contrast, binds tightly to fibrin, adjacent to a fibrin-bound plasminogen (PLGN), converting it to plasmin.*

duction of plasminogen concentration in ambient fluid compromises clot lysis.[17] Maintenance of the reservoir of plasminogen may therefore be necessary if optimal thrombolysis is to be achieved.

These potentially deleterious effects of nonspecific plasmin generation have made fibrin specificity an attractive therapeutic objective which has yet to be achieved. The natural plasminogen activators, t-PA and pro-UK, are both capable of selectively activating clot-bound plasminogen. However, at the high doses required for effective thrombolysis by monotherapy, at least with t-PA, nonspecific activation of plasma plasminogen is unavoidable. At lower doses, fibrin specificity is achieved, but with ineffective thrombolysis.

PROUROKINASE FIBRINOLYSIS

When pro-UK was isolated from urine, it was thought that pro-UK had a fibrin clot affinity similar to that of t-PA. This assumption was proved to be incorrect.[18] Certain properties of freshly voided urine were found to be required for binding, which occurred at an acid pH.[19] By contrast, in a plasma milieu, little or no binding to a fibrin clot occurred. Nevertheless, pro-UK was shown to induce fibrin specific clot lysis in plasma both in vitro and in vivo.[7, 8] This may be due in part to a conformational change in plasminogen when it binds to fibrin.[18] It also was postulated at one time

that dissociation of a presumed pro-UK–inhibitor complex in plasma was triggered by fibrin.[4] However, pro-UK does not form complexes with known inhibitors, and no alternative inhibitor has been identified. Regardless of the mechanism, there is a consensus that pro-UK is inert and stable in plasma for extended periods and, in contrast to UK, does not form SDS–stable inhibitor complexes. As a result, the fibrinolytic properties of pro-UK remain uncompromised when incubated for several days, and plasma plasminogen remains intact.[7,20]

The importance of this zymogenic property of pro-UK can be appreciated when contrasted to the enzymatic property of other activators. For example, t-PA is inactivated by several plasma inhibitors including PAI-1, C1-esterase inhibitor, α_2-antiplasmin, and α_2-macroglobulin. Hence, when t-PA is infused peripherally, binding by inhibitors reduces the amount of t-PA that reaches the clot, consuming important plasma defenses against plasmin and facilitating nonspecific proteolysis. In physiologic fibrinolysis, t-PA is released locally from the vessel wall endothelium at the site of a thrombus. The high fibrin specificity of t-PA then allows it to initiate fibrinolysis efficiently and to evade inhibition. In contrast, pro-UK can be infused peripherally without consuming plasma inhibitors and circulates to a clot intact.[5] The clinical usefulness of this property of pro-UK, which allows it to be infused for protracted periods without compromising hemostasis, has not yet been fully investigated.

Another difference between pro-UK and t-PA relates to the separate mechanisms by which they induce activation of fibrin-bound plasminogen. To appreciate the importance of this difference, it should be noted that lysine binding sites on plasminogen bind to two types of lysine residues in fibrin. One type of residue is situated internally and is therefore present on intact fibrin. The other residue is formed only after plasmin degradation of fibrin has been initiated, resulting in specific breaks in the alpha, beta, and gamma chains of fibrin. As a result, new lysine residues (carboxy-terminal lysines) are exposed at the carboxy-terminal ends of each of these chains. Pro-UK activates principally the plasminogen bound to the carboxy-terminal lysines which are present in fibrin only after limited digestion by plasmin. When plasminogen binds to any lysine residues in fibrin, it undergoes a conformational change.[21] The selective activation of plasminogen by pro-UK may be mediated by a particular conformational change which is induced only when plasminogen binds to carboxy-terminal lysines.[22] Single-chain pro-UK may be able to act as an enzyme on a special subset of plasminogen where the latter is bound to fibrin fragment E.[23] Tissue plasminogen activator, on the other hand, appears to activate plasminogen bound to the internal lysine residues which are present on intact fibrin.[24,25] Consequently, t-PA appears to be more effective in initiating lysis, priming the clot for pro-UK, which can then bring the thrombolytic process efficiently to completion.[26] These complementary mechanisms of action may explain the synergy in fibrinolysis found when t-PA and pro-UK are combined.[22] These complementary mechanisms also appear to explain why t-PA and pro-UK tend to be relatively ineffective when given alone, since neither efficiently activates the alternate plasminogen. Since pro-UK preferentially appears to activate plasminogen available only on partially degraded fibrin, the fibrinolytic effect of pro-UK should be potentiated by other plasminogen activators as well. And in fact, pro-UK–induced clot lysis in vitro[27] or in vivo in patients with acute myocardial infarction is potentiated by a small (but in suffi-

cient amount to overcome inhibitors), subtherapeutic bolus of UK.[28] Also, a bolus of heparin potentiates the thrombolytic effect of pro-UK, and this appears to be an in vivo effect. Heparin can bind to pro-UK and affect its properties. Additionally, heparin has been shown to release t-PA from the vessel wall endothelium,[29] and the potentiating effect of heparin on pro-UK–induced thrombolysis may be mediated by t-PA. Although no "priming" with streptokinase has been tested yet, streptokinase is also expected to potentiate thrombolysis by pro-UK.

EXPERIENCE WITH PROUROKINASE IN ACUTE MYOCARDIAL INFARCTION

Thrombolysis for acute myocardial infarction has been studied extensively in close to 100,000 patients in several randomized trials and has been shown to significantly reduce both short- and long-term mortality. Streptokinase (SK), tissue-type plasminogen activator (rt-PA), and anisoylated plasminogen-streptokinase activator complex (APSAC) are the most widely studied agents to date. Prourokinase (pro-UK), the precursor of urokinase, is undergoing clinical trials in Europe and the United States to establish the optimal dose regimen with respect to efficacy (early patency, reocclusion, recurrent ischemia) and safety. Mortality studies have yet to be conducted.

This overview focuses on current clinical experience with pro-UK in acute myocardial infarction. As reviewed earlier, pro-UK is obtained from various sources and through different manufacturing processes, resulting in differences in molecular structure and fibrinolytic potency. Whether these variations will result in major differences in clinical efficacy remains to be determined.

Throughout the overview, a coronary artery displaying TIMI grade 2 or 3 flow is considered a patent vessel.

Prourokinase and Heparin

In most clinical trials, anticoagulation with intravenous heparin was usually initiated prior to or concurrently with the pro-UK infusion and continued for at least 24 h. The importance of maintaining adequate anticoagulation levels during pro-UK–induced thrombolysis was demonstrated by Gulba et al.[30] Only 1 of 9 patients who did not receive heparin during the infusion of pro-UK had a patent coronary artery at the 90-min angiogram, while 7 of 9 patients who received heparin had a patent artery.

Prourokinase Dose-Ranging Studies

The early dose-ranging studies were reperfusion studies in small series of patients with acute myocardial infarction and angiographically documented coronary occlusion. In three trials using glycosylated pro-UK in 73 patients,[8,31,32] doses between 15 and 69 mg were studied. The administration occurred over 60 to 90 min, either as a straight infusion or as a combination of an infusion preceded by a bolus. Reperfusion rates at 90 min ranged from 25% to 83%. In the largest of these studies, Loscalzo et al.[32] reported a mean reperfusion range of 25% to 67% (Table 10-1) at 90 min in 40 patients.

Using a recombinant, nonglycosylated pro-UK (rpro-UK), Van de Werf et al.[33] found 60-min reperfusion rates of 75% and 79% following infusions of 40 and 70 mg, respectively, over 60 min in 17 patients. Diefenbach et al.,[34] using the same preparation, reported 90-min reperfusion rates of

50% after 40 mg and 91% after 80 mg administered over 60 min.

Although numbers of pro-UK–treated patients are too small to compare the recanalization rates of pro-UK and t-PA, data generated in the pro-UK reperfusion trials are comparable with observations in TIMI-1, where patients randomized to t-PA had a 70%[35] reperfusion rate at 90 min.

A substantially larger number of patients have been studied in so-called patency trials, where, in the absence of a baseline coronary angiogram, efficacy was assessed based on the status of the culprit coronary artery at 60 or 90 min after initiation of the infusion. Bode et al.[28] reported 60-min patency rates of 50% in 14 patients who received 48 mg over 60 min and 55% in 20 patients who received 74 mg of glycosylated pro-UK over 60 min (Table 10-2). In the PRIMI trial,[36] a randomized trial comparing nonglycosylated rpro-UK with streptokinase, 198 patients were given 80 mg rpro-UK intravenously over 60 min, with 20 mg given as a bolus. Streptokinase, 1.5 million IU, was administered to 203 patients over 60 min. The 60- and 90-min angiograms revealed patency rates of 72% and 71%, respectively, for rpro-UK and 48% and 64% for streptokinase (Table 10-3). These differences were statistically significant at 60 min ($p < 0.001$). More recently,

TABLE 10-1. Prourokinase in AMI:
A Dose-Ranging Multicenter Study

	I	II	III	IV	V	VI
Patients	2	11	6	4	5	12
Dosage (mg)	36	48	52	58	65	69
(MM IU)	4.73	6.25	6.75	7.5	8.5	9.0
Bolus (MM IU)	0.68	—	4.75	2.5	2.5	2.5
Infusion (MM IU)	4.05	6.25	2.0	5.0	6.0	6.5
Patency (90 min)	0	54%	33%	25%	60%	67%
Bleeding	1/40 = 2.5% significant bleed					
Hematologic	Fibrinogen decreased 10% FDP increased 63% Plasminogen decreased 36% α_2-Antiplasmin decreased 61%					

Created from data from ref. 32. Reprinted with permission from Sasahara AA. New developments in thrombolytic therapy. Adv Pharmacol 1992;23:227.

TABLE 10-2. Prourokinase versus Urokinase
Therapy in Patients with AMI

	Group I	Group II	Group III
Patients (within 5 h)	14	20	20
Regimen (60 min)			
Urokinase (IU)	0	0	250,000
Pro-UK (Bolus/ inf. mg.)	7.5/40.5	7.5/66.5	3.7/44.3
Patency (60 min), %	50	55	65
Bleeding, %	7	5	0
Fibrinogen change, %	−13	−42	−24
Plasminogen change, %	−39	−62	−33
α_2-Antiplasmin change, %	−41	−79	−53

Created from data from ref. 28. Reprinted with permission from Sasahara AA. Clinical experiences with urokinase and pruorokinase in patients with acute myocardial infarction. In: Haber, Braunwald, eds. Thrombolysis. St. Louis: Mosby-Year Book, 1991;293.

TABLE 10-3. The PRIMI Trial:
Prourokinase versus Streptokinase in AMI

	Pro-UK	SK
Patients (within 4 h)	198	203
Regimen (over 60 min)	B: 20 mg. I: 60 mg.	I: 1.5 MM
Patency, %		
90 min.	71	64
24–36 h	85	88
Reocclusion, %	4.9	4.4
Bleeding (all), %	14*	25
Intracranial, %	1.0	0.5
Fibrinogen, % of baseline	44%	17%

*Sig. = $p < 0.05$.
Reprinted with permission from Sasahara AA. Clinical experiences with urokinase and prourokinase in patients with acute myocardial infarction. In: Haber, Braunwald, eds. Thrombolysis. St. Louis: Mosby-Year Book, 1991;295.

Weaver et al.[37] reported a 60-min patency rate of 72% in 46 patients who had received 60 mg glycosylated rpro-UK over 60 or 90 mins; the 90-min angiogram showed a mean patency rate of 76%. In a further 31 patients, the administration of 80 mg resulted in patency rates of 59% at 60 min and 71% at 90 min.

Fibrin Specificity Is Dose-Related

An important finding in the dose-ranging trials was the observation of the gradual loss of fibrin specificity with increasing doses of pro-UK. The relative fibrin specificity of pro-UK, which had been demonstrated in animal studies,[7] was initially confirmed in humans by Trubestein et al.,[38] who compared 500,000 IU pro-UK with 500,000 IU UK, given intravenously over a 4-min period to 6 healthy subjects. There was only a slight decrease in plasminogen and α_2-antiplasmin levels and a minor elevation in fibrin (ogen) degradation products (FDPs) following pro-UK administration, indicating little systemic activation of the fibrinolytic system. In contrast, following UK administration, there was clear evidence of a systemic lytic state, as evidenced by marked decreases in plasminogen and α_2-antiplasmin levels and significant elevations in FDP levels.

In acute myocardial infarction, when the total dose did not exceed 48 mg, the fibrinogen drop

was limited to 25% of baseline values, and plasminogen consumption remained moderate, with nadir posttreatment values between 30% and 40% of baseline levels.[28,31,33]

Conversely, when doses between 70 and 80 mg were administered, the drop in fibrinogen and plasminogen levels tended to be more severe, resulting in a systemic lytic state.[28,36] In the PRIMI trial, where patients randomized to rpro-UK received 80 mg (20 mg as a bolus and 60 mg as an infusion) over 60 min, fibrinogen values dropped to 44% of baseline values (Fig. 10-3).

Preactivation Hastens Clot Lysis

In an attempt to identify an effective treatment regimen while preserving the relative fibrin specificity of pro-UK, several authors studied the effects of "preactivation" of pro-UK with a small, nonlytic dose of urokinase (200,000 to 250,000 IU). This regimen was based on animal studies which showed that pro-UK had a "lag phase" prior to effective lysis which could be overcome by prior administration of t-PA or urokinase in small doses as the "preactivator."[39]

Bode et al.[36] compared 48 mg pro-UK preactivated with 250,000 IU urokinase to 74 mg as monotherapy administered in 60 min to 40 patients with acute myocardial infarction. Sixty-minute patency rates were 55% in the mono-

FIGURE 10-3. Fibrinogen levels in patients entered into the PRIMI study showing the significant drop in those patients who received 80 mg of pro-UK. As expected, the fibrinogen level was significantly lower in the streptokinase group.

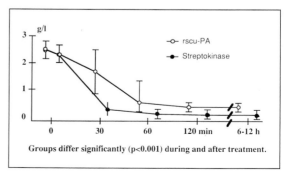

Groups differ significantly (p<0.001) during and after treatment.

therapy group, compared with 65% in the preactivated therapy group. Fibrinogen dropped to 58% of baseline values in the monotherapy group, compared with only 76% in the combined therapy group (see Table 10-2, groups II and III). Similar observations were made by Gurewich,[40] Loscalzo et al.,[32] and Gulba et al.,[30] using urokinase as the activator. In a series of 9 patients, Collen et al.[41] studied the effects of the combined administration of 10 mg rt-PA and 10 mg pro-UK IV over 1 h on coronary reperfusion and the fibrinolytic system. Activation with rt-PA produced complete recanalization in 7 patients and transient recanalization in 1. The fibrinogen level remained unchanged, and no fibrin(ogen) degradation products were generated.

Prourokinase and Reocclusion

One of the salient features of pro-UK appears to be the low incidence of reocclusion/reinfarction following successful thrombolysis. In the PRIMI trial,[36] reocclusion at 24 to 36 h occurred in less than 1% (1 of 108) in the absence of angioplasty, while the incidence was 4.8% (5 of 105) in the streptokinase group. Weaver et al.[37] reported a reocclusion rate of 1.5% in 64 patients who were restudied at 24 h.

These data suggest that the reocclusion rate following thrombolysis with pro-UK may be substantially lower than following t-PA administration. In a meta-analysis on 1173 patients with patent coronary arteries at acute angiography and comparing t-PA with either streptokinase, anistreplase, or urokinase, Granger et al.[42] found reocclusion rates of 13.5% (95% CI 11 to 16%) for t-PA and a combined mean incidence of reocclusion of 8% (95% CI 3 to 10%) for the non-fibrin-specific agents ($p = 0.002$). These data suggest that the anticoagulant effect of FDPs generated as a result of the plasmin-fueled conversion of pro-UK to urokinase may partly protect the coronary artery from acute reocclusion. More recently, it was noted that about 20% of the endogenous pro-UK in normal blood is inside platelets and that when exogenous pro-UK is added, a significant portion is further incorporated into platelets and persists there.[43] This property may give pro-UK a prolonged thrombolytic effect at a reduced level, but sufficient to minimize acute reocclusion.

To date, the largest report of patients with acute myocardial infarction treated with recombinant, nonglycosylated pro-UK includes 1197 patients treated within 6 h of onset of symptoms. Approximately 80% of these patients were on concurrent heparin therapy. Overall, the reported 90-min patency rate was 72%. In-hospital mortality was 4.9%, hemorrhagic stroke occurred in 0.7%, and severe bleeding complications occurred in 3.1%.[44]

SUMMARY

In summary, prourokinase is a relatively fibrin specific zymogen. Preliminary clinical data in patients with acute myocardial infarction indicate that the compound achieves coronary reperfusion rates which compare favorably with t-PA, while reocclusion rates appear to be lower than rates reported following thrombolysis with t-PA.[43]

Severe bleeding complications seem to be confined to currently accepted ranges in the treatment of patients with acute myocardial infarction. Whether pro-UK confers a survival advantage over other available thrombolytic agents will have to be determined in adequately designed mortality trials.

REFERENCES

1. Nolli ML, Sarubbi E, Corti A, et al. Production and characterization of human recombinant single chain urokinase type plasminogen activator from mouse cells. Fibrinolysis 1989;3:101.
2. DeMunk GAW, Rijken DC. Fibrinolytic properties of single chain urokinase type plasminogen activator (prourokinase). Fibrinolysis 1990;4:1.
3. Patthy L, Texler M, Vali Z, et al. Kringles: modules specialized for protein binding. Homology of the gelatin binding region of fibronectin with the kringle structures of proteins. FEBS Lett 1984; 171:131.
4. Lijnen HR, Zamarron C, Blaber M, et al. Activation of plasminogen by pro-urokinase: I. Mechanism. J Biol Chem 1986;261:1253.
5. Gurewich V. Pro-urokinase, an experimental

thrombolytic. In: Anderson JL, ed. Modern management of acute myocardial infarction in the community hospital. New York: Marcel Dekker, 1991:289.

6. Gurewich V, Pannell R. The fibrin specificity of single chain urokinase (sc-UK) induced proteolysis is not dependent on fibrin binding. Thromb Haemost 1986;50:386.

7. Gurewich V, Pannell R, Louis S, et al. Effective and fibrin-specific clot lysis by a zymogen precursor form of urokinase (pro-urokinase): a study in vitro and in two animal species. J Clin Invest 1984;73:1731–1739.

8. Van de Werf F, Nobuhara M, Collen D. Coronary thrombolysis with human single chain urokinase type plasminogen activator (pro-urokinase) in patients with acute myocardial infarction. Ann Intern Med 1986;104:345.

9. Pannell R, Gurewich V. The activation of plasminogen by single chain urokinase or by two-chain urokinase—a demonstration that single chain urokinase has a low catalytic activity (pro-urokinase). Blood 1987;69:22.

10. Petersen LC, Lund LR, Dano K, et al. One chain urokinase type plasminogen activator from human sarcoma cells is a proenzyme with little or no intrinsic activity. J Biol Chem 1988;111:89.

11. Gurewich V. Characterization and thrombolytic properties of pro-urokinase. In: Verstraete M, Collen D, eds. Thrombolysis: biological and therapeutic properties of new thrombolytic agents. London: Churchill Livingstone 1985:92.

12. Gurewich V, Pannell R, Broeze RJ, Mao J-I. Characterization of the intrinsic fibrinolytic properties of pro-urokinase through a study of plasmin resistant mutant forms produced by site specific mutagenesis of lysine-158. J Clin Invest 1988;82:1956.

13. Lijnen HR, Van Hoef B, DeCock F, Collen D. The mechanism of plasminogen activation and fibrin dissolution by single chain urokinase-type plasminogen activator in a plasma milieu in vitro. Blood 1989;73:1864.

14. Pannell R, Gurewich V. Activation of plasminogen by single chain urokinase or by two chain urokinase—a demonstration that single chain urokinase has a low catalytic activity (pro-urokinase). Blood 1987;69:22.

15. Petersen L, Lund L, Nielsen L, et al. One-chain urokinase type plasminogen activator from human sarcoma cells is a proenzyme with little or no intrinsic activity. J. Biol Chem 1988;263:11189.

16. Niewiarowski S, Senyi AF, Gillies P. Plasmin induced platelet aggregation and platelet release reaction: effects on hemostasis. J Clin Invest 1973;52:1647.

17. Chesterman CN, Allington AJ, Sharp AA. Relationship of plasminogen activator to fibrin. Nature 1972;238:15.

18. Pannell R, Gurewich V. Pro-urokinase: a study of its stability in plasma and a mechanism for its selective fibrinolytic effect. Blood 1986;67:1215.

19. Pannell R, Angles-Cano E, Gurewich V. The pH dependence of the binding of pro-urokinase to fibrin-celite. Thromb Haemost 1990;64:556.

20. Gurewich V, Pannell R. A comparative study of the efficacy and specificity of tissue plasminogen activator and pro-urokinase: demonstration of synergism and of different thresholds of nonselectivity. Thromb Res 1986;44:217.

21. Violand BN, Sodetz JM, Castellino FJ. The effect of epsilon aminocaproic acid on the gross conformation of plasminogen and plasmin. Arch Biochem Biophys 1975;170:300.

22. Pannell R, Black J, Gurewich V. The complementary modes of action of tissue plasminogen activator (t-PA) and pro-urokinase (pro-UK) by which their synergistic effect on clot lysis may be explained. J Clin Invest 1988;81:853.

23. Liu J, Pannell R, Gurewich V. A transitional state of pro-urokinase that has a higher catalytic efficiency against Glu-plasminogen than urokinase. J Biol Chem 1992;267(22):15289.

24. Nieuwenhuizen W, Vermond A, Voskuilen M, et al. Identification of a site in fibrin(ogen) which is involved in the acceleration of plasminogen activation by tissue plasminogen activator. Biochem Biophys Acta 1983;748:86.

25. Nieuwenhuizen W, Voskuilen M, Vermond A, et al. Lysine residue A-157 of fibrinogen plays a crucial role in the acceleration of the plasminogen activation by tissue plasminogen activator (t-PA) (abstract). Fibrinolysis 1986;1(suppl 1):9.

26. Gurewich V. The sequential, complementary and synergistic activation of fibrin-bound plasminogen by tissue plasminogen activator and pro-urokinase. Fibrinolysis 1989;3:59.

27. Gurewich V. Experiences with pro-urokinase and potentiation of its fibrinolytic effect by urokinase and by tissue plasminogen activator. J Am Coll Cardiol 1987;10:16B.

28. Bode C, Schoenermark S, Schuller G, et al. Efficacy of intravenous prourokinase and a combination of prourokinase and urokinase in acute myocardial infarction. Am J Cardiol 1988;61:971.

29. Fareed J, Walenga J, Hoppensteadt D, Messmore H. Studies on the profibrinolytic action of heparin and its fractions. Semin Thromb Haemost 1985;11:199.

30. Gulba DC, Fischer K, Barthels M, et al. Potentative effect of heparin in thrombolytic therapy of evolving myocardial infarction with natural prourokinase. Fibrinolysis 1989;3:165.

31. Kasper W, Meinertz T, Hohnloser S, et al. Coronary thrombolysis in man with prourokinase: improved efficacy with low dose urokinase. Klin Wochenschr 1988;66(suppl XII):109.

32. Loscalzo J, Wharton TP, Kirschenbaum JM, et al. Clot-selective coronary thrombolysis with prourokinase. Circulation 1989;79:776.

33. Van de Werf F, Vanhaecke J, De Geest H, et al. Coronary thrombolysis with recombinant single-chain urokinase-type plasminogen activator in patients with acute myocardial infarction. Circulation 1986;74:1066.

34. Diefenbach C, Erbel R, Pop T, et al. Recombinant single-chain urokinase-type plasminogen activator during acute myocardial infarction. Am J Cardiol 1988;61:966.

35. The TIMI Study Group. The thrombolysis in myocardial infarction trial: phase I findings. N Engl J Med 1985;312:932.

36. PRIMI Trial Study Group. Randomized double-blind trial of recombinant prourokinase against streptokinase in acute myocardial infarction. Lancet 1989;22:863.

37. Weaver WD, Hartman JK, Reddy PS, Anderson J. Prourokinase achieves rapid and sustained patency for treatment of acute myocardial infarction (abstract). J Am Coll Cardiol 1993;21:397A.

38. Trubestein G, Popov S, Wolf H, Welzel D. Effects of prourokinase and urokinase on the fibrinolytic system in man. Haemostasis 1987;17:238.

39. Collen D, Stassen JM, Stump DC, Verstraete M. In vivo synergism of thrombolytic agents. Circulation 1986;74:838.

40. Gurewich V. Experiences with prourokinase and potentiation of its fibrinolytic effect by urokinase and by tissue plasminogen activator. J Am Coll Cardiol 1987;10:16B.

41. Collen D, Van de Werf F. Coronary arterial thrombolysis with low-dose synergistic combinations of recombinant tissue-type plasminogen activator (rt-PA) and recombinant single-chain urokinase-type plasminogen activator (rscu-PA) for acute myocardial infarction. Am J Cardiol 1987;60:431.

42. Granger CB, Califf RM, Topol EJ. Thrombolytic therapy for acute myocardial infarction. Drugs 1992;44:293.

43. Gurewich V, Johnstone M, Loza JP, Pannell R. Pro-urokinase and prekallikrein are both associated with platelets: implications for the intrinsic pathway of fibrinolysis and for therapeutic thrombolysis. FEBS Lett 1993;318:317.

44. Vermeer F, Massberg I, Meyer J, et al. Saruplase, a new fibrin specific lytic agent: efficacy and safety data on 1200 patients (abstract). Eur Heart J 1991;12:29.

Anthony J. Comerota (Ed.). *Thrombolytic Therapy for Peripheral Vascular Disease.* Copyright © 1995 J. B. Lippincott Company.

11

CURRENT THROMBOLYTIC AGENTS: COMPARATIVE ANALYSIS

William R. Bell

The efficacy of thrombolytic therapy depends on the capacity of the thrombolytic agent to interact with and activate the human fibrinolytic system. The components of the fibrinolytic system—the plasminogen-plasmin proteolytic enzyme system—include proactivator, activator, plasminogen, and plasmin. The end product of this system, plasmin, is a nonspecific proteolytic enzyme that will interact with, degrade, and digest any proteinaceous material containing an arginyl-lysyl amino acid sequence. The therapeutic strategy with the various thrombolytic agents is to convert the inert single-chain 791 amino acid plasminogen molecule, with a molecular mass of 92 K Daltons, to the two-chain plasmin molecule (a heavy chain and a light chain). In the light-chain moiety of the molecule there occurs the formation of a proteolytic center at serine 740. It is this serine center that confers on this plasmin molecule the property of proteolysis. All known thrombolytic agents function by promoting this conversion from the single-chain to the two-chain structure by the introduction of the enzymatic clip at the 560–561 amino acid (Arg-Val) address in the plasminogen molecule.

There are different pathways within the human body whereby plasminogen can be converted to plasmin. In the intrinsic pathway, which is comprised of components that normally circulate in the blood, high- and low-molecular-weight kininogen, kallikrein, and components of the complement and coagulation systems can interact and generate plasmin. Also, in the extrinsic system, consisting of components not present in circulating blood but found intracellularly, in the extravascular compartment, vascular endothelial cells (tissue plasminogen activator), renal parenchymal cells (urokinase), pulmonary parenchymal cells (tissue factor), and pancreatic acinar cells (chymotrypsin) can migrate into circulating blood, take on activator status, and promote plasminogen to plasmin. Although these two pathways can result in activation of the human fibrinolytic system, the quantity of plasmin generated by either or both pathways is inadequate to satisfactorily induce resolution of pathologic thrombus formation. Utilization of the exogenous pathways by obtaining both endogenous compounds (urokinase, tissue plasminogen activator) and exogenous compounds (streptokinase, staphylokinase) in sufficient quantities, in purified form, and in a controlled manner and infusing them into the vascular compartment can directly induce activation of the fibrinolytic system sufficient in magnitude to induce dissolution and resolution of intravascular thrombi and emboli.

PLASMINOGEN

The central component of the fibrinolytic system, plasminogen, is a 791 amino acid single-chain structure with a molecular mass of 92 K Daltons synthesized by hepatocytes. Plasminogen is the circulating zymogen which, upon activation, yields the fibrinolytic enzyme plasmin. The major production site of plasminogen, like most other plasma proteins, is the liver.[1,2]

The plasma concentration of plasminogen in adult humans remains constant at approximately 200 µg/mL, or 2.2 µM.[3] The plasma concentration varies depending on the assay technique employed, but with most technique currently employed, the plasma concentration ranges between 6 and 11.0 mg/dL. Native plasminogen has a plasma half-life of about 2 days and disappears primarily through catabolic degradation rather than conversion to plasmin or intravascular consumption.[4]

Plasminogen is inherited as two codominant autosomal alleles.[5,6] Fetal synthesis and absence of transplacental passage have been demonstrated.[6] In newborns, there is both a decrease in plasma-plasminogen concentration[3] and a decrease in functional plasminogen activity suggestive of a fetal dysfunctional plasminogen molecule.[7] Several hereditary dysfunctional plasminogen molecules have been described in adults with recurrent thromboembolic disease.[8-10] The defects in these molecules include abnormal sites, impaired activator binding, and defective activation.

The isolation of human plasminogen has demonstrated a remarkable degree of microheterogeneity of the molecule. Plasminogen is usually purified from serum or plasma using the technique of affinity chromatography first described by Deutsch and Mertz in 1970.[11] Plasminogen is absorbed onto a column of lysine-sepharose and eluted with ε-aminocaproic acid. Using this technique, two plasminogen variants having different amino termini have been isolated: a "native" form containing glutamine at its NH₂ terminus (Glu-plasminogen)[12-14] and a "modified" form containing lysine at its NH₂ terminus (Lys-plasminogen).[15] The modified Lys-plasminogen has been shown to be a partial degradation product of native Glu-plasminogen that is formed during the isolation process by contaminating plasmin.[16] The lysine residue at the amino terminus of Lys-plasminogen corresponds to Lys_{77} in the amino acid sequence of Glu-plasminogen.[17] The properties of Lys-plasminogen and Glu-plasminogen differ markedly. The plasma half-life of Glu-plasminogen is 2 days, while the half-life of Lys-plasminogen is 0.8 day.[18]

Additional isolation techniques can separate plasminogen into many microheterogeneous forms. Using either polyacrylamide gel electrophoresis at acidic pH[19] or affinity chromatography,[20] two different forms of plasminogen, type 1 and type 2, can be distinguished. Polyacrylamide gel electrophoresis at alkaline pH further separates plasminogen types 1 and 2 into at least five subtypes.[14] Using isoelectric focusing, Gly-plasminogen can be further separated into four isoelectric forms with isoelectric points ranging from 6.2 to 6.6. Lys-plasminogen can be further separated into five isoelectric forms with isoelectric points from 6.7 to 8.5.[21]

Isolation of native human plasminogen also has led to determination of its molecular structure and biochemical properties. The plasminogen molecule is a single-chain glycoprotein having a molecular weight of between 83,000 and 93,000 and the electrophoretic mobility of a β-globulin.[22] The primary amino acid sequence of the molecule has been elucidated by Wiman[23] and Magnusson et al.[24] It is 790 amino acids long, with glutamine at its amino terminus and asparagine at its carboxy terminus. There are a total of 48 cysteine residues forming 24 disulfide bridges. Sixteen of these bridges are located in five oblate elipsoid looped structures known as *kringles*. These structures, numbered K1 through K5, contain about 80 residues each and are held together by triple disulfide bonds.[25] Homologous kringles can be found in the nonthrombin part of the prothrombin molecule.[26,27]

The carbohydrate portion of plasminogen, which comprises about 2% of the molecule,[24] accounts, at least in part, for its microheterogeneity. Plasminogen type 1 contains two oligosaccharide side chains, a glucosamine-based chain at Asn_{288} and a galactosamine-based chain at Thr_{345}. Plasminogen type 2, however, contains only the single galactosamine-based chain at Thr_{345}. In addition, the proportion of various sugars differs between the two types: Type 1 contains more sialic acid, galactose, mannose, and N-acetylglucosamine than type 2.[28]

The secondary structure of the plasminogen molecule, as determined by circular dichroism spectra, is 80% random coil, 20% beta structure, and 0% alpha helix.[29] Electron microscopy has demonstrated the tertiary structure of plasminogen to be a 22- to 24-nm-long spiral filament with a diameter of 2.2 to 2.4 nm.[30]

PLASMIN

The conversion of plasminogen to plasmin by plasminogen activators is accomplished by proteolytic cleavage of a single bond, Arg_{560}-Val_{561}. Two chains are thus formed. The A, or heavy, chain is derived from the NH_2 terminus of plasminogen, while the B, or light, chain originates from the COOH terminus. The molecular weights of the A and B chains are 65,000 and 25,000, respectively.[31,32] The A chain has only one isoelectric form (pH 4.9), while the B chain has three isoelectric forms ranging between pH 5.8 and 6.0. The A and B chains are connected by two disulfide bridges at Cys_{547}-Cys_{665} and Cys_{557}-Cys_{565}. The Cys_{547}-Cys_{665} bond is homologous to the interchain disulfide bonds of chymotrypsin, thrombin, and factor X.[25] The activator-sensitive Arg_{560}-Val_{561} bond is located within the Cys_{557}-Cys_{665} disulfide bridge, which is unique to plasmin and appears to facilitate the interaction between activator and cleavage sites.[25,28]

Although the precise mechanism of plasminogen activation is unknown, three major theories have developed based on studies of the in vitro activation of native human plasminogen. Activation of native Glu-plasminogen in the absence of any plasmin inhibitor yields Lys_{77}-plasmin plus the so-called preactivation peptides (PAPs) formed by cleavage at Lys_{62}-Ser_{63}, Arg_{67}-Met_{68}, or Lys_{76}-Lys_{77}.[33,34] Wiman and Wallen[35] propose, therefore, that activation takes place by a two-step mechanism in which both the release of the PAPs from the NH_2 terminal of Glu-plasminogen and the subsequent cleavage of the Arg_{560}-Val_{561} bond are catalyzed by the activator. Robbins and coworkers[36] showed, however, that when aprotinin, a synthetic plasmin inhibitor, is present to prevent any plasmic autodigestion, Glu-plasmin is the final end product.[36] They thus favor a one-step transformation of Glu-plasminogen to Glu-plasmin. Subsequent PAP fragment removal could occur by excess plasmic autodigestion. Finally, Violand and Castellino[37] proposed that the PAPs are first released by plasmic autodigestion to form the intermediate Lys_{77}-plasminogen, which is subsequently cleaved by activator at the Arg_{560}-Val_{561} bond to form Lys_{77}-plasmin. This pathway is, because of the precise and thoughtful design of the studies performed, correct and demonstrates that the PAPs do not occur before the generation of plasmin. The three possible mechanisms of plasmin formation are summarized in Figure 11-1.

The plasminogen molecule contains several sites which specifically bind a number of antifibrinolytic amino acids, such as lysine ε-aminocaproic acid (EACA). These sites are known as *lysine binding sites* (LBSs) and are localized mainly to the A, or heavy, chain of the molecule, the location of five kringles (K)[38,39] (Fig. 11-2). One is located in K4 and at least one more is in K1 through K3. One LBS, which is believed to reside in K1,[40] has a stronger affinity for EACA, while the others have weaker affinity.[41] The LBSs are important for the interaction of plasminogen with several components of the endogenous fibrinolytic system.

The weak LBSs are involved in the interaction of plasminogen with plasminogen activators. Both loss of the preactivation peptides from Glu-plasminogen and binding of the antifibrinolytic amino acids cause a conformational change in the plasminogen molecule which makes the Arg_{560}-Val_{561} bond more easily accessible for cleavage by

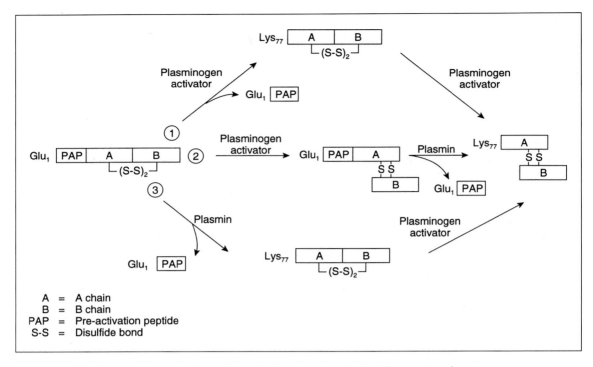

FIGURE 11-1. Three possible mechanisms of plasmin formation. Reprinted with permission from Baxter Diagnostics, Inc.

activator.[42,43] Kinetic data on the activation of both native Glu-plasminogen and modified Lys-plasminogen are consistent with facilitation of activation by removal of the PAP. Although the Michaelis constants for both forms are similar (K_m = 23 mM for Glu-plasminogen and K_m = 40 mM for Lys-plasminogen), the catalytic constant is 10 times greater for Lys-plasminogen (0.26 s^{-1} versus 2.6 s^{-1}).[44,45]

The high-affinity LBS, on the other hand, is involved in plasminogen's interaction with fibrin,[39,40,46,47] α_2-antiplasmin,[48] and a plasmin inhibitor called *histidine-rich glycoprotein*.[49] It has been observed that plasminogen activation takes place on the surface of fibrin and that α_2-antiplasmin competitively inhibits the plasminogen-fibrin interaction at the high-affinity LBS.[48]

The B, or light, chain of plasmin contains the proteolytic active site of the molecule and is ho-

mologous in both structure and mode of action to other proteases, including thrombin, factor Xa, and the pancreatic proteases.[50] The active center is formed by three amino acid residues, His$_{602}$, Asp$_{645}$, and Ser$_{740}$.[51,52] The serine residue is sensitive to diisopropyl fluorophosphate (DFP), while the histidine residue is sensitive to tosyl lysine chloromethyl ketone (TLCK).[53] Plasmin functions as an endopeptidase with an optimal pH of about 7.0.[54] It acts specifically as a serine protease, cleaving only synthetic esters and amides of lysine and arginine and peptide bonds having either lysine or arginine on the carboxyl side[55] of the molecule.

The kinetic data for the action of plasmin on different substrates under various conditions have been summarized. The Michaelis constant (K_m) varies between 10 and 1000 mM and the catalytic constant (k_{cat}) between 1 and 75 s^{-1}.[22]

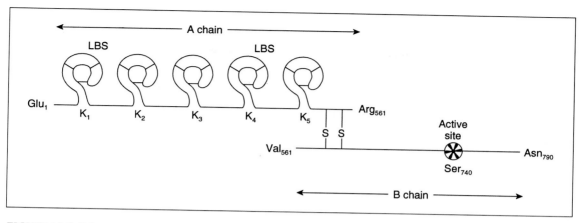

FIGURE 11-2. *Schematic representation of the plasmin molecule. The A and B chains are held together by two disulfide bridges. The five kringles are all located on the A chain and contain the lysine binding sites (LBSs). The active site of the plasmin molecule is located on the B chain and is responsible for plasmin's proteolytic activity. Reprinted with permission from Baxter Diagnostics, Inc.*

THROMBOLYTIC AGENTS

Streptokinase (SK)

Therapeutic utilization and enhancement of the fibrinolytic system was made possible in 1933 by Tillet and Garner,[56] who first described the exogenous plasminogen activator isolated from β-hemolytic streptococci. This activator subsequently was named *streptokinase* by Christensen and MacLeod[57] in 1945 and was found to react stoichiometrically with human plasminogen by Ratnoff[58] in 1948. Further work by Sherry and colleagues[59,60] and Johnson and McCarty[61] resulted in the introduction of streptokinase for thrombolytic purposes.

Streptokinase is a single-chain glycoprotein having a molecular weight of 45,000 to 50,000 and a very low carbohydrate content.[62,63] Primary structure determination reveals isoleucine at the amino terminus, lysine at the carboxyl terminus, and the absence of any intrachain disulfide bridges.[64] The secondary structure is mainly random coil, with only about 10% alpha helix.[62,63] Streptokinase has one major isoelectric point at pH 4.7.[61,65]

Unlike the other known activators of the plasminogen-plasmin system, streptokinase is not an enzyme. This compound within this complex is transformed into an activated plasminogen possessing a proteolytic active serine site.[66,67] The streptokinase-plasminogen activator complex is then able to cleave the Arg_{560}-Val_{561} "activator bond," converting both complexed and free plasminogen to plasmin. The streptokinase-plasmin complex thus formed also acts as an activator.[68,69]

While plasminogen is being converted to plasmin, the streptokinase molecule within the activator complex undergoes proteolytic degradation. Streptokinase fragments ranging in size from 40,000 to 10,000 Da are formed,[70,71] all of which retain some degree of activator activity.[72]

Streptokinase interacts with various forms of the plasmin(ogen) molecule, including Glu-plasminogen, Lys_{77}-plasminogen, Val_{442}-plasminogen, and the beta chain of plasmin.[73] In vitro studies show that activity of the activator complex varies with both the size of the streptokinase fragment and the form of plasmin(ogen) within the complex.[74-77] The amount of activator activity is proportional to the size of the streptokinase fragment and inversely proportional to the form of plasmin(ogen), with the streptokinase–beta chain complex having the highest degree of activator activity.

In vivo, the situation is more complex. The binding of the fibrinogen degradation product fragments Y and B to plasminogen enhances the interaction with streptokinase.[78] In addition, the binding of plasminogen to streptokinase prevents inhibition by α_2-antiplasmin. The plasmin-streptokinase complex is 10^5 times less reactive toward α_2-antiplasmin than plasmin itself.[78]

Since streptokinase is not produced by human tissue, it is antigenic and can induce the production of antistreptokinase antibodies. The metabolism and excretion of streptokinase are unclear because its clearance rate depends on the availability of plasminogen substrate. In the human body, two half-lives have been identified.[79] The first is 18 minutes and represents clearance after binding with antibodies or inhibitors (representing about 80% to 85% of a single dose given intravenously), and a second half-life is approximately 83 minutes (representing about 10% to 15% of an administered dose).

Urokinase (UK)

In the 1950s, febrile reactions associated with streptokinase prompted the search for another thrombolytic agent. Human urine was known to contain a fibrinolytic agent.[80] This agent was identified as a plasminogen activator by Williams[81] in 1951 and subsequently was named *urokinase* by Sobel and colleagues[82] in 1952. Major advances in the purification of urokinase from human urine were made by Plough and Kjeldgaard[83] and Lesuk et al.[84] Detailed studies by Sherry and coworkers[59,85] on the physicochemical properties of urokinase implemented its introduction for therapeutic purposes.

Purification of urokinase, the first tissue (from renal parenchymal cells) plasminogen activating agent, has revealed several forms of varying molecular weights.[86,87] The two major species are a 54,000-Da high-molecular-weight (HMW) form and a 33,000-Da low-molecular-weight (LMW) form, both having similar plasminogen activating activity.[88] The HMW form is the native form of the molecule and is probably degraded to the LMW form through limited proteolysis by either autodigestion or other proteases found in the urine.[89,90]

High-molecular-weight urokinase is a glycoprotein consisting of two polypeptide chains (33,000 and 18,000 Da) connected by disulfide bonds.[91,92] The molecule contains 6% carbohydrate, mainly mannose, N-acetylglucosamine, and N-acetylneuraminic acid.[93] The 33,000-Da chain contains the serine active site.[94,95] There is one major isoelectric form of HMW urokinase at pH 8.6 and three LMW forms at pH 8.35, 8.6, and 8.7.[96]

Urokinase is a serine protease[97] that hydrolyzes synthetic esters containing arginine and lysine.[98] Unlike streptokinase, urokinase directly activates plasminogen by cleaving the Arg_{560}-Val_{561} "activation bond."

Although kinetic data comparing the two forms of urokinase are essentially the same,[77] the HMW form appears to have a greater thrombolytic effect.[97] The fibrinogen degradation products X, Y, D, and E all enhance urokinase activity by binding to plasminogen.[78] Specific urokinase inhibitors have been isolated from human plasma[100,101] and human placenta.[102]

Urokinase is distinguished from extrinsic plasminogen activator both immunochemically[103–106] and by its ability to bind to fibrin.[107–109] The ability of human kidney cells in tissue culture to produce urokinase[110,111] indicates that urokinase is probably synthesized by the kidney. Plasminogen activators immunochemically identical to urokinase, however, also have been isolated from normal heart tissue[112] and human plasma,[113–115] as well as from several human malignant neoplasms grown in tissue culture, including ovary,[116] pancreas,[117] lung,[118] and breast.[119] The plasma half-life of urokinase is approximately 15 minutes.[79]

Since normal human urine contains only a small amount of urokinase (a few micrograms per milliliter), about 1500 L of urine is required to produce enough urokinase for a single thrombolytic treatment for one patient.[115] Fortunately, methods of producing large quantities of urokinase from human fetal kidney cell culture have been developed.[110,120] Both urinary and tissue culture urokinase are available for clinical use and are biochemically similar in producing a fibrinolytic state.[121] Recently, recombinant DNA techniques with *E. coli* have resulted in the preparation of this agent.[122] This may be the future source of urokinase.

Tissue Plasminogen Activator (t-PA)

Human t-PA is endogenously synthesized and secreted by vascular endothelial cells as a glycosylated protein of 68,000 Da and under regulation of a gene located one chromosome 8. Tissue plasminogen activator as it is released by the endothelial cell is 562 amino acids in a single chain and organized into five discrete domains linked in various locations by 17 disulfide bridges initiated by an amino terminus and ending with a carboxy terminus.[123] From the amino terminus inward, residues 4 to 50 possess homology with fibronectin and together are called the *finger domain*. Residues 51 to 87 share homology with the precursor of epidermal growth factor, also found in urokinase, protein C, coagulation factors IX and X, and the receptor for low-density lipoprotein. Residues 88 to 175 and 176 to 263 form two sequential kringle domains each with 3 disulfide linkages. These kringle domains are also found in urokinase, prourokinase, Factor XIII, vampire bat plasminogen activator, prothrombin, hepatocyte growth factor, plasminogen, and apolipoprotein-A. From residue 264 to residue 562 is the catalytic portion of the molecule containing the triad of histidine, asparagine, and serine. The recombinant molecule (rt-PA) employed therapeutically is 527 amino acids in length and is morphologically different from the naturally occurring molecule with respect to spatial arrangement of the kringle domains. Binding of the rt-PA to fibrin (in vitro) is mediated via the finger and second kringle domains. Activation of the rt-PA molecule takes place when Arg_{275}-Ile_{276} is cleaved. When activated, it now can activate its substrate plasminogen at the identical site acted on by SK and UK.

Prourokinase (Single-Chain Urokinase Plasminogen Activator)

Single-chain urokinase plasminogen activator (scu-PA) is a single-chain glycoprotein containing 411 amino acids with 24 cysteine residues with a molecular weight of 54,000.[124,125] After limited hydrolysis by plasmin or kallikrein of the Lys_{157}-

Ile_{159} peptide bond, the molecule is converted to a two-chain derivative whose catalytic center is located in the C-terminal chain and is composed of His_{204}, Asx_{255}, and Ser_{356}. The N-terminal chain contains domains homologous to epidermal growth factor and one region homologous to the plasminogen kringles. Single-chain urokinase plasminogen activator has a very low reactivity toward low-molecular-weight synthetic substrates that are negative toward urokinase. Recent studies have indicated that scu-PA does not directly bind to fibrin and is degraded to urokinase before it can activate plasminogen to plasmin.[126,127]

Anisoylated Lys-Plasminogen–Streptokinase Activator Complex (APSAC)

APSAC, *p*-anisoylated or acylated Lys-plasminogen streptokinase activator complex (anistreplase, Eminase), is a 1:1 stoichiometric inert complex of streptokinase with plasminogen in which the active serine center is protected by a *p*-anisoyl (acyl) group placed directly on Ser_{740} of the plasminogen molecule. The acylation process is performed with methodology so as not to alter or disturb the five convex discoid kringle structures on the opposite side of the molecule.[128] These five kringle structures are critical because they possess the lysine binding sites necessary for the binding of this compound to fibrin strands. When this complex, with a molecular weight of 131,000, is placed in an aqueous phase, deacylation occurs by simple ester hydrolysis, which follows pseudo-first-order kinetics in a temperature-dependent manner. Products of the deacylation reaction are *p*-anisic acid and the free Lys-plasminogen–streptokinase complex in equimolar quantities. Deacylation occurs at approximately equal rates in the free plasma and when bound to a fibrin clot. The free activator complex displays potent enzymatic activity in prompting the formation of the active fibrinolytic enzyme plasmin from its proenzyme plasminogen. The biologic half-life in the circulation varies between 40 and 90 minutes, and some metabolites may be present for close to 24 hours. The biologic activity of APSAC is expressed in units selected in a manner

TABLE 11-1. *Properties of Thrombolytic Agents*

	SK	UK	rt-PA	APSAC	Plasminogen
Source	Streptococcal culture	Heterologous mammalian tissue culture	Heterologous mammalian tissue culture	Streptococcal culture	Human hepatocytes
Molecular weight	47,000	32,000–54,000	70,000	131,000	92,000
Type of agent	Bacterial proactivator	Tissue plasminogen activator	Tissue plasminogen activator	Bacterial proactivator	Plasma substrate
Plasma clearance, min	12–18	15–20	2–6	40–60	53 h
Fibrinolytic activation	Systemic	Systemic	Systemic	Systemic	—
Fibrin binding	Minimal	Moderate	Moderate	Minimal	—
Antigenic	Yes	No	No	Yes	—
Allergic reactions	Yes	No	No	Yes	—
Gene (kb)	—	6.4	36.6	—	30
Chromosome location	—	10	8	—	6

where 1 mg of the compound equals 1 unit. The commonly employed clinical dose of 30 units of APSAC approximates 1.1 million units of streptokinase.[129,130]

The properties of the commercially available thrombolytic agents are listed in Table 11-1.

ALTERATIONS IN CIRCULATING BLOOD PROTEINS BY THROMBOLYTIC AGENTS

When the first-generation thrombolytic agents urokinase (UK) and streptokinase (SK) are administered in the standard doses universally employed to treat pulmonary emboli, deep vein thrombosis (spontaneous or catheter-associated), arterial thrombosis or emboli, or acute myocardial infarction and measurements are made of various circulating plasma proteins before infusion of the agent, at various times during the infusion and again following discontinuation of the infusion the following observations can be made: Plasma fibrinogen progressively declines from time zero, undergoing degradation by generated plasmin to reach nadir low values at between 5 and 7 hours (lower values with SK than observed with UK) at 100 ± 30 mg/dL (mean values). These values remain low for the duration of the infusion and then, following discontinuation of the infusion, progressively increase. Between 36 and 48 hours after discontinuation, the fibrinogen levels are back to baseline normal concentrations. This re-

duction in plasma fibrinogen results from plasmin lysis of the fibrinogen dimer into fragments X, Y, 2D, and E. Both UK and SK in their active forms only in a very minimal and limited way have the capacity to alter fibrinogen in the absence of plasminogen. These agents have almost no affect on plasminogen-free fibrinogen. The degradation products resulting from the lysis of fibrinogen or fibrin actually have the capacity to stimulate the hepatocyte to synthesize fibrinogen. Thus, even during continuation of the thrombolytic agent during the last 6 to 8 hours of the infusion, there can be observed a slight to modest increase in plasma fibrinogen concentration (Fig. 11-3).

Likewise, plasma plasminogen progressively declines in concentration following the institution of SK and UK. This decline is directly related to the conversion of the inert proenzyme plasminogen that circulates in the euglobulin fraction of the blood to the patent nonspecific proteolytic enzyme plasmin. The concentration of plasma plasminogen is considerably lower when SK or any SK-containing compound is being given (since SK must form a 1:1 stoichiometric complex with plasminogen before it has the property to convert plasminogen to plasmin). Thus, in facilitating the SK-plasminogen complex, plasma plasminogen per se is reduced in concentration. Thus, when the SK-plasminogen complex promotes plasminogen to plasmin, the plasminogen concentration is further reduced. When employing

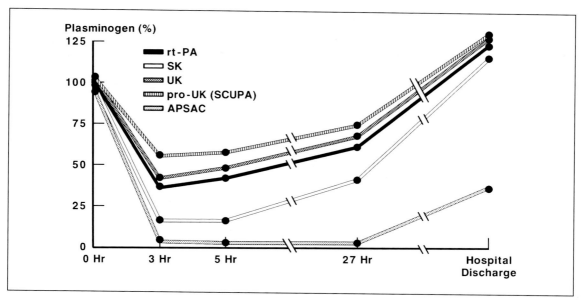

FIGURE 11-3. Mean plasma fibrinogen. Each point plotted is the mean value of fibrinogen determined by a non-rate-dependent thrombin-clottable technique in 2129 patients with SK, 2010 patients with UK, 437 patients with rt-PA, 285 patients with APSAC, and 167 patients with pro-UK.

SK, one must be cautious so as not to deplete the circulating blood of plasminogen, for if this occurs, there will not be sufficient plasminogen from which to generate plasmin. Such a state may indeed lead to the induction of thrombus formation (Fig. 11-4).

Degradation products of fibrinogen or fibrin (FDP) are the absolute index to the activity of the fibrinolytic system in humans. The only known pathway by which the FDPs are present in circulating blood is via the fibrinolytic system in humans. These degradation products result from the digestion of fibrinogen and/or fibrin by plasmin. Thus, when these FDPs reach excessive quantities in the circulating blood, they are easily detected and unequivocally establish intense activation on a systemic level of the plasminogen-plasmin proteolytic enzyme system. When both SK and UK are administered in the standard doses, large quantities of FDPs are detected. The quantity detected associated with SK is considerably greater than that observed when UK is administered (Fig. 11-5).

These data concerning the alterations in fi-brinogen-plasminogen and FDPs observed in the circulating blood following the administration of SK and UK unequivocally establish the presence of systemic activation of the fibrinolytic system.

Since there was considered an association between systemic activation of the fibrinolytic system and bleeding observed during treatment with thrombolytic therapy, emphasis was placed on the identification or design of agents that would activate the fibrinolytic system locally at the site of thrombus formation and therefore not give rise to systemic activation of the fibrinolytic system. As a result of considerable work, a second generation of thrombolytic agents became available and are as follows:

1. Recombinant tissue plasminogen activator (rt-PA)
2. Anisoylated (acylated) plasminogen-streptokinase activator complex (APSAC)
3. Prourokinase (scu-PA)
4. FAB-urokinase
5. FAB-streptokinase
6. FAB–rt-PA

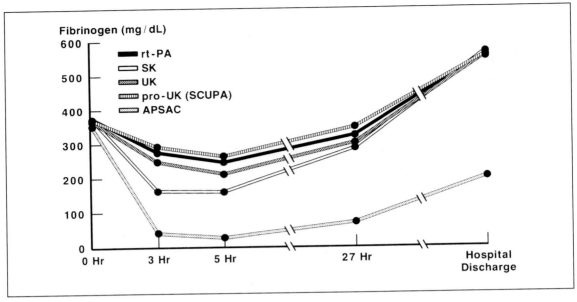

FIGURE 11-4. Mean plasma fibrinogen. Each point plotted is the mean value of plasminogen determined by an immunologic technique in the number of patients for each agent as indicated in Fig. 11-3.

The biochemical properties of rt-PA, APSAC, and scu-PA were described earlier. FAB-urokinase, FAB-streptokinase, and FAB–rt-PA are designated *antibody-directed thrombolytic agents.* The strategy behind the design of these was to prepare a highly purified monospecific monoclonal antibody against human fibrin (that would not interact with fibrinogen). The FAB portion of the whole anti-human fibrinogen IgG is then coupled to the respective thrombolytic agent, UK, SK or rt-PA. When any of these compounds is infused into the circulation, the FAB portion of the IgG molecule should avidly bind to the fibrin network of the thrombus (emboli) and thus transport the thrombolytic agent into the environment of the fibrin net and activate the fibrin-bound plasminogen. In this manner there would not be systemic activation of the plasminogen-plasmin fibrinolytic system, and all thrombi-emboli should undergo local dissolution.

However, to prepare the monospecific antibody against human fibrin, there must be employed a nonhuman species or a nonhuman cell line to generate this antibody (IgG). Thus this foreign IgG, when placed inside the human body, is capable of acting as an antigen and gives rise to an antibody. The antibody produced is a class I antibody that induces complement binding and anaphylactic antigen-antibody interaction, resulting immune complexes in the circulating blood. For these reasons, these antibody-directed thrombolytic agents are not able to be employed in humans at present.

In view of the availability of rt-PA, APSAC, and prourokinase, the data must be examined and the question asked: Are these agents of the second-generation category capable, as initially designed and advertised, of activating the fibrinolytic system only at the site of thrombus formation and thereby not inducing systemic fibrinolysis? Also, it is reasonable to examine whether it is good strategy to design or identify an agent that acts only at the site of thrombus formation? Having studied the activity of newer agents in vivo, is it reasonable to expect a reduction or an elimination of the undesirable problem of bleeding? Are these second-generation thrombolytic agents thrombus-specific, target-specific, or fibrin-specific?

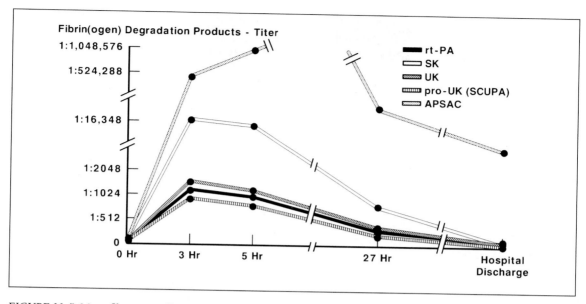

FIGURE 11-5. *Mean fibrinogen–fibrin degradation product titer. Each point plotted is the mean value of FDPs determined by the tanned red cell hemagglutination immunologic inhibition assay in the number of patients for each agent indicated in Fig. 11-3.*

As shown in Figure 11-3, when plasma fibrinogen is quantified, eliminate during the infusion of each of the second-generation thrombolytic agents (each agent is given in the standard dose for treatment of myocardial infarction and infused over a 3-hour interval for rt-PA, 60 minutes for SK and UK, and 5 to 10 minutes for APSAC), there is easily observed a progressive reduction in the plasma fibrinogen concentration. The decline is greatest for APSAC and SK. The degree of decline is very similar for UK, rt-PA, and pro-UK. With APSAC, SK, pro-UK, and UK, the decline in fibrinogen is due to the generation of plasmin and degradation of fibrinogen to fragments X, Y, 2D, and E. In the presence of rt-PA, in addition to the generation of plasmin, rt-PA can directly degrade purified fibrinogen in the absence of plasminogen.[131] If the thrombolytic agents rt-PA, APSAC, or pro-UK were "fibrin-specific" in their action, there would not be any interaction with circulating fibrinogen, but this is not what was found following the institution of these thrombolytic agents.

As is clearly evident in Figure 11-4, plasma plasminogen also undergoes a progressive reduction in concentration following the institution of APSAC, rt-PA, and pro-UK. The reduction is most pronounced for APSAC and SK. If the agents rt-PA, pro-UK, and APSAC were fibrin-specific, they would activate the plasminogen associated with fibrin. However, as evident in Figure 11-2, plasma plasminogen freely circulating in the blood is significantly reduced below the normal concentration. If these agents interacted only with fibrin-associated plasminogen, there would be no reduction in circulating plasma plasminogen.

As shown in Figure 11-5, enormous quantities of FDPs are generated by all available thrombolytic agents, including APSAC, rt-PA, and pro-UK. These data establish without question that none of the second-generation thrombolytic agents are capable of specifically activating the fibrinolytic system at the site of thrombus formation and that they all induce systemic activation of the entire fibrinolytic system. The most systemically active agent known at the present time is APSAC.

In addition, we observed, following the institution of rt-PA, a progressive increase in the plasma level of the adhesive von Willebrand protein, as determined by the immunologic Laurell rocket technique.[132] The increase was linear during the 3-hour infusion of the rt-PA compound. Increases were not observed in association with the infusion of SK, UK, APSAC, or pro-UK.

In the TIMI phase I study,[133,134] it was observed that approximately 10% of potential screening rt-PA became thrombocytopenic in contrast to <1% of patients receiving SK. This problem associated with rt-PA has been observed by others.[135] In an attempt to identify how the rt-PA compound was interacting with platelets, we observed, employing in vitro studies, that rt-PA inhibited platelet aggregation to ristocetin. The degree of inhibition progressively was more severe as the concentration of rt-PA was increased.[136] We also observed that the synthesis of thromboxane A_2 was inhibited and ^{14}C-serotonin release was increased above controls in the presence of rt-PA.[136] These alterations in platelet aggregation, thromboxane A_2 synthesis, and ^{14}C-serotonin release were not observed in the presence of a variety of concentrations of UK and SK. Bennet et al.[137] have observed in association with infusions of rt-PA but not invasive manipulatory procedures of cardiac catheterization a prominent increase in the activation of C3a, C4a, and C5a components of the complement system. We have not seen these changes in association with UK or SK.

It is apparent from these studies that the rt-PA agent is not appreciably fibrin- or thrombus-specific but in addition, in a rather promiscuous manner, activates the complement system and binds to and damages the membranes of platelets and vascular endothelial cells.[138,139]

Even though there are no currently available thrombolytic agents that possess fibrin, thrombus, or target specificity, the question must be raised, is it good strategy to try and design such an agent that would not give rise to systemic activation of the fibrinolytic system? When studies of whole blood and plasma viscosity were performed before and during infusions of SK and UK as well as in patients receiving rt-PA, it was observed that in association with SK, whole-blood viscosity at

shear rates of 50 and 0.5 s^{-1} was reduced from 5.1 to 3.8 cP and from 3.8 to 1.9 cP, respectively. Plasma viscosity in association with SK was reduced significantly from 1.4 to 0.86 cP. No significant reductions in identical studies could be observed in patients receiving rt-PA. Although not established, reduction in blood and plasma viscosity at the time of left ventricular insult, myocardial infarction, or severe ischemia may be beneficial. At this time of myocardial damage, the ejection force and ejection fraction are reduced, thereby resulting in a reduction of normal blood flow. If, however, there is a simultaneous reduction in viscosity at the time of left ventricular insult with a lower ejection force, it is possible to maintain normal or near-normal blood flow. This is clearly important to facilitate more rapid recovery via nutrition and oxygenation to the myocardium. With a normal or near-normal rate of blood flow, a thrombogenic environment will be less likely than at blood flow reduced below normal. Such a thrombogenic environment associated with a reduction in blood flow may more frequently predispose to reocclusion of the coronary vessels following patency induced by thrombolytic therapy.

Bleeding associated with thrombolytic therapy, regardless of the thrombolytic agent employed, is greatest in frequency at invaded sites (sites used for cardiac catheterization, arterial blood gas studies, intracath insertion for IV infusion, venipuncture for blood studies of any type, etc.). At any invaded site the vascular endothelium is disrupted, and there takes place an inflammatory reaction. The major components of an inflammatory reaction are fibrin and two different cell types that form the hemostatic plug. It has been established that the fibrin in the hemostatic plug is identical to the fibrin in a pathologic thrombus. The hemostatic plug in this instance, in contrast to the pathologic thrombus, is very freshly (recently) formed and much more susceptible to dissolution. Thus, if a "fibrin-specific" thrombolytic agent is infused into the circulation, it will interact with molecularly identical fibrin in both the hemostatic plug and the pathologic thrombus and may promptly bring about dissolution of the hemostatic plug, thereby inducing bleeding. This may be the reason why in all recently completed studies comparing first- and second-generation thrombolytic agents there is certainly not less bleeding with the newer second-generation agents, but in actual fact there may be more bleeding with these in contrast to the first-generation agents SK and UK.

With respect to clinical efficacy of the newer thrombolytic agents in comparison with the first-generation thrombolytic agents, this can best be viewed by evaluation of studies performed in treatment of myocardial infarction. In the treatment of myocardial infarction, all currently available thrombolytic agents have been employed. A large number of well-designed prospective, randomized, blinded, and appropriately controlled studies have been conducted employing thrombolytic therapy in the treatment of myocardial infarction.

Concerning opening of the coronary artery or infarct-related coronary arteries, this has been observed, as shown in Table 11-2, to occur with all agents in the range of approximately 50% to 85% of patients and not different with one agent versus the others with one exception, i.e., the TIMI phase I study, which demonstrated greater patency with rt-PA compared with SK. With respect to hemorrhage, there is no question that bleeding frequency is not less with the newer agents, and as more studies are being completed, there may be more bleeding seen with the newer agents compared with UK and SK. This was particularly evident in the recently completed ISIS-3 study, with statistically significant more hemorrhage seen in patients receiving rt-PA and APSAC than in those who received SK. In those studies which have examined the frequency of reocclusion, it appears to

be greatest in those patients receiving the rt-PA compound. In all very large population studies (10,000 or more patients), there has been demonstrated a reduction in mortality associated with thrombolytic therapy in contrast with placebo control therapy. This reduction has been observed with all thrombolytic agents and is not greater with one thrombolytic agent versus any other thrombolytic agent. With respect to the one exception mentioned above, i.e., the TIMI phase I study,[133,134] this is the only one of these studies that was not carried out to completion, since it was stopped before the predesigned patient accession number was achieved. It is the only one of all the comparative studies that have been conducted whose results have not been able to be reproduced by any other study.

The current physician, being aware of the preceding facts, can recognize that thrombolytic therapy can induce dissolution and complete resolution of thrombi and emboli. With knowledge of the properties of the various thrombolytic agents available today, giving attention to the safety records of each agent, the current physician can intelligently select an optimal agent for a given patient problem.

Acknowledgment

This work was supported in part by NIH research grant HL 36260 from the NHLBI of the National Institutes of Health.

TABLE 11-2. Thrombolytic Therapy for Acute Myocardial Infarction

	SK	UK	APSAC	rt-PA
Patency, %	50–85	50–85	50–80	50–85
Hemorrhage	+	+	+	+++
CNS Hemorrhage, %	0.1	<0.1	0.3	1.5
Reocclusion	+	+	+	3–4+
Mortality reduction, %	53	50	55	51

REFERENCES

1. Bohmfalk JF, Fuller GM. Plasminogen is synthesized by primary cultures of rat hepatocytes. Science 1980;209:408.
2. Raum D, Marcus D, Alper CA, et al. Synthesis of human plasminogen by the liver. Science 1980; 208:1036.
3. Rabiner SF, Goldfine ID, Hart A, et al. Radioimmunoassay of human plasminogen and plasmin. J Lab Clin Med 1969;74:265.
4. Collen D, Tytgat G, Claeys H, et al. Metabolism of plasminogen in healthy subjects: effects of tranexamic acid. J Clin Invest 1972;51:1310.

5. Hobart MJ. Genetic polymorphism of human plasminogen. Annu J Hum Genet 1979;42:419.

6. Raum D, Marcus D, Alper C. Genetic polymorphism of human plasminogen. Am J Hum Genet 1980;32:681.

7. Estelles A, Aznar J, Gilabert J, et al. Dysfunctional plasminogen in full-term newborn. Pediatr Res 1980;14:1180.

8. Miyata T, Iwanaga S, Sakata Y, et al. Plasminogen Tochigi inactive plasmin resulting from alanine-600 by threonine in the active site. Proc Natl Acad Sci USA 1982;79:6132.

9. Wohl RC, Sammaria L, Robbins KC. Physiological activation of the human fibrinolytic system: isolation and characterization of human plasminogen variants, Chicago I and Chicago II. J Biol Chem 1979;254:9063.

10. Wohl RC, Summaria L, Chediak J. Human plasminogen variant Chicago III. Thromb Haemost 1982;48:146.

11. Deutsch DG, Mertz ET. Plasminogen: purification from human plasma by affinity chromatography. Science 1970;170:1095.

12. Wallen P, Wilman B. Characterization of human plasminogen: I. On the relationship between different molecular forms of plasminogen demonstrated in plasma and found in purified preparations. Biochim Biophys Acta 1970;221:20.

13. Rickli EE, Cuendet PA. Isolation of plasmin-free human plasminogen with N-terminal glutamic acid. Biochim Biophys Acta 1971;250:447.

14. Wallen P, Wiman B: Characterization of human plasminogen: II. Separation and partial characterization of different molecular forms of human plasminogen. Biochim Biophys Acta 1972;257:122.

15. Robbins KC, Summaria L, Elwyn O, et al. Further studies on the purification and characterization of human plasminogen and plasmin. J Biol Chem 1965;240:541.

16. Claeys H, Molla A, Verstraete M. Conversion of NH2-terminal lysine human plasminogen by plasmin. Thromb Res 1973;3:513.

17. Wilman B, Wallen P. Structural relationship between "glutamic acid" and "lysine" forms of human plasminogen and their interaction with the NH2-terminal activation peptide as studies by affinity chromatography. Eur J Biochem 1975;50:489.

18. Collen D, Verstraete M. Molecular biology of human plasminogen: II. Metabolism in physiological and some pathological conditions in man. Thromb Diathem Haemorrh 1975;34:403.

19. Wallen P. Electrophoretic properties of purified human plasminogen. Fed Proc 1963;22:609.

20. Brockway WJ, Castellino FJ. Measurement of the binding of antifibrinolytic amino acids to various plasminogens. Arch Biochem Biophys 1972;151:194.

21. Summaria L, Arzadon L, Bernabe P, et al. Studies on the isolation of the multiple molecular forms of human plasminogen and plasmin by isoelectric focusing methods. J Biol Chem 1972;247:4691.

22. Robbins KC. The plasminogen-plasmin enzyme system. In: Coleman RW, Hirsh J, Marder VJ, Salzman EW, eds. Hemostasis and thrombis: basic principles and clinical practice. Philadelphia: JB Lippincott, 1982:623.

23. Wiman B, Wallen P. On the primary structure of human plasminogen and plasmin: purification and characterization of cyanogen-bromide fragments. Eur J Biochem 1975;57:387.

24. Sottrup-Jensen L, Claeys H, Zajdel M, et al. The primary structure of human plasminogen: isolation of two lysine-binding fragments and one "mini"-plasminogen (MW 38000) by elastase-catalyzed-specific limited proteolysis. In: Rowan JF, Samama RM, Desnoyers PC, eds. Progress in chemical fibrinolysis, vol 3. New York: Raven Press, 1978:191.

25. Magnusson S, Sottrup-Jensen L, Petersen TE, et al. Homologous "kringle" structures common to prothrombin and plasminogen. In: Ribbons DW, Brew K, eds. Proteolysis and physiological regulation. New York: Academic Press, 1976:203.

26. Sottrup-Jensen L, Zaidel M, Claeys H, et al. Amino acid sequence of activation cleavage site in plasminogen: homology with "pro" part of prothrombin. Proc Natl Acad Sci USA 1975;72:2577.

27. Wiman B, Wallen P. Amino acid sequence of the cyanogen-bromide fragment from human plasminogen that forms the linkage between the plasmin chains. Eur J Biochem 1975;58:539.

28. Hayes ML, Castellino FJ. Carbohydrate of the human plasminogen variants: I. Carbohydrate composition, glycopeptide isolation and characterization. J Biol Chem 1979;254:8768.

29. Sjoholm I, Wiman B, Wallen P. Studies on the conformational changes of plasminogen induced during activation to plasmin and by 5-aminohexanoic acid. Eur Biochem 1973;39:471.

30. Tranqui L, Prandini MH, Chapel A. The structure of plasminogen studied by electron microscopy. Biol Cell 1979;34:39.

31. Robbins KC, Summaria L, Hsieh B, et al. The peptide chains of human plasmin: mechanism of activation of human plasminogen to plasmin. J Biol Chem 1967;242:2333.

32. Summaria L, Hsieh B, Robbins KC. The specific mechanism of activation of human plasminogen to plasmin. J Biol Chem 1967;242:4279.

33. Rickli EE, Otavsky WL. Release of an N-terminal

peptide from human plasminogen during activation with urokinase. Biochim Biophys Acta 1973; 295:381.

34. Wiman B. Primary structure of peptide released during activation of human plasminogen by urokinase. Eur J Biochem 1973;39:1.

35. Wiman B, Wallen P. Activation of human plasminogen by an insoluble-derivative of urokinase: structural changes of plasminogen in the course of activation to plasmin and demonstration of possible intermediate compound. Eur J Biochem 1973;36:25.

36. Summaria L, Arzadon L, Bernabe P, et al. The activation of plasminogen to plasmin by urokinase in the presence of the plasmin inhibitor Trasylol: the preparation of plasmin with the same NH_2-terminal heavy (A) chain sequence as the parent zymogen. J Biol Chem 1975;250:3988.

37. Vloland BN, Castellino FJ. Mechanism of the urokinase-catalyzed activation of human plasminogen. J Biol Chem 1976;251:3906.

38. Rickli EE, Otavsky WJ. A new method of isolation and some properties of the heavy chain of human plasmin. Eur J Biochem 1975;59:441.

39. Wiman B, Wallen P. The specific interaction between plasminogen and fibrin: a physiological role of the lysine binding site in plasminogen. Thromb Res 1977;10:213.

40. Lerch PG, Rickli EE, Lergier W, et al. Localization of individual lysine-binding regions in human plasminogen and investigations of their complex-forming properties. Eur J Biochem 1980;107:7.

41. Markus G, DePasquale JL, Wissler FC. Quantitative determination of the binding of α-aminocaprooic acid to native plasminogen. J Biol Chem 1978;253:727.

42. Claeys H, Vermylen J. Physicochemical and proenzyme properties of NH_2-terminal glutamic acid and NH_2-terminal lysine human plasminogen: influence of 6-aminohexanoic acid. Biochim Biophys Acta 1974;342:351.

43. Walther PJ, Hill RL, McKee PA: The importance of the preactivation peptide in the two-stage mechanism of human plasminogen activation. J Biol Chem 1975;250:5926.

44. Christensen U, Mullertz S. Kinetic studies on the urokinase catalyzed conversion of NH_2-terminal lysine plasminogen to plasmin. Biochim Biophys Acta 1977;480:275.

45. Christensen U. Kinetic studies of the urokinase catalyzed conversion of NH_2-terminal glutamic acid plasminogen to plasmin. Biochim Biophys Acta 1977;481:638.

46. Thorsen S. Differences in the binding to fibrin of native plasminogen and plasminogen modified by proteolytic degradation: influence of ω-amino-

carboxylic acids. Biochim Biophys Acta 1975;393: 55.

47. Hoylaerts M, Linjen HR, Collen D. Studies on the mechanism of the antifibrinolytic action of transexamic acid. Biochim Biophys Acta 1981; 673:75.

48. Moroi M, Aoki N. Inhibition of plasminogen binding to fibrin by alpha$_2$-plasmin inhibitor. Thromb Res 1977;10:851.

49. Lijnen HR, Hoylaerts M, Collen D. Isolation and chemaeterization of human plasma protein with affinity for the lysine binding sites in plasminogen: role in the regulation of fibrinolysis and identification as histidine-rich glycoprotein. J Biol Chem 1980;255:10214.

50. Summaria L, Ksieh B, Groskopf WR. The isolation and characterization of the S-carboxyl-methyl B (light) chain derivative of human plasmin: the localization of the active site on the B (light) chain. J Biol Chem 1967;242:5046.

51. Groskopf WR, Summaria L, Robbins KC. Studies on the active center of human plasmin: partial amino acid sequence of a peptide containing the active center serine residue. J Biol Chem 1969; 244:3590.

52. Robbins K, Bernabe P, Arzadon L, et al. The primary structure of human plasminogen: II. The histidine loop of human plasmin: light (B) chain active center histidine sequence. J Biol Chem 1973; 248:1631.

53. Groskopf WF, Hsieh B, Summaria L, et al. Studies on the active center of human plasmin: the serine and histidine residues. J Biol Chem 1969;244:359.

54. Christessen LR, MacLeod CM. A proteolytic enzyme of serum: characterization, activation, and reaction with inhibitors. J Gen Physiol 1945;28: 363.

55. Weinstein MJ, Doolittle RF. Differential specification of thrombin, plasmin, and trypsin with regard to synthetic and natural substrates and inhibitors. Biochim Biophys Acta 1972;258:577.

56. Tillet WS, Garner RL. The fibrinolytic activity of hemolytic streptococci. J Exp Med 1933;58:485.

57. Christensen LR, MacLeod CM. A proteolytic enzyme of serum: characterization, activation and reaction with inhibitors. J Gen Physiol 1945;28: 559.

58. Ratnoff OD. Studies on a proteolytic enzyme in human plasma: I. The probable identity of the enzymes activated by chloroform and by filtrates of cultures of beta hemolytic streptococci. J Exp Med 1948;87:199.

59. Sherry S. The fibrinolytic activity of streptokinase activated human plasmin. J Clin Invest 1954; 33:1054.

60. Fletcher AP, Alkjaersig N, Sherry S. The mainte-

nance of a sustained thrombolytic state in man: I. Induction and effects. J Clin Invest 1959;38:1096.

61. Johnson AJ, McCarty WR. The lysis of artificially induced intravascular clots in man by intravenous infusions of streptokinase. J Clin Invest 1959; 38:1627.

62. Taylor FB Jr, Botts J. Purification and characterization of streptokinase with studies of streptokinase activation of plasminogen. Biochemistry 1968;7: 232.

63. Castellino FJ, Sodetz JM, Brockway WJ, et al. Streptokinase. Methods Enzymol 1976;45:244.

64. Morgan FJ, Henschen A. The structure of streptokinase, cyanogen bromide fragmentation, amino acid composition, and partial amino acid sequences. Biochim Biophys Acta 1969;181:93.

65. Loch T, Bilinski T, Zakrzewski K. Studies on streptokinase: the conformation. Acta Biochim Pol 1968;15:129.

66. McClintock DK, Bell PH. The mechanism of activation of human plasminogen by streptokinase. Biochem Biophys Res Commun 1971;43:694.

67. Reddy KNN, Markus G. Mechanism of activation of human plasminogen by streptokinase: presence of an active center in streptokinase-plasminogen complex. J Biol Chem 1972;247:1683.

68. McClintock DK, Englert ME, Dziobkowski C, et al. Two distinct pathways of the streptokinase-mediated activation of highly purified human plasminogen. Biochemistry 1974;13:5334.

69. Summaria L, Arzadon L, Bernabe P, et al. The interaction of streptokinase with human, cat, dog, and rabbit plasminogen: the fragmentation of streptokinase in the equimolar plasminogen-streptokinase complexes. J Biol Chem 1974;249: 4760.

70. Brockway WJ, Castellino FJ. A characterization of native streptokinase isolated from a human plasminogen activator complex. Biochemistry 1974; 13:2063.

71. Siefring GE, Castellino FJ. Interaction of streptokinase with plasminogen: isolation and characterization of a streptokinase degradation product. J Biol Chem 1976;251:3913.

72. Chesterman CN, Cederholm-Williams SA, Allington MJ. The degradation of streptokinase during the production of plasminogen activator. Thromb Res 1974;5:413.

73. Summaria L, Robbins KC. Isolation of a human plasmin-derived functionally active, light (B) chain capable of forming with streptokinase an equimolar light (B) chain-streptokinase complex with plasminogen activator activity. J Biol Chem 1976;251:5810.

74. Markus G, Evers JL, Hobika GH. Activator activities of the human plasminogen-streptokinase complex during its proteolytic conversion to the stable activator complexes. J Biol Chem 1976; 251:6495.

75. Wohl RC, Summaria L, Arzadon L, et al. Steady state kinetics of activation of human and bovine plasminogens by streptokinase and its equimolar complexes with various activated forms of human plasminogen. J Biol Chem 1978;253:1402.

76. Robbins KC, Wohl RC, Summaria L. Plasmin and plasminogen activators: kinetics and kinetics of plasminogen activation. Ann NY Acad Sci 1981; 370:588.

77. Takada A, Takada Y. Potentiation of the activation of Glu-plasminogen by streptokinase and urokinase in the presence of fibrinogen degradation products. Thromb Res 1982;25:229.

78. Cederholm-Williams SA, DeCock F, Lijnen HR, et al. Kinetics of the reactions between streptokinase, plasmin, and alpha₂-antiplasmin. Eur J Biochem 1979;100:125.

79. Urokinase Pulmonary Embolism Trial. Phase I results: a cooperative study. JAMA 1970;214:2163.

80. MacFarlane RG, Pilling J. Fibrinolytic activity of normal urine. Nature 1947;159:779.

81. Williams JRB. The fibrinolytic activity of the urine. Br J Exp Pathol 1951;32:530.

82. Sobel GW, Mohler SR, Jones NW, et al. Urokinase: an activator of plasma profibrinolysin extracted from urine. Am J Physiol 1952;171:768.

83. Ploug J, Kjelgaard NO. Urokinase: an activator of plasminogen from human urine: I. Isolation and properties. Biochim Biophys Acta 1957;24:278.

84. Lesuk A, Terminiello L, Traver JH. Crystalline human urokinase: some properties. Science 1965; 147:880.

85. Sherry S, Lindemeyer RI, Fletcher AP, et al. Studies on enhanced fibrinolytic activity in man. J Clin Invest 1959;38:810.

86. Burges RA, Brammer KW, Coombes JD. Molecular weight of urokinase. Nature 1965;208:894.

87. Lesuk A, Terminiello M, Traver JH. Crystalline human urokinase: some properties. Science 1965; 147:880.

88. White WF, Barlow GH, Mozen MM. The isolation and characterization of plasminogen activators (urokinase) from human urine. Biochemistry 1966;5:2160.

89. von Doleschel W. Isolierung einer dritten humanen urokinase. Wien Klin Wochenschr 1975;87: 282.

90. Murano G, Aronson DL. High and low molecular weight urokinase. Thromb Haemost 1979;42: 1066.

91. Lesuk A, Terminiello L, Traver JH, et al. Biochemical and biphysical studies of human urokinase. Thromb Diatherm Haemorrh 1967;18:293.

92. Soberano ME, Ong EB, Johnson AJ. The effects of inhibitors on the catalytic conversion of urokinase. Thromb Res 1976;9:675.

93. Holmberg L, Bladh B, Astedt B. Purification of urokinase by affinity chromatography. Biochim Biophys Acta 1976;445:215.

94. Soberano ME, Ong EB, Johnson AJ, et al. Purification and characterization of two forms of urokinase. Biochim Biophys Acta 1976;445:763.

95. McLellan WL, Vetterlein D, Roblin R. The glycoprotein nature of human plasminogen activators. FEBS Lett 1980;115:181.

96. Landmann H, Markwardt F. Irreversible synthetische inhibitoren der urokinase. Experientia 1970; 26:145.

97. Sherry S, Alkjaersig N, Fletcher AP. Assay of urokinase preparation with the synthetic substrate acetyl-L-lysine methyl ester. J Lab Clin Med 1964; 64:145.

98. Suyama T, Nishida M, Iga Y, et al. Difference in thrombolytic effect between higher and lower molecular weight forms of urokinase. Thromb Haemost 1977;38:48.

99. Beattie AG, Ogston D, Bennett B, et al. Inhibitors of plasminogen activation in human blood. Br J Haematol 1976;32:135.

100. Brakeman P, Mohler E, Astrup T. A group of patients with impaired plasma fibrinolytic system and selective inhibition of tissue activator-induced fibrinolysis. Scand J Haematol 1966;3:389.

101. Kacinski CS, Fletcher AP, Sherry S. Effect of urokinase antiserum on plasminogen activators: demonstration of immunologic dissimilarity between plasma plasminogen activator and urokinase. J Clin Invest 1968;47:1238.

102. Uszynski M. Isolation of peptides with antiurokinase activity from the human placenta. Thromb Haemost 1980;42:1411.

103. Rijken DC, Collen D. Purification and characterization of the plasminogen activator secreted by human melanoma cells in culture. J Biol Chem 1981;256:7035.

104. Mackie M, Booth NA, Bennett B. Comparative studies on human activators of plasminogen. Br J Haematol 1981;47:77.

105. Rijken DC, Wijngaards G, Welbergen J. Relationship between tissue plasminogen activator and the activators in blood and vascular wall. Thromb Res 1980;18:815.

106. Bernik MB, Kwaan HC. Origin of fibrinolytic activity in cultures from human tissue. J Lab Clin Med 1967;70:650.

107. Mullertz S. Plasminogen activator is spontaneously active human blood. Proc Soc Exp Biol Med 1953;82:291.

108. Camiolo SM, Thorsen S, Astrup T. Fibrongenolysis and fibrinolysis with tissue plasminogen activator, urokinase, streptokinase-activated human globulin and plasmin. Proc Soc Exp Biol Med 1971;138:277.

109. Thorsen S, Glas-Greenwalt P, Astrup T. Differences in the binding to fibrin of urokinase and tissue plasminogen activator. Thromb Diatherm Haemorrh 1972;28:65.

110. Barlow GH, Lazer L. Characterization of the plasminogen activator isolated from human embryo kidney cells: comparison with urokinase. Thromb Res 1972;1:201.

111. Bernik MB, Whiate WF, Oiler EP, et al. Immunologic identity of plasminogen activator in human urine, heart, blood vessels and tissue culture. J Lab Clin Med 1974;84:546.

112. Tissot JD, Schneider P, Hawert J, et al. Isolation from human plasma of a plasminogen activator identical to urinary high molecular weight urokinase. J Clin Invest 1982;70:1320.

113. Wijagaards G, Kluft C, Greenveld E. Demonstration of urokinase-related fibrinolytic activity in human plasma. Br J Haematol 1982;51:165.

114. Wun TC, Schleuning WD, Reich E. Isolation and characterization of urokinase from human plasma. J Biol Chem 1982;257:3276.

115. Verstraete M: Biochemical and clinical aspects of thrombolysis. Semin Haematol 1978;15:35.

116. Astedt B, Holmberg L. Immunological identity of urokinase and ovarian carcinoma plasminogen activator released in tissue culture. Nature 1976; 261:595.

117. Wu MC, Adel AY. Comparative studies on urokinase and plasminogen activator from cultured pancreatic carcinoma. Int J Biochem 1979;10: 1001.

118. Markus G, Takita H, Cumiolo SM, et al. Content and characterization of plasminogen activators in human lung tumors and normal lung tissue. Cancer Res 1980;40:841.

119. Evers JL, Patel J, Madeja JM. Plasminogen activator activity and composition in human breast cancer. Cancer Res 1982;42:219.

120. Lewis LJ. Plasminogen activator (urokinase) from cultured cells. Thromb Haemost 1979;42:895.

121. Marder VJ, Donahoe JF, Bell WR, et al. Changes in the plasma fibrinolytic system during urokinase therapy: comparison of tissue culture urokinase with urinary source urokinase in patients with pulmonary embolism. J Lab Clin Med 1978;92:721.

122. Genton E, Claman HN. Urokinase antigenic studies in patients following thrombolytic therapy. J Lab Clin Med 1970;75:619.

123. Gerard RD, Chien KR, Meidell RS. Molecular biology of tissue plasminogen activator and endogenous inhibitors. Mol Biol Med 1986;3:449.

124. Husain SS, Gurewich V, Lipinski B. Purification and partial characterization of a single-chain high molecular-weight form of urokinase from human urine. Arch Biochem Biophys 1983;20:31.

125. Gurewich V, Pannell R. Inactivation of single-chain urokinase (prourokinase) by thrombin and thrombin-like enzymes. Blood 1987;69:769.

126. Liknen HR, Van Hoef B, DeCock F, et al. The mechanism of plasminogen activation and fibrin dissolution by single chain urokinase-type plasminogen activator in a plasma millieu in vitro. Blood 1989;73:1864.

127. DeMunk GAW, Rijken DC. Fibrinolytic properties of single chain urokinase-type plasminogen activator (prourokinase). Fibrinolysis 1990;4:1.

128. Smith RAS, Dupe RJ, English PD, et al. Fibrinolysis with acyl-enzymes: a new approach to thrombolytic therapy. Nature 1981;290:505.

129. Ferres H. Pre-clinical pharmacological evaluation of anisoylated plasminogen streptokinase activator complex. Drugs 1987;33(suppl 3):33.

130. Crabbe SJ, Grimm AM, Hopkins LE. Acylated plasminogen-streptokinase activator complex: a new approach to thrombolytic therapy. Pharmacotherapy 1990;10:115.

131. Weitz JI, Cruickshank MK, Thong B, et al. Human tissue-type plasminogen activator releases fibrinopeptides A and B from fibrinogen. J Clin Invest 1988;82:1700.

132. Topol EJ, Bell WR, Weisfeldt ML. Coronary thrombolysis with recombinant tissue-type plasminogen activator. Ann Intern Med 1985;103:837.

133. TIMI-Study Group. The thrombolysis in myocardial infarction (TIMI) trial: phase I findings. N Engl J Med 1985;312:932.

134. Rao AK, Pratt C, Bell WR, et al. Thrombolysis in myocardial infarction (TIMI) trial—phase I. J Am Coll Cardiol 1988;11:1.

135. Bovill EG, Terrin ML, Strump DC. Hemorrhagic events during therapy with recombinant tissue-type plasminogen activator, heparin, and aspirin for acute myocardial infarction. Ann Intern Med 1991;115:256.

136. Bell WR. Complications of thrombolytic therapy-bleeding and rethrombosis. In: Sherry S, Schroeder R, Kluft C, eds. Contraversies in coronary thrombolysis. London: Current Medical Literature, Ltd., 1989:59.

137. Bennett WR, Yawn DH, Migliore PJ, et al. Activation of the complement system by recombinant tissue plasminogen activator. J Am Coll Cardiol 1987;10:627.

138. Hajjar KA, Nachman RL. Endothelial cell-mediated conversion of glu-plasminogen to lys-plasminogen: further evidence for assembly of the fibrinolytic system on the endothelial cell surface. J Clin Invest 1988;82:1769.

139. Vaughan DE, Mendelsohn MC, Declerck PJ, et al. Characterization of the binding of human tissue-type plasminogen activator to platelets. J Biol Chem 1989;264:15869.

Anthony J. Comerota (Ed.). *Thrombolytic Therapy for Peripheral Vascular Disease.* Copyright © 1995 J. B. Lippincott Company.

12

THROMBOLYTIC THERAPY FOR PULMONARY EMBOLISM

Samuel Z. Goldhaber

Pulmonary embolism (PE) and deep venous thrombosis account for more than 250,000 hospitalizations[1] and approximately 50,000 deaths annually in the United States. The immediate cause of death from PE is usually acute right-sided heart failure. When nonfatal, PE can cause chronic pulmonary hypertension.

The death rate from PE in the United States is higher in men than in women and in nonwhites than in whites. Death from PE occurs more frequently with increasing age. Unfortunately, over the past 30 years, the fatality rate from PE has not declined[2] (Fig. 12-1). This is not too surprising because the standard treatment of PE with anticoagulation alone has essentially remained unchanged since the 1960s. The lack of progress in improving outcome from PE may be due to insufficient use of thrombolysis, which appears to have several proven and potential advantages among properly selected patients with PE (Table 12-1).

For patients with massive PE (Fig. 12-2), it seems evident that thrombolysis followed by anticoagulation should be more effective than anticoagulation alone. Nevertheless, lack of familiarity with PE thrombolysis is pervasive, and most hospitals have just a few patients each year who present with recognized massive PE. Current estimates are that no more than 10% of PE patients are treated with thrombolysis in the United States.

PATHOPHYSIOLOGY

The hemodynamic response to PE depends on the size of the embolus, coexisting cardiopulmonary disease, and neurohumoral responses. Pulmonary artery obstruction and circulating vasoconstrictive and bronchospastic neurohumoral substances reduce the pulmonary vascular bed and cause an increase in right ventricular afterload. The two most important humoral factors appear to be serotonin and thromboxane A_2 (TxA_2). Serotonin, a potent neural and smooth-muscle agonist, is stored primarily in the dense bodies of platelets and mediates bronchospasm in the small airways. Activated platelets also secrete TxA_2, a potent vasoconstrictor and bronchoconstrictor. By dissolving thrombus rapidly, thrombolytic agents

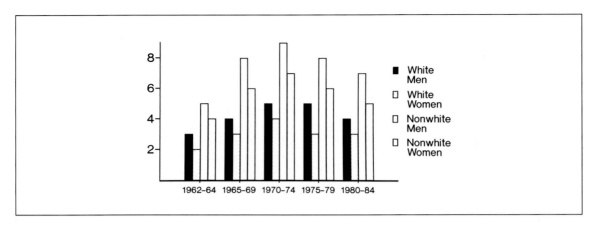

FIGURE 12-1. Death rate from PE per 100,000 in the United States from 1962 through 1984, based on data from the National Hospital Discharge Survey. (Reprinted with permission from Lilienfeld DE, Chan E, Ehland J, et al: Mortality from pulmonary embolism in the United States: 1962 to 1984. Chest 98:1067, 1990.

might minimize the potentially adverse impact of the neurohumoral response to PE.

As right ventricular and pulmonary artery pressures rise, the right ventricle dilates, becomes hypokinetic, and ultimately fails. Right ventricular failure adversely affects left ventricular function because of the anatomic juxtaposition of the two ventricles and *ventricular interdependency.* The dilated right ventricle can displace the interventricular septum toward the left ventricle, resulting in decreased left ventricular diastolic filling and end-diastolic volume (Fig. 12-3). Thrombolysis often can relieve obstruction to pulmonary artery blood flow, reduce pulmonary artery pressure, and thus improve right ventricular function. Because of ventricular interdependen-

dency, improved right ventricular function often leads to better left ventricular function, which should help to reverse cardiogenic shock and reduce mortality from PE.

When major PE is treated with anticoagulation alone, pulmonary artery clots may fail to resolve completely in 75% of patients after 1 to 4 weeks[3] (Fig. 12-4) and in 50% after 4 months of follow-up[4] (Fig. 12-5). Dissolution of the thrombus should improve pulmonary tissue perfusion, which, in turn, should prevent chronic pulmonary hypertension as a late effect of PE. PE thrombolysis also might reduce the rate of recurrent PE by lysing the source of the PE in situ, usually thrombus in the pelvic or deep leg veins.

PROGNOSIS WITH ANTICOAGULATION ALONE

Among patients treated with anticoagulation alone, the rate of death or recurrent PE within 2 weeks of diagnosis is approximately 10%. The Prospective Investigation of Pulmonary Embolism Diagnosis (PIOPED) group reported on the clinical course of PE among 399 patients.[5] Only 2.5% died, and most deaths were caused by recurrent PE. Overall, the rate of PE recurrence was 8.3%. This report on 399 PE patients was based

TABLE 12-1. *Advantages of Thrombolysis*

Proven
1. Accelerate clot lysis
2. Accelerate pulmonary tissue reperfusion
3. Accelerate reversal of right heart failure
4. Improve pulmonary capillary blood volume

Possible
1. Reduce mortality
2. Reduce recurrent PE
3. Minimize adverse neurohumoral effects
4. Reduce chronic pulmonary hypertension
5. Improve the quality of life.

Reprinted with permission from Goldhaber SZ. Prog Cardiovasc Dis 1992;34:113.

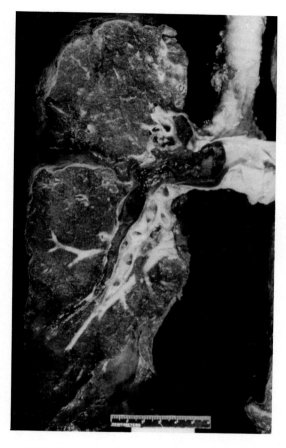

FIGURE 12-2. This 67-year-old man collapsed suddenly and suffered a cardiopulmonary arrest. Massive bilateral (right lung shown in figure) pulmonary emboli were documented at autopsy. (Reprinted with permission from Goldhaber SZ. Prog Cardiovasc Dis 1992;34:113.)

on a highly selected patient population. Of 5587 patients who underwent lung scans, 1523 refused to participate in PIOPED, and an additional 1032 were excluded because pulmonary angiography was contraindicated. Another 1539 patients were ineligible for PIOPED for other reasons. Undoubtedly, the recruitment process for PIOPED excluded many patients with large PEs who were considered too ill to participate (Fig. 12-6). This selection process may have skewed the report toward the inclusion of patients with less life-threatening PE than those who were omitted.

Overall, only 6% of the 399 PE patients received thrombolytic therapy. When 1-year mor-

tality rates from all causes were assessed in the PIOPED cohort, patients who had received anticoagulation alone had a 19% mortality rate. In contrast, the lowest all-cause mortality rate—9%—was in the group treated with thrombolytic therapy (Fig. 12-7). Thus, even in this nonrandomized observational report of patients with PE, a hint exists that thrombolysis administered acutely may improve long-term prognosis.

INITIAL CLINICAL TRIALS

Urokinase (UK) was compared with heparin alone in phase I of the Urokinase Pulmonary Embolism Trial (UPET).[6] Urokinase was shown to dissolve pulmonary arterial clot more rapidly than heparin alone and, in certain instances, to reverse clinical shock. In the UPET, it appeared that thrombolytic therapy followed by heparin might reduce the mortality and recurrent PE rate when compared with heparin alone. However, the differences did not attain statistical significance, possibly due to a relatively small sample size. Furthermore, among PE patients who survived for 1 week, there was no significant difference in lung scan improvement between the two treatments.

In the Urokinase-Streptokinase Pulmonary Embolism Trial, acute thrombolysis of PE followed by heparin improved pulmonary capillary blood volume at 2 weeks and at 1 year more than treatment with heparin alone.[7] When a subgroup of these patients was followed for an average of 7 years, those assigned initially to thrombolysis appeared to have a more complete resolution of PE, as assessed by preservation of the normal pulmonary vascular response to exercise.[8] Patients treated with heparin alone demonstrated a markedly abnormal rise in pulmonary artery pressure and pulmonary vascular resistance when undergoing supine bicycle exercise in the cardiac catheterization laboratory. In addition, those PE patients randomly allocated to heparin alone and followed for an average of 7 years had more functional disability than those who had initially received thrombolysis followed by heparin.[8] This suggests that thrombolysis given at the time of acute PE may improve the long-term quality of life.

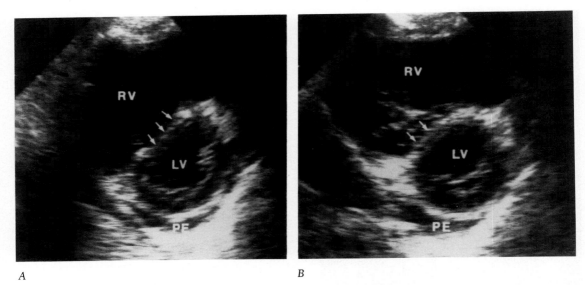

A   B

FIGURE 12-3. Parasternal short-axis views of the right ventricle (RV) and left ventricle (LV) in
diastole (A) and systole (B). There is diastolic and systolic bowing of the interventricular septum
(arrows) into the left ventricle compatible with right ventricular volume and pressure overloads,
respectively. The right ventricle is appreciably dilated and markedly hypokinetic, with little change in
apparent right ventricular area from diastole to systole (PE = small pericardial effusion). (Reprinted
with permission from Come PC: Echocardiographic evaluation of pulmonary embolism and its response to therapeutic interventions. Chest 101:151S, 1992.)

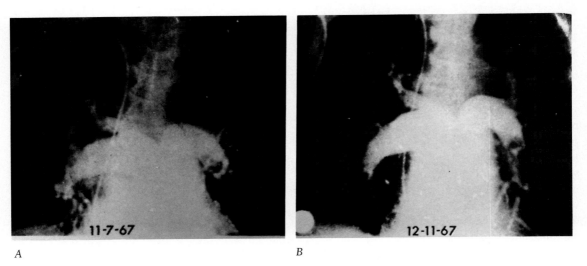

A   B

FIGURE 12-4. Massive bilateral pulmonary embolism is documented angiographically (A). After
34 days of anticoagulation alone, the angiogram is repeated (B), and only minimal resolution is observed. (Reprinted with permission from Dalen JE, et al: Resolution rate of acute pulmonary embolism
in man. N Engl J Med 280:1197, 1969.)

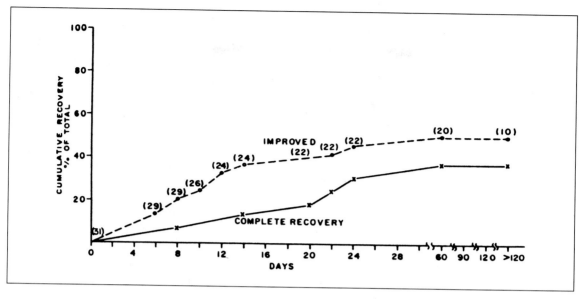

FIGURE 12-5. The rate of recovery of the pulmonary circulation is expressed as a percentage of the total number of patients with pulmonary embolism who were observed. Figures in parentheses indicate the number of patients observed at the time indicated after pulmonary embolism. A patient was considered to have recovered completely when no region of the lung had a less than normal concentration of radioactivity. If at least 50% of the regions of decreased radioactivity became normal but the lung scan was still abnormal, the patient was classified as improved. Results in this figure are among patients considered to have pulmonary embolism of intermediate size, defined as 16% to 30% of the lung involved. They were treated with anticoagulation alone. (Reprinted with permission from Tow DE, et al: Recovery of pulmonary arterial blood flow in patients with pulmonary embolism. N Engl J Med 276:1055, 1967.)

CONTEMPORARY CLINICAL TRIALS

In the 1980s, recombinant tissue plasminogen activator (rt-PA) was developed for PE treatment because initial animal studies were promising. In experimental studies of venous thromboembolism, tissue plasminogen activator (t-PA) appeared more potent than UK or streptokinase (SK) and possibly safer.[9–13] Unlike SK, rt-PA has not been reported to be antigenic[14] and has not been causally linked to allergic reactions.

Plasminogen Activator Italian Multicenter Study 2 (PAIMS-2) investigators[15] randomized 36 patients with angiographically proven PE to 100 mg rt-PA over 2 h or to heparin. Clot lysis at post-treatment angiography, assessed by the Miller index, occurred in the rt-PA group (with the Miller index improving from 28.3 ± 2.9 to 24.8 ± 5.2) but not in the patients who received heparin alone. Mean pulmonary artery pressure decreased from 30.2 ± 7.8 to 21.4 ± 6.7 mmHg in the rt-PA group but increased in patients who received heparin alone. Two rt-PA patients died (one from renal failure following cardiac tamponade and one from intracranial bleeding), and one patient who received heparin alone died from recurrent PE.

European Cooperative Study Group investigators compared 100 mg rt-PA over 2 h with a 12-h weight-adjusted infusion of urokinase (4400 U/kg bolus, followed by 4400 U/kg per hour for 12 h).[16] The principal endpoint was reduction in total pulmonary resistance, defined as pulmonary artery mean pressure divided by cardiac index. At 2 h, total pulmonary resistance decreased by 36%

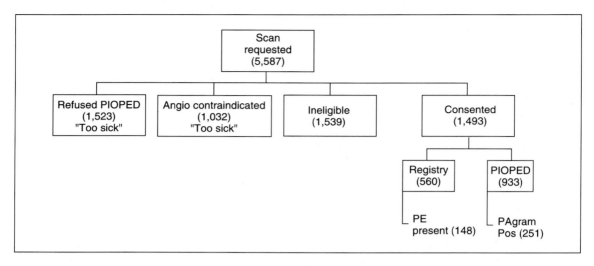

FIGURE 12-6. The PIOPED study followed 399 patients with PE: 148 from the registry and 251 who actually participated in the diagnostic protocol. Many patients refused to participate. Others were excluded from PIOPED because pulmonary angiography was contraindicated. Some of these nonparticipants probably had anatomically large or hemodynamically compromising PEs and could have benefited from thrombolytic therapy. The omission of these patients from the PIOPED cohort may have resulted in a relatively low rate of death and recurrent PE in this observational report.

in the rt-PA group, compared with a decrease of 18% in the urokinase-treated patients ($p = 0.0009$). However, by 6 h, urokinase appeared to "catch up" to rt-PA, and hemodynamic differences between the two groups did not persist.

In Boston, we have coordinated five trials of PE thrombolysis: four completed and one in progress. The most recent trial (PE Trial No. 5) is international and includes investigators from Italy, Canada, and the United States.

FIGURE 12-7. All-cause 1-year mortality rates in the PIOPED cohort of 399 patients with PE. The group that received thrombolytic therapy had the lowest mortality rate (8.7%), compared with 19.2% for those patients who received anticoagulation alone.

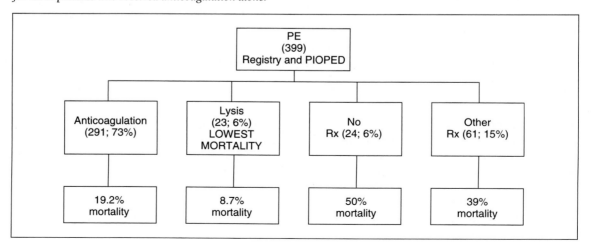

PE Trial No.1[17-19] was an open-label study of 47 patients with angiographically documented PE that showed that 50 to 90 mg rt-PA administered over 2 to 6 h caused clot lysis in 94% of patients. All patients received 50 mg rt-PA over 2 h, followed immediately by a research angiogram (Fig. 12-8). If clot lysis had not occurred, as judged by the investigator at the time of the angiogram, an additional 40 mg rt-PA was administered over the subsequent 4 h and was followed immediately by a third angiogram. Two-thirds of the patients received more than 2 h of rt-PA. During the third and subsequent hours of rt-PA therapy, however, an increased frequency of bleeding, particularly at the femoral vein puncture site used for pulmonary angiography, caused us to shorten the dura-tion and raise the rt-PA dose in our subsequent trials.

Clot lysis was graded as moderate or marked in 83% and slight in an additional 11%. Among patients with pulmonary artery hypertension, the pulmonary artery pressures decreased during the acute treatment period from 43/17 (27) to 31/13 (19) mmHg without any change in systemic arterial pressure.

Hemodynamic and angiographic improvement was accompanied by recovery in pulmonary perfusion.[20] One day after rt-PA, there was a 57% increase in perfusion among the 19 patients who had follow-up lung scans.

Right ventricular function also improved. Come and colleagues[21] performed Doppler echo-

FIGURE 12-8. (A) *A large embolus is present in the right pulmonary artery (arrow).* (B) *After a 2-h infusion of rt-PA through a peripheral vein, there is pronounced resolution, with only a small amount of residual thrombus in segmental branches. (Reprinted with permission from Goldhaber SZ, et al: Acute pulmonary embolism treated with tissue plasminogen activator. Lancet 2:886, 1986.)*

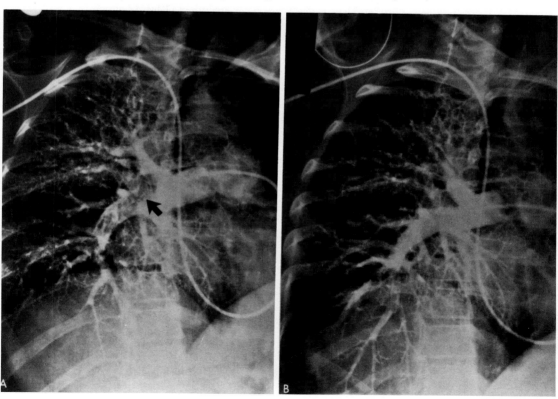

cardiography on seven patients with PE before and after they received rt-PA (Fig. 12-9). Within a day of treatment, the right ventricular end-diastolic diameter was halved from an average of 3.9 to 2.0 cm. Right ventricular wall motion normalized in five and improved in two patients. Tricuspid regurgitation was present before lytic therapy in six patients but was detected after the completion of lytic therapy in only two patients. The early reversal of the hallmarks of right-sided heart failure—right ventricular dysfunction, right ventricular dilatation, and tricuspid regurgitation—suggests that thrombolytic agents might reduce the mortality from acute PE.

PE Trial No.2 was a randomized trial comparing 100 mg rt-PA over 2 h with 2000 U/lb of UK as a bolus followed by 2000 U/lb per hour for up to 24 h.[22] The Food and Drug Administration (FDA) considered this trial to be a pivotal study when it approved rt-PA for PE treatment. The principal endpoints were improvement on the 2-h angiogram and 24-h lung scan compared with the baseline studies. All 45 patients received the full dose of rt-PA, but UK infusions were terminated prematurely in 9 of 23 patients because of allergy in 1 and uncontrollable bleeding in 8. By 2 h, 82% of rt-PA–treated patients showed clot lysis compared with 48% of UK-treated patients ($p = 0.0008$). Thrombolysis at angiography was associated with a return of elevated pulmonary arterial pressures toward normal. Thus, in the dosing regimens employed, rt-PA was more rapid and safer than UK. However, at 24 h, there was no difference in scintigraphic improvement between rt-PA– and UK-

FIGURE 12-9. *Subcostal two-dimensional images at end-diastole in a PE patient from our PE Trial No. 1 who presented with syncope and "heart failure." Before rt-PA (**A**), the right ventricle (RV) is markedly enlarged and the left ventricular (LV) diameter is reduced. After rt-PA (**B**), a remarkable decrease in RV size and a corresponding increase in LV size are apparent (RA = right atrium; SEP = septum; PW = posterior wall). (Reprinted with permission from the American College of Cardiology and Come PC, et al: Early reversal of right ventricular dysfunction in patients with acute pulmonary embolism after treatment with intravenous tissue plasminogen activator. J Am Coll Cardiol 10:971, 1987.)*

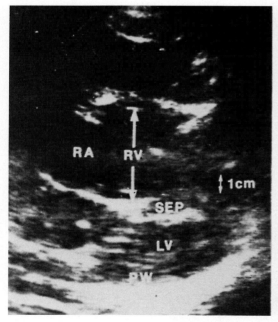

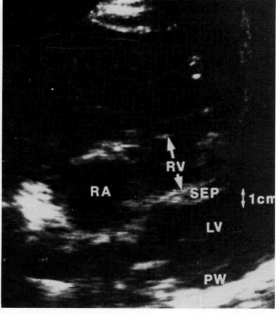

A   B

treated patients. Furthermore, at 2 and 24 h after initiation of thrombolysis, the fibrinogen levels were similar in both treatment groups.

PE Trial No. 3 compressed the 24-h dose of UK to make it more comparable with the high concentration and short infusion period that was used for rt-PA.[23] The novel UK dose was 3 million U over 2 h, with the first 1 million U given as a bolus over 10 minutes. This trial enrolled 90 patients. Repeat pulmonary angiograms at 2 h were performed in 87 patients and then graded by a blinded panel. The results indicated that a 2-h regimen of rt-PA and the novel concentrated dosing regimen of UK exhibit similar efficacy and safety for treatment of acute PE. The one substantive difference between the two agents was that 8 of 46 UK-treated patients, compared with 0 of 44 rt-PA–treated patients, suffered rigors ($p = 0.004$), even though all UK-treated patients were pretreated with hydrocortisone, diphenhydramine, and acetaminophen. In contrast, rt-PA–treated patients received no premedication. (More recent information suggests that the rigors from urokinase can be averted if 1,500 mg [rather than 1,000 mg] of acetaminophen premedication is utilized.)

PE Trial No. 4 was a multicenter randomized, controlled trial in which 101 patients were randomized: 46 to rt-PA 100 mg over 2 h, followed by heparin, and 55 to heparin alone.[24] Thus PE Trial No. 4 is the largest thrombolysis followed by heparin versus heparin alone trial that has been undertaken since phase I of the Urokinase Pulmonary Embolism Trial.[6] The hypothesis was that rt-PA accelerates the improvement of right ventricular dysfunction and pulmonary perfusion after PE more rapidly than anticoagulation alone. The principal endpoints were improvement (or worsening) on the 3-h echocardiogram, 24-h echocardiogram, and 24-h lung scan compared with the baseline echocardiogram and lung scan. Subsequent analyses reveal that rt-PA provides striking improvement in right ventricular function and pulmonary perfusion compared with heparin anticoagulation alone.[24]

We have observed in our previous trials that shorter thrombolytic infusion times of both rt-PA and UK have been accompanied by fewer bleeding complications. PE Trial No. 5 compares 100 mg rt-PA as a continuous infusion over 2 h against a weight-adjusted bolus of rt-PA, 0.6 mg/kg with a maximum dose of 50 mg, administered over 15 minutes. The hypothesis is that a smaller bolus of rt-PA is safer than a larger dose administered over several hours.[25]

We believe that expensive and potentially risky therapy for PE will not gain widespread application unless properly conducted clinical trials are carried out. Therefore, our research group is planning to undertake PE Trial No. 6. The objective is *to determine whether routine use of thrombolysis will reduce the frequency of adverse clinical outcomes compared with heparin alone.* In this future trial, which might encompass as many as 400 patients, the principal endpoint will be a combination of death and recurrent PE. The proposed PE Trial No. 6 will enroll more patients but will collect less data per patient than our previous trials. The only required research test will be an echocardiogram obtained prior to randomization.

BOLUS THROMBOLYSIS

The concept of *bolus thrombolysis* is not new and was employed by Dickie et al.[26] in 1974 when 9 patients received local pulmonary artery infusions of UK in an initial bolus dose of 15,000 U/kg. A similar bolus UK regimen was employed by Petitpretz and colleagues[27] and was associated with rapid clinical improvement in 12 of the 14 patients who were described.

Agnelli[25] has proposed a rationale for bolus rt-PA as a safer alternative than continuous-infusion rt-PA (Fig. 12-10). PEs are rich in fibrin and are likely to release large amounts of cross-linked fibrin degradation products (XL-FDPs) when being lysed. Circulating XL-FDPs from a lysed PE can activate rt-PA when it is continuously present in the circulation due to a prolonged rt-PA infusion. This interaction of XL-FDPs with a prolonged rt-PA infusion could cause the undesirable activation of circulating (not fibrin-bound) plasminogen to circulating plasmin and thus, in turn, could induce a systemic lytic state. The rationale supporting bolus rt-PA is that rapid clearance pre-

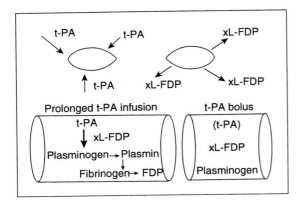

FIGURE 12-10. Schematic representation of the differences between a prolonged t-PA infusion versus a t-PA bolus. (Adapted with permission from Agnelli G: Rationale for bolus t-PA therapy to improve efficacy and safety. Chest 97:164S, 1990.)

vents large amounts of continuously infused, circulating rt-PA from interacting with the XL-FDPs of the PE being lysed. Therefore, bolus rt-PA should be able to limit the potential of the circulating XL-FDPs to promote fibrinogenolysis.

To test the concept of bolus rt-PA, Levine et al.,[28] from McMaster University, enrolled 57 PE patients in a randomized trial of 2-minute bolus rt-PA (0.6 mg/kg over 2 minutes) versus heparin. The principal endpoint was improvement on the 24-h perfusion lung scan compared with the baseline scan. They found that rt-PA causes more resolution of abnormal lung scans than heparin alone. Importantly, none of the patients who received bolus rt-PA experienced major bleeding.

French investigators from Tours have recently reported a pilot study of rt-PA, 50 mg over 10 minutes, to treat massive PE. None of their 21 patients died or suffered a serious bleeding complication.[29]

Another trial of bolus rt-PA for PE treatment has been carried out by Parisian investigators at Laennec Hospital.[30] They enrolled 54 patients with massive PE in a prospective, open study of bolus rt-PA administered in a dose of 1 mg/kg. Improvement in pulmonary perfusion compared with baseline lung scans was similar to the results reported by Levine et al.[28] These French investigators have now completed a trial of bolus

rt-PA, 0.6 mg/kg over 15 minutes, versus rt-PA, 100 mg over 2 h. Their inclusion and exclusion criteria are virtually identical to those in our PE Trial No. 5. Importantly, the French investigators will measure changes in total pulmonary resistance in the two groups of patients, thus providing important hemodynamic information which will complement the echocardiographic and angiographic data that we have collected.

Practical Points

The U.S. Food and Drug Administration (FDA) approved the use of streptokinase (SK) in 1977 and urokinase (UK) in 1978 for treatment of pulmonary embolism. rt-PA was approved for this use in 1990. All three regimens (Table 12-2) utilize fixed or weight-adjusted doses of thrombolytic agents. Therefore, there is no need to obtain laboratory tests during the thrombolytic infusion because no dosage adjustments are made.

Peripheral intravenous and local pulmonary arterial infusion of rt-PA were compared among patients with angiographically documented PE.[31] In a randomized, controlled trial, both routes of administration caused similar rates of lysis, bleeding, and induction of a systemic lytic state. Therefore, locally delivered rt-PA appears to confer no advantage over peripheral administration of the drug.

For patients with a high clinical suspicion for PE and high-probability ventilation-perfusion lung scans, the likelihood of PE exceeds 95%.[32] Therefore, thrombolytic therapy can be administered without angiographic confirmation of the diagnosis. However, angiography should be performed among patients with non-high-proba-

TABLE 12-2. FDA-Approved Thrombolytic Regimens for PE

Streptokinase: 250,000 IU as a loading dose over 30 minutes, followed by 100,000 U/h for 24 h—approved in 1977

Urokinase: 4400 IU/kg as a loading dose over 10 minutes, followed by 4400 IU/kg per hour for 12–24 h—approved in 1978

rt-PA: 100 mg as a continuous peripheral intravenous infusion administered over 2 h—approved in 1990

Reprinted with permission from Goldhaber SE. Prog Cardiovasc Dis 1992;34:113.

bility scans prior to administering thrombolytic therapy. For hemodynamically stable patients admitted in the evening or at night, our group defers angiography until the next morning and empirically initiates heparin. Heparin is usually held for 1 or 2 hours prior to angiography. Angiography is performed using a Cordis sheath with a sidearm (for blood sampling) that is usually placed in the right femoral vein.[33]

When considering PE thrombolysis, our group does not have an arbitrary upper age limit. Additionally, we do not consider the presence of cancer an exclusion criterion. We have found that PE patients have a wide "window" for effective use of thrombolysis. Specifically, patients who receive thrombolysis 6 to 14 days after new symptoms or signs have as effective a response as patients who receive thrombolytic therapy within 5 days after the onset of PE. Therefore, we consider patients suspected of PE as potentially eligible for thrombolysis if they have had any new symptoms or signs within the 2 weeks prior to presentation.

None of the FDA-approved regimens for PE thrombolysis employs concomitant heparin therapy, an important difference when compared with the usual approach to thrombolysis in myocardial infarction. At the conclusion of the thrombolytic infusion, a partial thromboplastin time (PTT) should be obtained. As long as the test result is less than twice the upper limit of normal, heparin therapy can be initiated (or resumed) as a continuous intravenous infusion, without a loading dose. Occasionally, after termination of the thrombolytic infusion, the PTT will exceed twice the upper limit of normal. In this circumstance, the test should be repeated every 4 h until it declines into the range in which heparin therapy is safe. We leave the Cordis sheath in place until the next morning and discontinue the heparin infusion for several hours before removing the sheath. Heparin administration is resumed without a bolus after adequate hemostasis is achieved at the catheterization site.

Contemporary PE thrombolysis should not require an intensive care unit (ICU) bed unless the patient is unstable and needs the ICU for reasons other than thrombolysis. For example, a patient who has a PE and is respirator-dependent warrants an ICU bed, as does a patient who requires Swan-Ganz monitoring. However, even with a Swan-Ganz line in place, thrombolytics should be administered through a peripheral vein. The McMaster group treated all 57 patients in their trial of 2-minute rt-PA (or placebo) infusion either in the emergency department or in the general medical ward.[28]

Complications

Of greatest concern is the risk of intracranial bleeding, which occurs in 2 to 6 of every 1000 patients treated with thrombolytic therapy. If intracranial bleeding is suspected, thrombolytic therapy or heparin should be discontinued immediately, and both neurologic and neurosurgical consultation should be obtained. Retroperitoneal hemorrhage also can be life-threatening because the bleeding is often sustained, brisk, and difficult to diagnose. This complication can occur during the femoral vein catheterization for pulmonary angiography if the femoral artery is inadvertently punctured above the inguinal ligament.

If bleeding is brisk or potentially life-threatening, 10 units of cryoprecipitate should be ordered from the blood bank. Each unit contains 200 to 500 mg fibrinogen and 80 units of factor VIII in a volume of 10 to 15 mL. A dose of 10 units will increase the fibrinogen level by about 70 mg/dL and the factor VIII level by about 30% of normally circulating levels. Cryoprecipitate can be thawed rapidly and should be available within 10 minutes of a request. In addition, 2 units of fresh frozen plasma (FFP) should be ordered. FFP, which may take 45 minutes to thaw, is a source of factors V and VIII as well as α_2-antiplasmin, fibrinogen, and other active coagulation factors.[34]

During the past decade, appropriate patient selection and minimization of the "handling" of patients during the thrombolytic infusion have lessened the bleeding rate. Gross hematuria and other internal bleeding generally can be well managed by discontinuing therapy. Trivial superficial oozing at venipuncture or arterial catheter insertion sites can be controlled with manual compression followed by a pressure dressing.[35]

Allergic reactions due to SK or, less often, UK occur occasionally and are manifested by fever and chills. In an attempt to suppress this reaction, intravenous steroids, diphenhydramine, cimetidine, and oral acetaminophen can be administered prophylactically. Anecdotally, 1,500 mg of acetaminophen premedication is usually effective.

ALTERNATIVE MECHANICAL INTERVENTIONS TO DISLODGE/ REMOVE THROMBUS

For patients who have contraindications to thrombolytic therapy or who do not improve despite its use, surgical pulmonary embolectomy can be considered. If patients have already suffered an episode of cardiac arrest, the prognosis is grim, with only about one-third of patients surviving.[36] Conversely, the prognosis is much improved for those who undergo surgery without preoperative asystole or ventricular fibrillation. The overall survival rate with this heroic intervention is about 60% to 70%.[37,38]

Some patients with massive PE are too unstable to be transported from the catheterization laboratory to the operating room. For this small group of patients, suction catheter embolectomy can be attempted,[39] with a survival rate of 72% in one case series.[40]

Surgical or catheterization laboratory intervention for these desperately ill patients ordinarily occurs in tertiary-care hospitals, where the minority of patients with massive PE will be treated. A promising "low technology" approach is to undertake percutaneous catheter fragmentation and distal dispersion of the proximal PE. This approach can be utilized in any hospital equipped to undertake temporary cardiac pacing because standard percutaneous transvenous catheters are utilized.[41, 42] These patients also can receive combined mechanical clot fragmentation and thrombolytic therapy.[43]

Some patients who suffer PE, particularly a subgroup treated initially with anticoagulation alone, will not succumb to the acute embolism but will develop intractable pulmonary hypertension. Among carefully selected patients with chronic pulmonary hypertension due to PE, elective pulmonary thromboendarterectomy can be undertaken, with a reported mortality rate of 13% at one center with a great amount of experience.[44]

PREVENTION

The estimated direct cost of diagnosing and treating deep venous thrombosis and PE in the United States is $2.9 billion annually. For every 1 million patients who receive prophylaxis against venous thrombosis, approximately $60 million could be saved in direct health care costs.[45] Fortunately, effective mechanical and pharmacologic modalities are available to prevent venous thrombosis among most hospitalized patients.[46] However, at most institutions, these preventive approaches are underutilized.[47]

FUTURE PERSPECTIVES

Many clinicians who practiced in the early and middle 1970s remember PE thrombolysis as a heroic measure that consumed hospital resources and physicians' time round the clock for at least several days. Indeed, more than one in every four patients suffered a major hemorrhagic complication when a 24-h thrombolysis dosing regimen was utilized.[6] This unfavorable experience soured some physicians, who have been reluctant to reconsider PE thrombolysis in the 1990s. Fortunately, recently completed clinical trials have taught us many ways to make thrombolytic therapy safer, more streamlined, and more economical.

At this point, no trial has proven the benefit of thrombolytic therapy in saving lives or in reducing clinically evident morbidity.[48] Future studies will require international collaboration and must focus on relevant clinical endpoints such as reduction of mortality, recurrent PE, and chronic pulmonary hypertension.[49] It is now time for a large trial not only in patients with massive embolism but also among those with smaller emboli that so often herald catastrophic events.[50]

REFERENCES

1. Anderson FA Jr, Wheeler HB, Goldberg RJ, et al. A population-based perspective of the hospital incidence and case-fatality rates of venous thrombosis and pulmonary embolism: the Worcester DVT Study. Arch Intern Med 1991;151:933.

2. Lilienfeld DE, Chan E, Ehland J, et al. Mortality from pulmonary embolism in the United States: 1962 to 1984. Chest 1990;98:1067.

3. Dalen JE, Banas JS Jr, Brooks HL, et al. Resolution rate of acute pulmonary embolism in man. N Engl J Med 1969;280:1194.

4. Tow DE, Wagner NH Jr. Recovery of pulmonary arterial blood flow in patients with pulmonary embolism. N Engl J Med 1967;276:1053.

5. Carson JL, Kelley MA, Duff A, et al. The clinical course of pulmonary embolism. N Engl J Med 1992;326:1240.

6. The Urokinase Pulmonary Embolism Trial. A national cooperative study. Circulation 1973;47:II-1.

7. Sharma GVRK, Burleson VA, Sasahara AA. Effect of thrombolytic therapy on pulmonary-capillary blood volume in patients with pulmonary embolism. N Engl J Med 1980;303:842.

8. Sharma GVRK, Folland ED, McIntyre KM, Sasahara AA. Long-term hemodynamic benefit of thrombolytic therapy in pulmonary embolic disease (abstract). J Am Coll Cardiol 1990;15:65A.

9. Korninger C, Matsuo O, Suy R, et al. Thrombolysis with human extrinsic (tissue-type) plasminogen activator in dogs with femoral vein thrombosis. J Clin Invest 1982;69:573.

10. Collen D, Stassen JM, Verstraete M. Thrombolysis with human extrinsic (tissue-type) plasminogen activator in rabbits with experimental jugular vein thrombosis: effect of molecular form and dose of activator, age of the thrombus, and route of administration. J Clin Invest 1983;71:368.

11. Agnelli G, Buchanan MR, Fernandez F, et al. A comparison of the thrombolytic and hemorrhagic effects of tissue-type plasminogen activator and streptokinase in rabbits. Circulation 1985;72:178.

12. Matsuo O, Rijken DC, Collen D. Thrombolysis by human tissue plasminogen activator and urokinase in rabbits with experimental pulmonary embolus. Nature 1981;291:590.

13. Prewitt RM, Hoy C, Kong A, et al. Thrombolytic therapy in canine pulmonary embolism. Am Rev Respir Dis 1990;141:290.

14. Jang I-K, Vanhaecke J, De Geest H, et al. Coronary thrombolysis with recombinant tissue-type plasminogen activator: patency rate and regional wall motion after 3 months. J Am Coll Cardiol 1985;8:1455.

15. Dalla-Volta S, Palla A, Santolicandro A, et al. PAIMS 2: alteplase combined with heparin versus heparin in the treatment of acute pulmonary embolism. Plasminogen Activator Italian Multicenter Study 2. J Am Coll Cardiol 1992;20:520.

16. Meyer G, Sors H, Charbonnier B, et al. on behalf of the European Cooperative Study Group for Pulmonary Embolism. Effects of intravenous urokinase versus alteplase on total pulmonary resistance in acute massive pulmonary embolism: a European multicenter double-blind trial. J Am Coll Cardiol 1992;19:239.

17. Goldhaber SZ, Vaughan DE, Markis JE, et al. Acute pulmonary embolism treated with tissue plasminogen activator. Lancet 1986;2:886.

18. Goldhaber SZ, Markis JE, Kessler CM, et al. Perspectives on treatment of acute pulmonary embolism with tissue plasminogen activator. Semin Thromb Hemost 1987;13:221.

19. Goldhaber SZ, Meyerovitz MF, Markis JE, et al. on behalf of the participating investigators. Thrombolytic therapy of acute pulmonary embolism: current status and future potential. J Am Coll Cardiol 1987;10:96B.

20. Parker JA, Markis JE, Palla A, et al. on behalf of the participating investigators. Early improvement in pulmonary perfusion after rt-PA therapy for acute embolism: segmental perfusion scan analysis. Radiology 1988;166:441.

21. Come PC, Kim D, Parker JA, et al. on behalf of the participating investigators. Early reversal of right ventricular dysfunction in patients with acute pulmonary embolism after treatment with intravenous tissue plasminogen activator. J Am Coll Cardiol 1987;10:971.

22. Goldhaber SZ, Kessler CM, Heit J, et al. A randomized, controlled trial of recombinant tissue plasminogen activator versus urokinase in the treatment of acute pulmonary embolism. Lancet 1988;2:293.

23. Goldhaber SZ, Kessler CM, Heit JA, et al. Recombinant tissue-type plasminogen activator versus a novel dosing regimen of urokinase in acute pulmonary embolism: a randomized, controlled multicenter trial. J Am Coll Cardiol 1992;20:24.

24. Goldhaber SZ, Haire WD, Feldstein ML, et al. Alteplase versus heparin in acute pulmonary embolism: randomized trial assessing right ventricular function and pulmonary perfusion. Lancet 1993;341:507.

25. Agnelli G. Rationale for bolus t-PA therapy to improve efficacy and safety. Chest 1990;97:161S.

26. Dickie KJ, deGroot WJ, Cooley RN, et al. Hemodynamic effects of bolus infusion of urokinase in pulmonary thromboembolism. Am Rev Respir Dis 1974;109:48.

27. Petitpretz P, Simmoneau G, Cerrina J, et al. Effects of a single bolus of urokinase in patients with life-

threatening pulmonary emboli: a descriptive trial. Circulation 1984;70:861.

28. Levine MN, Hirsh J, Weitz J, et al. A randomized trial of a single bolus dosage regimen of recombinant tissue plasminogen activator in patients with acute pulmonary embolism. Chest 1990;98:1473.

29. Pacouret G, Charbonnier B, Delahousse B, Fournier P. Pilot study of a 50 mg over 10 minutes Alteplase regimen in massive pulmonary embolism (abstract). J Am Coll Cardiol 1992;19: 315A.

30. Diehl J-L, Meyer G, Igual J, et al. Effectiveness and safety of bolus administration of alteplase in massive pulmonary embolism. Am J Cardiol, 1992; 70:1477.

31. Verstraete M, Miller GAH, Bounameaux H, et al. Intravenous and intrapulmonary recombinant tissue-type plasminogen activator in the treatment of acute massive pulmonary embolism. Circulation 1988;77:353.

32. PIOPED Investigators. Value of the ventilation/perfusion scan in acute pulmonary embolism: results of the Prospective Investigation of Pulmonary Embolism Diagnosis (PIOPED). JAMA 1990; 263:2753.

33. Meyerovitz M. How to maximize the safety of coronary and pulmonary angiography in patients receiving thrombolytic therapy. Chest 1990;97: 132S.

34. Sane DC, Califf RM, Topol EJ, et al. Bleeding during thrombolytic therapy for acute myocardial infarction: mechanisms and management. Ann Intern Med 1989;111:1010.

35. Goldhaber SZ. What role for thrombolysis in patients with pulmonary embolism? J Crit Illness 1992;7:192.

36. Clarke DB, Abrams LD. Pulmonary embolectomy: a 25-year experience. J Thorac Cardiovasc Surg 1986;92:442.

37. Gray HH, Morgan JM, Paneth M, Miller GAH. Pulmonary embolectomy for acute massive pulmonary embolism: an analysis of 71 cases. Br Heart J 1988;60:196.

38. Meyer G, Tamisier D, Sors H, et al. Pulmonary embolectomy: a 20-year experience at one center. Ann Thorac Surg 1991;51:232.

39. Feitelberg SP, Kahn SE, Kotler MN, et al. Transfemoral embolectomy for massive pulmonary embolus and associated myocardial infarction. Am Heart J 1987;113:819.

40. Timsit J-F, Reynaud P, Meyer G, Sors H. Pulmonary embolectomy by catheter device in massive pulmonary embolectomy. Chest 1991;100: 655.

41. Brady AJB, Crake T, Oakley CM. Percutaneous catheter fragmentation and distal dispersion of proximal pulmonary embolus. Lancet 1991;338: 1186.

42. Brady AJB, Crake T, Oakley CM. Simultaneous mechanical clot fragmentation and pharmacologic thrombolysis in acute massive pulmonary embolism. Am J Cardiol 1992;70:836.

43. Essop MR, Middlemost S, Skoularigis J, Sareli P. Simultaneous mechanical clot fragmentation and pharmacologic thrombolysis in acute massive pulmonary embolism. Am J Cardiol 1992;69:427.

44. Daily PO, Dembitsky WP, Iversen S, et al. Risk factors for pulmonary thromboendarterectomy. J Thorac Cardiovasc Surg 1990;99:670.

45. Landefeld CS, Hanus P. Economic burden of venous thromboembolism. In: Goldhaber SZ, ed. Prevention of venous thromboembolism. New York: Marcel Dekker, 1993:69.

46. Goldhaber SZ, Morpurgo M, for the WHO/ISFC Task Force on Pulmonary Embolism. Diagnosis, treatment, and prevention of pulmonary embolism. Report of the WHO/International Society and Federation of Cardiology Task Force. JAMA 1992;268:1727.

47. Anderson FA Jr, Wheeler HB, Goldberg RJ, et al. Physician practices in the prevention of venous thromboembolism. Ann Intern Med 1991;115: 591.

48. Anderson DR, Levine MN. Thrombolytic therapy for the treatment of acute pulmonary embolism. Can Med Assoc J 1992;146:1317.

49. Goldhaber SZ. Pulmonary embolism thrombolysis: a clarion call for international collaboration. J Am Coll Cardiol 1992;19:246.

50. Thrombolysis for pulmonary embolism. Lancet 1992;2:21.

13

THROMBOLYTIC THERAPY FOR ACUTE DEEP VEIN THROMBOSIS

Anthony J. Comerota

Although the early complication of acute deep vein thrombosis (DVT), which is pulmonary embolism, is recognized by most physicians today, the potential severity of the postthrombotic syndrome is frequently not appreciated when the acute DVT is treated initially. In general, physicians have conceptually unified "deep vein thrombosis" as a single entity and have considered patients with extensive, multisegment venous thrombosis similar to those having short-segment superficial femoral vein thrombosis. The acute and long-term sequelae are quite different in these two groups of patients, but treatment is identical in most medical communities. Unfortunately, in many medical centers, the treatment of acute deep vein thrombosis has not changed in the past 35 years.

Restoring patency by eliminating thrombus in the deep venous system is an ideal goal of therapy for acute DVT, although pharmacologic and mechanical methods designed to clear the deep venous system remain controversial. Reports have shown that lysis can be achieved and patency restored with thrombolytic therapy and that the long-term postthrombotic sequelae can be reduced if lytic therapy is successful in clearing the deep venous system. However, these observations are not uniformly appreciated, and many physicians are unwilling to risk the potential complications or pay the additional expense associated with thrombolytic therapy. Although accumulated data[1–15] demonstrate that significantly more patients have patency of their venous system restored after treatment with thrombolytic therapy compared with standard anticoagulation, in absolute terms, there is a substantial number of lytic failures. Therefore, a physician may not appreciate the advantages of lytic therapy based on his or her anecdotal experience, especially since certain patients tolerate acute DVT quite well. This is particularly true when only a single segment of the venous system is involved and if the valves remain competent above and/or below the site of thrombosis. When patients suffer severe postthrombotic consequences, it is usually attributed to "patient's disease" rather than admission of inadequate treatment of the acute disease.

Preservation of venous function is the long-term goal of thombolysis for acute DVT, which includes restoring patency and maintaining valvular function. Those who argue against the use of lytic agents point to the risk involved, the cost of therapy, the limited application when considering all patients with acute DVT, and the low success rate from selected studies. However, proponents of lytic therapy reiterate that treatment today is less risky than suggested by earlier reports and emphasize that the cost of the postthrombotic syndrome is high, although spread over many years.[16] Although many patients with acute DVT are not candidates for lytic therapy (i.e., those in the early postoperative period or those with a history of intracranial disease), many eligible patients are young and therefore will enjoy the benefit from thrombolysis, if successful, for many years.

Reports of the results of thrombolytic therapy are potentially biased, since many centers reserve lytic therapy for the most severe disease (extensive iliofemoral DVT/phlegmasia cerulea dolens). Patients with less troublesome DVT, however, who are likely to have less severe postthrombotic sequelae, are generally treated with anticoagulation alone.

NATURAL HISTORY

The natural history of DVT has been of increasing interest during the past several decades. Current technology offers important information on patency, recanalization, and valvular function which can be obtained quickly and easily in an objective fashion.

The underlying pathophysiology of the postthrombotic syndrome is ambulatory venous hypertension. The two important components producing ambulatory venous hypertension are residual venous obstruction and valvular incompetence. As recanalization of the thrombosed venous segment occurs, patency is restored. With recanalization and development of collateral venous drainage, noninvasive studies of maximal venous outflow are likely to be normal. The fact that recanalization has occurred or that maximal venous outflow (with the patient at rest) is normal does not mean that the vein is free of luminal

obstruction. Figure 13-1 demonstrates this concept. The ascending phlebogram (Fig. 13-1A) was performed in a patient with chronic venous insufficiency and venous ulceration due to the postthrombotic syndrome. The phlebogram demonstrates the classic appearance of a recanalized common and superficial femoral vein approximately 15 years after acute DVT. The official angiographic reading described a "chronically diseased but patent superficial femoral vein with no evidence of obstruction." A maximal venous outflow test (impedance plethysmography) was normal. This patient subsequently underwent a classic Linton procedure, at which time the superficial femoral vein was ligated and divided below the profunda femoris vein. A cross section of the superficial femoral vein high in the thigh is shown in Figure 13-1B. While multiple channels due to recanalization can be observed, a large percentage of the normal luminal area remains obstructed. One can easily appreciate the extensive destruction of the venous valves and therefore the natural progression to the postthrombotic syndrome. Shull and Nicolaides[17] demonstrated the additive effects of residual venous obstruction and valvular incompetence on ambulatory venous hypertension in postthrombotic patients in their long-term follow-up evaluation of such patients. In addition to physical examination, they performed ambulatory venous pressures, ascending phlebography, and Doppler evaluation of the popliteal valve. Their data indicate that venous obstruction was associated with higher ambulatory pressures for any degree of valvular function. They also showed that the combination of obstruction and incompetence produced the most severe ambulatory venous hypertension.

Recent studies demonstrate that valvular reflux develops progressively from the time of acute venous thrombosis. Markel and colleagues[18] followed 268 patients with acute deep venous thrombosis with venous duplex imaging. At initial presentation, 14% had valvular reflux. Patients were then restudied sequentially at 1 week, 1 month, 3 months, and 1 year. Reflux developed in 17% of patients by the end of the first week, 40% at 1 month, and 66% at 1 year. In a cohort of over 1000 patients who had symptoms but did

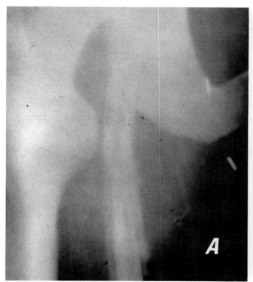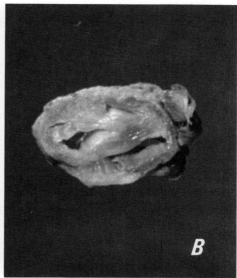

FIGURE 13-1. (**A**) *The ascending phlebogram of a patient suffering from postthrombotic syndrome and venous ulceration. The phlebographic interpretation was that this patient had a patent deep venous system characteristic of the chronically diseased postthrombotic vein without evidence of obstruction.* (**B**) *This is a cross section of the proximal superficial femoral vein visualized by ascending phlebography. It demonstrates the multiple channels of recanalization; however, it also demonstrates the significant amount of residual luminal obstruction.*

not have DVT, only 6% demonstrated reflux at 1 year. Valvular insufficiency was more common in patients suffering occlusive thrombosis compared with those with nonocclusive venous thrombosis. This study demonstrates that increasing amounts of time are required for some valves to become incompetent. In an earlier analysis it was shown that incompetent valves developed in vein segments not involved in the thrombotic process.[19] This new observation suggests that the mechanisms by which valvular incompetence occurs following deep venous thrombosis must involve more than a physical effect of the thrombus on the valve. Another important observation was that 38% did not develop valvular incompetence during the study, and the majority who maintained good valve function long term had complete recanalization of the vein within 30 days. Such observations suggest that early lysis of the thrombus preserves valvular function. These early conclusions were strengthened by their larger follow-up report on the relationship between re-

canalization and valve competence in 113 patients with acute DVT.[20] Meissner and associates[20] found that early recanalization was important in preserving valve integrity and that 85% to 90% of vein segments not developing reflux had complete lysis by 12 months. These natural history studies indicate that persistent obstruction increases the severity of the postthrombotic syndrome and that early lysis preserves valve function. It is intuitive that treatment specifically designed to eliminate thrombus should reduce the severity of the postthrombotic symptoms by avoiding obstruction and maintaining valve function.

Systemic Thrombolysis for Acute DVT

In light of our understanding of the pathophysiology of the postthrombotic syndrome and the results of recently published natural history studies, the ideal management of patients presenting with acute DVT should include the following: (1) supportive care of the patient, (2) prevention of extension and embolization of the thrombus, (3) restoring patency to the deep venous system, and (4) maintaining venous valvular function. Successfully eliminating the thrombus can achieve the last three of these goals. Thrombolytic agents have been used in patients with acute DVT to this end. However, it might be worthwhile to address several important issues, allowing the efficacy of thrombolytic therapy to be put into proper perspective. These issues include (1) evaluating the natural history of anticoagulant therapy, (2) assessing whether venous thrombi can be lysed, and (3) determining whether lysis of venous thrombi is important for long-term valvular function.

Thirteen studies have been reported comparing anticoagulant therapy with thrombolytic therapy for acute DVT (Table 13-1). The diagnosis was established with ascending phlebography, which was repeated after treatment to assess the result. Pooled analysis (Table 13-2) indicates that only 4% of patients treated with anticoagulants had significant or complete lysis, and an additional 14% had partial lysis. The majority (82%) had either no objective phlebographic clearing or actually had extension of their thrombi. Therefore, only a minority of patients had sufficient clearing of thrombus to expect return of normal venous valvular function. In patients treated with thrombolytic therapy, 45% had significant or complete clearing of the clot and 18% had partial clearing. Thirty-seven percent failed to improve or worsened. Although 10 times as many patients had significant or complete clearing with lytic therapy compared with anticoagulation, less than half had a good to excellent phlebographic outcome.

Four additional studies described the results of thrombolytic therapy for deep venous thrombosis but were considered unsuitable for inclusion in the collective data.[21–24] Two studies failed to include an anticoagulation cohort,[21–22] and therefore, comparative data were not available. In another series, Kakkar and Lawrence[23] reported venous hemodynamic changes in patients followed for 24 months after initial randomization to treatment with streptokinase or heparin for acute DVT. Unfortunately, the patients included in the final report represent less than one-third of those initially randomized. Since the initial response to therapy was not clarified in all patients, one cannot assume that the outcome of the subset followed for 2 years is representative of all patients initially randomized. Symptomatic patients are more likely to seek continued care than those who feel well; therefore, this report probably represents a pessimistic bias due to patient self-selection.

The fourth study excluded from the preceding analysis described the response of calf vein thrombosis to treatment with either heparin or streptokinase.[24] Although the authors reported treatment group response with an average quantitative venographic score, they failed to report individual patient response to therapy.

Two studies reported long-term symptomatic results following randomization to either anticoagulation or thrombolytic therapy for acute DVT[11,25] (Table 13-3). Although the follow-up period was shorter in Elliot's study than in Arnesen's study, 1.6 versus 6.5 years, respectively, both treatment protocols were similar, and the same drug (SK) was used. Posttreatment evaluation indicates that the majority of patients who were free of postthrombotic symptoms were treated with streptokinase (SK), whereas the majority with severe symptoms of the postthrombotic syndrome received anticoagulation alone.

The most important question is whether lysis of deep venous thrombi preserves venous valvular function. In a long-term follow-up of a prospective, randomized study, Jeffrey et al.[13] have shown significant functional benefit 5 to 10 years after therapy of acute DVT in patients following successful lysis. Early recanalization (55% for SK versus 5% for heparin) was similar to that in the pooled data reviewed previously. Patients were then followed long term (5 years) for popliteal valve incompetence and venous insufficiency of the involved limb using photophlethysmography, foot volumetry, and direct Doppler examination of the popliteal valve. Patients who had initially successful lysis were compared with patients who did not lyse. Patients who lysed demonstrated normal venous function tests compared with patients who did not lyse ($p < 0.001$). Nine percent

TABLE 13-1. *Review of Anticoagulation versus Lytic Therapy for Deep Vein Thrombosis*

Author, Year	Investigation Type/Total No. of Pts.[a]	Treatment Groups	Results — Significant/Complete Resolution	Results — Partial Resolution	Results — No Resolution/Propagation	Complications — Bleeding Minor	Complications — Bleeding Major	Complications — PE	Death Due to Rx
Browse et al., 1968	PR/10	SK/5	3 (60%)	1 (20%)	1 (20%)	0 (0%)	0 (0%)	None	None
		Hep/5	0 (0%)	0 (0%)	5 (100%)	0 (0%)	0 (0%)	None	None
Robertson et al., 1968	PRB/16	SK/8	5 (63%)	2 (25%)	1 (12%)	2 (25%)	2 (25%)	NA	None
		Hep/8	1 (12%)	2 (25%)	5 (63%)	1 (12%)	1 (12%)[b]	NA	1 (12%)[b]
Kakkar et al., 1969	PR/18	SK/9	6 (67%)	1 (11%)	2 (22%)	0 (0%)	3 (33%)	None	None
		Hep/9	2 (22%)	2 (22%)	5 (56%)	0 (0%)	2 (22%)	None	1 (11%)
Tsapogas et al., 1973	PR/34	SK/19	10 (53%)	0 (0%)	9 (47%)	0 (0%)	4 (21%)	NA	None
		Hep/15	0 (0%)	1 (7%)	14 (93%)	NA	NA	NA	None
Duckert et al., 1975	PNRB/134	SK/92	39 (42%)	23 (25%)	30 (33%)	24 (26%)	58 (62%)	7	None
		Hep/42	0 (0%)	4 (10%)	38 (90%)	4 (10%)	2 (5%)	5	None
Porter et al., 1975[c] Seaman et al., 1976[e] Rosch et al., 1976[e]	PR/48	SK/22	9 (40%)	1 (5%)	12 (55%)	4 (17%)	6 (25%)[b]	1	1 (4%)[b]
		Hep/26	2 (8%)	5 (19%)	19 (73%)	1 (0.4%)	7 (27%)	None	None
Marder et al., 1977	PR/24	SK/12	5 (42%)	2 (16%)	5 (42%)	NA	NA	NA	1 (8%)[b]
		Hep/12	0 (0%)	3 (25%)	9 (75%)	NA	NA	NA	None
Arneson et al., 1978	PR/42	SK/21	11 (52%)	4 (19%)	6 (29%)	1 (5%)	2 (10%)	1[c]	None
		Hep/21	2 (10%)	3 (14%)	16 (76%)	1 (5%)	2 (10%)	None	None
Elliot et al., 1979	PR/51	SK/26	17 (65%)	1 (4%)	8 (31%)	1 (4%)	2 (8%)	None	None
		Hep/25	0 (0%)	0 (0%)	25 (100%)	0 (0%)	0 (0%)	None	None
Watz and Savage, 1979	PR/35	SK/18	8 (44%)	4 (22%)	6 (34%)	3 (12%)	0 (0%)	2[d]	None
		Hep/17	1 (6%)	5 (29%)	11 (65%)	2 (12%)	0 (0%)	1	None
Jeffery et al., 1986	PR/40	SK/20	11 (55%)	0 (0%)	9 (45%)	NA	NA	1	None
		Hep/20	1 (5%)	0 (0%)	19 (95%)	NA	NA	NA	None
Turpie et al., 1990	PRB/82	rt-PA/40	13 (33%)	9 (22%)	18 (45%)	3 (8%)	2 (5%)	NA	None
		Hep/42	2 (5%)	7 (17%)	33 (78%)	1 (2%)	1 (2%)	NA	None
Goldhaber et al., 1990	PRB/67	rt-PA/45	15 (33%)	14 (31%)	16 (36%)	11 (24%)	1 (2%)[b]	NA	None
		Hep/12	0 (0%)	2 (17%)	10 (83%)	0 (0%)	0 (0%)	NA	None

[a] PR, prospective, randomized; PRB, prospective, randomized, blinded interpretation; PNRB, prospective, nonrandomized, blinded interpretation; SK, streptokinase; Hep, heparin; rt-PA, recombinant tissue plasminogen activator; PE, pulmonary embolism; NA, not available.
[b] Intracranial hemorrhage.
[c] Nonfatal pulmonary embolus prior to therapy.
[d] Fatal pulmonary embolus during therapy.
[e] Same study population.

TABLE 13-2. *Phlebographic Outcome of Anticoagulation versus Thrombolytic Therapy for Acute DVT: Results of 13 Studies**

	Lysis		
Rx (No.)	None/ Worse	Partial	Significant/ Complete
Heparin (254)	82%	14%	4%
Lytic Rx (337)	37%	18%	45%

* References 1 to 15 (references 6 to 8 report the same patient group and therefore, for tabulation purposes, are considered as one report).

of patients successfully lysed had an incompetent popliteal valve compared with 77% of those who failed to lyse ($p < 0.001$). Therefore, it appears that in patients without a contraindication to thrombolytic therapy, systemic thrombolysis is preferred, especially when deep venous thrombosis is limited to the infrainguinal venous system. Another important issue currently being evaluated is whether lytic therapy for acute DVT reduces the incidence of recurrent DVT.

Failure of Thrombolytic Therapy

Failure of thrombolytic therapy occurs for a number of reasons, which include (1) poor patient selection, (2) an inadequate fibrinolytic response, (3) premature termination of therapy, and (4) failure of the plasminogen activator to contact the venous thrombus. Patients selected for lytic therapy usually are those with the most extensive venous thrombosis, namely, patients with iliofemoral venous thrombosis or phlegmasia cerulea dolens. Since patients with extensive deep vein thrombosis have the most severe postthrombotic seque-

TABLE 13-3. *Heparin versus Thrombolytic Therapy for Proximal DVT: Long-Term Symptomatic Results (Follow-Up 1.6 to 5.0 Years)*

		Postthrombolytic Symptoms		
Rx	Pts.	Severe	Moderate	None
Heparin	39	8 (21%)	23 (59%)	8 (21%)
SK	39	2 (5%)	12 (31%)	25 (64%)

Data from references 11 and 25.

lae,[27] outcome reports are likely influenced by an inherent selection bias unless randomized studies are performed.

Most patients selected for lytic therapy have extensive, occlusive venous thrombosis, which means that the involved veins do not have luminal blood flow. Therefore, plasminogen activators infused systemically do not reach the thrombus and are unlikely to restore patency.

Selecting patients with older thrombi leads to failure, especially in patients receiving systemic infusions. Successful lysis is related to the amount of plasminogen bound to fibrin (within the thrombus), which diminishes with age. Successful systemic therapy correlates with the age of the thrombus and is unlikely to dissolve a thrombus more than a week old. Unfortunately, clinicians cannot accurately age thrombi and must rely on patient symptoms, which in many instances may not correlate with thrombus age.

Thrombolytic therapy depends on activation of plasminogen; therefore, systemic lytic therapy must be accompanied by a systemic fibrinolytic response. Failure to achieve adequate plasmin production invariably leads to a poor outcome. Streptokinase has been the most frequently used plasminogen activator for the treatment of acute DVT. Circulating antistreptococcal antibodies neutralize SK and minimize its fibrinolytic activity. Likewise, urokinase inhibitors also have been demonstrated.[26] It is important that patients treated with systemic lytic therapy demonstrate appropriate plasminogen activation. Current practice is to obtain baseline coagulation studies, including fibrinogen. After beginning a systemic infusion, the partial thromboplastin time (PTT) and fibrinogen determinations are repeated at 6 and 12 h, expecting a 25% or more drop in fibrinogen and a prolongation of the PTT. This indicates that the drug is activating plasminogen and that a lytic effect is present. Infusion is continued, monitoring the PTT and fibrinogen at 12-h intervals. While bleeding complications do not always correlate with laboratory studies of blood coagulation, we have found that patients demonstrating the most severe induced coagulopathy (i.e., fibrinogen less than 100 mg%) had the greatest likelihood of severe bleeding complications. If profound hypofibrinogenemia occurs, the lytic infusion can be temporarily halted.

Although the goal of thrombolytic therapy is clot dissolution, few physicians monitor the target thrombus as an endpoint of therapy. Many patients have lytic infusions discontinued prior to thrombus resolution, thereby leaving a residual thrombus burden and the continued risk of postthrombotic sequelae. In a prospective evaluation of 28 patients receiving thrombolytic therapy for acute DVT at Temple University Hospital, 33% had their lytic therapy terminated while their clot demonstrated lysis but had not resolved. In patients who had partial lysis, 64% had the lytic agent discontinued while the clot was lysing, prior to complete dissolution. These data indicate that many patients have treatment discontinued prior to maximal lysis, which contributes to the high number of therapeutic failures. The duration of therapy is frequently determined arbitrarily by the attending physician. A predetermined duration of therapy may place the patient at a higher risk of a bleeding complication if lysis occurs early and treatment is continued beyond that time period required for a maximal response. If the clot shows no lysis after 24 h or if the clot completely resolves during this period, lytic therapy should be discontinued. On the other hand, if lysis occurs but is incomplete, lytic therapy should be continued until maximal lysis or resolution is documented. It is the practice in our unit to follow patients during lytic therapy with venous duplex imaging at 12- to 24-h intervals in order to assess thrombus resolution. If no benefit occurs after 24 h, the lytic agent is discontinued. If the thrombus continues to resolve, lytic infusion continues until complete clearing occurs or until no change is apparent on two successive duplex examinations.

ILIOFEMORAL DVT

Many patients with iliofemoral deep vein thrombosis are categorized as having phlegmasia cerulea dolens and have a high risk of acute pulmonary emboli, suffer significant acute morbidity, and are likely to have severe postthrombotic sequelae.[16,27] Physicians observing the morbid natural history of iliofemoral DVT have an intuitive desire to eliminate the thrombus and restore venous drainage from the involved leg. Historically, this was initially attempted with venous thrombectomy. Although preliminary reports were encouraging,[28,29] long-term follow-up of operated patients failed to demonstrate objective benefit.[30,31] Operative morbidity also became an issue, with patients suffering pulmonary emboli, blood loss often requiring transfusion, prolonged hospitalization, and an appreciable operative mortality.[30] As a result, venous thrombectomy has not been widely accepted in the United States as a reasonable treatment for these patients despite more recent reports indicating substantially better outcome.[32-34]

Thrombolytic therapy is a treatment alternative which has the potential for pharmacologically restoring patency to the affected veins. Although systemic therapy for acute DVT is not widely accepted, when used, it is generally reserved for patients with phlegmasia cerulea dolens. Although our unit adopted a similar policy in these patients who had no contraindication to lytic therapy, the results of treatment were marginal in some patients and poor in most. Since extreme postthrombotic morbidity from iliofemoral DVT was observed frequently despite aggressive anticoagulation, and because our experience with systemic lytic therapy had been disappointing, we adopted an aggressive regional approach for the treatment of these patients.

The goal of this approach is to provide unobstructed venous return to the affected limb, primarily by restoring patency to the iliofemoral venous system by taking advantage of the more efficient delivery of thrombolytic agents via regional (intrathrombus) infusion and the improved techniques of contemporary venous thrombectomy. Integrating thrombolytic therapy with the other available options can maximize favorable patient outcome.

Using a multimodality approach, the severe acute morbidity can be reduced or eliminated and the long-term postthrombotic sequelae avoided in most patients. Since treatment options are expanded and concepts unified, long-term favorable results can be anticipated.

METHODS

All patients should have the diagnosis confirmed objectively with venous duplex imaging and iliofemoral phlebography. Venous duplex imaging is used to evaluate the infrainguinal deep venous system and as much of the ipsilateral iliac venous system as possible. An iliofemoral phlebogram should be obtained to assess the proximal extent of thrombus, and a routine contralateral iliocavagram should be performed to evaluate the contralateral iliofemoral venous system and the vena cava. If a patient has suffered a pulmonary embolus during the acute thrombotic episode, a vena caval filter can be inserted at the discretion of the physician. If patients have large, irregular, and nonocclusive vena caval clots, a vena caval filter is recommended prior to catheter-directed thrombolysis. It is not our practice to routinely place vena caval filters preoperatively or prior to catheter-directed thrombolysis if the thrombus is limited to the iliofemoral venous system.

Patients who have no contraindication to thrombolytic therapy are initially offered catheter-directed thrombolysis. Those patients who fail the catheter-directed approach and those who have an absolute contraindication to thrombolytic therapy or multiple relative contraindications are offered venous thrombectomy and an arteriovenous fistula (AVF) under general anesthesia. A crosspubic venous bypass is constructed if unobstructed ipsilateral iliofemoral venous patency cannot be restored. A transluminal dilation with iliac venous stenting is an alternative to crosspubic venous bypass and is currently considered as an alternative in patients with segmental stenosis of the involved iliac vein.

During the past 5 years, 12 patients presenting with occlusive iliofemoral venous thrombosis have been treated according to the approach summarized in Figure 13-2. Their ages ranged from 20 to 58 years, with the mean of 40 years. All patients had the diagnosis confirmed objectively as described. All patients had thrombus extending from their popliteal vein through their iliofemoral venous system, and 5 patients had thrombosis of their vena cava. The etiology for acute venous thrombosis was established in all patients. Postoperative/posttraumatic thrombosis occurred in

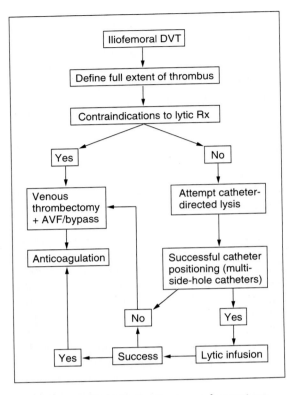

FIGURE 13-2. Algorithm for the approach to patients with iliofemoral venous thrombosis.

7, malignancy was found in 4, and 1 patient had an underlying hypercoagulable state. Patients were followed for a mean of 25 months. One patient was lost to follow-up after 36 months, and 2 patients died due to metastatic cancer 2 weeks and 8 months after therapy.

Catheter-Directed Thrombolysis Technique

Direct intraclot infusion is achieved by placing a catheter from the contralateral femoral vein or from the right jugular vein or both (Fig. 13-3). An alternative access through an ipsilateral femoral vein catheter can be used at the discretion of the physician (Table 13-4). Using the contralateral femoral vein or the jugular vein allows placement of a vena caval filter, if indicated, prior to infusion. While we have not routinely inserted vena caval filters prior to catheter-directed lytic therapy, they were placed in three patients; two had pulmonary

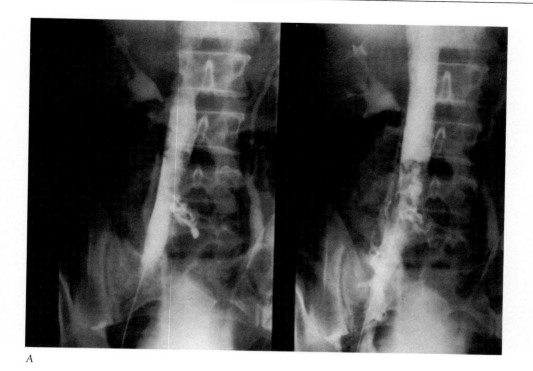

A

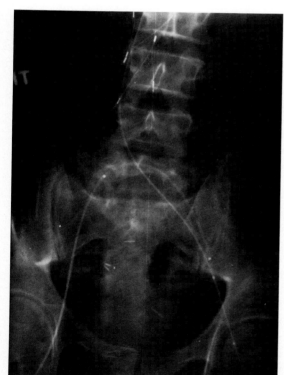

B

FIGURE 13-3. An example of catheter thrombolysis for acute iliofemoral venous thrombosis which is extending to the popliteal vein in a 40-year-old man presenting 9 days after a total colectomy for ulcerative colitis. (**A**) The ilio-cavagram (anteroposterior and oblique views) demonstrating thrombus extending from the left iliac vein and partially occluding the distal vena cava. (**B**) Because of the large volume of partially occluding thrombus in the vena cava, a "bird's nest" vena caval filter was placed above the thrombus. Two multisidehole catheters were inserted into the clot, one from the right jugular vein and one from the contralateral femoral vein. Bolus rt-PA and a continuous infusion of UK were given through both catheters to restore venous patency. (**C**) After 72 h, patency was restored with an excellent clinical response. Note the embolus trapped by the vena caval filter (arrow). At 1 year, the superficial femoral and iliofemoral veins remained patent. (Figure continues)

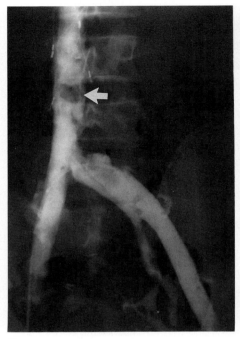
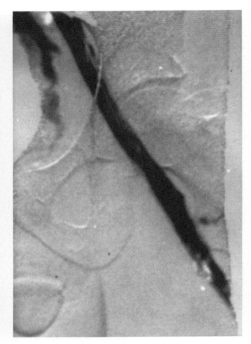

C

FIGURE 13-3. (Continued).

TABLE 13-4. Technical Aspects of Successful
Catheter-Directed Thrombolysis

1. Use right jugular vein, contralateral femoral vein, and occasionally ipsilateral femoral approach to access thrombus.

2. Use multisidehole catheters, infusing as much of the thrombus as possible. Multiple catheters should be considered with extensive thrombosis.

3. Consider caval filter prior to thrombolysis if patient had pulmonary embolus with current episode of DVT or if vena cava has large, partially occluding thrombus. (Caval filter creates problems if patient requires subsequent venous thrombectomy.)

4. Consider bolus of rt-PA (5–10 mg) followed by continuous UK infusion to take advantage of synergistic lysis. Bolus rt-PA may be repeated at 12–24-h intervals.

5. Repeat contrast evaluation every 12–24 h to follow lysis, and reposition catheters as indicated.

6. Follow PT/PTT and fibrinogen levels at 8–12-h intervals. If fibrinogen falls below 100 mg%, stop lytic infusion for 8–12 h, increase heparin, and allow fibrinogen levels and clotting factors to return.

7. If lysis fails (failure to properly position catheters), prepare patient for venous thrombectomy.

embolism as part of their current presentation, and one had large, nonocclusive vena caval thrombus. The indications for vena caval filtration in this setting are currently evolving. However, patients requiring thrombectomy subsequent to vena caval filtration present technical limitations which can compromise operative results.

Once a guidewire is appropriately positioned in the thrombus, multisidehole catheters are advanced into the thrombus to ensure maximal delivery of the lytic agent to the fibrin-bound plasminogen. Systemic doses of plasminogen activators are used. We have chosen to use urokinase delivered as a 250,000- to 500,000-U bolus followed by continuous infusion of 250,000 U/h. In two patients, bolus doses of rt-PA (10 mg) followed by urokinase infusion (250,000 U/h) were used to take advantage of potential synergistic fibrinolysis[35–37] Venous duplex imaging is used to follow lysis of the infrainguinal clot and as much of the iliac venous system as can be visualized. Repeat phlebography through the infusion catheters is performed at 12- to 24-h intervals, and therapy is continued until maximal lysis is achieved. Routine coagulation studies are performed before treatment. During treatment, prothrombin times, partial thromboplastin times, fibrinogen, and fibrin(ogen) split products are monitored and followed at 12-h intervals. If the fibrinogen falls below 100 mg/dL, the lytic agent is stopped for 6 to 12 h, and additional heparin is given. The lytic infusion is resumed when the fibrinogen rises above 100 mg/dL. After completion of the lytic infusion, patients remain anticoagulated with heparin and are converted to oral anticoagulation. If infusion catheters cannot be appropriately positioned within the iliac vein thrombus, a venous thrombectomy is performed.

Venous Thrombectomy Technique

Although a venous thrombectomy can be performed under local anesthesia, regional or general anesthesia is preferred. Since most patients are receiving heparin and remain anticoagulated postoperatively, regional (spinal or epidural) anesthesia is contraindicated. Our preference is general endotracheal anesthesia with at least 10 cmH$_2$O of positive end-expiratory pressure applied. Patients have 2 units of blood cross-matched, and autotransfusion devices are used routinely to minimize transfusion requirements.

A vertical inguinal incision is made over the femoral vessels and the common, superficial femoral, deep femoral, and saphenous veins are mobilized and controlled. Patients are systemically anticoagulated with heparin at 100 U/kg (or more). A transverse or slightly oblique venotomy is made in the distal common femoral vein just proximal to the saphenofemoral junction (Fig. 13-4). The proximal thrombus is removed with passage of a no. 8 to 10 venous thrombectomy catheter. A balloon catheter is not passed from the contralateral femoral vein to occlude the vena cava prior to thrombectomy, since the incidence of pulmonary embolism during iliofemoral venous thrombectomy is low.[32–34] Positive end-expiratory pressure is applied during the thrombectomy, further minimizing the likelihood of pulmonary em-

boli. In an awake patient, the Valsalva maneuver can be performed. If the patient has a vena caval filter in place, fluoroscopy guides the passage of the thrombectomy catheter, and liquid contrast material is used to inflate the balloon.

The proximal venous segment is always assessed by completion phlebography, obtained with an injection of 25 to 30 mL of contrast material through the common femoral venotomy. In light of the inflow occlusion, this technique generally gives good visualization of the entire iliac venous system (see Fig. 13-4D). An alternative is to use direct venoscopy with an angioscope, as reported by Loeprecht.[38] We have not been successful with venous angioscopy due to our inability to adequately clear the lumen of blood draining from collateral veins.

If patency cannot be restored to the proximal venous segment, or if it is found to be extrinsically compressed, a cross-pubic venous bypass is performed using an 8- to 10-mm externally supported PTFE graft. A 3- to 4-mm in-line arteriovenous fistula is created approximately 4 to 6 cm distal to the origin of the superficial femoral artery (Fig. 13-5).

Following the proximal thrombectomy, the distal thrombus is removed. As much clot as possible is extracted by the extrusion technique, either by stroking along the course of the distal veins or by use of a tight rubber bandage wrapped from the foot proximally. Attempts can be made to pass a Fogerty venous thrombectomy catheter distally, although its passage is usually prohibited by venous valves. Others have reported exploration of the posterior tibial vein, into which a catheter is introduced and advanced to the common femoral vein. A thrombectomy catheter can then be attached and guided distally, at which time a thrombectomy of the entire leg can be performed.[33] Although I have no experience with this technique, it may represent an improvement over what can be achieved by compression/extrusion alone; however, the endothelial damage created by balloon catheters is always a concern. Venography can be performed through the distal point of access to assess the adequacy of thrombectomy.

An arteriovenous fistula (AVF) is constructed

(*Text continued on page 188*)

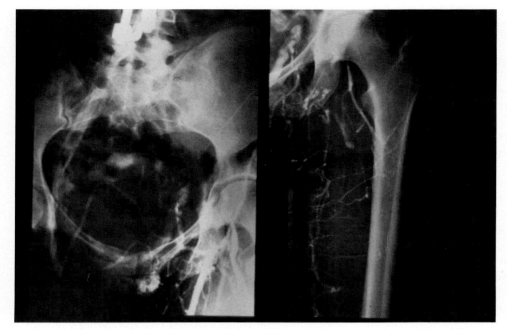

A

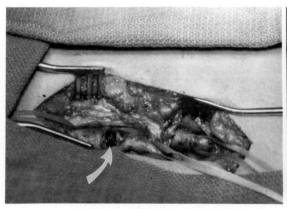

B

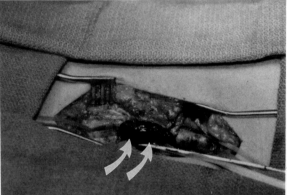

FIGURE 13-4. Technique of venous thrombectomy with arteriovenous fistula. (A) This ascending phlebogram of a young woman following lumbar spine reconstruction for scoliosis demonstrates extensive deep vein thrombosis. All named veins, from her foot to the vena cava, are occluded. (B) Through a longitudinal femoral incision, the common femoral, saphenous, and superficial femoral veins are exposed. A transverse venotomy is made in the common femoral vein (arrow), which is packed with thrombus (left). Within a short time, thrombus begins to extrude from the venotomy (double arrow) due to the high venous pressure (right). (C) The leg is raised and a rubber bandage wrapped tightly from the foot to the upper thigh to remove as much clot as possible from the infrainguinal venous system (above). After passage of a no. 10 venous thrombectomy catheter proximally, one can appreciate the extensive amount of thrombus retrieved (below). (D) A completion operative venogram demonstrates a patent iliofemoral venous system without residual thrombus or obstruction. (E) A small (4 mm) AV fistula (arrow) is created, sewing the end of the transected saphenous vein to the side of the superficial femoral artery (right). The proximal saphenous vein frequently requires thrombectomy prior to creating the AV fistula. A small cuff of 5-mm PTFE graft around the proximal saphenous vein segment is now used routinely. (F) A photograph taken at the 3-year follow-up visit. The patient has only mild intermittent swelling, controlled with low-pressure-gradient compression stockings.

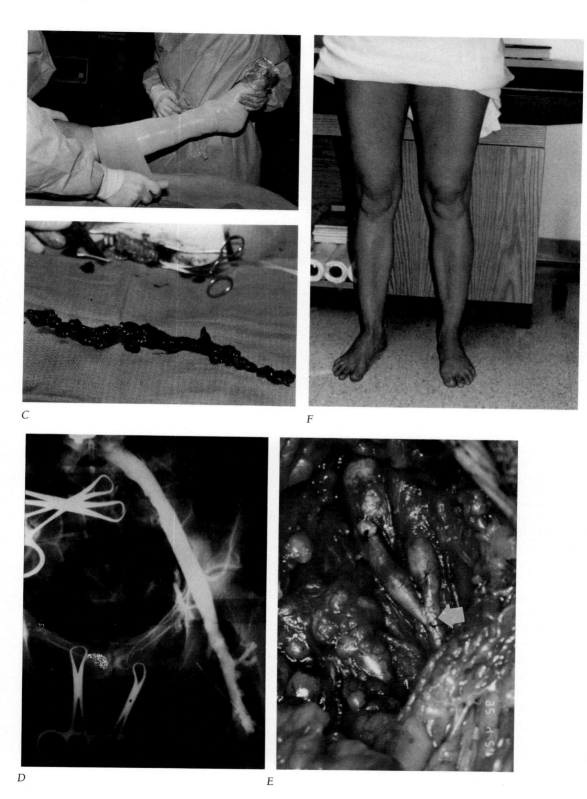

C

D

E

F

FIGURE 13-4. (Continued).

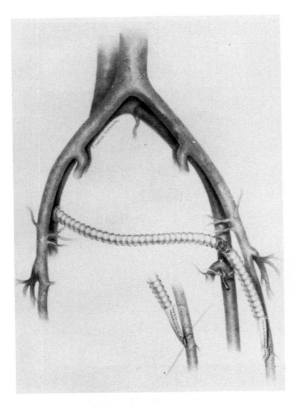

FIGURE 13-5. *Schematic of a preferred method of cross-pubic venous bypass with an 8- or 10-mm externally supported PTFE graft. Note small in-line AV fistula (≤4 mm) to the superficial femoral artery.*

using a large proximal branch of the greater saphenous vein or the proximal greater saphenous vein itself if a branch is not available. The proximal greater saphenous vein usually requires thrombectomy to restore patency; therefore, one does not "sacrifice" it for the AVF. If only the proximal saphenous is thrombosed, every effort is made to preserve it with a proximal thrombectomy and by creating the AVF to a branch of the saphenous vein, if available. A small piece of 4-mm PTFE graft is placed around the vein prior to anastomosis with the superficial femoral artery. This ensures that the arteriovenous communication will not enlarge to create a vascular steal. The superficial femoral artery is mobilized 4 to 6 cm

distal to its origin, and an end-to-side anastomosis, no greater than 4 mm in diameter, is performed. A double loop of Prolene suture is passed around the vein segment (PTFE graft) with a silver or titanium clip joining its ends and left in the subcutaneous tissue beneath the skin. This can be readily accessed in the future should one wish to close the AVF. Since the AVFs are only 3 to 4 mm in diameter, they do not cause hemodynamic consequences, and therefore, routine closure is not required.

Heparin is continued throughout the operative and postoperative period, and warfarin is begun on the first postoperative day. External pneumatic compression devices are applied in the recovery room to further accelerate venous return and prevent recurrent thrombosis.

Occasionally, a combined approach using catheter directed thrombolysis and operative thrombectomy, AVF and possibly bypass, may be required (Figure 13-6). These are complementary procedures and can be used to considerable advantage in selected patients.

RESULTS OF TREATMENT

The results of therapy have been categorized according to clinical outcome and the SVS/ISCVS clinical classification of chronic venous disease.[39] Clinical outcome was defined as excellent if patients had no postthrombotic signs or symptoms, did not require gradient compression stockings to control swelling, and were classified as grade 0 according to the SVS/ISCVS classification of chronic venous disease. A good result was defined as mild postthrombotic symptoms with gradient compression stockings required to control swelling and classified as SVS/ISCVS grade I. A poor result was defined as persistent pain, poorly controlled swelling despite gradient compression stockings, symptoms of venous claudication, and SVS/ISCVS grade II or III. Not surprisingly, outcome correlated directly with patency of the iliofemoral venous segment or the venous bypass. Twelve patients with occlusive iliofemoral venous thrombosis were treated in this manner. Eleven patients were treated with full anticoagulation and failed to improve prior to referral, and one patient had anticoagulation withheld due to an intracranial malignancy. Five patients failed previous systemic fibrinolysis.

Nine of the 12 patients had their iliofemoral thrombus treated successfully (3 involving the vena cava), with patency restored to the native iliofemoral venous system or a patent bypass providing unobstructed venous outflow from the affected limb. These patients had either a good or excellent clinical outcome. Two of the treatment failures had persistent occlusion of the iliofemoral veins and vena cava, and the patient with an intracranial malignancy developed vena caval thrombosis 2 months postoperatively.

Seven patients had catheter-directed lytic therapy attempted. In five of the seven the catheters were correctly positioned, and in each of these, successful lysis occurred with a good or excellent long-term clinical outcome. One patient had intraarterial thrombolysis with urokinase via the femoral artery for unilateral iliofemoral DVT with impending venous gangrene. The second patient developed a complex problem of massive phlegmasia cerulea dolens complicated by acute aortic thrombosis. Multiple catheters were positioned, two intraarterially (distal aorta and left iliac artery) and an intravenous catheter embedded into the intracaval thrombus. This patient was treated with bolus doses of rt-PA followed by a continuous infusion of UK through both the arterial and venous catheters. The two patients having intraarterial infusion had excellent and good clinical outcomes, respectively. Although both patients who had unsuccessful catheter placement were treated with UK, both failed fibrinolysis and underwent venous thrombectomy, which was successful in one and unsuccessful in the other.

Eight patients had venous thrombectomy, five as a primary procedure and three following catheter-directed lysis. Four had an arteriovenous fistula, and three underwent venous bypass to provide unobstructed venous drainage from the affected limb. Two of the eight patients operated on were catheter-directed lytic failures, and one had an adjunctive iliofemoral thrombectomy and bypass following successful lysis of infrainguinal thrombus. Two patients had residual obstruction

following iliofemoral thrombectomy, one in the proximal common iliac vein and one with residual iliocaval thrombus. The patient with the intracranial malignancy initially had a good outcome from thrombectomy with AVF but subsequently developed accelerated leg swelling due to vena caval thrombosis (anticoagulation was contraindicated), and the AVF was dismantled. These three patients were classified as poor clinical outcomes. In all five patients in whom unobstructed venous outflow was restored, a good or excellent result was obtained (mean follow-up of 38 months). No patient suffered symptomatic pulmonary embolism during therapy or hospitalization.

DISCUSSION

Unfortunately, our experience with systemic thrombolysis for iliofemoral venous thrombosis has been disappointing, and others have had similar results.[40] This is not surprising to physicians experienced in the care of these patients, since it is recognized that the iliofemoral venous system is completely filled with thrombus, blood flow is obliterated, the plasminogen activator cannot reach the thrombus, and therefore, lysis does not occur. The regional intrathrombus delivery of thrombolytic agents takes advantage of the basic principle of thrombolytic therapy, which is activation of fibrin-bound plasminogen.[41] All patients with appropriate intrathrombus catheter positioning had successful fibrinolysis and did not require additional intervention. One patient with intraarterial lytic infusion for thrombosis of all named veins in his leg and pelvis had successful clearing of the infrainguinal thrombus but required thrombectomy and venous bypass for persistent occlusion of his iliofemoral venous segment.

The pathophysiology of the postthrombotic syndrome is ambulatory venous hypertension, with its pathologic components being valvular incompetence and luminal obstruction. The most severe manifestations of the postthrombotic syndrome, associated with the highest ambulatory venous pressures, occur in patients who have both obstruction and valvular incompetence.[17] Recent studies demonstrate that valvular function can be preserved after physiologic lysis of deep vein thrombosis, especially if it occurs relatively quickly, i.e., within a month or so of diagnosis.[19,20] Extending these observations to therapeutic fibrinolysis, one could expect further preservation of long-term valvular function with successful lysis. This has been demonstrated in three prospective, randomized series.[11,13,25] In general, patients suffering postthrombotic sequelae following thrombolytic therapy are those who fail lysis or who have recurrent thrombosis, not those who enjoy successful lysis and remain patent.

Venous thrombectomy with contemporary techniques can be performed successfully as a rule rather than an exception. The historical perspective of venous thrombectomy has been reviewed,[42] with appropriate emphasis placed on the evolution of improved results in the more recent series.[32,33] The principles of contemporary venous thrombectomy are listed in Table 13-5 and include complete proximal clot removal, removal of as much distal thrombus as possible, assessment of the iliofemoral venous system for residual thrombus or an underlying lesion (proximal iliac vein web or extrinsic compression), the creation of a small arteriovenous fistula, or the construction of a cross-pubic venous bypass (also with a small AVF) to achieve adequate venous outflow. If patients are selected properly for thrombectomy (within 7 days), it should not be difficult to clear the iliofemoral venous system. After patency is restored, appropriate measures should be instituted to avoid rethrombosis. Completion iliofemoral phlebography is essential and demonstrates whether the thrombectomy is complete and if any residual lesion exists. Postoperative anticoagulation coupled with increasing flow velocity by a small arteriovenous fistula has significantly improved operative results.[32] Recurrent thrombosis has occurred following routine closure of arteriovenous fistulas; therefore, since a small AVF does not cause hemodynamic disturbances, we have not chosen to close AVFs routinely.

We also favor the application of external pneumatic compression garments postoperatively to further reduce the chance of recurrent thrombosis. The risk of causing a PE as a result of external pneumatic compression is unsubstantiated but is believed to be low, and the benefits of external pneumatic compression appear to far outweigh the risks. Intraluminal venous pressures

FIGURE 13-6. *An example of combined multimodality therapy with catheter-directed intraarterial thrombolysis, venous thrombectomy, and cross-pubic venous bypass with an AV fistula. (A) Ascending phlebography in a patient with advanced phlegmasia cerulea dolens whose condition clinically worsened on full anticoagulation. Concern about impending venous gangrene lead to consideration of alternative treatment. The phlebogram demonstrates thrombosis of every named vein of the right lower extremity. The left iliofemoral venous system and vena cava were patent and free of thrombus. (B) An arteriogram was performed to evaluate arterial inflow because of impending gangrene. There was no occlusive disease; however, due to severe venous hypertension, no contrast material was visualized distal to the popliteal artery despite delayed imaging. The catheter was left in place, and urokinase was infused into the common femoral artery at 4000 U/min. (C) A graph of the patient's venous pressure recorded via a dorsal foot vein indicates severe venous hypertension initially. There was a rapid drop in pressure in response to urokinase infusion, which plateaued at 78 cmH$_2$O. Although the patient's pain resolved, the swelling persisted. After 16 h without additional improvement, the urokinase was discontinued and the patient was taken to the operating room for venous thrombectomy. No thrombus was extracted from the veins below the inguinal ligament. Although thrombus was removed from the iliofemoral venous system, a persistent pelvic venous obstruction was appreciated; therefore, a cross-pubic bypass was performed. The patient's venous pressure returned to normal postoperatively, and the patient was anticoagulated. (D) A predischarge phlebogram demonstrates a patent deep venous system with multiple functional valves in the superficial femoral vein and a patent cross-pubic bypass (arrows). Physiologic studies have confirmed normal venous valve function. Although there was some degree of residual venous obstruction of the popliteal vein, the patient's physiologic studies returned to normal and after 3 years of follow-up demonstrated no evidence of venous insufficiency.*

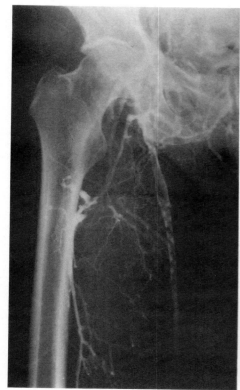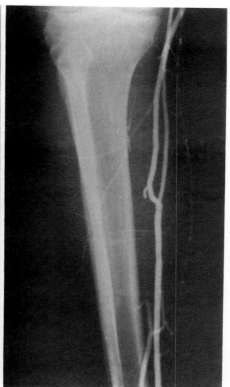

A

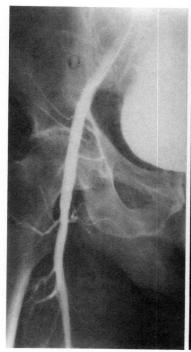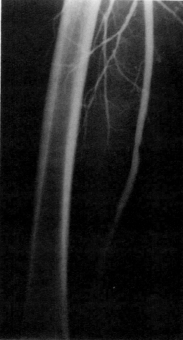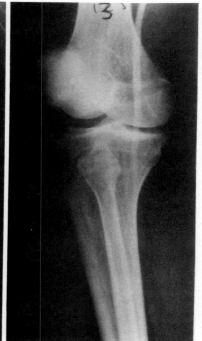

B

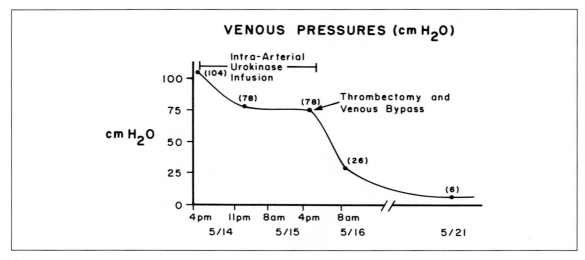

C

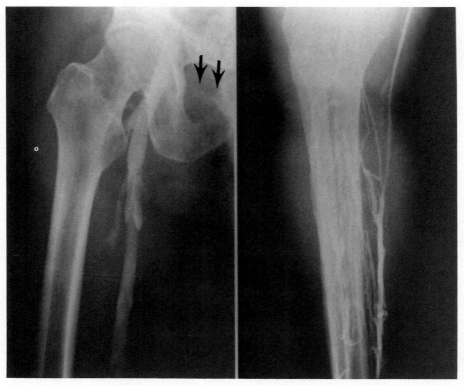

D

FIGURE 13-6. (Continued).

TABLE 13-5. Technical Aspects of Successful Venous Thrombectomy

1. Complete visualization of thrombus, including contralateral iliofemoral phlebography and cavagram.
2. Preferential use of general anesthesia with positive endexpiratory pressure.
3. Type and cross-match 2–3 units of blood.
4. Use autotransfusion device during procedure.
5. Use generous doses of heparin.
6. If caval filter is in place, fluoroscopy is used during thrombectomy, with liquid contrast material used to inflate balloon of thrombectomy catheter.
7. Consider intraoperative infusion of plasminogen activators after thrombectomy, with balloon occlusion of the iliac vein.
8. Use extrusion technique to remove distal thrombus.
9. Perform completion iliofemoral phlebography to assess adequacy of thrombectomy and to evaluate for residual iliac vein pathology.
10. If proximal thrombectomy is complete, a small AV fistula (approx. 4 mm) is constructed with the saphenous vein or one of its large proximal branches to the proximal superficial femoral artery. A short sleeve of 4-mm PTFE graft is placed around the saphenous vein to prevent dilation. An O polypropylene ligature is looped around the graft, tagged with metal clips, and left in the subcutaneous space.
11. If iliac system remains occluded or if external compression exists, a cross-pubic venous bypass is performed with an 8–10-mm externally supported PTFE graft with an associated AV fistula (see Fig. 13-3). Alternatively, transluminal dilation and stenting can be performed with fluoroscopic guidance.
12. Apply external pneumatic compression devices in recovery room.
13. Continue heparin throughout postoperative period, with early conversion to oral anticoagulation.
14. Leave AV fistula functional if anastomosis is small. Enlargement of the fistula is limited by the small size of the anastomosis and the PTFE cuff; therefore, hemodynamic complications of the AVF are avoided and hemodynamic sequelae are absent.

with simple foot dorsiflexion and plantar flexion are many-fold higher than those obtained with a 60- to 80-mmHg pneumatic pressure garment applied externally (personal observation during lower extremity venous pressure evaluation).

Two of the three thrombectomy failures did not have their venous system cleared during the thrombectomy. The third patient developed vena caval thrombosis 2 months postoperatively, as described above.

It is evident that the key to a successful outcome following thrombectomy is removal of the iliofemoral venous thrombus, restoration of unobstructed venous drainage from the involved leg, and prevention of recurrent thrombosis. Although our preference is to restore patency and preserve the native venous system, there are instances, such as chronic organized thrombus and intraluminal web or iliac vein compression, when this is not possible.

If the contralateral iliofemoral system and the vena cava are patent, unilateral obstruction is easily handled with a cross-pubic venous bypass. In our experience, the saphenous vein is often inadequate due to its small size relative to the deep venous system and frequently fails when used for cross-pubic venous bypass. Previous reports of successful cross-pubic venous bypasses with saphenous veins included many patients with chronic iliac vein obstruction.[43] In many patients, the pelvic vein obstruction was due to malignancy, frequently presenting as a preterminal event without associated iliofemoral thrombosis. Patients with malignant pelvic venous obstruction are different from those described in the present discussion in that obstruction is frequently gradual and other noninvolved veins remain patent. A recent report by Gruss[44] indicates improved patency with a PTFE cross-pubic venous bypass compared with saphenous vein. Our preferred bypass conduit is an externally supported PTFE graft at least 8 mm in diameter. When constructed with an inline 3- to 4-mm AVF (Fig. 13-6) combined with long-term anticoagulation, sustained patency can be anticipated. Balloon dilation of a residual iliac vein stenosis (with stenting, if appropriate) also can be considered if fluoroscopy is available.

Despite the extensive nature of the venous thrombosis in these patients, the acute relief of the iliofemoral venous occlusion eliminated early morbidity in 10 of the 12 patients (83%) and provided sustained benefit in 9 of 12 (75%).

These patients with iliofemoral venous thrombosis represent the most extensive acute venous thrombosis cases treated at our institution during a 5-year period. Each patient had multilevel venous occlusion with thrombus extending from the lower leg through the common iliac vein, and 33% involved the vena cava. I believe that this approach is conceptually unified and is designed to eliminate thrombus, restore patency, and provide unobstructed venous return, with ongoing anticoagulation to prevent rethrombosis.

Understanding the natural history of acute deep vein thrombosis and the pathophysiology of chronic venous insufficiency and the postthrombotic syndrome and an appreciation that all patients with DVT are not the same establish a foundation for an individualized approach to the patient with acute DVT. Judicious application of thrombolytic therapy can significantly reduce acute morbidity and postthrombotic sequelae. Inasmuch as possible, thrombolytic agents should be infused into the thrombus. As percutaneous techniques continue to improve, this is likely to become routine even for the infrainguinal forms of acute DVT. Hopefully, the guidelines set forth within this chapter will assist clinicians in the appropriate use of thrombolytic therapy for acute DVT.

REFERENCES

1. Browse NL, Thomas ML, Pim HP. Streptokinase and deep vein thrombosis. Br Med J 1968;3:717.
2. Robertson BR, Nilsson IM, Nylander G. Value of streptokinase and heparin in therapy of acute deep vein thrombosis. Acta Chir Scand 1968;134:203.
3. Kakkar VV, Franc C, Howe CT, et al. Treatment of deep vein thrombosis: a trial of heparin, streptokinase and arvin. Br Med J 1969;1:806.
4. Tsapogas MJ, Peabody RA, Wu KT, et al. Controlled study of thrombolytic therapy in deep vein thrombosis. Surgery 1973;74:973.
5. Duckert F, Muller G, Hyman D, et al. Treatment of deep vein thrombosis with streptokinase. Br Med J 1975;1:973.
6. Porter JM, Seaman AJ, Common HH, et al. Comparison of heparin and streptokinase in the treatment of venous thrombosis. Am Surg 1975;41:511.
7. Seaman JS, Common HH, Rosch J, et al. Deep vein thrombosis treated with streptokinase or heparin. Angiology 1976;27:549.
8. Rosch JJ, Dotter CT, Seaman AJ, et al. Healing of deep vein thrombosis: venographic findings in a randomized study comparing streptokinase and heparin. AJR 1976;127:533.
9. Marder VJ, Soulen RL, Atichartakarn V. Quantitative venographic assessment of deep vein thrombosis in the evaluation of streptokinase and heparin therapy. J Lab Clin Med 1977;89:1018.
10. Arnesen H, Heilo A, Jakobsen E, et al. A prospective study of streptokinase and heparin in the treatment of deep vein thrombosis. Acta Med Scand 1978;203:457.
11. Elliot MS, Immelman EJ, Jeffrey P, et al. A comparative randomized trial of heparin versus streptokinase in the treatment of acute proximal venous thrombosis: an interim report of a prospective trial. Br J Surg 1979;66:838.
12. Waltz R, Savidge GF. Rapid thrombolysis and preservation of venous valvular function in high deep vein thrombosis. Acta Med Scand 1979;205:293.
13. Jeffrey P, Immelman E, Amoore J. Treatment of deep vein thrombosis with heparin or streptokinase: long-term venous function assessment (abstract No. S20.3). In: Proceedings of the Second International Vascular Symposium, 1989.
14. Turpie AGG, Levine MN, Hirsh J, et al. Tissue plasminogen activator vs heparin in deep vein thrombosis. Chest 1990;97:172S.
15. Goldhaber SZ, Meyerrovitz MF, Green D, et al. Randomized controlled trial of tissue plasminogen activator in proximal deep venous thrombosis. Am J Med 1990;88:235.
16. O'Donnell TF, Browse NL, Burnand KG, et al. The socioeconomic effects of an iliofemoral thrombus. J Surg Res 1977;22:483.
17. Shull KC, Nicolaides AN, Fernandez JF, et al. Significance of popliteal reflux in relation to ambulatory venous pressure and ulceration. Arch Surg 1979;114:1304.
18. Markel A, Manzo R, Bergelin R, Strandness E. Valvular reflux after deep vein thrombosis: incidence and time of occurrence. J Vasc Surg 1992;15:377.
19. Killewich LA, Bedford GR, Beach KW, et al. Spontaneous lysis of deep vein thrombi: rate and outcome. J Vasc Surg 1989;9:89.
20. Meissner MH, Manzo RA, Bergelin RO, et al. Deep venous insufficiency: the relationship between lysis and subsequent reflux. J Vasc Surg 1993;18:596.
21. Albrechtsson U, Anderson J, Einarsson E, et al. Streptokinase treatment of deep venous thrombosis and the post-thrombotic syndrome. Arch Surg 1981;116:33.
22. van de Loo JCW, Kriessman A, Trubestein G, et al. Controlled multicenter pilot study of urokinase-heparin and streptokinase in deep vein thrombosis. Thromb Haemost 1983;50:660.
23. Kakkar VV, Lawrence D. Hemodynamic and clinical assessment after therapy for acute deep vein

thrombosis: a prospective study. Am J Surg 1985; 150:28.

24. Schulman S, Granqvist S, Juhlin-Danfelt A, et al. Long-term sequelae of calf vein thrombosis treated with heparin or low-dose streptokinase. Acta Med Scand 1986;219:349.

25. Arnesen H, Hoiseth A, Ly B. Streptokinase or heparin in the treatment of deep vein thrombosis: follow-up results of a prospective study. Acta Med Scand 1982;211:65.

26. Comerota AJ. Urokinase. In: Messerli F, ed. Current cardiovascular drug therapy, Philadelphia: WB Saunders, 1990.

27. Cockett FB, Thomas L. The iliac compression syndrome. Br J Surg 1965;52:816.

28. Haller JA, Abrams BL. Use of thrombectomy in the treatment of acute iliofemoral venous thrombosis in forty-five patients. Ann Surg 1963;158:561.

29. De Weese JA. Thrombectomy for acute iliofemoral venous thrombosis. J Cardiovasc Surg 1964;5:703.

30. Lansing AM, Davis WM. Five-year follow-up study of iliofemoral venous thrombectomy. Ann Surg 1968;168:620.

31. Karp RB, Wylie EJ. Recurrent thrombosis after iliofemoral venous thrombectomy. Surg Forum 1966;17:147.

32. Plate G, Einarsson E, Ohlin P, et al. Thrombectomy with temporary arteriovenous fistula: the treatment of choice in acute iliofemoral venous thrombosis. J Vasc Surg 1984;1:867.

33. Eklof B, Juhan C. Revival of thrombectomy in the management of acute iliofemoral venous thrombosis. Contemp Surg 1992;40:21.

34. Swedenborg J, Hagglof R, Jacobsson H, et al. Results of surgical treatment for iliofemoral venous thrombosis. Br J Surg 1968;73:871.

35. Gurewich V, Pannell R. A comparative study of the efficacy and specificity of tissue plasminogen activator and pro-urokinase: demonstration of synergism and of different thresholds of non-selectivity. Thromb Res 1986;44:217.

36. Collen D, Stump DL, Van de Werf F. Coronary thrombolysis in patients with myocardial infarction by intravenous infusion of synergic thrombolytic agents. Am Heart J 1986;11:1083.

37. Collen D, Stassen J, Stump D, Verstraete M. Synergism of thrombolytic agents in vivo. Circulation 1986;14:838.

38. Loeprecht H. Angiosopie veineuse. Phlebologie 1988;41:165.

39. Porter JM, Rutherford RB, Clagett GP, et al. Reporting standards in venous disease. J Vasc Surg 1988;8:172.

40. Hill SL, Martin D, Evans P. Massive vein thrombosis of the extremities. Am J Surg 1989;158:131.

41. Alkjaersig N, Fletcher AP, Sherry S. The mechanism of clot dissolution by plasmin. J Clin Invest 1959;38:1086.

42. Rutherford RB. The role of thrombectomy in the management of iliofemoral venous thrombosis. In: Rutherford RB, ed. Vascular surgery. 3rd ed. Philadelphia: WB Saunders, 1989:1569.

43. Dale WA. Crossover grafts iliofemoral venous occlusion. In: Bergan JJ, Yao JST, eds. Venous problems. Chicago: Year Book Medical Publishers, 1978:411.

44. Gruss J. Venous bypass for chronic venous insufficiency. In: Bergan JJ, Yao JST, eds. Venous disorders. Philadelphia: WB Saunders, 1991:316.

14

THROMBOLYTIC THERAPY FOR ACUTE PRIMARY AXILLOSUBCLAVIAN VEIN THROMBOSIS

Herbert I. Machleder

Concepts in the management of acute subclavian vein thrombosis have undergone considerable evolution since the initial review in the *International Abstracts of Surgery* in 1949.[1,2] From the first reported surgical thrombectomy in 1911 by Schepelmann to the present time, aggressive surgical therapy has been recommended to remove the occluding thrombus and restore normal upper extremity hemodynamics.[3-5] Unfortunately, surgical thrombectomy has a very high incidence of failure, limited as it is by the considerable thrombogenicity of the damaged vein segment and the difficulty in maintaining adequate anticoagulation in the early postoperative period.

Nevertheless, because of generally nonlethal consequences, relatively young age of onset, protracted (often permanent) disability, and the outcome being dependent on the effectiveness of initial therapy, early management of the thrombus remains a critical aspect of treatment for this disorder. Recent studies have emphasized that failure to achieve venous patency or failure to deal effectively with the underlying anatomic abnormality will have an adverse impact on regaining a functionally normal upper extremity. The consequences of ineffective therapy have led to rates of disability ranging from a low of 25% reported by Linblad et al.[9] from Sweden, to 40% reported by Gloviczki et al.[7] from the Mayo Clinic, to 47% reported by Donayre et al.[6] and 74% by Tilney et al.[8]

Recent advances in techniques of thrombolytic therapy, together with improved understanding of the pathophysiology and underlying morphologic disorder, have led to improved results of therapy.[10-12] Following a comprehensive multimodality approach to therapy, a long-term disability rate of 12% could be anticipated.[2]

The following discussion will emphasize early recognition and an effective algorithm for management of this increasingly recognized vascular disorder.

HISTORY

Spontaneous or effort-related thrombosis of the axillosubclavian vein is a disabling disorder of young, otherwise healthy individuals that was described independently over 100 years ago by Paget in England and Von Schroetter in Germany. In 1949, Hughes[1] analyzed 320 cases of spontaneous upper extremity venous thrombosis collected from the medical literature and recognized the first two descriptions by naming the entity the *Paget-Schroetter syndrome*. Over the course of subsequent investigations, it has become evident that in contrast to the apparent spontaneous nature of the event, there is an underlying chronic venous compressive anomaly at the thoracic outlet[13,14] (Fig. 14-1).

Despite increasing recognition of this syndrome and innovative approaches to management, there have been recurrent areas of disagreement with regard to optimal therapy.[4,15,16] The 167 reports in Hughes' literature review averaged 2 patients per article, with no series containing more than 10 patients. This paucity of concentrated experience, particularly in view of major improvements in pharmacologic, interventional radiologic, and surgical techniques, inhibited the development of a comprehensive and effective therapeutic approach.

In 1981, Zimmerman and colleagues[17] reported the results of urokinase therapy in a group of patients with axillosubclavian vein thrombosis. Steed and coworkers,[18] reporting from Pittsburgh, used streptokinase in the treatment of subclavian vein thrombosis and achieved complete clot lysis in only one of their patients. In 1986, Perler and Mitchell[19] reported the results in a single patient in whom the underlying compressive stricture at the thoracic outlet was demonstrated and treated by transaxillary first rib resection. They used balloon angioplasty to correct a residual stricture found on follow-up venography.

In 1985, a clinical management strategy based on contemporary concepts of pathophysiology and a multidisciplinary approach to therapy was initiated at the UCLA Medical Center, with final results published in 1992.[2,10]

PATHOLOGIC ANATOMY AND PHYSIOLOGY

The acute thrombosis is most often in an area of chronic compression and stricture of the axillo-subclavian vein at the thoracic outlet. The vein is compressed between a hypertrophied scalene or subclavius tendon and the first rib. A large exostosis is often found at the costoclavicular junction[20] (Fig. 14-1*A* and *B*).

The natural history of the disease reflects the development of venous hypertension due to chronic venous compression, with acute symptoms resulting from sudden thrombosis, and obstruction of collateral veins. Following resolution of acute thrombotic manifestations, patients may be relatively free of symptoms at rest, with edema resolving fairly promptly within 1 to 3 weeks.

From 1985 to 1989, 33 patients with classic Paget-Schroetter syndrome were treated at the UCLA Medical Center. The 20 men and 13 women, who otherwise were in excellent general health, had spontaneous or effort-related upper extremity axillary and subclavian venous thrombosis unrelated to intercurrent illness or iatrogenic manipulation.

Fifteen patients were engaged in occupations involving upper extremity labor. Eight were so-called white-collar workers or the equivalent, and 10 were engaged in competitive athletics. Twenty-five patients (76%) had been engaged in competitive sports or manual labor, with the thrombotic event following strenuous effort [20 males (100% of the men) and 4 females (31% of the women)]. Nine patients were engaged in relatively sedentary activity with no recognizable precipitating event (all females).

Bilateral venograms revealed a contralateral venous deformity at the thoracic outlet in 65% of the patients. We have come to recognize this deformity as a precursor to the thrombotic event. One patient presenting with acute thrombosis while working as a carpenter/framer presented 1 year later with spontaneous thrombosis in the contralateral axillosubclavian vein while working as a cashier in a record store. A second man had contralateral axillosubclavian vein thrombosis 18 months after the first episode under identical circumstances during a camping trip at the same campsite. A female patient had two contralateral episodes separated by 17 years.

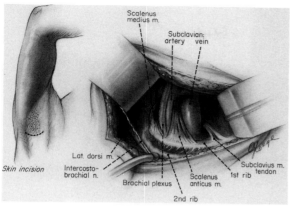

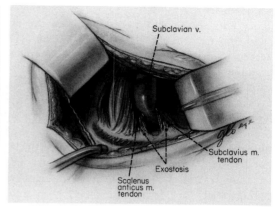

A

B

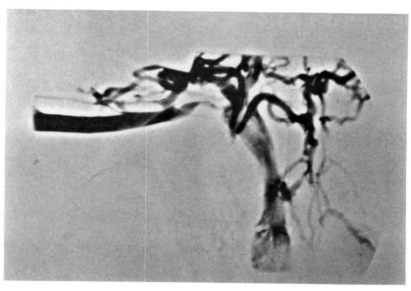

C

FIGURE 14-1. (**A**) *Transaxillary view of thoracic outlet anatomy. (Reprinted with permission from Machleder HI, ed: Vascular disorders of the upper extremity. 2nd ed. Mt. Kisco, NY: Futura Press, 1989.)* (**B**) *Transaxillary view of thoracic outlet anatomy in a patient with the typical abnormality seen in the Paget-Schroetter variant of thoracic outlet syndrome. (Reprinted with permission from Kunkel JM, Machleder HI: Treatment of Paget-Schroetter syndrome: a staged, multidisciplinary approach. Arch Surg 1989;124:1153.).* (**C**) *Venographic appearance of the compressive abnormality in a patient just having completed a successful course of thrombolytic therapy for acute occlusion.*

LABORATORY EVALUATION

All patients should have venography of the affected upper extremity to confirm the diagnosis. Thirty patients in our series (91%) had complete thrombotic obstruction, and 3 had evidence of external compression or stricture without evidence of residual thrombus (2 males and 1 female). This characteristic of high-grade stenosis with probable intermittent occlusion was suspected in 14 of Hughes' collected cases (where exploration of the vein failed to reveal any thrombus). This phenomenon was analyzed later in more detail by McLeery et al.[21]

After we encountered 3 patients with separate thrombotic events involving both upper extremities, bilateral upper extremity venography was included in the patient evaluation. In the 19 patients studied, abnormalities were found in the contralateral vein in 13 (65%). This included 11 of the 13 males studied (85%) and 2 of the 6 females studied (33%). The contralateral vein was found to be thrombosed in 3, normal in 6, and compressed at the thoracic outlet in 10. The occurrence of bilateral abnormalities corroborates the findings in other reports of Paget-Schroetter syndrome.[22]

TREATMENT

The algorithm for management that we have followed includes verification of the diagnosis by venography, followed by local thrombolytic therapy and anticoagulation for 3 months. After that time, patients with stable occlusion of the axillosubclavian vein are evaluated for residual symptoms. For those patients with significant residual disability or a persistent area of compression in either the neutral or stress position, thoracic outlet decompression via transaxillary first rib resection is recommended (Fig. 14-2).

Following first rib resection, percutaneous transluminal balloon angioplasty was utilized to correct residual venous stenosis or stricture when this was demonstrated on follow-up venogram.

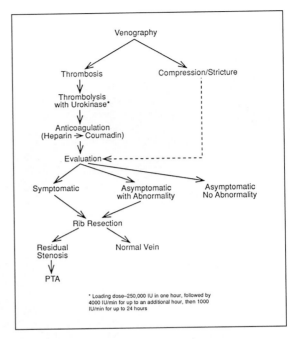

FIGURE 14-2. Management of suspected thrombosis of the axillosubclavian vein.

Local Thrombolytic Therapy

In recent years, the superiority of local thrombolytic therapy over systemic infusion of fibrinolytic agents has been demonstrated, particularly for the treatment of axillosubclavian vein thrombosis.[23–25] Venography should be performed via the basilic vein of the affected extremity. A separate retrograde innominate artery or superior vena caval injection from a transfemoral approach can be utilized in selected patients to obtain better visualization of the central veins (Fig. 14-3).

When thrombus is visualized in the brachial, axillary, or subclavian vein, a small catheter is positioned in the clot via the percutaneous basilic vein approach. An attempt is made to traverse the clot with either a guidewire or a catheter to establish a channel prior to infusion (Fig. 14-4).

A loading dose of 250,000 IU urokinase is infused into the clot over 1 h (4000 IU/min) (Fig. 14-5). Infusion at this rate can be continued for an additional hour and then changed to 1000 IU/min for up to 24 h[26] (Fig. 14-6).

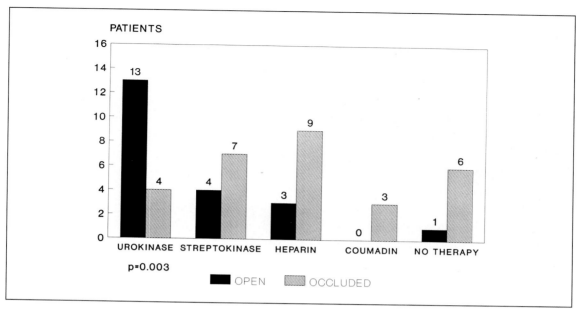

FIGURE 14-3. Status of the axillosubclavian vein after initial medical therapy in the use of urokinase (p = 0.003). (Reprinted with permission from Machleder HI: Evolution of a new treatment strategy for Paget-Schroetter syndrome: spontaneous thrombosis of the axillary-subclavian vein. J Vasc Surg 1993;17:305.)

Systemic heparinization sufficient to maintain the partial thromboplastin time at 1.5 times the control value is used if there is any evidence of thrombus formation in the segment of vein traversed by the catheter or if a prolonged thrombolytic infusion is anticipated. After discontinuation of the fibrinolytic agent, full heparinization is maintained until anticoagulation with Coumadin to a prothrombin time of 1.5 to 2 times the control value is established. Coumadin anticoagulation is continued for 3 months.

Following initial treatment, 22 patients were maintained on Coumadin for an average of 17 weeks. This regimen was planned to allow resolution of the thrombophlebitic process prior to a decision regarding definitive treatment of the underlying abnormality.

We found it particularly noteworthy that three patients had successful surgical thrombectomy (at a referring hospital) as part of their initial treatment, and all experienced rethrombosis of the vein in the early postoperative period, as verified by follow-up venography. Upon comple-

tion of thrombolytic therapy and visualization of the underlying compressive lesion, four patients had percutaneous transluminal balloon venoplasty as part of their initial therapy. These procedures, performed at the referring hospitals without prior surgical decompression, resulted in the thrombotic reocclusion of the previously patent but stenotic axillosubclavian vein in all patients (Fig. 14-7). The futility of this approach as a definitive procedure has been documented by others.[27]

At the conclusion of anticoagulation therapy, patients who had failed attempts at recanalization of the vein but had a stable, nonprogressing venous thrombus were advised to resume normal activity, intending to evaluate the severity of residual symptoms. Patients with disability which restricted them from their usual occupation or avocation were offered the option of surgical decompression of the thoracic outlet. The rationale for this therapy in patients with irremediable thrombosis is based in part on venographic evidence demonstrating compression of the collat-

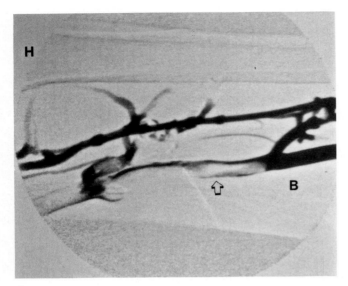

A

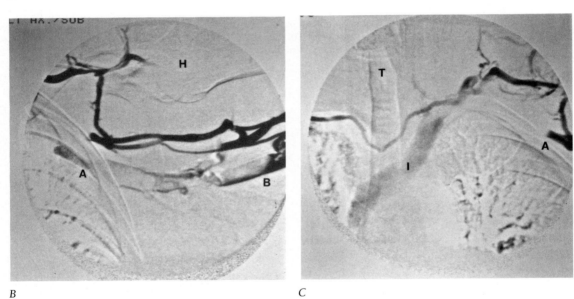

B   *C*

FIGURE 14-4. (A) Venographic appearance of acute effort thrombosis of axillosubclavian vein. Note the thrombus in the brachial and axillary veins (arrow). Humeral head (H), brachial vein (B). (B) Baseline venographic appearance of axillary vein (same patient). Head of humerus (H), brachial vein (B), axillary vein (A). (C) Proceeding centrally, note complete thrombosis of subclavian vein, with filling of innominate vein (I) from axillary vein (A) via first rib collaterals. The trachea is indicated (T).

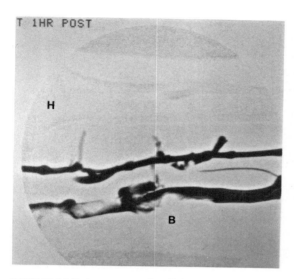

FIGURE 14-5. *Appearance of axillobrachial segment after 1 h of lytic therapy (compare with Fig. 14-2 and use the prominent collateral vein at left center for reference).*

eral veins at the thoracic outlet when the arm is placed in the elevated position.

COMPLICATIONS OF THERAPY

In a series of 50 consecutive patients, the following complications were attributed to therapy.[2]

Venography

One patient had an episode of phlebitis following venography, and three were treated for cutaneous allergic reactions.

Lytic Therapy

Two patients had systemic allergic reactions to streptokinase despite cortisone and diphenhydramine. A 23-year-old woman had an episode of disorientation and ataxia during urokinase therapy. This event was evaluated by MRI scan, lumbar puncture, and serial CT scans as part of a comprehensive neurologic evaluation. There was no evidence of an intracerebral bleed, and the

FIGURE 14-6. **(A)** *After 24 h of lytic therapy (note position of multiple sidehole infusion catheter).* **(B)** *After 28 h of lytic therapy.*

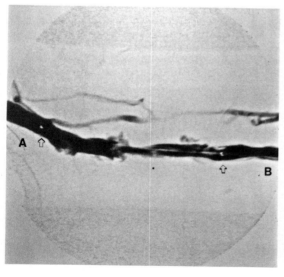

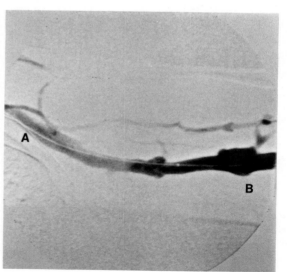

A   *B*

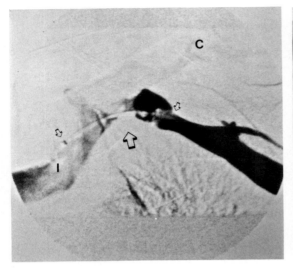

A

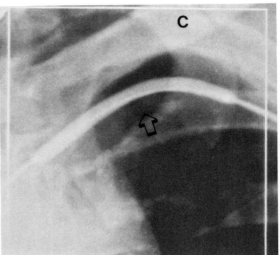

B

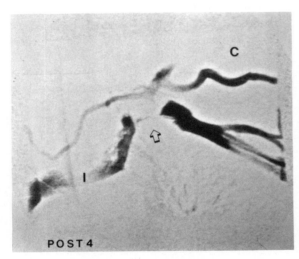

C

FIGURE 14-7. **(A)** *After lysis of all thrombus, the area of subclavian vein compression at the thoracic outlet is visualized (large arrow). This is the site where the vein passes between the clavicle (C) and the first thoracic rib. This deformity is often misinterpreted as residual thrombus, leading to prolonged lytic therapy without further change in the radiologic picture. The compressed area is being transversed by a guidewire to the innominate vein (I), demonstrating patency and continuity of subclavian vein [note markers (small arrows)].* **(C)** *After a fourth attempt at dilatation, the compressed area remains unchanged due to continued pressure from the first rib below and subclavius tendon above. Vein is tethered in position by the costoclavicular ligaments medially and the anterior scalene muscle laterally. This lesion will require surgical decompression if patency of the vein is to be maintained.*

episode was attributed to an idiosyncratic reaction to midazolam given as premedication. One patient developed an axillary hematoma after infusion of urokinase 3 days after first rib resection to treat residual vein occlusion.

Anticoagulation

One patient had transient gastrointestinal and urinary tract bleeding while on warfarin sodium. Two patients treated with inadequate warfarin sodium (normal prothrombin times) had thrombosis of the previously open axillosubclavian vein while awaiting surgery.

Surgery

Of patients undergoing first rib resection, one required thoracocentesis for a pneumothorax and pleural effusion recognized postoperatively. One patient received a blood transfusion.

Balloon Angioplasty

Seven of 12 balloon angioplasties performed after successful thrombolytic therapy but *prior* to surgery resulted in immediate rethrombosis of the vein. Technical failure occurred in 2 of 9 balloon angioplasties attempted after first rib resection due to failure to traverse the stenosis with a guidewire. One initially successful balloon angioplasty restenosed and required repeat angioplasty with a larger balloon (15 mm) and remained successful.

Results

At the last follow-up evaluation (mean of 33 months and median of 24 months), 23 patients had returned to their preillness work or activity. Four laborers were advised to undergo retraining, primarily because of untreated abnormalities of the contralateral thoracic outlet. One patient returned to school, two of the older women did not return to work, two patients were awaiting a favorable Workers' Compensation determination before consenting to first rib resection. One pa-

tient, a laborer referred after failure to achieve recanalization of the vein, continued to have symptoms after transaxillary first rib resection.

Summary

Patients suspected of having effort thrombosis of the axillosubclavian vein (Paget-Schroetter's syndrome) should have bilateral axillosubclavian venography via the basilic vein with arms in the neutral and overhead position. When demonstrated, the thrombus should be lysed with local urokinase infusion into the clot (see Fig. 14-5).

The residual compressive abnormality should be recognized and not confused with residual clot. This abnormality should not be dilated because it represents external compression and will recur immediately or when the patient abducts the arm (see Fig. 14-7). Occasionally, when there is a minimal lumen with precarious flow, a 2-mm balloon may be used to improve flow past the stenotic segment. This maneuver is occasionally successful. When the phlebitic process has resolved and the vein endothelium is restored, the patient should undergo correction of the underlying etiologic compressive abnormality (Fig. 14-8 and 14-9).

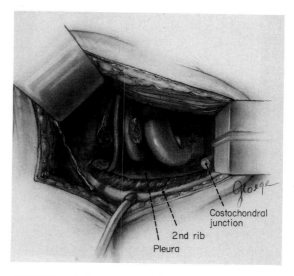

FIGURE 14-8. Appearance of the thoracic outlet after surgical removal of the first rib and the elements compressing the subclavian vein (compare with Fig. 14-1).

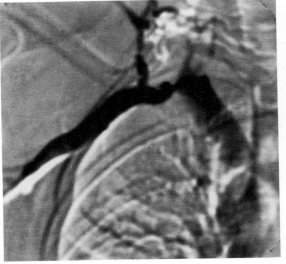

A

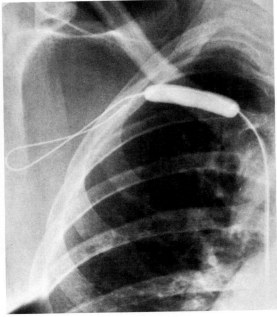

B

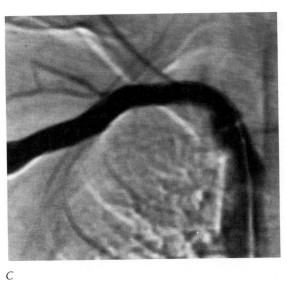

C

FIGURE 14-9. Correction of residual stenosis by balloon venoplasty after surgical removal of the first rib and relief of the external compression elements (1-year follow-up).

REFERENCES

1. Hughes ESR. Collective review: venous obstruction in the upper extremity (Paget-Schroetter's syndrome): a review of 320 cases. Int Abst Surg 1949;88:89.
2. Machleder HI. Evolution of a new treatment strategy for Paget-Schroeter syndrome: spontaneous thrombosis of the axillary-subclavian vein. J Vasc Surg 1992;17:305.
3. Schepelmann E. Muench Med Wochenschr 1910; 57:2444; as cited by Hughes.
4. DeWeese JA, Adams JT, Gaiser DL. Subclavian venous thrombectomy. Circulation 1970;42:159.
5. Aziz S, Straehley CJ, Whelan TJ. Effort-related axillosubclavian vein thrombosis: a new theory of pathogenesis and a plea for direct surgical intervention. Am J Surg 1986;152:57.
6. Donayre CE, White GH, Mehringer SM, Wilson SE. Pathogenesis determines late morbidity of axillosubclavian vein thrombosis. Am J Surg 1986; 152:179.
7. Gloviczki P, Kazmier FJ, Hollier LH. Axillary-subclavian venous occlusion: the morbidity of a nonlethal disease. J Vasc Surg 1986;4:333.
8. Tilney NL, Griffiths HJG, Edwards EA. Natural history of major venous thrombosis of the upper extremity. Arch Surg 1970;101:792.
9. Linblad B, Bornmyer S, Kullendorff B, Bergqvist D. Venous haemodynamics of the upper extremity after subclavian vein thrombosis. Vasa 1990;19: 218.
10. Kunkel JM, Machleder HI. Treatment of Paget-Schroetter syndrome: a staged, multidisciplinary approach. Arch Surg 1989;124:1153.
11. Machleder HI. Upper extremity venous thrombosis. Semin Vasc Surg 1990;3:219.
12. Machleder HI. Effort thrombosis of the axillosubclavian vein: a disabling vascular disorder. Compr Ther 1991;17:18.
13. Daskalakis E, Bouhoutsos J. Subclavian and axillary vein compression of musculoskeletal origin. Br J Surg 1980;67:573.
14. Machleder HI. Vaso-occlusive disorders of the upper extremity. Curr Probl Surg 1988;25(1):1.
15. Molina JE. Thrombolytic therapy of axillary-subclavian venous thrombosis. Arch Surg 1988;123: 662.
16. Taylor LM, McAllister WR, Dennis DL, Porter JM. Thrombolytic therapy followed by first rib resection for spontaneous ("effort") subclavian vein thrombosis. Am J Surg 1985;149:644.
17. Zimmerman R, Morl H, Harenberg J, et al. Urokinase therapy of subclavian-axillary vein thrombosis. Klin Wochenschr 1981;59:851.
18. Steed DL, Teodori MF, Peitzman AB, et al. Streptokinase in the treatment of subclavian vein thrombosis. J Vasc Surg 1986;4:28.
19. Perler BA, Mitchell SE. Percutaneous transluminal angioplasty and transaxillary first rib resection. Am Surg 1986;52:485.
20. Makhoul RG, Machleder HI. Developmental anomalies at the thoracic outlet: an analysis of 200 consecutive cases. J Vasc Surg 1992;16:534.
21. McCleery RS, Kesterson JE, Kirtley JA, et al. Subclavius and anterior scalene muscle compression as a cause of intermittent obstruction of the subclavian vein. Ann Surg 1951;133:588.
22. Stevenson IM, Parry EW. Radiological study of the etiological factors in venous obstruction of the upper limb. J Cardiovas Surg 1975;16:580.
23. Machleder HI. The role of thrombolytic agents for acute subclavian vein thrombosis. Semin Vasc Surg 1992;5:82.
24. Becker GJ, Holden RW, Rabe FE, et al. Local thrombolytic therapy for subclavian and axillary vein thrombosis. Radiology 1983;149:419.
25. Machleder HI. Venous disorders. In: Machleder HI, ed. Vascular disorders of the upper extremity. 2nd ed. Mt Kisco, NY: Futura, 1989:269.
26. McNamara TO, Fischer JR. Thrombolysis of peripheral arterial and graft occlusions: improved results using high-dose urokinase. AJR 1985;144: 769.
27. Glanz S, Gordon DH, Lipkowitz, et al. Axillary and subclavian vein stenosis: percutaneous angioplasty. Radiology 1988;168(2):371.

15

THROMBOLYTIC THERAPY FOR SECONDARY AXILLOSUBCLAVIAN VEIN THROMBOSIS

Edward M. Druy

Long-term central venous access is required for treatment of many chronic disorders. Upper extremity veins are the preferred sites of access, with the external jugular, internal jugular, and subclavian veins being the most commonly used structures. Some patients may require venous access for years, either for hyperalimentation, antibiotic administration, chemotherapy, or dialysis. While the initial morbidity of central venous catheterization has remained acceptably low, many of the long-term consequences are only beginning to be appreciated. A complication of central venous catheterization which is receiving increasing recognition is axillosubclavian vein thrombosis. However, there is little consensus about its overall incidence, morbidity, or proper therapy. This chapter summarizes the extent of current knowledge of this disorder and presents my approach to its therapy.

ETIOLOGY OF SECONDARY SUBCLAVIAN VEIN THROMBOSIS

The apparent incidence of subclavian vein thrombosis has been increasing over the past two decades. While increased recognition of the disorder is partly responsible for the reported increase, it is likely that the growing number of central vein catheterizations may play an even larger role.[1] There are a host of factors leading to the development of catheter-induced or secondary axillosubclavian vein thrombosis. Some are related to the nature of the underlying disease being treated, while others are related to physical properties of the access catheter and to the insertion technique. Central venous catheterization has a major role in the therapy of patients with a variety of chronic, often malignant, disorders where a hypercoagulable state may be present. Reduced protein C and S levels are often seen in patients undergoing adjuvant treatment for breast cancer.[2,3] Patients with a history of intrathoracic neoplasms may have compression of mediastinal veins (i.e., the superior vena cava, the innominate vein, or the azygous vein) by enlarged nodes. A significant percentage of patients have a past history of mediastinal radiation or surgery.[4] The trauma of catheter insertion, leading to mechanical disruption of the endothelial surface of the vein, may be responsible for the initial environment conducive to thrombosis. Subsequent contact between the catheter and the vein wall may continue to activate clotting factors. The nature of the catheter material, size of the catheter, location of the infusion holes, duration of catheter placement, and nature of the infusate have all been implicated as additional cofactors.[5–7] Larger catheters are known to have greater thrombotic potential than smaller ones, probably by causing a greater degree of vascular stasis. Catheter manufacturers initially fabricated chronic access catheters from Teflon, polyethylene, polyurethane, and polyvinyl. Follow-up evaluation of patients with these devices demonstrated thrombotic complications as high as 42%.[8–10] It was hoped that constructing these catheters from silicone would lower the incidence of thrombosis, but this has been only partly achieved. A venographic follow-up study of patients with centrally placed silicone catheters demonstrated that only 30% of catheters were free of thrombotic complications, with a tendency for the smaller catheters to cause fewer complications.[11]

Venous stenosis following catheterization is a likely precursor to venous thrombosis, since any lesion sufficiently stenotic to cause stasis will promote thrombosis. Both the site and side of insertion of central venous catheters are known factors in the development of axillosubclavian vein stenosis. Schillinger et al.[12] reported on 100 patients undergoing catheterization for hemodialysis access. Patients were divided into two groups according to access site: subclavian vein or internal jugular vein. Angiographic evaluation was performed at least 3 weeks following removal of the catheter. The authors found that 42% of the catheterized subclavian veins developed a stenotic lesion, while only 10% of the jugular veins became stenotic.[12] This observation also has been reported by other investigators.[13–15] While these studies were performed primarily in patients who underwent temporary venous access for hemodialysis, there is little reason to doubt that the results are not applicable to patients undergoing catheterization for other reasons. Patients who are

receiving drug infusions are more susceptible to the irritating effects of these infusions if a venous stenosis is present. There will be increased contact time of the drug with the vein wall, and there will be less dilution of the drug. This environment tends to potentiate the thrombotic potential of the infusate (Fig. 15-1).

The side of catheter insertion is also implicated in thrombotic complications. Horattas et al.[16] noted that two-thirds of their catheter-induced thromboses were related to left-sided catheter insertions. I have seen this as well and think that it may be related to the role of the innominate vein in initiating the thrombotic state. This will be discussed more fully later.

MORBIDITY OF SECONDARY SUBCLAVIAN VEIN THROMBOSIS

Conventional wisdom, gleaned from the older literature, has maintained that axillosubclavian vein thrombosis does not carry a significant morbidity and may be asymptomatic.[17,18] Many authors today still persist in this belief.[19] Some authors have suggested that the lack of symptoms implies spontaneous recanalization of the thrombosed vein. Given the lack of consensus concerning the clinical findings of the disorder, it is reasonable that its natural history is poorly defined. Only a few studies have obtained long-term venographic follow-up in this group of patients. These studies indicated that few veins spontaneously recanalize when treated conservatively.[20] More careful clinical follow-up of patients has lead to the realization that this disorder has the potential for significant morbidity. An upper extremity venous hypertension syndrome exits which consists of swelling, fatigability, and weakness of the affected arm. A potentially devastating consequence of axillosubclavian vein thrombosis is the development of the superior vena caval (SVC) syndrome.[21] While minor episodes of thrombosis usually do not lead to this complication, if thrombosis extends to the superior vena cava in patients with already limited collateral flow into compromised mediastinal veins, this may become a distinct possibility. Patients who appear to be at

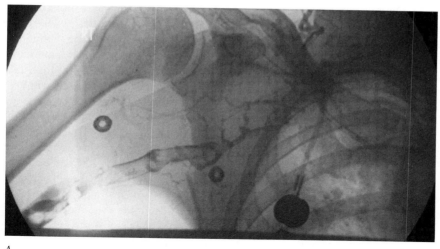

A

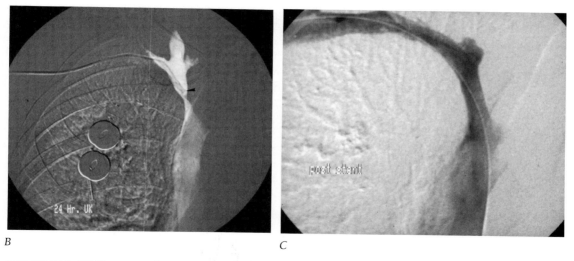

B

C

FIGURE 15-1. **(A)** *Venogram of a 45-year-old man with non-Hodgkin's lymphoma who developed extensive catheter-induced axillosubclavian vein thrombosis. An Infusaid catheter is in place.* **(B)** *Following successful lytic therapy, repeat venography and cavography demonstrate a venous stenosis at the tip of the infusion catheter (arrowhead). The thrombosis extended to this level.* **(C)** *An expandable stent was placed across the venous stenosis to maintain a normal luminal diameter.*

greatest risk for this devastating complication are those with underlying mediastinal tumor, mediastinal lymphadenopathy, or a history of mediastinal radiation. The SVC syndrome is commonly thought to be a primary complication of extensive mediastinal disease, but it is likely that underlying secondary subclavian vein thrombosis may potentiate the effect of malignancy.

Pulmonary embolism is becoming a more frequently recognized complication of secondary subclavian vein thrombosis. Upper extremity venous thrombosis is now recognized as leading to pulmonary embolism in 12% to 25% of cases.[22] Massive pulmonary emboli arising from axillosubclavian veins have been reported.[23,24] Aside from these direct consequences of axillosubclavian vein thrombosis, a potentially devastating consequence of the disorder is loss of venous access in patients in whom it may be required for long-term therapy. Standard anticoagulation is not associated with sufficient recanalization of thrombosed veins to allow for future vascular access.

DIAGNOSIS OF SECONDARY SUBCLAVIAN VEIN THROMBOSIS

In the appropriate clinical setting, the diagnosis of axillosubclavian vein thrombosis secondary to venous catheterization should not be difficult. The obvious clinical findings are painful neck and shoulder swelling, mottling of the skin, and dilated superficial veins. Once the diagnosis is suspected clinically, appropriate imaging studies should be performed not only to confirm the diagnosis but also to determine the extent of the thrombus.

Imaging Studies

Because duplex ultrasound and, more recently, color flow duplex ultrasound have been found to be useful tools in the evaluation of patients with suspected lower extremity deep venous thrombosis, it has been hoped by many that their usefulness would extend to the upper extremity as well. Unfortunately, there are too many false-negative studies for these modalities to be truly accurate screening methods. Even occlusive subclavian vein thrombi may not be visualized with ultrasound.[25] Although the technique is accurate in demonstrating thrombosis of the axillary vein and distal subclavian vein, the ultrasound beam cannot penetrate the clavicle or other bony structures of the thorax, thus making it an ill-suited technique for evaluating the patency of the central third of the subclavian vein, the brachiocephalic veins, or the superior vena cava.

Catheter Injections

Nonobstructing thromboses which extend from the site of catheter insertion to the tip of the catheter may cause the catheter to malfunction in such a manner that infusions are possible but withdrawal of blood is not. In order to determine vein patency in this clinical setting, clinicians may request that radiopaque contrast material or a radiolabeled tracer be injected through the catheter. This technique will usually show flow of contrast material or tracer out the tip of the catheter into the superior vena cava or right atrium. This demonstration of contrast flow may give rise to the erroneous impression that no thrombosis exists. Clinicians may infer from the results of this type of study that the vein is patent and that the catheter can continue to be used. If this is the only study done, the chance to make the diagnosis of subclavian vein thrombosis may be lost. If the catheter has continued use, it is likely that the thrombus will continue to propagate centrally due to stasis and lack of dilution of the infusate. With continued thrombus propagation, function of the catheter will soon be lost. Only a peripheral injection of contrast material will adequately visualize entire course of the axillosubclavian vein.

Venography

Contrast venography should represent a thorough examination of the entire affected upper extremity, with demonstration of the proximal and distal extent of the thrombus. Documentation of patency or occlusion of the brachiocephalic vein and the superior vena cava also must be provided. While contrast venography remains the "gold standard" of diagnosis of axillosubclavian vein thrombosis, little attention has been paid in the literature to the proper method of performing the study. Although the diagnosis of axillosubclavian vein thrombosis can be made with certainty via a distal injection of contrast material into a wrist vein, this technique rarely provides anything more than visual confirmation of a clinical impression. Thrombus will rarely be seen in this type of study. What is usually demonstrated are multiple collateral veins bypassing the obstructed area and reconstituting flow into a jugular or thoracic vein (Fig. 15-2A). If, instead, the venapuncture is made into the median basilic vein, a more realistic assessment of the extent of the thrombosis can be made (Fig. 15-2B). The reason for this

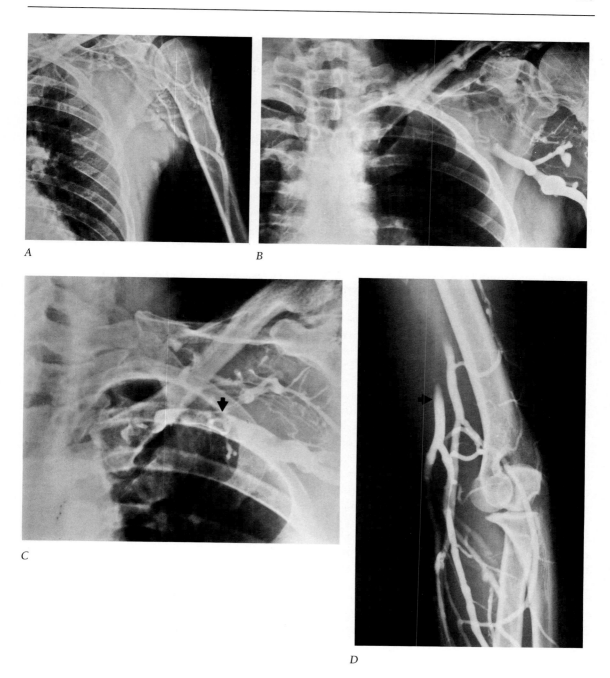

FIGURE 15-2. (A) Venogram of the left upper extremity with a distal contrast material infusion. All flow is in collateral veins, and it is impossible to determine the actual site of thrombus. No contrast material is seen in the brachial, axillary, or subclavian veins. (B) Contrast material is injected via the median basilic vein. Brachial and axillary veins are patent, although thrombus is not identified. (C) A catheter has been advanced into the axillary vein. Contrast material injection at this site shows trailing edge of thrombus (arrow). With definition of extent of thrombus, a decision to attempt local lytic therapy can be made. (D) Spot film of antecubital fossa showing position of median basilic vein (arrow), which could not be palpated. An angiocath can be positioned fluoroscopically into the vein.

disparity is best understood by realizing that the venous circulation in the extremity is a parallel system, composed of a deep and a superficial circulation, each exposed to the same pressure gradient. Obstruction of any component of the deep system will raise the pressure in that circuit and cause blood to flow into the relatively lower pressure superficial circulation. When axillosubclavian vein thrombosis is present and contrast material is injected into a superficial vein in the wrist, contrast material will remain in the lower-pressure superficial system and move from the site of injection to a site central to the occlusion. Not only will the thrombus not be demonstrated, but neither will patent deep veins distal to the thrombus, since the pressure in these veins also will be greater than the pressure in the superficial veins which serve as collateral vessels.

If contrast material is injected into the median basilic vein, which is part of the deep venous system in the upper extremity, much of the injected contrast material will stay in the basilic vein to the level of the thrombosis. The closer the injection is to the thrombus, the more likely that the true extent of the thrombosis can be assessed accurately (Fig. 15-2C). Even if the arm is so edematous that the median basilic vein cannot be palpated, it usually can be punctured by road-mapping techniques. The easiest technique is to opacify the basilic vein from an injection into a wrist vein. Then, under fluoroscopic guidance, the opacified median basilic vein can be punctured directly (Fig. 15-2D). If an 18-gauge angio-cath is used, a 0.035-in guidewire can be passed through it in order to exchange for an angiographic catheter.

The venogram also should demonstrate the central extent of the thrombus and make the determination of whether or not the brachiocephalic veins and superior vena cava are patent. This may be a difficult determination with standard venographic techniques, and if necessary, a contrast material injection into the contralateral, unaffected extremity should be performed. In patients with superior vena caval or brachiocephalic vein obstruction, it is necessary to obtain a CT scan of the mediastinum to determine the presence or absence of mediastinal tumor or other

changes which may predispose to central venous obstruction (Fig. 15-3).

TREATMENT OF AXILLOSUBCLAVIAN VEIN THROMBOSIS

Traditional Therapy

Standard therapy of axillosubclavian vein thrombosis has traditionally been catheter removal, bed rest, heat, limb elevation, and anticoagulation. With conservative therapy, acute symptoms usually resolve within several days, although if a careful history and physical examination are performed, it is possible to elicit symptoms of swelling, pain, or other forms of disability in up to 70% of patients.[26] Conservative measures, including heparinization, may not eliminate the development of pulmonary embolism.[27] While chronic venous hypertension may be more common in patients with the primary form of the disorder than in those with the secondary form,[28] the most significant disability faced by patients with secondary axillosubclavian vein thrombosis is potential loss of venous access. None of the usual conservative treatments available are likely to restore luminal patency. Symptomatic improvement observed after conservative therapy results from recruitment of collaterals to bypass the occluded primary vein.

Newer Therapies

The failure of conservative measures to prevent the sequelae of axillosubclavian vein thrombosis has prompted investigation of more aggressive forms of therapy which may restore luminal patency of the vein, prevent pulmonary embolism, and preserve venous access. Thrombectomy, lytic therapy, first rib resection, and angioplasty all have been utilized with varying estimates of success.[29-31] These therapies have been directed mainly toward the primary form of axillosubclavian vein thrombosis, but many can be applied to the secondary form as well. Primary axillosubclavian vein thrombosis is distinguished from the secondary form by assuming that, in the former, there is a natural (inherent) abnormality present

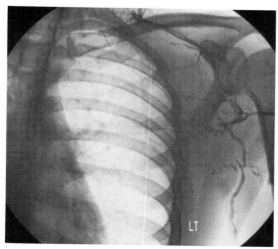

A

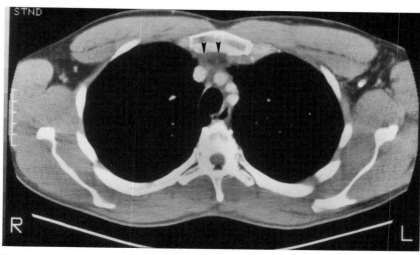

B

FIGURE 15-3. **(A)** *There is extensive thrombosis of the veins of the left upper extremity. Only chest wall veins serving as collaterals can be identified.* **(B)** *CT scan of the mediastinum shows streaking of fat in the anterior mediastinum at the level of the innominate vein, secondary to radiation (arrowhead). Radiation changes presumably predisposed the innominate vein to thrombosis.*

predisposing the patient to thrombosis. Often there is both extrinsic compression of the vein by surrounding ligamentous structures and an intrinsic venous structural abnormality resulting from long-standing external compression. In secondary axillosubclavian vein thrombosis, the presumption has been that perivenous pathology is not present and that thrombosis was the result of

the venous catheterization or other direct insult to the vein. If this is true, and if the underlying vein is essentially normal, then lytic therapy alone should be sufficient to restore patency. Thus aggressive therapy in the secondary form of the disorder has been directed solely toward the thrombus and not toward correction of other abnormalities extrinsic to the vein. In those instances where the underlying vein is intrinsically abnormal, other measures, such as angioplasty and venous stenting, may be necessary to maintain long-term patency.[32–35] Mediastinal pathology secondary to tumor, fibrosis, nodal compression, or radiation changes may sufficiently compromise the integrity of the central veins to make this necessary (Fig. 15-1C).

The initial therapy necessary to restore luminal patency in axillosubclavian vein thrombosis is thrombolytic therapy. Without eliminating the thrombus, all other measures are only palliative. Although the results of lytic therapy are well-documented in the literature, there is little agreement as to the appropriate drug, correct dosage, or method of delivery.[36–39] Most reports concerning the use of lytic agents in upper extremity venous thrombosis describe peripheral administration of drug in dosages high enough to induce a lytic state. The reason for these necessarily high doses is because of the disadvantageous pharmacokinetics of the systemic route of administration. Peripherally administered drugs will tend to bypass thrombosed veins, similar to the way peripherally injected contrast material tends to flow through patent collateral veins. Thus, in order to maintain a sufficient concentration of drug at the surface of the thrombus, high doses are required. While successful venous thrombolysis often can be achieved in this manner, there is sufficient potential for significant bleeding complications, and systemic lytic therapy may be contraindicated in many patients who could otherwise benefit from this therapy. Difficulties and complications associated with the peripherally administered, systemic use of lytic agents have prompted evaluation of the local "low-dose" concept of fibrinolytic therapy. This form of therapy has been used successfully in the arterial system for the past 10 years.[40] The basic concept behind this form of therapy is that a sufficient amount of lytic agent can be delivered directly into the thrombus via a percutaneously placed catheter so that with the appropriate dose, thrombus can be lysed without systemic fibrinolysis. Although local thrombolysis rarely occurs without a "systemic effect," the speed of thrombus resolution and overall success are considerably greater with catheter-directed

lysis compared with systemic infusion. This is due primarily to efficient activation of fibrin-bound plasminogen and the absence of inhibitors (of the plasminogen activator and plasmin) in the thrombus. Reports concerning the use of lytic agents for the treatment of axillosubclavian vein thrombosis are still largely anecdotal. No prospective, randomized studies comparing lytic therapy with anticoagulation have been performed. However, the impressions from anecdotal reports of lytic therapy have been largely favorable.[41–43]

TECHNIQUE OF CATHETER-BASED THROMBOLYSIS

Successful catheter-based thrombolytic therapy is hinged on venographic documentation of the total extent of the thrombus. The severity or extent of symptoms and findings is not a reliable guide to the extent of the thrombosis, which can only be determined by venography. The technique of venography was described earlier. Once percutaneous access is achieved into the median basilic vein, a no. 5 French vascular sheath is placed to maintain access. An angiographic catheter with either a headhunter or cobra configuration is advanced to the thrombus. A hydrophilic guidewire such as a Glide-wire (Medi-Tech, Inc., Watertown, Mass.) or a Road-Runner (Cook, Inc., Bloomington, Ind.) is then manipulated through the thrombus into the superior vena cava central to the leading edge of the thrombus. The total length of the thrombus is determined by estimating the length of catheter necessary to traverse the thrombosed vein. The angiographic catheter is then replaced with an appropriately long infusion catheter by using standard exchange techniques.

Catheter Types

There are numerous catheters available for delivery of thrombolytic agents. They are divided into three basic types: *end-hole*, *coaxial*, or *multiport*. End-hole catheters were initially used for delivery of thrombolytic agents but suffer from the disadvantage of supplying the drug only to the part of the thrombus in contact with the tip of the catheter. This usually necessitated constant advancement of the catheter to ensure that the drug continued to be delivered into the thrombus rather than into patent, peripheral portions of the vein and thus into the systemic circulation. End-hole catheters also have a tendency to migrate and advance into the orifices of collateral veins, again delivering the lytic agent into the systemic circulation rather than into the thrombus. Coaxial catheters are designed to deliver the drug at the trailing and leading edges of the thrombus, while multiport catheters are designed to deliver the drug throughout the thrombus. Shorter lengths of thrombus can be treated easily with a coaxial catheter system. The simplest system to use is to advance an infusion wire through the angiographic catheter previously placed. By using a Touhey-Bourst catheter adapter, drug can be delivered through both catheters. The only precaution that is necessary with this arrangement is to ensure that the infusion catheter or wire is small enough to permit the drug to be infused through the outer catheter. Any of the commercially available infusion catheters will permit this. For longer thromboses, I favor use of the multiport infusion catheter (EDM catheter, Peripheral Systems Group, Mountain View, Calif.). This is a no. 4 French catheter which is tapered to an 0.018-in guidewire. In order to exchange it with the initial angiographic catheter used to traverse the thrombus, the initial guidewire needs first to be exchanged for the 0.018-in guide. The infusion catheter is manufactured in multiple infusion lengths so that the infusion ports are spaced appropriately over the length of thrombus to be treated (Fig. 15-4A and B).

Lytic Agents and Dose Schedules

Streptokinase (SK) and urokinase (UK) have both been used, systemically and locally, to achieve venous thrombolysis. The only advantage of SK is the lower cost of the drug, but this may be masked when taking into account longer duration of treatment and the increased complication rate associated with SK.[44] SK, being both antigenic and pyrogenic, may cause serious side effects.[45-47] The

safety, efficacy, tolerance, and freedom from serious side effects of UK currently favor its use over SK. There is little experience with the use of tissue plasminogen activator (t-PA).

The dosage of UK has been determined empirically and is similar to that used for intraarterial thrombolysis: a 250,000 U/h infusion is begun for 2 h, followed by a 60,000 U/h infusion until clot lysis has been achieved. If a coaxial system is used, the total dose delivered is the same, but it is divided between the two catheters used. It is my practice to evaluate the progression of the lytic therapy after the initial 2-h infusion and every 12 h thereafter. The site of the contrast material injection on the follow-up examinations will vary depending with the type of infusion catheter. If a multiport catheter is used, the side ports should be injected. If a coaxial system is used, then the distal (peripheral) port is injected. Most thrombi will show early lysis at 2 h, but complete lysis generally will take 12 to 24 h. Prior to removal of the catheter, a complete venogram is again performed with contrast material injected into the access sheath in the median basilic vein. This determines whether there is residual thrombus in the upper arm and demonstrates intrinsic venous abnormalities or stenoses which may need additional therapy.

Concurrent Heparinization

In order to prevent rethrombosis of the lysed segment of vein, it has been my practice to begin heparinization at the onset of lytic therapy. A 5000-U bolus is first given, followed by 500 to 800 U/h, or sufficient to maintain the PTT at 70 s.

Postlysis Management

While most thrombosed veins will recanalize within 24 h, the subsequent management is a key determinant of long-term success. If the venographic appearance of the vein is normal, then only a short-term period of heparinization is warranted. A 48-h course of anticoagulation will usually maintain venous patency (see Fig. 15-4C). Frequently, however, the underlying vein is abnormal, with irregularities and stenoses of the

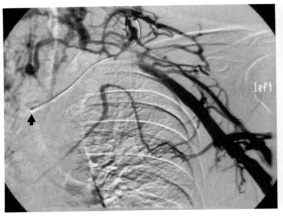

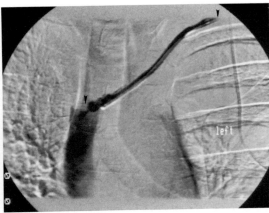

A   B

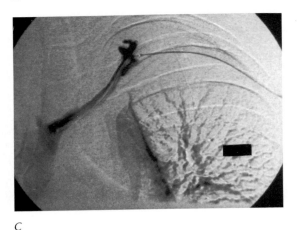

C

FIGURE 15-4. **(A)** Thrombosis of the innominate and subclavian veins secondary to central venous catheter. The tip of the catheter is in the innominate vein (arrow). **(B)** A multihole infusion catheter has been placed through the entire length of thrombus from the subclavian vein through the innominate vein and into the superior vena cava (infusion catheter between arrows). Early lysis of the innominate vein has occurred. **(C)** Progressive lysis has occurred, and the innominate vein appears normal.

lumen. When the vein has this appearance, our group has advocated a 10 to 12-week course of oral anticoagulation (Fig. 15-5). If the underlying vein appears normal at the conclusion of lytic therapy, the central infusion catheter is left in place as long as the patient is anticoagulated. If the vein appears abnormal following thrombolytic therapy, we advocate removal of the catheter, since either the catheter or the infusate may be the stimulus for thrombosis. Without anticoagulation and catheter removal, our experience has been one of early rethrombosis. In instances where there is no other venous access, the central catheter should remain in place if it is still therapeutically useful.

RESULTS

There are very few series of patients with secondary axillosubclavian vein thrombosis that have been reported in the literature. Fraschini et al.[48] reported on 31 patients who underwent 36 local UK infusions. They infused UK both peripherally and via the central venous catheter, a technique that did not always allow for intrathrombic administration of drug. When optimal catheter position and drug delivery were possible, they were able to achieve a 78% lysis rate. When they were unable to position the catheter in the thrombus, they were able to lyse only the thrombus that was directly exposed to the drug. Rethrom-

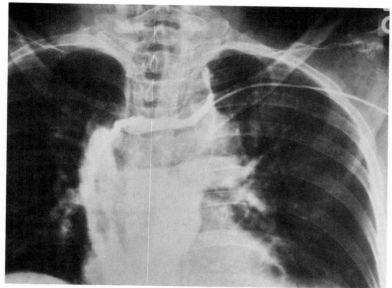

A

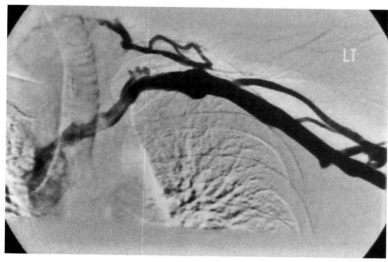

B

FIGURE 15-5. (A) *Abnormal appearance of innominate vein after 24 h of lytic therapy. There are residual stenoses and wall irregularities which require 8 to 10 weeks of anticoagulation if patency is to be maintained.* (B) *After 10 weeks of anticoagulation, the innominate vein appears normal.*

bosis was most commonly associated with incomplete lysis and retention of the central venous catheter in patients with an underlying venous abnormality.

In our experience, thromboses present for less than 72 h will virtually always lyse within 24 h of lytic therapy.[49] Those thromboses which have been present longer than 7 days appear more resistant to lytic therapy, and the infusion time necessary to achieve total lysis may be longer than 48 h. By this time, many patients will approach a lytic state, thus obviating the advantages of local "low-dose" therapy. For this reason, unless there are no alternatives for future venous access, we do not commit these patients to lytic therapy.

Thromboses affecting the right upper extremity are usually shorter than those affecting the left, which often involve the innominate vein as well. Venous thromboses affecting the left brachiocephalic vein and which extend to the axillosubclavian vein have, in our experience, required longer infusion times and may be more prone to rethrombosis. The longer infusion times are a result of the greater clot burden, but the tendency toward rethrombosis is a result of many factors. The left innominate vein is not well suited for central venous catheterization for several reasons. If the tip of the catheter does not extend to the superior vena cava, infusions will take place in the relatively smaller caliber innominate vein. In-

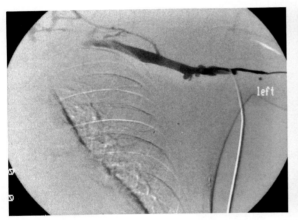

A

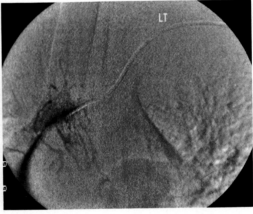

B

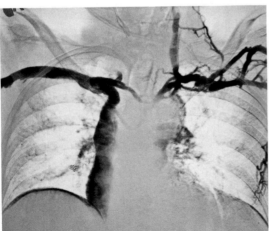

C

FIGURE 15-6. **(A)** *Same patient as Fig. 15-3. Lytic therapy is successful in restoring patency of the axillosubclavian vein.* **(B)** *Contrast material injected into the innominate vein demonstrates marked luminal narrowing of the structure with flow into network of abnormal collateral structures. This appearance of the innominate vein suggests that long-term patency will not be achieved, although anticoagulation may maintain patency of the axillosubclavian venous system until sufficient collateral veins develop.* **(C)** *Follow-up at 6 weeks shows continued patency of the axillosubclavian vein with occlusion just distal to the internal jugular vein, which serves as a collateral. The patient is asymptomatic.*

fusate will be less diluted, and the effects of the infusate on the vein wall will be correspondingly greater than had the tip been positioned in the superior vena cava. Mechanical irritation of the vein wall by the catheter is greater in the innominate vein than in the superior vena cava, again because of the former's relatively smaller caliber. The innominate vein, coursing as it does in the anterior mediastinum, is affected to a greater degree by mediastinal pathology, such as acute or chronic radiation effects, lymphadenopathy, or tumor, than is the superior vena cava. The tendency of the innominate vein to rethrombosis is an argument against left-sided central venous catheterization if other routes are available. We also have determined that even though the innominate vein may rethrombose, it is possible to maintain patency of the axillosubclavian veins as long as the patient is anticoagulated until collateral veins have a chance to develop. This may leave the patient asymptomatic, although the left upper extremity will no longer be able to be utilized for further access (Fig. 15-6).

Complications of Lytic Therapy

The local low-dose administration of UK for upper extremity venous thrombosis has been associated with a low complication rate in all reported series. The most common complication has been bleeding at the venotomy site. Fibrinogen levels vary with the duration of therapy and usually remain normal for the first 24 h at the doses currently used.

CONCLUSIONS

Axillosubclavian vein thrombosis is becoming increasingly recognized as a significant complication of central venous catheterization. The morbidity of upper extremity venous thrombosis consists of chronic extremity edema, pulmonary embolism, and loss of use of central catheters. Lytic therapy, given via a catheter placed directly into the thrombus, appears to represent a worthwhile therapeutic approach. When begun early,

lytic therapy is highly effective, has a low rate of complications, and will eliminate most of the sequelae of the disorder. Rethrombosis can be prevented by achieving complete thrombolysis, removing catheters from abnormal-appearing veins, and short-term anticoagulation. Mediastinal abnormalities which affect central venous structures may prevent therapy from being totally successful, but clinical trials involving the placement of venous stents appear promising.

REFERENCES

1. Aburahma AF, Sadler DL, Robinson PT. Axillary-subclavian vein thrombosis: changing patterns of etiology, diagnostic, and therapeutic modalities. Am Surg 1991;57(2):101.
2. Levine MN, Gent M, Hirsh J, et al. The thrombogenic effect of anticancer drug therapy in women with stage II breast cancer. N Engl J Med 1988; 318:404.
3. Rogers JSII, Murgo AJ, Fontana JA, Raich PC. Chemotherapy for breast cancer decreases plasma protein C and protein S. J Clin Oncol 1988;6:276.
4. Hill SL, Berry RE. Subclavian vein thrombosis: a continuing challenge. Surgery 1990;108(1):1.
5. DiCostanzo J, Sastre B, Choux R, et al. Experimental approach to prevention of catheter-related central venous thrombosis. JPEN 1984;8:293.
6. Welch GW, McKeel DW, Silverstein P, Walker H. The role of catheter composition in the development of thrombophlebitis. Surg Gynecol Obstet 1974;138:421.
7. Ross AH, Griffith CD, Anderson JR, Grieve DC. Thromboembolic complications with silicone elastomer subclavian catheters. JPEN 1982;6:61.
8. Cheung AK, Gregory MC. Subclavian vein thrombosis in hemodialysis patients. Trans Am Soc Artif Internal Organs 1985;31:131.
9. Brismar B, Hardstedt C, Jacobson S. Diagnosis of thrombosis by catheter phlebography after prolonged central venous catheterization. Ann Surg 1981;194:779.
10. Lokich JJ, Becker B. Subclavian vein thrombosis in patients treated with infusion chemotherapy for advanced malignancy. Cancer 1983;52:1586.
11. Haire WD, Leberman RP, Lund GB, et al. Thrombotic complications of silicone rubber catheters during autologous marrow and peripheral stem cell transplantation: prospective comparison of Hickman and Groshong catheters. Bone Marrow Transplant 1991;7:57.
12. Schillinger F, Schillinger D, Montagnac R, Milcent

T. Post-catheterization venous stenosis in hemodialysis: comparative angiographic study of 50 subclavian and 50 jugular accesses. Nephrologie 1992;13(3):127.

13. Lee SJ, Neiberger R. Subclavian vein stenosis: complication of subclavian vein catheterization for hemodialysis. Child Nephrol Urol 1991;11(4):212.

14. Surratt RS, Picus D, Hicks ME, et al. The importance of preoperative evaluation of the subclavian vein in dialysis access planning. AJR 1991;154(3):623.

15. Cussenot O, Barral V, Bourquelot P. Central venous stenoses after using a Hickman catheter in hemodialysis in children: apropos of 4 cases. Ann Urol 1989;23(5):395.

16. Horattas MC, Wright DJ, Fenton AH, et al. Changing concepts of deep venous thrombosis of the upper extremity: report of a series and review of the literature. Surgery 1988;104(3):561.

17. Kleinsasser LJ. "Effort" thrombosis of the axillary and subclavian veins. Arch Surg 1949;59:258.

18. Smith VC, Hallett JW Jr. Subclavian vein thrombosis during prolonged catheterization for parenteral nutrition: early management and long-term follow-up. South Med J 1983;76(5):603.

19. Hill SL, Berry RE. Subclavian vein thrombosis: a continuing challenge. Surgery 1990;108(1):1.

20. Axelsson K, Efsen F. Phlebography in long-term catheterization of the subclavian vein. Scan J Gastroenterol 1978;13:933.

21. Theriault RL, Buzdar AU. Acute superior vena caval thrombosis after central venous catheter removal: successful treatment with thrombolytic therapy. Med Pediatr Oncol 1990;18(1):77.

22. Monreal M, Lafoz E, Ruiz J, et al. Upper-extremity deep venous thrombosis and pulmonary embolism. Chest 1991;99(2):280.

23. Horattas MC, Wright DJ, Fenton AH, et al. Changing concepts of deep venous thrombosis of the upper extremity: report of a series and review of the literature. Surgery 1988;104(3):561.

24. Martin EC, Koser M, Gordon DH. Venography in axillary-subclavian vein thrombosis. Cardiovasc Radiol 1979;2:261.

25. Haire WD, Lynch TG, Lieberman RP, et al. Utility of duplex ultrasound in the diagnosis of asymptomatic catheter-induced subclavian vein thrombosis. J Ultrasound Med 1991;10(9):493.

26. Adams JT, DeWeese JA, McEvoy RK. Primary deep venous thrombosis of the upper extremity. Arch Surg 1965;91:29.

27. Campbell CB, Chandler JG, Tegtmeyer CJ, Bernstein EF. Axillary, subclavian, and brachiocephalic vein obstruction. Surgery 1977;82:816.

28. Donayre CE, White GH, Mehringer SM, Wilson SE. Pathogenesis determines late morbidity of axillosubclavian vein thrombosis. Am J Surg 1986;152:179.

29. Zimmermann R, Morl H, Harenberg J, et al. Urokinase therapy of subclavian-axillary vein thrombosis. Klin Wochenschr 1981;59:851.

30. Fankuchen EI, Neff RA, Collins RA, et al. Urokinase perfusion for axillary-subclavian vein thrombosis. Cardiovasc Intervent Radiol 1984;7:90.

31. Taylor LM, McAllister WR, Dennis DL, Porter JM. Thrombolytic therapy followed by first rib resection for spontaneous ("effort") subclavian vein thrombosis. Am J Surg 1985;149:644.

32. Edwards RD, Cassidy J, Taylor A. Case report: superior vena cava obstruction complicated by central venous thrombosis—treatment with thrombolysis and Gianturco-Z stents. Clin Radiol 1992;45:278.

33. Charnsangavej C, Carrasco CH, Wallace S, et al. Stenosis of the vena cava: preliminary assessment of treatment with expandable metallic stents. Radiology 1986;161:295.

34. Elson JD, Becker GJ, Wholey MH, Ehrman KO. Vena caval and central venous stenoses: management with Palmaz balloon-expandable intraluminal stents. JVIR 1991;2:215.

35. Putnam J, Uchida BS, Anbtonovic R, Rosch J. Superior vena cava syndrome associated with massive thrombosis: treatment with expandable wire stents. Radiology 1988;167:727.

36. Wilson JJ, Lesk D, Newman H. Subclavian-axillary vein thrombosis: successful treatment with streptokinase. Can Med Assoc J 1984;130:891.

37. Appleby DH, Heller MS. Low-dose streptokinase therapy for subclavian vein thrombosis. South Med J 1984;77:536.

38. Rubenstein M, Creger WP. Successful streptokinase therapy for catheter-induced subclavian vein thrombosis. Arch Intern Med 1980;140:1370.

39. Herrera JL, Willis HM, Williams TH. Successful streptokinase therapy of acute idiopathic superior vena cava thrombosis. Am Heart J 1981;102(8):1063.

40. Katzen B, van Breda A. Low dose streptokinase in the treatment of arterial occlusion. AJR 1981;136:1171.

41. Becker GJ, Holder RW, Rabe FE, et al. Local thrombolytic therapy for subclavian and axillary vein thrombosis. Radiology 1983;149:419.

42. Fraschini G, Jadeja J, Lawson M, et al. Local Infusion of urokinase for the lysis of thrombosis associated with permanent central venous catheters in cancer patients. J Clin Oncol 1987;5:672.

43. Druy EM, Trout HH III, Giordano JM, Hix WR. Lytic therapy in the treatment of axillary and subclavian vein thrombosis. J Vascular Surg 1985;6(2):821.

44. Graor RA, Young JR, Risius B, Ruschaupt WF.

Comparison of cost-effectiveness of streptokinase and urokinase in the treatment of deep venous thrombosis. Ann Vasc Surg 1987;1:524.

45. Sharma GVRK, Cella G, Parisi AF, et al. Thrombolytic therapy. N Engl J Med 1982;306:1268.

46. Totty WG, Romano T, Bnian GM, et al. Serum sickness following streptokinase therapy. AJR 1982;138:143.

47. Sallen MK, Efrusy ME, Kniaz JL, et al. Streptokinase induced hepatic dysfunction. Am J Gastroenterol 1983;78:523.

48. Fraschini G, Jadeja J, Lawson M, et al. Local infusion of urokinase for the lysis of thrombosis associated with permanent central venous catheters in cancer patients. J Clin Oncol 1987;5(4):672.

49. Druy EM, Trout HH III, Giordano JM, Hix WR. Lytic therapy in the treatment of axillary and subclavian vein thrombosis. J Vasc Surg. 1985; 6(2):821.

16

OVERVIEW OF CATHETER-DIRECTED THROMBOLYTIC THERAPY FOR ARTERIAL AND GRAFT OCCLUSION

Anthony J. Comerota

John V. White

The intraarterial infusion of fibrinolytic agents has become a valuable adjunct for the treatment of acute arterial and graft occlusion. Although the initial attempt at regional delivery of fibrinolytic agents was made over 30 years ago, only in the 1980s did it become routinely accepted. The evolution in therapy is the result of increasing interest in thrombolysis for all forms of thromboembolic vascular disease, an improved understanding of the technique of delivery, and continuing technical improvement by the interventionalists and catheter delivery systems.

Since the most effective means of dissolving clot is the activation of plasminogen bound to fibrin within the matrix of the clot,[1] it is intuitive that delivery of the plasminogen activator into the thrombus should maximize lysis (Fig. 16-1).

When the plasminogen activator is delivered into the thrombus, it is protected from plasminogen activator inhibitors. Upon activation of plasminogen, plasmin acts efficiently within the thrombus, effecting lysis while being protected from plasmin inhibitors. As regional or intrathrombus infusion continues, systemic activation of plasminogen occurs, resulting in breakdown of fibrinogen, clotting factors, and other plasma proteins.

The first attempt at the direct local delivery of a fibrinolytic agent for arterial thrombosis was made by McNicol and colleagues[2] over 30 years ago. The technique of catheter-directed intraarterial delivery of thrombolytic agents was promoted by Dotter and associates,[3] and the good results of low-dose streptokinase infusion reported by Katzen and van Breda[4] drew the attention of interventional radiologists and vascular surgeons. Techniques for the intraarterial delivery of thrombolytic agents have been refined over the past decade,[2–39] to the point where arterial occlusions can be assessed to predict the likelihood of clot lysis and to ensure the most efficient delivery of the lytic agent to the occluding thrombus. Katzen reviewed important developments in catheter technology (Chap. 20), and Bookstein, Valji, and Roberts summarize the potential advantages of the Pulse-Spray technique (Chap. 21).

The issues that remain regarding catheter-directed lytic therapy include (1) whether patency

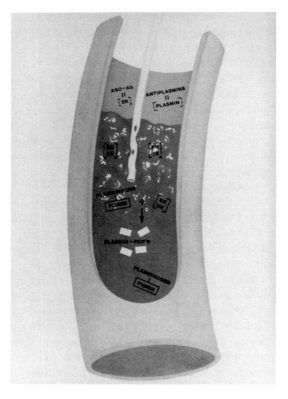

FIGURE 16-1. A schematic illustration of the principle of intraarterial delivery of thrombolytic agents into the occluding thrombus. The lytic agent interacts with the fibrin-bound plasminogen. The active agent, plasmin, dissolves fibrin with the release of fibrin degradation products. If SK is used and escapes into the systemic circulation, it will be bound (at least in part) by antistreptococcal antibodies, thereby inactivating the SK molecule. If small amounts of plasmin escape into the circulation, it will be bound by circulating antiplasmins, thereby inactivating its systemic effect. If, however, appreciable amounts of the lytic agent or appreciable amounts of plasmin escape into the systemic circulation, a systemic fibrinolytic effect will occur.

of the occluded vessel or graft can be restored, (2) whether the risk of thrombolysis has been substantially reduced during recent years, making it a reasonable treatment alternative, and (3) whether there is long-term benefit from lysis in terms of the patients' ultimate revascularization. While many patients have enjoyed the benefit of catheter-directed thrombolysis and many physicians have witnessed favorable outcomes (Table 16-1), the

risks of treatment and substantial failure rates persist; therefore, appropriate patient selection has become perhaps the most critical issue.

OBJECTIVES

The primary objectives of catheter-directed thrombolysis are to dissolve the occluding thrombus, restore perfusion, and identify the underlying cause of arterial or graft thrombosis, thereby allowing definitive correction. Important additional goals of therapy are to

1. Convert an urgent surgical procedure to an elective one.
2. Gain patency of an occluded but nondiseased inflow source for subsequent bypass.
3. Lyse thrombi in the distal vasculature, thereby opening the outflow tract.
4. Convert a major vascular reconstruction to a limited, less extensive procedure.
5. Prevent arterial intimal injury from balloon catheter thrombectomy.
6. Restore patency of branch vessels that are inaccessible to mechanical thrombectomy.
7. Reduce the extent of amputation in patients in whom complete success cannot be achieved.

Although these are desirable goals, the likelihood of achieving them in any given patient requires an understanding of the underlying problem, knowledge of the risks and benefits of alternative therapeutic options, and familiarity with the techniques and potential complications of intraarterial thrombolytic therapy.

PATIENT SELECTION

Proper identification of patients appropriate for catheter-directed thrombolysis is the key to successful treatment and minimizing complications. Results of ongoing and recently completed prospective, randomized trials will invariably assist in proper patient identification. The initial step in patient selection is recognizing that elimi-

TABLE 16-1. *Short-Term Efficacy and Safety of Catheter-Directed Intraarterial Thrombolysis*

Drug	Number	Refs.	Average Duration of Infusion	Success	Major Complications
SK	542	3–21	41 h	354 (65%)	112 (21%)
UK	277	15–23	28 h	222 (80%)	32 (12%)
rt-PA	137	23–25	7 h	117 (85%)	11 (8%)

Pooled data from representative studies (retrospective reports).

nating the occluding thrombus will be of benefit in ultimate therapy. The observation that long segments of the vascular tree can be obliterated by acute thrombus precipitated by severe but relatively segmental atherosclerotic disease is the underlying rationale for catheter-directed thrombolytic therapy. This applies to segmental disease in native arteries as well as bypass grafts. Therefore, the ability to identify and correct segmental pathology following successful thrombolysis is the key to long-term benefit.

Good Candidates for Lytic Therapy

Patients who have a higher likelihood of successful reperfusion or a potentially lower complication rate with catheter-directed lysis are considered good candidates for therapy.

- *Acute embolic or thrombotic occlusions of vessels inaccessible to mechanical thrombectomy.*
- *Patients with wound complications in whom another wound is associated with substantial morbidity.* These patients are candidates for intraarterial fibrinolytic therapy not because catheter-directed thrombolysis is likely to be highly successful, but rather because the risk of complications and failure of alternative approaches are considerable.
- *Acute thrombosis of a popliteal aneurysm causing significant foot ischemia.* Such severe ischemia occurs most frequently when the popliteal trifurcation is occluded. Emergent operative reconstruction in such patients is associated with a high amputation rate. Reestablishing patency of infrapopliteal vessels with the regional delivery of fibrinolytic agents significantly increases the chance of successful aneurysm repair with concomitant limb salvage. On the other hand, patients tolerating popliteal aneurysm thrombosis without limb jeopardy do not require catheter-directed thrombolysis and may not require operative repair.

- *Acute embolic occlusion.* This can usually be treated successfully with catheter-directed thrombolysis (Fig. 16-2). Lytic therapy appears especially appropriate in patients with clinical conditions in which operative thromboembolectomy would be associated with substantial additional morbidity.
- *Acute thrombosis.* Especially if proximally located and easily accessible with infusion guidewires and catheters, this should be considered for catheter-directed thrombolysis (Fig. 16-3).
- *Thrombosed saphenous vein grafts.* Although the treatment of patients with occluded bypass grafts is controversial, patients presenting with thrombosed saphenous vein grafts which have been functioning well for a year or more should have catheter-directed thrombolysis offered as primary therapy. These are patients in whom a segmental, underlying lesion is likely to be responsible for graft failure (Fig. 16-4).

Poor Candidates for Lytic Therapy

Patients whose underlying condition is associated with a low likelihood of success or a high complication rate or who have better surgical options should not be offered fibrinolytic therapy.

- *Acute embolic occlusion of large arteries easily accessible via a limited operative procedure.*

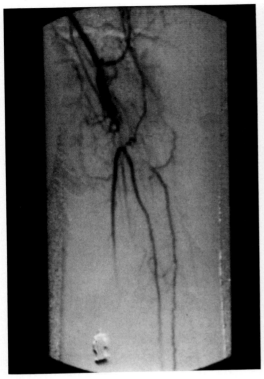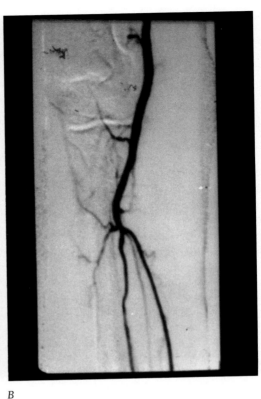

A   B

FIGURE 16-2. *This patient illustrates rapid thrombolysis of an acute embolus to the left brachial artery with subsequent demonstration of the embolic source from an axillosubclavian aneurysm.* (A) *Acute embolic occlusion of the left brachial artery in a young woman presenting with an acutely ischemic arm and hand.* (B) *Following 8 h of catheter-directed thrombolysis, all the embolic occlusion is dissolved.* (C) *The axillosubclavian artery appeared normal in the neutral position.* (D) *In the abduction position, however, two areas of occlusion were demonstrated with an associated aneurysm, which was the source of the embolus. This was electively resected.*

These patients can be quickly and efficiently treated with standard operative thromboembolectomy. However, these individuals are best selected following arteriography, since fragmentation with distal embolization cannot be reliably identified by clinical examination alone.

- *Severely ischemic limb in which viability is imminently threatened.* This is usually due to multisegment occlusion and is associated with a high failure rate. Choosing between catheter-directed thrombolysis and primary operative reconstruction is frequently a difficult decision, since both can be associated with considerable morbidity and mortality in these patients. However, if a major arterial segment can have patency restored with reperfusion of a major collateral, marked improvement is frequently observed (Fig. 16-5). If the limb is no longer threatened (i.e., correcting ischemic rest pain to tolerable claudication), a potentially high-risk operative revascularization can be avoided.

- *Acute postoperative bypass graft thrombosis.* These patients face an excessive risk of hemorrhage with little chance of success from catheter-directed thrombolysis. Early postoperative thrombosis is usually associated

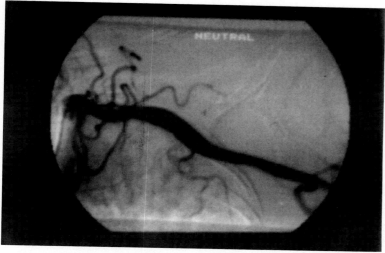

C

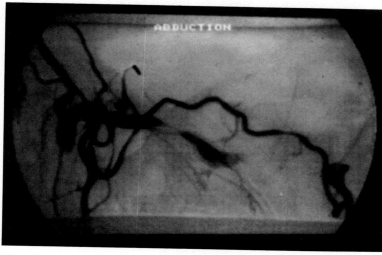

D

FIGURE 16-2. (Continued).

with a technical error or poor patient selection. For the former, operative thrombectomy should be performed concurrently with correction of the technical problem. For the latter, rethrombosis is certain following either mechanical or pharmacologic thrombectomy; therefore, any additional intervention with lytic agents would pose a needless risk without potential gain. The combined complication and failure rate of thrombolysis in these patients is considerable.

- *Modest ischemia, producing tolerable symptoms (intermittent claudication).* Such patients are ordinarily not offered angiography or operative intervention. Likewise, these patients should not be treated with catheter-directed thrombolysis for the same reasons

(Text continued on page 232)

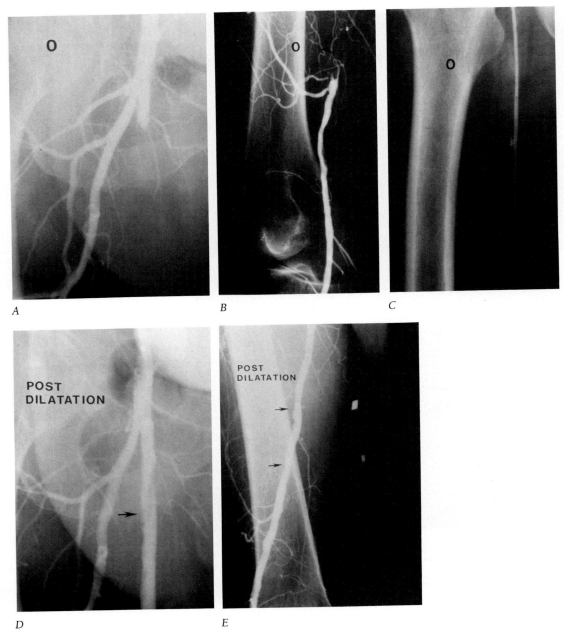

FIGURE 16-3. *This case illustrates successful lysis of an acutely thrombosed superficial femoral artery causing intolerable intermittent claudication.* (A) *The arteriogram demonstrating acute occlusion of the proximal superficial femoral artery.* (B) *A patent popliteal artery reconstituted via profunda collaterals.* (C) *The infusion catheter was placed into the occluded superficial femoral artery.* (D, E) *Following successful thrombolysis of the occluding thrombus, three areas of stenosis were dilated with 8-mm balloon catheters demonstrating an excellent short-term result. Eleven years later the patient continues to walk without symptoms, with palpable distal pulses and with an ankle brachial index of 0.95.*

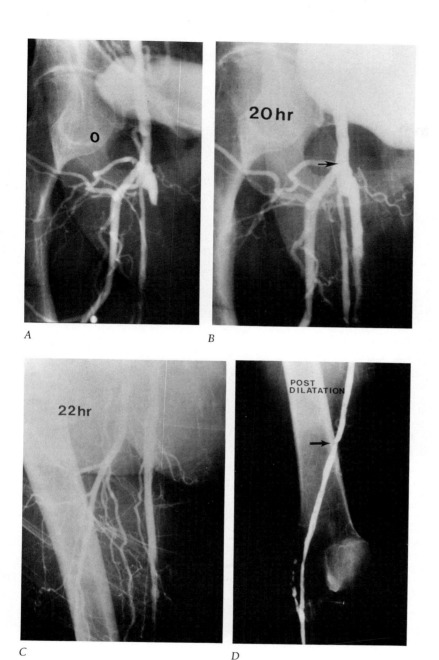

FIGURE 16-4. This case illustrates the importance of proper catheter position and also illustrates salvage of a patient's primary autogenous bypass graft. This patient presented with a 1-week history of ischemic rest pain following occlusion of her femoral-popliteal saphenous vein bypass graft. (A) The catheter was positioned just above the proximal anastomosis at the origin of the profunda femoris artery (arrow). (B) After 20 h of infusion, only 3 in of the proximal thrombus had lysed. The catheter was then advanced into the saphenous vein graft and positioned at the level of the thrombus. Following an additional 2 h of infusion (22 h), significant lysis occurred. (C) After continuing the infusion, the entire thrombus lysed, and the graft regained patency. The distal graft fibrosis responded well to percutaneous balloon dilation. (D) The sclerotic venous valve (arrow) did not respond to dilation, but was easily excised, and a small vein patch angioplasty performed. This graft remained patent and functioning normally until the patient died of an acute myocardial infarction 3½ years later.

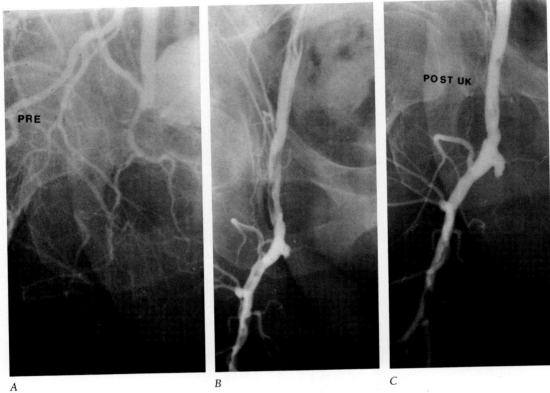

A   *B*   *C*

*FIGURE 16-5. This case is an example of a severely ischemic limb due to multiple segment thrombo-
sis. Thrombolysis successfully restored perfusion to a major collateral (the profunda femoris artery)
with marked improvement of the patient's perfusion. The thrombosed femoral anterior tibial bypass
was not successfully opened. The patient was anticoagulated and had 2- to 3-block intermittent claudication which extended to 3 to 4 blocks after 1 year. (A) Arteriogram demonstrating iliac artery
thrombosis and occlusion of the patient's femoral arteries and femoral–anterior tibial–saphenous
vein bypass. (B) Partial lysis of iliac and femoral arteries. (C) Lysis of thrombus in iliac, femoral,
and profunda femoris arteries. There is persistent occlusion of the femoral anterior tibial bypass.*

that bypass procedures are not considered, since the natural history of their disease is quite favorable with noninterventional therapy. Although the likelihood of success with any intervention in claudicants is high, there is a finite complication and amputation rate, and each patient treated should be so informed. The attitude of "lets treat the lesion and see what happens since we have nothing to loose" should be avoided.

TECHNIQUE

The first step in successful technique is anticipating that intraarterial lytic therapy is a treatment alternative prior to angiography. The approach is usually from the contralateral femoral artery, threading the catheter around the aortic bifurcation. Vessels considered for thrombolysis should have an attempt at guidewire penetration of the occlusion. If a guidewire can be passed well into or through the occlusion, successful thrombolysis is likely. Conversely, if a guidewire cannot be passed, then neointimal fibroplasia, atherosclerotic disease, or highly organized thrombus is the probable cause of the occlusion which will not respond to a lytic agent, and primary operative reconstruction should be recommended. If guidewire passage is successful, the infusion catheter should be embedded well into the occluded vessel. Lytic therapy is usually not successful if the catheter tip remains above the occlusion (see Fig. 16-4).

Once catheters are appropriately positioned, either urokinase (UK) or recombinant tissue-type plasminogen activator (rt-PA) is the recommended agent. Our prior experience with streptokinase (SK) resulted in unacceptably high bleeding complications. The initial dose of UK is 4000 units per minute until recanalization is achieved, at which point the dose can be reduced to 1000 to 2000 units per minute. If rt-PA is chosen, a dose of 0.05 mg/kg per minute is used for a period of up to 12 h. These generic recommendations can be modified by using higher doses if more rapid lysis is required. Patients are generally given broad-spectrum intravenous antibiotics while the catheter is in place. Routine blood studies are performed prior to and during treatment and include a complete coagulation profile. A guaiac test on a stool specimen is performed prior to treatment for documentation. All patients remain at absolute bed rest, most of them in the intensive care unit. Puncture sites are frequently observed, and the circulatory status of the infused extremity is monitored with ankle pressures every 1 to 2 h.

Periodic arteriography is performed to follow the therapeutic response and guide positioning of the catheter. The initial 2 to 4 h of infusion is generally performed in the radiology suite. Catheters are then advanced into the thrombus as required, appreciating that inappropriate catheter position frequently leads to failure.

If one is faced with multisegment occlusion and infusion guidewires can be advanced into the distal segment, infusion of lytic agents is performed through a coaxial system. The dose of the lytic agent is then split between the two catheters, with relatively higher doses delivered to the distal occlusion.

The concurrent administration of heparin with SK has been associated with excessively high hemorrhagic complication rates. The severity of bleeding complications by adding heparin to UK has not been similarly observed; however, most physicians agree that the concurrent use of heparin with all thrombolytic agents increases the risk of bleeding. Heparin is used to reduce the risk of pericatheter thrombosis. If a catheter is placed into a long, static arterial segment or if the catheter traverses a high-grade stenosis to reach the occluding thrombus, we would recommend the use of intravenous heparin. However, if the catheter is placed through relatively disease-free arterial segments, the risk of pericatheter thrombosis is small, and the added risk of a hemorrhagic complication with concomitant heparin outweighs the potential benefit.

The fibrinogen level, prothrombin time, partial thromboplastin time, and fibrin degradation products are monitored during infusion to document the presence of a systemic lytic effect. If the fibrinogen level falls below 100 mg/dL, the infusion is slowed or stopped to allow restoration of circulating fibrinogen and clotting factors. On rare occasions, fresh frozen plasma or cryoprecipitate can be given. Plasmin inhibitors such as aprotinin can be used and have corrected abnormal bleeding times caused by tissue plasminogen activator.[34]

After successful infusion, a completion arteriogram is performed, and blood studies are repeated. The catheter is removed after the fibrinogen level returns to 100 mg/dL or more. After successful lysis, the underlying cause of the occlusion must be identified and corrected by means of standard interventional techniques. If percutaneous correction is not possible or appropriate, systemic anticoagulation is continued until definitive operative repair is performed.

The technique chosen to repair the underlying lesion may have substantial impact on long-term success. In general, operative repair is more durable than percutaneous techniques. This has been demonstrated by several studies evaluating the threatened femoral-popliteal/tibial-saphenous vein bypass graft (Table 16-2). Since neointimal fibroplasia is important in the etiology of prosthetic graft failure, operative revision is recommended.

Taking advantage of collective previous experience, one can identify patients who are likely to have initially successful (or unsuccessful) lysis (Table 16-3). The most important factors are whether the guidewire can pass into or through the thrombus (Fig. 16-6) and whether the catheter is appropriately positioned within the thrombus during infusion. If the guidewire cannot be passed or if the catheter is not properly positioned, intraarterial thrombolytic therapy should not be attempted. Patients presenting with proximal large-vessel occlusion of short duration whose distal vessels are visualized and have audible Doppler signals are likely to have a successful response without the risk of suffering additional ischemia during infusion (see Fig. 16-3). Those patients who have distal vessel occlusion, no audible Doppler signal, and no visible distal vessels angiographically generally have more significant ischemia and less chance of a favorable outcome.

With appropriate patient selection, if the guidewire passes and the catheter is positioned properly, one can expect a 75% to 85% chance of successful lysis. It is incumbent on the physician to then identify the underlying cause of the occlusion and correct the lesion in a timely fashion.[30] When this is possible, enviable patency rates can

TABLE 16-3. Parameters Predictive of Successful Lysis

Parameter	Success	
	Likely	Unlikely
Guidewire	Passes	Does not pass
Catheter position	In thrombus	Not in thrombus
Occluded vessel	Proximal	Distal
Duration of occlusion	Hours/days	Weeks
Distal Doppler signal	Present	Absent
Visualization of distal vessels	Yes	No

be obtained. However, if an underlying stenosis is not identified and corrected, rethrombosis is the rule.[18,30] If a single-plane arteriogram does not identify the causative lesion, additional oblique views or arterial duplex imaging is indicated (Figs. 16-7 and 16-8).

Graor et al.[24] have shown that catheter-directed thrombolysis followed by operative correction is preferred to primary operative thrombectomy and graft revision. Significantly better patency rates and fewer amputations were re-

FIGURE 16-6. Diagram of thrombus-dominant and plaque-dominant arterial occlusion. Both would look the same on arteriography, but the thrombus-dominant occlusion (gray shading) would allow guidewire passage and appropriate catheter positioning, whereas the plaque-dominant occlusion (stippled shading) would not allow guidewire passage or appropriate catheter positioning.

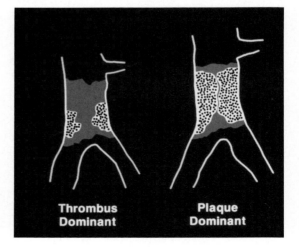

TABLE 16-2. The Threatened Femoropopliteal/Tibial Autogenous Bypass: Comparison of the Durability of Techniques of Graft Revision

Author	5-Year Durability	
	Balloon Dilation	Operative Revision
Bandyk et al.[35] (1991)	50% (9/18)	86% (55/64)
Perler et al.[36] (1990)	22% (4/18)*	62% (5/19)
Cohen et al.[37] (1986)	43% (3/7)	82% (18/22)
TOTAL	37% (16/43)	82% (78/95)

* 3-year durability.

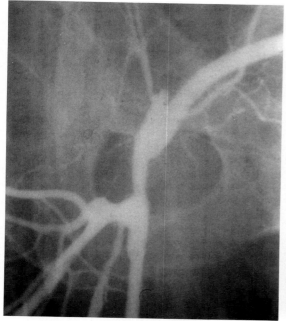

A

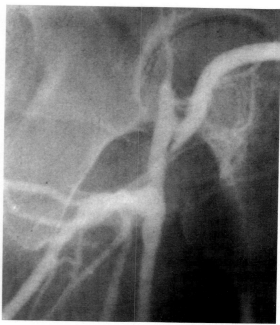

B

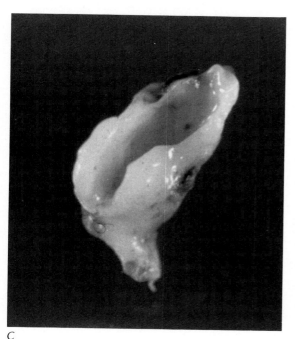

C

FIGURE 16-7. (A) *The completion arteriogram following successful lysis of an acutely thrombosed iliofemoral by-pass graft. There is no evidence of an underlying stenosis.* (B) *Repeat arteriogram in an extended oblique position demonstrates high-grade stenosis at the anastomosis. Attempts at percutaneous dilation failed, most likely due to neointimal fibroplasia.* (C) *The neointimal fibroplastic lesion is seen following operative excision. It is easily understood why percutaneous balloon dilation is not successful for these lesions.*

quired in patients treated with preoperative thrombolysis (Table 16-4). This is probably due to more precise definition of the underlying lesion that caused graft thrombosis resulting in a more definitive repair. A less thrombogenic luminal surface and lysis of thrombi in the runoff bed are also potential advantages.

OUTCOME OF CATHETER-DIRECTED THROMBOLYSIS

The most critical question when assessing intraarterial delivery of lytic agents for the treatment of occluded arteries and/or bypass grafts is whether lysis of the occluded vessel is of significant benefit to a patient's ultimate revascularization? Regaining patency for short periods of time only to have a patient reocclude appears short-sighted and is of no lasting benefit. On the other hand, if lysis can be achieved and perfusion restored with identification and correction of a focal underlying lesion, thereby salvaging the patient's native artery or primary bypass graft, few would argue that dissolving the underlying thrombus is of benefit. Belkin et al.,[28] Wolfson et al.,[10] and Sicard et al.[29] have reported poor long-term patency following lysis of occluded arteries and grafts. Others, however, have reported substantially better long-term results.[18,22]

As mentioned previously, sustained success of catheter-directed thrombolysis depends on identifying and correcting the underlying lesion causing thrombosis. While intuitively obvious, this was initially substantiated by McNamara and Bomberger[30] when they showed that after thrombolysis, patients who left the hospital without a persistent stenosis had enviable 6-month patency rates compared with those who had uncorrected disease. This was true both for native arteries and for bypass grafts. These observations were confirmed by Sullivan and associates.[38]

When treating patients with graft failure, it is also important to appreciate the higher incidence of an underlying hypercoagulable disorder.[40] If an underlying coagulopathy exists but is not identified and treated, rethrombosis is inevitable. Reviewing the literature following intraarterial thrombolytic therapy, patients are variously

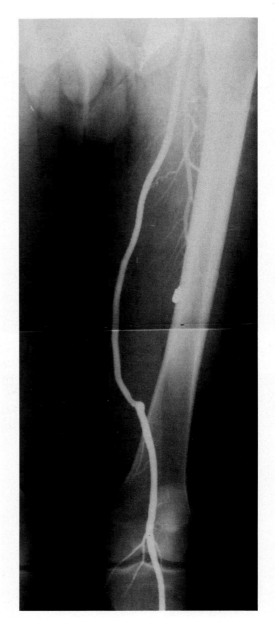

A

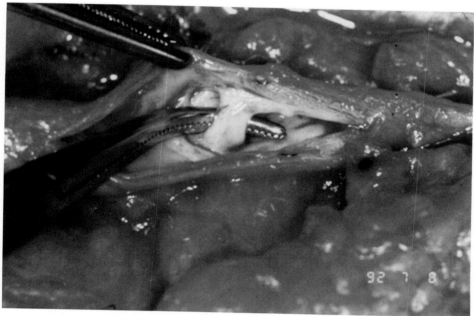

B

FIGURE 16-8. (A) *The completion arteriogram following successful thrombolysis of an occluded femoral-popliteal bypass graft. The arteriogram fails to demonstrate any significant lesion responsible for graft failure. A subsequent arterial duplex of the graft demonstrated high velocities at the distal anastomosis and raised suspicion of a lesion in that location.* (B) *At exploration, a column of neointimal fibroplasia extended through the middle of the anastomosis. This was not visible angiographically, since contrast material flowed on each side of the lesion. This was resected and replaced by a small segment of interpositional graft placed end-to-end.*

treated either with anticoagulation and platelet inhibitors or without any attention to modifying the hemostatic process. We believe that in the absence of contraindications, all patients having graft failure require anticoagulation unless uncompromised revascularization can be achieved with autogenous tissue and patients are free of an underlying coagulopathy.

COMPLICATIONS

The major disincentive to the use of catheter-directed thrombolysis is the risk of additional complications. Complications encountered with catheter-directed delivery of thrombolytic agents can be categorized as those secondary to the drug and its subsequent effects on the fibrinolytic and

TABLE 16-4. *Thrombolysis versus Thrombectomy for Acute Graft Thrombosis: Follow-Up of 84 Patients*

	No.	500-Day Patency	Operative Revision	Eventual Amputation
Lytic therapy (rt-PA)	43	35%	91%	24%
Operative thrombectomy	43	25%	89%	40%
p Value		<0.05		0.05

Updated from Graor RA, Risius B, Young JR, et al. Thrombolysis of peripheral arterial bypass grafts: Surgical thrombectomy compared with thrombolysis. J Vasc Surg 1988;7:347. (Updated data provided by Dr. Graor via personal communication.)

coagulation system and those mechanical (arteriographic) complications associated with the technique (Table 16-5). Each clinical situation should be individually assessed, with the potential adverse complications weighted against the benefit of lytic therapy, and placed in the context of the risk of therapeutic alternatives versus their likelihood of success.

Allergic Reactions

Allergic reactions to SK have been appreciated since its initial use. Because bacteria are the source of SK, foreign antigen accounts for much of the allergic and pyretic side effects, although with the present-day refined preparations these allergic reactions are less frequent and mild. Pretreatment doses of hydrocortisone, 100 mg IV, have been used to blunt the pyretic response, and acetaminophen also has been used during treatment to control the febrile reactions. Severe anaphylactic reactions and bronchospasm have been reported infrequently with SK preparations and usually are unaffected by pretreatment with hydrocortisone. Treatment consists of stopping the infusion and administering antihistamines and additional steroids. We have observed a serum sickness reaction, which has previously been reported with SK infusion,[41] with the characteristic

TABLE 16-5. Complications of Intraarterial Lytic Therapy

I. Drug-associated complications
  A. Hemorrhage
    1. Due to lysis of hemostatic fibrin
    2. Due to the induced coagulopathy
  B. Distal emboli
  C. Allergic reaction
  D. Pyretic reaction
  E. Serum sickness (SK)
  F. Transgraft extravasation (Hemorrhage)
II. Technique-associated complications
  A. Pericatheter thrombosis
  B. Catheter-induced thrombosis
  C. Toxic complications of contrast
  D. Pseudoaneurysm at puncture site
  E. Arteriogram complications

multiarticular joint involvement, macular rash, and associated drop in serum compliment. Our patient was treated with the regional infusion of SK, and interestingly, the rash remained localized to only the infused leg.

Allergic complications with UK are substantially less, since it is a derivative of human protein. However, significant pyretic reactions have been observed increasingly with UK and in one study resulted in he termination of therapy in 22%[42] when it was used systemically for the treatment of pulmonary embolism. While we have observed such severe allergic and pyretic responses in patients treated systemically for deep venous thrombosis and/or pulmonary embolism, such side effects have been infrequent when using UK intraarterially. The pyretic reaction observed with UK is thought to be due to the carrier substance, which stimulates production of interleukin 6 (Sasahara AA: Personal communication).

Hemorrhage

Bleeding is the most common and most feared complication of thrombolytic therapy, which can occur as a result of the active lytic state or the coagulopathy (fibrinogen and clotting factor depletion) caused by the lytic agent. It is often difficult to distinguish the incidence of the major bleeding complications from the less serious ones in many reports, since definitions frequently vary. Major bleeding complications should be defined as those which cause permanent disability or which prolong hospital stay. Blood transfusion requirement is an unsatisfactory criterion because indications for blood replacement vary regionally, institutionally, and individually.

There is little doubt that patients who have major invasive procedures, especially arterial cannulation, have higher rates of bleeding complications than those who do not. This has been observed in myocardial infarction trials, where patients with arterial interventions had a 30% bleeding complication rate compared with 5% or less in those without.[43] Intracerebral bleeding is the most dreaded of all hemorrhagic events, and its incidence is probably an inescapable 1% to 2%. Voluminous data generated from numerous myocardial infarction trials demonstrate that the risk of intracerebral bleeding is increased by age, hypertension, low body weight, coincident head injury, previous stroke, and previous Coumadin anticoagulation.[43]

The mechanisms for bleeding during thrombolytic therapy can be categorized as (1) lysis of hemostatic thrombi, (2) consequences of clotting factor and fibrinogen depletion, and (3) continued anticoagulation. Most of the bleeding during the infusion of lytic agents is not caused by the biochemical changes created by the lytic agents but rather by the lysis of hemostatic clot. Patients treated with lytic agents who have complete vascular integrity have a smooth therapeutic course, without bleeding complications. Most bleeding problems are due to the trauma of invasive diagnostic or therapeutic procedures. By definition, invasive procedures are required for catheter-directed thrombolysis; therefore, an unavoidable minimal number of bleeding complications occur. However, if lytic therapy is anticipated prior to diagnostic arteriography, the appropriate entry site can be chosen using a single-wall puncture technique, permitting appropriate catheter or sheath placement with minimal or no additional trauma. The hemorrhagic complication from lysis of hemostatic thrombi are minimized by proper patient selection, good technique, short duration of therapy, and avoidance of unnecessary vascular intervention.

Initially, it was hoped that the intraarterial delivery of lytic agents would diminish the systemic activation of plasminogen, thereby decreasing hemorrhagic complications. While regional arterial delivery of lytic agents appears to increase efficacy, and selected patients will have rapid clot lysis with a minimal systemic effect, there is usually a substantial systemic fibrinolytic response. We have observed an increased severity of bleeding and more frequent bleeding complications when catheter-directed lytic therapy was accompanied by marked fibrinogen depletion and therefore prefer to maintain fibrinogen levels greater than 100 mg/dL. Intracranial hemorrhagic complications are rare; however, 1% to 2% is likely to be the minimal achievable level despite appropriate screening, no matter what the lytic agent. In our experience with catheter-directed thrombolysis, bleeding complications were more frequent with SK than with UK or rt-PA.

The purpose of laboratory monitoring of thrombolytic therapy is to document that the agent is effectively producing a lytic state. While this is a necessary part of systemic thrombolysis, efficacy of catheter-directed thrombolysis is evaluated clinically and angiographically and does not depend on laboratory markers of systemic fibrinolysis. In general, laboratory values do not correlate with hemorrhagic complications or efficacy of lysis.

Early in the clinical experience with thrombolysis, the importance of fibrinogen depletion was probably overrated, and subsequent analyses demonstrated that there was no correlation with bleeding complications.[44] The majority of these observations were made in patients treated for venous thromboembolism or acute myocardial infarction. On the other hand, the clinical experience with catheter-directed thrombolysis for peripheral arterial and graft occlusion suggested that fibrinogen depletion was linked to bleeding complications. A number of factors are relevant to these observations, including (1) patients treated for peripheral arterial or graft occlusion require arterial puncture and prolonged cannulation, (2) the duration of therapy extends far beyond that required for acute myocardial infarction and may exceed that required for venous thromboembolism, (3) the fibrinogen concentration measured may detect hemostatically ineffective fibrinogen,[45] (4) certain individuals with low fibrinogen concentrations (those treated with thrombolytic agents and those with hereditary afibrinogenemia) do not uniformly have hemorrhagic complications[46] and (5) the fibrinogen associated with platelets may be as important hemostatically as circulating fibrinogen.[47]

Thrombolytic agents have a marked effect on platelet function, causing both activation and inhibition. Platelet activation tends to occur early in the course of lytic therapy, and inhibition occurs later.[48] Platelet inhibition occurs because of plasmin's inhibition of arachidonic acid metabolism, lysis of platelet-bound fibrinogen, and interference of fibrinogen binding to platelets by fibrin degradation products liberated during thrombolysis.[47]

There is an increased risk of hemorrhage with concurrent heparin administration. The need to treat all patients with concurrent anticoagulation is controversial. Anticoagulation is given concurrently to diminish the risk of pericatheter thrombus formation and, following thrombolysis, to reduce reocclusion. Pericatheter thrombosis is usually not a problem, since the lytic effect of the infused plasminogen activator lyses fibrin as it is deposited around the catheters. If a catheter traverses a high-grade stenosis to reach the target occlusion, concurrent heparin is indicated. Heparin bound to the surface of infusion catheters appears to be a more logical solution to this problem.

Transgraft Extravasation

Extravasation of contrast material and blood has been reported in patients treated with SK or UK who have arterial prostheses in place.[49,50] Extravasation has been observed mostly through knitted Dacron grafts. The larger mesh of the knitted graft is the likely explanation for this observation. Plasmin lyses the fibrin sealing the graft, which opens the interstices, allowing subsequent extravasation of dye and blood. Reports of extravasation from grafts in place for over a year indicate that the fibrin meshwork is continually susceptible to lysis despite a long graft implant time. Therefore, patients with knitted prostheses in place have a major added hemorrhagic potential when treated with lytic agents, and in our opinion, these patients are also considered to have a relative contraindication to thrombolytic therapy. If a knitted prosthesis is in a central location (chest or abdomen), we believe that if hemorrhage occurs, it can be life-threatening; therefore, alternative therapy is suggested. Since many patients with aortic aneurysmal and occlusive disease subsequently suffer acute myocardial infarction (MI), the vascular surgeon must be cognizant that using a knitted Dacron graft material in a central location may exclude the patient from being offered thrombolytic therapy for the acute MI.

Transgraft extravasation is not equivalent to an anastomotic leak. If contrast material extravasates from an anastomosis, fibrin dissolution at the suture line generally occurs, and a major hemorrhagic complication can be expected. Treating a thrombosed graft in the early postoperative period with lytic agents is likely to be associated with hemorrhagic complications, since the "hemostatic fibrin" at the anastomosis will lyse along with the intraluminal thrombus, the two being of relatively the same age. Since graft thrombosis in the early postoperative period is most commonly due to poor patient selection or technical error, lytic therapy will not affect either of these causes, and operative intervention is required for long-term success.

We have observed transgraft extravasation in three patients undergoing intraarterial thrombolytic therapy for thrombosed polytetrafluoroethylene (PTFE) grafts. In none of these patients was contrast extravasation associated with a drop in hemoglobin or other evidence of blood loss. This observation (Fig. 16-9) was noted only while the grafts were obstructed distally. After outflow was reestablished, contrast extravasation was no longer observed. It appears that transgraft extravasation can occur through PTFE grafts due to prolonged contact of the lytic agent with the graft in the presence of outflow obstruction. One of our patients underwent amputation following immediate rethrombosis of his graft due to unreconstructable distal disease, and no blood was observed in the perigraft tissues. Therefore, the radiologic finding of extravasation through PTFE grafts appears to have different meaning compared with knitted Dacron grafts.

Distal Emboli

Embolic complications distal to the occluded artery or graft being treated can occur during intraarterial thrombolytic therapy, which usually is the result of either partial lysis of thrombus, with fragments carried distally during reperfusion, or less frequently, a mechanical complication due to catheter manipulation or volume of infusate.

In our experience, distal embolic occlusion is observed infrequently during treatment of throm-

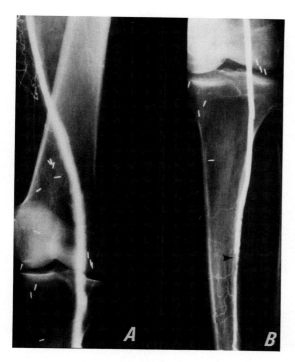

FIGURE 16-9. *A patient underwent lysis of an occluded femoral–anterior tibial artery PTFE graft which was placed 1.5 years earlier. After 2.5 h of catheter-directed thrombolysis, the patient's ischemia was not improved. (A) An arteriogram was repeated which demonstrated transgraft extravasation of contrast material through the PTFE graft. The graft remained occluded distally. (B) With continued infusion, the graft opened distally, and transgraft extravasation was no longer observed. The patient had a badly diseased anterior tibial artery (arrow) which led to rapid rethrombosis. A below-knee amputation failed to demonstrate any blood in the perigraft tissue, and the patient had no drop in hematocrit.*

bosed arteries or saphenous vein grafts. It has been observed occasionally during treatment of acute arterial emboli; however, most occur during treatment of thrombosed PTFE grafts. An example of distal embolic occlusion during catheter-directed thrombolysis is illustrated in Figure 16-10. In this instance, the patient presented with acute thrombosis of a femoral-popliteal PTFE graft. The distal popliteal artery was patent. After several hours of infusion, the patient's ischemia suddenly worsened. Repeat angiography demonstrated em-

bolic occlusion of all vessels of the popliteal trifurcation and distal embolic occlusion of the posterior tibial artery at the level of the ankle. The severity of the patient's ischemia prompted an urgent operative thrombectomy, which resulted in perforation of the peroneal artery and vein with a subsequent AV fistula.

Appropriate treatment of distal emboli that occur during catheter-directed thrombolysis is catheter advancement and continued infusion, perhaps with an increased dose. While this usually lyses distal emboli, occasionally, occlusions of the smaller arteries are resistant to lysis. If lysis does not occur in the face of sudden progressive ischemia, the risk of irreversible ischemic damage rapidly escalates, and clinical judgment as to appropriate treatment can be difficult.

Technical Complications

Technique-related complications are those associated with arteriography and catheter placement. Intimal dissection, thrombosis, allergic and toxic reactions to contrast agents, and femoral neuropathy also have been encountered. If a patient suffers a technique-related complication prior to the infusion of the lytic agent, thrombolysis will often be deferred; hence these complications are usually not included in reports of intraarterial thrombolytic therapy. Since many patients who are candidates for lytic therapy have additional associated vascular disease, selective catheterization may be difficult. This has been appreciated recently in the prospective, randomized STILE study, where 40% of patients with occluded grafts and 21% of patients with occluded arteries failed to achieve proper catheter position.[51] Such technical problems must be considered in the overall management of patients.

Pericathiter thrombosis was addressed earlier. However, whenever the catheter passes through a stenosis to treat an occlusion, the risk increases, and concurrent anticoagulation should be given (Fig. 16-11). Repeated arteriography associated with thrombolytic therapy may lead to large contrast loads and subsequent renal failure. Since

(Text continued on page 244)

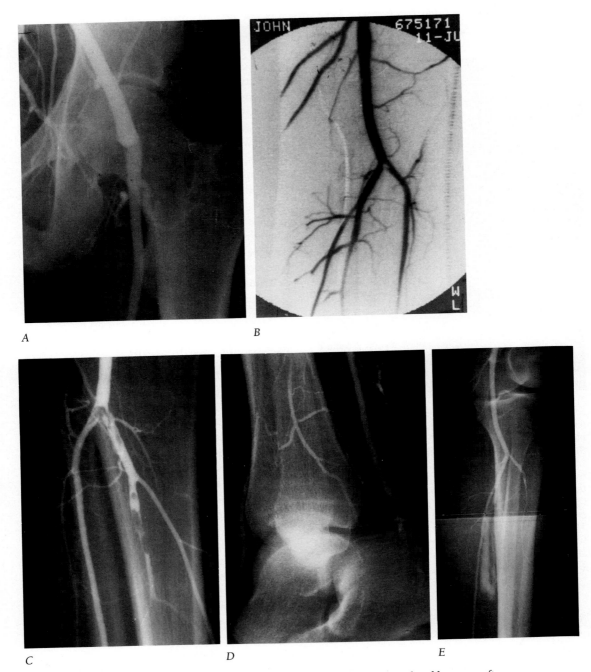

A

B

C

D

E

FIGURE 16-10. (A) Arteriogram demonstrating occlusion of a PTFE femoral-popliteal bypass graft. (B) Distal popliteal artery is patent via reconstitution from profunda collaterals with a patent trifurcation. A catheter was placed into the occluded PTFE graft. Within 3 h the patient's symptoms became acutely worse with the rapid onset of motor and sensory loss and loss of Doppler signals. (C) A repeat arteriogram demonstrates embolic occlusion of the distal popliteal artery and trifurcation vessels with further embolic occlusion of the posterior tibial artery at the ankle. (D) Thrombolysis was discontinued, and the patient was taken urgently to the operating room, where a thromboembolectomy was performed. The patient sustained injury from the balloon catheter to the peroneal artery–peroneal vein resulting in a traumatic AV fistula (E).

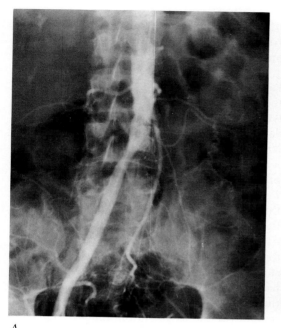

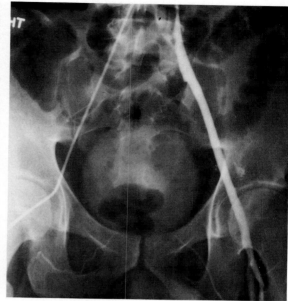

A

B

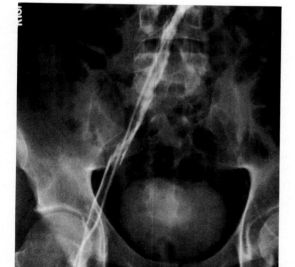

C

FIGURE 16-11. This is an example of pericatheter thrombosis in a patient undergoing thrombolysis of an occluded left iliac artery. (A) Initial arteriogram demonstrated occluded left iliofemoral arterial segment. Although a stenosis of the right common iliac was appreciated, it was assumed to be nonsignificant. (B) Completion arteriogram demonstrates successful thrombolysis of left iliofemoral segment with high-grade stenosis at the origin of the left common iliac artery. However, the patient's right foot became ischemic, and he lost his right femoral pulse. (C) A repeat arteriogram demonstrates acute thrombosis of the right iliofemoral segment around the infusion catheter.

compromised renal function frequently accompanies patients with peripheral arterial disease, the volume of contrast material required for diagnosis and to follow therapy may be a limiting factor. Arterial digital subtraction angiography is valuable in the management of these patients, since the required information is obtained with marked reduction in volume and concentration of contrast material compared with that required for standard arteriography.

PROSPECTIVE, RANDOMIZED TRIALS

The initial question, "Can occluded arteries or grafts have patency restored with catheter-directed thrombolytic therapy?" has been undeniably affirmed. Both occluded native arteries and bypass grafts can have patency restored with the appropriate delivery of catheter-directed thrombolysis. Clinical experience has demonstrated that early success rates are predicted by the ability to pass a guidewire through the occlusion and properly place an infusion catheter into the occluded artery or graft. However, reports of high complication rates and recurrent thromboses have diminished enthusiasm for catheter-directed thrombolysis in some centers and have challenged the medical community to define selection criteria that can appropriately identify patients who should be treated operatively and who should be treated with catheter-directed thrombolysis. While many physicians consider these treatment modalities as "either/or," it is our view that catheter-directed thrombolysis is an adjunct to operative reconstruction and other mechanical procedures and frequently needs to be combined with these other procedures for a successful outcome. Information from prospective, randomized studies evaluating catheter-directed thrombolytic therapy compared with operative revascularization in patients with lower extremity ischemia will be valuable for designing appropriate patient care plans in the future. Two prospective, randomized studies have been completed and one is ongoing, with preliminary results available. A brief discussion of each study follows.

A Randomized Trial of Catheter-Directed Thrombolysis for the Treatment of Acute Arterial and Graft Occlusion[52]

Purpose. This study was performed to evaluate the efficacy and safety of intraarterial thrombolytic therapy for acute limb ischemia (less than 7 days) compared with routine operative revascularization.

Design. One-hundred and fourteen patients presenting with acute limb ischemia of less than 7 days' duration were randomized to either thrombolytic therapy or operative reconstruction. Patients with embolic and thrombotic occlusion, native arterial and bypass graft occlusion, and autogenous bypass graft or prosthetic graft occlusion were included. Patients were excluded if they had a contraindication to either thrombolytic therapy or operative revascularization, if the extremity was thought to be nonfunctional prior to the ischemic event, or if irreversible ischemia was present.

Patients randomized to receive intraarterial lytic therapy were given UK 4000 IU/min × 2 h, 2000 IU/min × 2 h, and subsequently 1000 IU/min continuously. Aspirin, 325 mg, was given. Systemic heparin anticoagulation was not used.

Patients who were randomized to operative revascularization usually underwent diagnostic arteriography, except at the discretion of the attending surgeon. Operation was performed as soon as feasible in each patient.

Endpoints. Amputation-free survival to 1 year.

Results. Randomization was equal in both groups (57 per group). The ratio of patients suffering thrombotic occlusion compared with embolic occlusion was 79:21. Native arterial occlusion occurred in 45%, while 55% had occluded bypass grafts.

Arteriographically successful thrombolysis was defined as greater than 80% thrombus resolution and was achieved in 70% (40 of 57) of the patients randomized to the thrombolytic arm. The mean duration of UK infusion was 36 h. A defect responsible for either arterial or bypass graft occlusion was identified in only 37% (21 of 57) of

TABLE 16-6. Long-Term Results of a Prospective, Randomized Study
of Catheter-Directed Thrombolysis versus Surgery for Acute Limb Ischemia: Results

	Thrombolysis	Surgery	p Value
Early results			
Initial revascularization	70% (40/57)	NA	
Primary amputation	4% (2/57)	5% (3/57)	NS
In-hospital mortality	14% (8/57)	18% (10/57)	NS
Major amputation	11% (6/57)	12% (7/57)	NS
Major bleeding	9% (5/57)	2% (1/57)	0.09
Length of stay (median)	11 days	11 days	NS
Cost of care	$15,672	$12,253	NS
Long-Term Results (1 year)			
Event-free survival	75%	52%	0.03
Mortality	16%	42%	0.02
Amputation	18%	20%	NS

the patients, and each underwent correction of the lesion either by percutaneous balloon dilation (2 patients) or operative revision (19 patients). We do not know how many of the successfully treated patients had embolic occlusion or thrombotic occlusion. It is our impression that acute emboli lyse much more rapidly and completely than thrombosed arteries. Thirty-three percent (19 of 57) had no anatomic defect found and had systemic anticoagulation with heparin which was converted to long-term oral anticoagulation. In the 30% with unsuccessful thrombolysis (17 patients), 15 subsequently underwent operative revascularization, and 2 patients had primary amputation. The early and long-term results (1 year) are summarized in Table 16-6.

Discussion

The results of this single-center study indicate that patients with acute peripheral arterial occlusion have a significant benefit of "event-free survival for 1 year with intraarterial UK." *Event-free survival* is defined as patients who survive without a major amputation. The difference in outcome favoring thrombolysis was due to a reduction in mortality in the UK-treated patients rather than improvement in limb salvage. Both groups had similar 12-month amputation rates; however, the 1-year mortality of patients receiving thrombolytic therapy was significantly better compared

with those randomized to operative therapy. This was not a primary endpoint of the study; however, it was an interesting observation. A similar and unexpected observation was made in the prospective, randomized trial of intraoperative UK infusion[52] (see Chap. 20). Table 16-7 reviews the mortality reduction associated with intraarterial UK infusion in these two prospective, randomized trials. These data appear to justify a prospective clinical trial designed to evaluate whether this survival benefit is real in patients with advanced arterial occlusive disease.

Catheter-directed UK infusion eliminated the need for operative intervention in approximately one-third of patients presenting with acute limb ischemia, many of whom had acute embolic occlusion. This benefit was achieved without in-

TABLE 16-7. Mortality Reduction Associated
with Intraarterial Urokinase in Two Prospective,
Randomized Studies

Author	No. of Patients	Method	Mortality*
Ouriel (ref. 51)	114	Percutaneous catheter-directed	16% vs 42% $p \leq 0.02$
Comerota et al. (ref. 52)	134	Intraoperative	2% vs 12% $p = 0.034$

* Incidental observation, not a primary endpoint.

crements in length of hospital stay at a cost of approximately $3400 per patient. Whether this benefit would be observed equally in all patients with nonembolic limb ischemia is being evaluated by other trials.

These preliminary results indicate that catheter-directed thrombolysis appears justified in patients with acute limb-threatening ischemia who have no contraindications to thrombolytic agents. Unfortunately, patency rates and limb-salvage rates are not different from surgery, but the mortality benefit observed is an intriguing observation.

Surgery versus Thrombolysis for the Ischemic Lower Extremity: The STILE Study[51]

Purpose. The purpose of this study was to evaluate the role of catheter-directed thrombolysis compared with routine operative revascularization in the management of nonembolic lower extremity ischemia.

Design. This was a prospective trial, randomizing patients with nonembolic lower extremity ischemia who had progression of ischemic symptoms within 6 months. It was designed as an "all-inclusive" study of patients with nonembolic limb ischemia. Randomization followed angiographic documentation of obstruction of either a native artery or a bypass graft. Patients were randomized to either rt-PA infusion (0.05 mg/kg/h) or UK infusion (4000 IU/min × 4h, followed by 2000 IU/min for up to 36 h) versus operative intervention. The randomization ratio was 2:1:2 respectively, with approximately 1000 patients projected for entry into the study (Fig. 16-12).

Endpoints. The primary endpoint was a composite clinical outcome consisting of death, amputation, ongoing or recurrent ischemia, and defined major morbidity. The defined major morbidity included major hemorrhage, perioperative complications, renal failure, anesthesia complications, vascular complications, and postintervention wound complications.

FIGURE 16-12. *Algorithm of the STILE study design (surgery versus thrombolysis for ischemia of the lower extremity).*

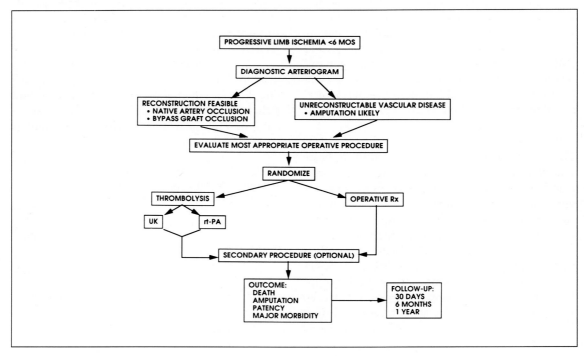

Results. Randomization was stopped and the study terminated after the first interim analysis, which occurred after 393 patients were randomized. The O'Brien-Flemming boundary rule was applied and indicated that the primary conclusions would not change if patient entry continued to the target of 1000. The primary conclusion was that lower limb ischemia was treated more effectively with operative revascularization compared with catheter-directed thrombolysis (Table 16-8).

Among the patients randomized, 68% were male and 32% female, with 68% native arterial and 32% bypass graft occlusion. Rest pain was present in 56% and ulceration or tissue necrosis in 33%.

Catheter placement was not achieved in 28% randomized to lysis (40% with graft occlusion and 21% with native arterial occlusion). Although significant outcome differences were observed between the surgery and thrombolysis groups, results with rt-PA and UK were similar. Recurrent and ongoing ischemia strongly predicted additional morbidity ($p < 0.001$). When delivered, lysis was more successful for restoring patency to bypass grafts compared with native arteries (81% versus 69% p = N.S.) and reduced the need for or magnitude of a subsequent surgical procedure ($p < 0.001$).

The outcome was stratified by duration of ischemia (Fig. 16-13). Acutely ischemic patients were defined as those who were treated within 14 days of worsening ischemia, whereas chronically ischemic patients were defined as those who were treated more than 14 days after their symptoms worsened. There was no difference in overall composite clinical outcome in patients with acute ischemia (0–14 days); however, operated patients had significantly more limb loss (18%) than patients treated with catheter-directed thrombolysis (6%) p = 0.052. In the group of acutely ischemic patients, there was a high rate of ongoing/recurrent ischemia in both the surgical and thrombolysis groups, 39% and 49% respectively (p = N.S.). On the other hand, in the patients with more chronic ischemia, operative revascularization had significantly less ongoing/recurrent ischemia (20% versus 58% $p < 0.001$) and a trend toward a reduction in major amputation.

Six month follow-up was reported for the major endpoints of death and amputation. Interestingly, there was no difference between overall data comparing the two treatment groups. However, when the treatment strategies were stratified by duration of ischemia, once again differences were observed. In the more acutely ischemic patients, there was significantly better amputation-free survival in patients treated with catheter-directed thrombolysis, due predominantly to a

TABLE 16-8. *30-Day Results of Surgery versus Thrombolysis for the Ischemic Lower Extremity: The STILE Trial*

Stratum	Event	Surgery (n = 144)	Lysis (n = 248)	p Value
Overall (n = 392)	Composite clinical outcome	36%	61%	< 0.001
	Death	5%	4%	0.698
	Amputation	6%	5%	0.673
	Ongoing/recurrent ischemia	26%	53%	< 0.001
	Major morbidity	15%	20%	0.229
Native artery (n = 268)	Composite clinical outcome	35%	62%	< 0.001
	Death	7%	4%	0.285
	Amputation	2%*	4%	0.364
	Ongoing/recurrent ischemia	24%	54%	< 0.001
	Major morbidity	17%	21%	0.449
Bypass graft (n = 124)	Composite clinical outcome	39%	60%	0.023
	Death	0%	4%	0.180
	Amputation	15%*	8%	0.188
	Ongoing/recurrent ischemia	30%	53%	0.017
	Major morbidity	11%	18%	0.292

* $p < 0.05$ for comparison of native artery versus bypass graft for amputation within surgical group; $p > 0.05$ for all other comparisons of native artery versus bypass graft.

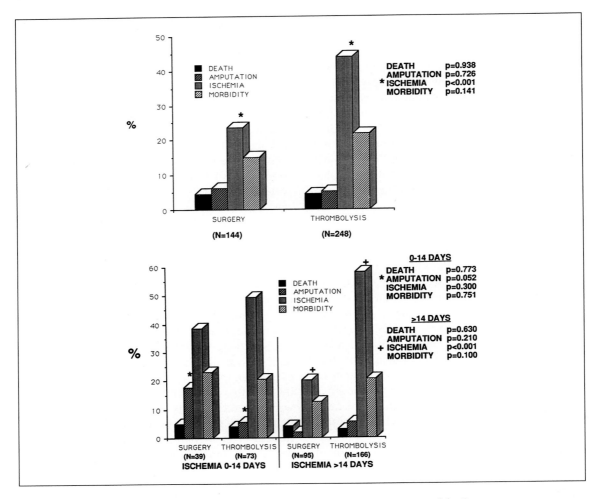

FIGURE 16-13. (A) Results of the STILE trial at 30 days, analyzed for the components of the Composite Clinical Outcome. There is significantly greater ongoing/recurrent ischemia in patients treated with thrombolysis. (B) Results of the STILE trial at 30 days stratified by duration of ischemia. Acutely ischemic patients (0–14 days) have a better outcome when treated with catheter directed thrombolysis, whereas patients with chronic ischemia (> 14 days) are more effectively treated with operative revascularization.

significant reduction in major amputation. However, surgical revascularization was more effective in chronically ischemic patients demonstrating a significantly lower amputation rate compared to those treated with catheter-directed thrombolysis. (Fig. 16-14).

Discussion

The STILE study attempted to define the role of catheter-directed thrombolysis in patients with the ischemic lower extremity. The design of the

protocol was all inclusive, in that it randomized patients with chronic limb ischemia as well as those with acute limb ischemia. However, acute embolic occlusions were excluded, since the treatment outcome and natural history of these patients is quite different from individuals with occlusive vascular disease.

Within the STILE study, there were 2.5 times as many patients with chronic limb ischemia as those with acute limb ischemia. Therefore, whatever the result in the chronic group, it would have the most impact on the primary results.

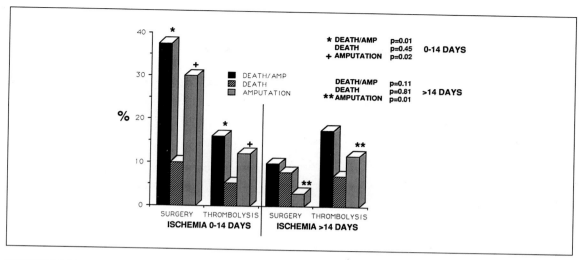

FIGURE 16-14. Bar graph of 6 month outcome by duration of ischemia. Overall results of death and amputation rates are no different between surgical and thrombolysis patients. However, stratified by duration of ischemia, there is significantly better amputation-free survival in acutely ischemic patients treated with catheter-directed thrombolysis, whereas patients with chronic limb ischemia treated surgically had significantly lower amputation rates than thrombolysis patients.

It is instructive to appreciate that ongoing/recurrent ischemia is associated with significantly more adverse events, which emphasizes the need for successful primary treatment.

The 6-month follow-up data are particularly instructive when evaluating patients who received the treatment to which they were randomized, especially in the patients in whom primary treatment failed. In acutely ischemic patients who failed surgical therapy, there was a 22% mortality and 68% major limb amputation compared to 10% and 30% respectively for patients who failed thrombolysis. In chronically ischemic patients, those who failed surgical intervention had a 17% mortality and 17% major amputation at 6 months, compared to 8% and 20% respectively for patients failing catheter-directed thrombolysis. Of course these results need to be interpreted with caution, since patients who failed catheter-directed thrombolysis can be subsequently salvaged by a surgical procedure, whereas patients who failed the best operative procedure have few other options.

On the basis of the results of the STILE study, it appears that a treatment strategy which combines catheter-directed thrombolysis for patients with acute limb ischemia with operative revascularization for patients with chronic ischemia will offer the best overall results.

Thrombolysis or Peripheral Artery Surgery: TOPAS Study [A Prospective Study Evaluating Catheter-Directed Thrombolysis with Recombinant Urokinase (r-UK) versus Operative Intervention in Patients with Acute Limb Ischemia]

The single-center, prospective, randomized study for patients with acute limb ischemia[51] has generated interest in evaluating these results as part of a multicenter trial, as well as establishing the efficacy of r-UK. Recombinant DNA technology has produced rt-PA, which has been used successfully in restoring patency in acutely occluded arteries and bypass grafts.[23–25] Currently, research has shown that UK can be produced more efficiently and with higher purity using recombinant DNA technology. In so doing, reliance on human sources for UK can be eliminated.

Purpose. The purpose of this study is to compare intraarterial r-UK versus operative interven-

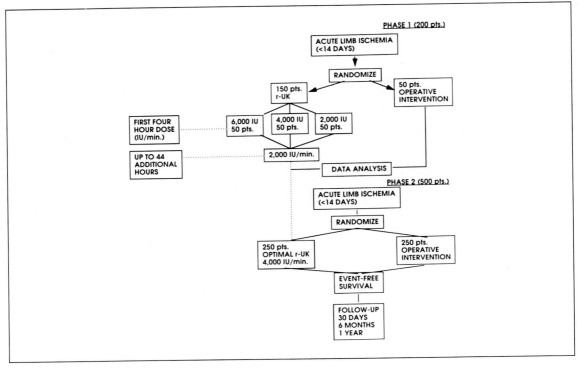

FIGURE 16-15. Algorithm of the TOPAS study design (thrombolysis or peripheral arterial surgery).

tion as the initial treatment of acute limb-threatening ischemia due to acute (< 14 days) arterial or graft thrombosis and acute embolic occlusion of the lower extremity.

Design. Seven-hundred patients will be entered into this two-phase study. The first phase was a dose-ranging study to identify the optimal r-UK dose. Two-hundred patients were entered during phase I, 50 randomized to each of three r-UK dosage regimens and 50 to surgical reconstruction. The r-UK doses tested were those used for the initial 4-h treatment, either 2000 IU/min, 4000 IU/min, or 6000 IU/min, followed by a continuous infusion of 2000 IU for up to 44 additional hours.

In phase II, 500 patients will be entered, 250 randomized to the optimal r-UK dosage regimen (4000 IU/min) and 250 randomized to surgical reconstruction.

Patients who present with acute lower limb ischemia of less than 14 days' duration are eligible for randomization. Following angiographically demonstrated occlusion of a lower extremity artery or bypass graft, patients will be randomized to either catheter-directed r-UK or operative intervention (Fig. 16-15).

Endpoints. The primary endpoint of the study is amputation-free survival at 6 months. Other secondary endpoints include a composite in-hospital adverse outcome index composed of ongoing/recurrent ischemia, major hemorrhage, operative complications, vascular complications, etc. All patients will be followed for a period of 1 year.

While the study is ongoing, the preliminary results indicate that demographic distribution of patients is similar in the operated group compared with the r-UK group. Although the results are preliminary and the analysis incomplete, there is an outcome trend similar to the STILE study, with more major hemorrhagic complications with r-UK, a slightly higher mortality in the surgical patients, and a higher amputation rate in r-UK patients.

Following complete analysis of these prospective, randomized trials, subgroups of patients will be identified who undoubtedly will benefit from catheter-directed thrombolysis. Likewise, subgroups will be identified in whom operative revascularization offers the most effective short- and long-term benefit. Such selection information is vital to optimal outcome, since substantial morbidity and mortality are associated with failure of revascularization.

REFERENCES

1. Alkjaersig N, Fletcher AP, Sherry S. The mechanism of clot dissolution of plasmin. J Clin Invest 1959;38:1086.
2. McNicol GP, Reid W, Bain WH, Douglas AS. Treatment of peripheral arterial occlusion by streptokinase perfusion. Br Med J 1963;1:1508.
3. Dotter CT, Rosch J, Seamen AJ. Selective clot lysis with low dose streptokinase. Radiology 1974;111:31.
4. Katzen BT, van Breda A. Low dose streptokinase in the treatment of arterial occlusions. AJR 1981;36:1171.
5. Totty WG, Gilula LA, McClennan BL, et al. Low dose intravascular fibrinolytic therapy. Radiology 1982;143:59.
6. Berni GA, Bandyk DF, Zierler E, et al. Streptokinase treatment of acute arterial occlusion. Ann Surg 1983;198:185.
7. Mori KW, Bookstein JJ, Heeney DJ, et al. Selective streptokinase infusion: clinical and laboratory correlates. Radiology 1983;148:677.
8. Becker GJ, Rabe FE, Richmond BD, et al. Low dose fibrinolytic therapy: results and new concepts. Radiology 1983;148:663.
9. Katzen BT, Edwards KC, Albert AS, et al. Low dose fibrinolysis in peripheral vascular disease. J Vasc Surg 1984;1:718.
10. Wolfson RH, Kumpe DA, Rutherford RB. Role of intraarterial streptokinase in the treatment of arterial thromboembolism. Arch Surg 1984;119:697.
11. van Breda A, Robinson JC, Feldman L, et al. Local thrombolysis in the treatment of arterial graft occlusion. J Vasc Surg 1984;1:103.
12. Kakkasseril JS, Cranley JJ, Arbaugh JJ, et al. Efficacy of low dose streptokinase in acute arterial occlusion and graft thrombosis. Arch Surg 1985;120:427.
13. Graor RA, Risius B, Denny KD, et al. Local thrombolysis in the treatment of thrombosed arteries: bypass grafts and arteriovenous fistulae. J Vasc Surg 1985;2:406.
14. Fong H, Downs A, Lye C, Morrow I. Low dose intra-arterial streptokinase infusion therapy of peripheral arterial occlusions and occluded vein grafts. Can J Surg 1986;29(4):259.
15. van Breda A, Katzen BT, Deutsch AF. Urokinase vs streptokinase in local thrombolysis. Radiology 1987;165:109.
16. Koltun WA, Gardiner GA, Harrington DP, et al. Thrombolysis in the treatment of peripheral arterial vascular occlusions. Arch Surg 1987;122:901.
17. Belkin M, Belkin B, Buckman CA, et al. Intra-arterial fibrinolytic therapy: efficacy of streptokinase vs urokinase. Arch Surg 1986;121:7659.
18. Gardiner GA, Harrington DP, Koltun W, et al. Salvage of occluded bypass grafts by means of thrombolysis. J Vasc Surg 1989;9:426.
19. Traughber PD, Cook PS, Micklos TJ, Miller FJ. Intraarterial fibrinolytic therapy for popliteal and tibial artery obstruction: comparison of streptokinase and urokinase. AJR 1987;149:453.
20. Price C, Jacocks MA, Tytle T. Thrombolytic therapy in acute arterial thrombosis. Am J Surg 1988;156:488.
21. O'Donnell TF, Coleman JC, Sentissi J, et al. Comparison of direct intraarterial streptokinase to urokinase infusion in the management of failed infrainguinal e-PTFE grafts. Symposium: medical and surgical management of peripheral vascular disease, Colorado Springs, Colorado, April 20–22, 1990.
22. McNamara TA, Fischer FR. Thrombolysis of peripheral arterial and graft occlusions: improved results using high dose urokinase. AJR 1985;144:769.
23. Myerovitz MR, Goldhaber SZ, Reagan K, et al. Recombinant tissue-type plasminogen activator versus urokinase in peripheral arterial and graft occlusions: a randomized trial. Radiology 1990;175:75.
24. Graor RA, Risius B, Lucas FV, et al. Thrombolysis with recombinant human tissue-type plasminogen activators in patients with peripheral artery and bypass thrombosis. Circulation 1986;74(suppl I):115.
25. Verstraete M, Hess H, Mahler F, et al. Femoropopliteal artery thrombolysis with intraarterial infusion of recombinant tissue-type plasminogen activator report of a pilot trial. Eur J Vasc Surg 1988;2:155.
26. van Breda A, Katzen BT. Radiologic aspects of intra-arterial thrombolytic therapy. In: Comerota AJ, ed. Thrombolytic therapy. Orlando: Grune & Stratton, 1988:99.
27. Comerota AJ. Urokinase. In: Messerli FH, ed. Cardiovascular drug therapy. Philadelphia: WB Saunders, 1990:1470.
28. Belkin M, Donaldson MC, Wittemore AD, et al. Observations on the use of thrombolytic agents for

thrombotic occlusion of infrainguinal vein grafts. J Vasc Surg 1990;11:289.

29. Sicard G, Schier JJ, Totty WG, et al. Thrombolytic therapy for acute arterial occlusion. J Vasc Surg 1985;2:65.

30. McNamara TO, Bomberger RA. Factors affecting initial and six month patency rates after intraarterial thrombolysis with high dose urokinase. Am J Surg 1986;152:709.

31. Graor RA, Risius B, Young JR, et al. Peripheral artery and bypass graft thrombolysis with recombinant human tissue-type plasminogen activator. J Vasc Surg 1986;3:115.

32. Comerota AJ, Rubin R, Tyson R, et al. Intraarterial thrombolytic therapy in peripheral vascular disease. Surg Gynecol Obstet 1987;165:1.

33. Graor RA, Risius B, Young JR, et al. Thrombolysis of peripheral arterial bypass grafts: surgical thrombectomy compared with thrombolysis. J Vasc Surg 1988;7:347.

34. de Bono DP, Pringle S, Underwood I. Differential effects of aprotinin and tranexamic acid on cerebral bleeding and cutaneous bleeding time during rt-PA infusion. Thromb Res 1991;61:159.

35. Bandyk DF, Bergamini TM, Towne JB, et al. Durability of vein graft revisions: the outcome of secondary procedures. J Vasc Surg 1991;13:200.

36. Perler BA, Osterman FA, Mitchell SE, et al. Balloon dilation versus surgical revision of infra-inguinal autogenous vein graft stenoses: long-term follow-up. J Cardiovasc Surg 1990;31(5):656.

37. Cohen FR, Mannick JA, Couch NP, Whittemore AD. Recognition and management of impending vein-graft failure. Arch Surg 1986;121:758.

38. Sullivan KL, Gardiner GA, Kandarpa K, et al. Efficacy of thrombolysis in infrainguinal bypass grafts. Circulation 1991;83(suppl I):I-99.

39. McNamara TA, Bomberger RA, Merchant RF. Intraarterial urokinase as the initial therapy for acutely ischemic lower limbs. Circulation 1991;83 (suppl I):I-106.

40. Whittemore AD, Donaldson MC, Mannick JA. Detection and treatment of hypercoagulable states: can they improve infrainguinal bypass results: In: Veith FJ, ed. Current critical problems in vascular surgery. Vol 3. St Louis: Quality Medical Publishing, 1991:81.

41. Comerota AJ. Complications with systemic and localized fibrinolytic therapy. In: Bernhard VM, Towne JB, eds. Complications in vascular surgery. Orlando: Grune & Stratton, 1985:421.

42. Goldhaber SZ, Kessler CM, Heit J, et al. A randomized, controlled trial of recombinant tissue plasminogen activator versus urokinase in the treatment of pulmonary embolism. Lancet 1988;2:293.

43. deBono DP, More RS. Prevention and management of bleeding complications after thrombolysis. Int J Cardiol 1993;38:1.

44. Marder VJ. The use of thrombolytic agents: choice of patient, drug administration, laboratory monitoring. Ann Intern Med 1973;90:802.

45. Ranjadayalan K, Stevenson R, Marchant B, et al. Streptokinase-induced defibrination assessed by thrombin time: effects on residual coronary stenosis and left ventricular ejection fraction. Br Hear J 1992;68:171.

46. Sharp RA, Forbes CD. Congenital coagulation disorders. In: Ludlam CA, ed. Clinical haemotology. Edinburgh: Churchill Livingstone, 1990:351.

47. Coller BS. Platelets and thrombolytic therapy. N Engl J Med 1990;322:33.

48. Rudd MA, Amarante P, Smick D, et al. Temporal effects of tissue plasminogen activator infusion on platelet aggregation ex vivo (abstract). Blood 1988;78(suppl I):374A.

49. Hargrove WC, Barker CF, Berkowitz HD, et al. Treatment of acute peripheral arterial and graft thromboses with low-dose streptokinase. Surgery 1982;92:981.

50. Rabe FE, Becker GJ, Richmond BD, et al. Contrast extravasation through Dacron grafts: a sequela of low-dose streptokinase therapy. AJR 1982;138:917.

51. The STILE Investigators. Results of a prospective trial of surgery vs thrombolysis for the ischemic lower extremity: the STILE trial. Ann Surg (in press).

52. Ouriel K. Comparison of results: surgery, PTA and thrombolysis. In: Proceedings: thrombolytic therapy in the management of vascular disease, Los Angeles, October 2, 1993.

53. Comerota AJ, Rao AK, Throm RC, et al. A prospective, randomized, blinded and placebo-controlled trial of intraoperative urokinase infusion during lower extremity revascularization: regional and systemic effects. Ann Surg 1993;218(4):534.

17

Thrombolysis as the Initial Treatment for Acute Lower Limb Ischemia

Thomas O. McNamara

Despite over 80 years of experience with various methods of treating acute lower limb ischemia (ALLI), the reported mortality continues to be in the 10% to 30% range, as does the incidence of amputation in the survivors.[1-4] As would be expected, these results have prompted recurrent proposals for change in the method of treatment.

Background

The initial form of interventional treatment was that of direct embolectomy. It was reportedly first performed by Labey in 1911.[5] This gradually caught on, but the results plus the morbidity restricted the use to a minority of patients with ALLI. The location and extent of the occlusion required that, in many instances, either abdominal laparotomy or extensive leg dissection be performed to remove all the occluding clot. The more extensive surgery was associated with higher morbidity. Several modifications were then developed to try to minimize the extent of surgical incisions, and they were applied primarily to leg occlusions. The first was retrograde flushing, introduced in 1930, as an attempt to force distal clot proximally to facilitate removal from a femoral arteriotomy.[6] Thus only two short incisions were required. Another attempt to further minimize surgical incisions was described in 1951. This utilized rubberized bandages to produce retrograde milking of distal clot, either propagated thrombus or embolus fragments, to facilitate removal through a proximal arteriotomy.[7] A corkscrew-type wire was developed by Shaw in 1960 and utilized to retrieve clot distal to the arteriotomy.[8] A special vein stripper with an olive-shaped head was described by Oeconomus in 1961.[9] This also was introduced in the femoral region and advanced through distal occlusions to try to pull that clot back to the arteriotomy.

None of these techniques was particularly effective in addressing iliac occlusions. They also were not uniformly successful in removing all the clot distal to a femoral arteriotomy.

OPERATIVE THROMBOEMBOLECTOMY

The Fogarty balloon-tip catheter, introduced in 1963, represented a significant advance over the previous devices and techniques.[10] In addition to being able to be introduced at the femoral artery site with a minimum of surgical exposure, the device was soft, thin, and relatively atraumatic, and the tip could be inflated to varying diameters in an attempt to match the changing diameters of the vessel segments during withdrawal. The device could be modified to reach and extract clot as far proximally as the aortoiliac junction and as far distal as the pedal vessels. The procedure could be performed under local anesthesia. These features markedly decreased the extent and severity of surgery for ALLI. Theoretically, the combination of these features would be expected to be associated with less surgical "stress" to the patient, reduced anesthesia risk, less operative morbidity, more complete clot removal, and lower perioperative mortality than experienced with direct embolectomy. The initial reports contained excellent results, and the procedure quickly became the procedure of choice for ALLI.[11,12] The acceptance of and enthusiasm for this procedure/catheter are exemplified by Thompson's description of it in 1974 as the "single most important advance in the management of embolism in the last decade."[13] Surgical treatment of ALLI increased significantly following the introduction of the Fogarty procedure/catheter.[14]

The efficacy of this new "gold standard"— emergency performance of thromboembolectomy with the Fogarty catheter—for the treatment of ALLI was challenged in 1978 by Blaisdell et al.[4] They reviewed the published results of 3345 patients who had undergone such treatment of ALLI since introduction of the Fogarty procedure/catheter in 1963. The review yielded a cumulative mortality rate of approximately 25% and a 30% amputation rate in the survivors. These investigators stressed the high mortality rate and developed an alternative treatment algorithm to reduce it.

They proposed that patients with ALLI receive massive doses of heparin rather than emergency surgery. If the limb ischemia subsided during the ensuing days, heparinization was continued until the improvement seemed to stabilize, and then the patient underwent reconstructive surgery. If, on the other hand, the limb deteriorated, primary amputation was performed.

In their experience, this algorithm yielded a substantially lower mortality rate without an attendant higher amputation rate. They postulated that this reduction in mortality was partly due to better preparation of these patients prior to the "stress" of surgery.

Similar reports from widely separate institutions appeared at approximately the same time.[15-22] These articles also reported mortality rates of 15% to 20% associated with emergency thromboembolectomy for ALLI, "even higher for aortoiliac or aortic bifurcation occlusions," and amputation rates of 3% to 25% in the survivors. These studies confirmed the earlier observation by Blaisdell and associates that the risk of death was much higher after emergency surgery for ALLI than after elective revascularization surgery for chronically ischemic limbs (3% to 4%).[23]

It was thought by some that this surprisingly high mortality rate reflected the extension of surgical treatment for ALLI to patients who would not have been considered candidates for surgery prior to the availability of the Fogarty technique/catheter. Support for this hypothesis was provided by Abbott et al. in 1982.[14] They reviewed the type and results of treatment of ALLI at the Massachusetts General Hospital over a 44-year period (1937–1981). They noted that during the period 1937–1964, only 23% of patients with emboli to the upper or lower extremity had undergone surgical treatment. In contrast, during the period 1964–1981, after introduction of the Fogarty procedure/catheter, 88% had undergone embolectomy.

In addition to confirming the marked increase in the use of surgery for acute upper and lower limb ischemia, they demonstrated a lack of significant improvement in both mortality and amputation rates despite the use of this presumably safer and more effective method of treatment. They documented that through the 44-year period, the limb-salvage rate after surgical treatment in 498 patients was 83% versus 77% in the

235 patients treated conservatively. They also noted, however, that the surgical limb-salvage rates after introduction of the Fogarty procedure/catheter were not significantly improved: 83% after versus 82% prior. The mortality rate decreased only 5%, from 24% to 19%.

Most of the decrease in mortality was associated with the surgical treatment of arm emboli, a decrease from 21% to 6%. The mortality rate associated with surgical treatment of ALLI remained at approximately 20% despite the extensive use of the Fogarty procedure/catheter after 1963.

The authors postulated that the lack of change in limb-salvage rates and the lack of a marked decrease in mortality rates after introduction of the Fogarty procedure/catheter were due to extension of the procedure to patients of more advanced age or more extensive underlying vascular disease or with more severe ischemia or more advanced associated coronary disease than would have undergone surgery prior to introduction of the procedure/device. An explanation was not offered to account for the improvement in results of treating the upper extremity in contrast to the lack of similar improvement in results for treating ALLI. This author would explain that difference as due to the Fogarty procedure/catheter being most efficacious when used to extract clot from an otherwise normal vascular tree. The arteries in the upper extremity are usually free of underlying atherosclerotic disease, and acute arm occlusions are almost invariably due to emboli. In contrast, the arteries in the lower extremities are frequently diseased and narrowed by diffuse atherosclerotic disease. Additionally, acute occlusions in the lower extremity are most commonly due to spontaneous thrombosis rather than to emboli. The Fogarty procedure/catheter can remove much of this fresh thrombus from the main vessels, but it does not clear the underlying flow-limiting atherosclerotic lesions. Furthermore, use of the device may cause spasm, intimal tearing, and intimal flaps and make the system thrombogenic without making it free of flow-limiting lesions. Thus reocclusions, repeated operations, limb loss, and recurrent "stress" to the patient with associated risk of cardiac failure or myocardial infarction can occur despite initially successful restoration of flow with balloon catheter thromboembolectomy.

EMBOLIC VERSUS THROMBOTIC OCCLUSION

These reports prompted some, including Fogarty, to suggest that the best application of the procedure/catheter for emergency clot removal was in relatively normal vessels occluded by an acute embolus that might also have an associated distal secondary thrombus.[24] It was advised that use of the procedure/catheter for thrombectomy, as opposed to embolectomy, could result in "blind endarterectomy" in an atherosclerotic vessel, and despite successful removal of clot, one could expect more complications than when using the procedure/catheter in a relatively normal vessel that was acutely occluded with an embolus. Fogarty described the possible complications associated with the use of his procedure/catheter in thrombosed atherosclerotic vessels as including perforation, dissection, arterial rupture, plaque avulsion, intimal damage, and retention of a broken catheter part.[25,26]

In accord with these concepts, McPhail et al.[27] reported improved results by performing emergency clot extraction surgery only on embolic occlusions, while utilizing Blaisdell's approach of immediate high-dose heparinization and delayed surgery for thrombotic occlusions in atherosclerotic vessels.[27] This approach supported Fogarty's contention that Blaisdell's results reflected the common, but inappropriate, use of his procedure/catheter for thrombotic occlusions rather than for only embolic occlusions. McPhail's results demonstrated that emergency embolectomy was accompanied by an 8.7% mortality and 7.5% amputation rate. This was considerably better than the results reported in series in which emergency surgery had been performed on both embolic and thrombotic occlusions without an effort to discriminate between the etiologies. McPhail's experience with delayed surgery for thrombotic occlusions yielded a mortality rate of 12% and an amputation rate of 22%, which approximated the results reported by others, in which both acute embolic and thrombotic occlusions were treated with emergency clot extraction. To differentiate between embolic versus thrombotic occlusions, McPhail utilized the criteria suggested by Fogarty.[24,26] These consisted of a history of atrial fibrillation and/or the absence of antecedent claudication and the presence of normal pulses in the unaffected limb to indicate that the occlusion was embolic in etiology. Fogarty stated that these criteria could enable accurate differentiation between embolic and thrombotic occlusions in 85% of cases.

In response to this suggestion, Blaisdell et al.[4] have countered that such clinical differentiation is more difficult than stated by Fogarty. Cambria and Abbott[28] have stated that atrial fibrillation is the only reliable clinical predictor of an embolic etiology.

One of the few analyses of the accuracy of clinically diagnosing an embolic etiology for ALLI was published in 1986 by Jivegard et al.[3] They had the policy of performing acute clot extraction for ALLI only in those patients with a clinical diagnosis of acute embolism. In a series of 122 patients, they experienced a misdiagnosis rate of 29%.

They also confirmed the previously reported poor results with use of the Fogarty procedure/catheter to remove spontaneous in situ thrombosis superimposed on atherosclerosis. In the 29% of their patients with ALLI due to thrombosis, they experienced a 50% surgical failure rate versus 13% for the true embolic occlusions. One-half the surgical failures in the thrombotic group involved the development of gangrene, with many patients dying of sepsis, versus only a 14% incidence of gangrene in the failed embolic group. The thrombotic occlusion group experienced a 30-day mortality rate of 27% and a 50% amputation rate in the survivors as opposed to a 25% mortality and a 6% amputation rate in those correctly diagnosed as having an embolic occlusion.

It is worth pointing out that the diagnosis of an embolic versus a thrombotic etiology was made solely on clinical grounds rather than with the aid of arteriography. It is this author's experience that the additional information provided with arteriography can significantly improve one's ability to differentiate between embolism and spontaneous in situ thrombosis.

One of the earliest published reports of the value of preoperative arteriography in patients with ALLI was by Haimovici et al. in 1975.[29] They recommended it because they had found it to be valuable both in treatment planning and as an aid to prognosis. They noted that the demonstration of associated significant atherosclerotic disease predicted a markedly poorer outcome. This confirmed the experience of Freund et al.,[30] who had reported a 52% mortality in ALLI patients with underlying atherosclerosis versus 18% in those without.

These results, as well as the previously cited results, continue to indicate that the most efficacious application of the Fogarty procedure/catheter is for removal of acute embolus from relatively disease-free vessels. To date, the best results for limb salvage are with embolectomy, reported by Fogarty to be 95%.[31] Even in his series, however, this continues to be associated with a substantial mortality (16%).

Thus it is not surprising that further revision of the surgical algorithm continues to take place. In 1986, Jivegard et al.[3] partially refuted the dismal results reported by Blaisdell and suggested including primary reconstructive surgery as a treatment option for the patient with ALLI. They had reviewed the surgical literature from 1978 to 1984, which included reports of 2495 cases of ALLI treated with emergency thromboembolectomy. This yielded a cumulative 30-day mortality rate of 18% and an amputation rate of 16% in the survivors. This contrasted with the 30-day mortality rate of 25% and amputation rate of 30% in the survivors reported by Blaisdell et al.[4] in a review of earlier reports. The Jivegard report bolstered the view of those who believed that the results reported by Blaisdell et al. reflected outmoded surgical and postoperative treatment. Jivegard et al. also proposed that the results could be further improved by delaying surgery, if necessary, so that the surgeon could be the one to perform reconstructive surgery if the simpler restorative (thromboembolectomy) approach failed. This was controversial in that it raised the concern that both delay and the application of more extensive surgery in this group of patients, with an already high mortality rate, would yield even higher mortality and amputation rates.

Jivegard's suggestion was based, in part, on the already published experience of Field et al.[32] (1982), who reported their experience with 61 patients with ALLI who underwent delayed surgery an average of 37 h after the onset of symptoms. In 18 patients (30%), restorative surgical attempts (thromboembolectomy) had failed. This led them to perform reconstructive surgery immediately. Although the reconstructive surgery was not always successful, it was not associated with a rise in the mortality rate. They cited a 14% mortality rate and 12% amputation rate in those undergoing only thromboembolectomy versus 0% and 12% in the 18 patients who were treated with additional reconstructive surgery.

This trend toward increased utilization of reconstructive surgery for ALLI has resulted in one group using this as their preferred approach. In 1992, Yeager et al.[1] reported the use of reconstructive surgery in 84% of 74 patients with ALLI. They utilized thrombectomy or embolectomy in only 12%. This was based in part on their assessment that only 8% of the occlusions were due to emboli. Although they recommend this more aggressive approach, it is noteworthy that it was associated with a 30-day mortality rate of 15% (8% due to myocardial infarction, 7% due to cancer) and a major amputation rate of 30% in the survivors.

In addition to the ongoing controversy regarding the type of surgical procedure, there is lack of agreement regarding the timing. In contrast to Blaisdell's recommendation against immediate surgery, most investigators have stressed the importance of operating as early as possible for ALLI. In a 1933 review of the early experience with direct embolectomy, Pearse[33] reported on a series of 282 cases collected from the literature; when embolectomy was performed within 10 h, the limb was saved in 40% of these patients; after 10 to 15 h, in only 16%; and after 30 h, in none. Similar statistics were reported by others.[34–37] In 1941, Linton[38] demonstrated that this phenomenon was due to persistent occlusion by distal thrombus despite successful proximal embolectomy. He postulated that the distal vessels were protected from secondary thrombosis and clot propagation by an initial reflex of vasospasm which would last approximately 6 h. Conse-

quently, he urged that direct embolectomy be performed within 6 h of the onset of occlusion.

Early reports suggested that mortality rates also rise with an increasing interval between the onset of ischemia and successful surgical treatment. In 1963, Sterling et al.[39] demonstrated a mortality rate of 19% in patients treated within 6 h of onset of ischemia versus 67% in those treated 24 h or more following onset of ischemia. A similar pattern of increasing incidence of both mortality and amputation with increasing lapse of time from onset of symptoms to successful restoration of flow has been reported with the use of the Fogarty technique/catheter.[14,40]

Despite this well-established trend, these and other studies have determined that duration of symptoms alone should not be used as a criterion to exclude patients from either direct or indirect thromboembolectomy.[14,39,40] Field et al.,[32] Fogarty,[31] and Spencer and Eisman[41] all cite excellent results after delayed embolectomy for occlusions up to 90 days in duration. Jivegard et al.[2] found that thromboembolectomies performed in the time period of 13 to 24 h after the onset of ALLI carried the greatest risk of mortality (48%), a threefold greater risk than when surgery was performed within 3 or beyond 72 h after the onset of ischemia.

ARTERIOGRAPHY FOR ACUTE LIMB ISCHEMIA

These paradoxical observations probably reflect the varying degrees of collateral blood flow and patency of distal vessels. This was suggested by early investigators, who speculated that their success with late embolectomies was due to adequate collateral flow despite the presence of pain, pallor, and decreased sensorimotor function.[14,31,39,41,42] Arteriography would have been expected to clarify the issue and aid in treatment planning; however, it was invariably not performed because of concern that the attendant delay would prejudice a good surgical outcome.

In the absence of arteriographic definition of the location and extent of the occlusive process, surgeons have had to rely on physical findings. These have the disadvantage of being subjective, as is evidenced by the following terms used to identify limbs with a poor likelihood of success for revascularization: *early rigor, stiff joints,* and *extreme tenderness of the muscles*[43] and the proximal extension of skin discoloration to involve the thigh.[4,44] The question of patency of the collateral and distal vessels was answered indirectly by the operative finding of back bleeding following thromboembolectomy.[3,38] It is this author's belief that a good deal of the confusion regarding the duration of the so-called grace period stems from reliance on physical findings rather than on arteriographic demonstration of the presence and quality of collateral flow and the degree of patency of distal vessels.

The author and associates have demonstrated a very strong correlation between the angiographic pattern of occlusion, the clinical degree of ischemia, and the ultimate outcome.[45,46] We performed a retrospective analysis of 72 cases of ALLI in which the angiographic pattern of vascular occlusion(s) and the clinical degree of ischemia, as described by the Ad Hoc Committee on Reporting Standards of the Society for Vascular Surgery (North American Chapter) and the International Society for Cardiovascular Surgery, were correlated.[47] The results demonstrated a very strong correlation, as shown in Table 17-1. For inclusion in the study, the patients had to have had ischemia for less than 7 days and persistent pallor, pulselessness (pedal), and coolness. We found that the angiographic findings could be divided into three separate patterns of occlusion (I to III).

Angiographic occlusion category I consisted of a single-segment occlusion with normal inflow, normal collaterals, and patent vessels distal to the occlusion. These patients all had normal sensorimotor function despite persistent pallor, pulselessness, and coolness. They also had an audible Doppler signal in a pedal vessel. Angiographic pattern I corresponded with the viable clinical classification of ischemia, as suggested by the ad hoc committee referred to earlier, chaired by Dr. Robert Rutherford.[45–47]

Angiographic occlusion category II most commonly consisted of tandem occlusions of contiguous vascular segments such as the superficial femoral and popliteal arteries but normal inflow, normal collaterals, and at least one patent major distal vessel. Functionally equivalent flow-limiting patterns are shown in Table 17-1, but basically this category consisted of more than a single segmental occlusion with patent collaterals and distal vessel(s). In this category, in contrast to category I, the flow was required to go through two contiguous collateral beds before supplying the distal vessels, thereby encountering more resistance with consequent complete loss of pulsatility and a marked reduction of flow. This is presumably the explanation for the absence of arterial Doppler signal in the foot or ankle despite the vessels having been demonstrated to be patent on the arteriogram. All these patients had impairment of sensorimotor function. This ranged from only hypesthesia (loss of sensation to light touch) to an inability to feel anything less than vigorous

TABLE 17-1. *Correlation Between Angiographic Acute Occlusion Categories, Functionally Equivalent Patterns, and the Clinical Degree of Ischemia*

Clinical Degree of Ischemia	Angiographic Category	Occluded Segments	Status of Inflow	Status of Collateral	Distal Vessels Seen to be Patent?
Viable	I	Single	Normal	Normal	Yes
Threatened	II	Tandem	Normal	Normal	Yes
		Single	Stenotic	Normal	Yes
		Single	Normal	Stenotic	Yes
		Single	Stenotic	Stenotic	Yes
Irreversible	III	Multiple	Normal	Normal	No
		Multiple	Normal	Occluded	No*

*The lack of flow through the collateral vessels may yield a false impression of thrombus of the distal vessels.

squeezing pressure. These clinical findings were classified by Rutherford et al.[47] as "threatened."

Angiographic occlusion category III consisted of multiple occluded segments with normal inflow and absence of visualization of the distal vessels due either to thrombosis (despite the presence of patent collateral channels) or to lack of filling of the distal vessels due to occlusion of all the collaterals. This angiographic pattern correlated with the clinical findings of anesthesia and paralysis. In the SVS/ISCVS clinical classification of ischemia, these findings would result in the limb being termed as having "irreversible ischemia."[47]

PERCUTANEOUS INTRAARTERIAL THROMBOLYSIS

These angiographic patterns correlated well not only with the clinical degree of ischemia but also with the outcome of treatment with percutaneous intraarterial thrombolysis (PIAT). The results of a correlation between the outcome of PIAT and the initial angiographic occlusion pattern are shown in Table 17-2. The results demonstrated in the table are from a retrospective review of the first 72 consecutive patients treated with PIAT for ALLI.[45,46] The previously mentioned criteria for inclusion in the study (persistent pallor, pulselessness, coolness, and ischemia duration of less than 7 days) were applied to the initial 298 consecutively treated ischemic limbs. This yielded 72 applications of PIAT for ALLI. Using standard clinical and angiographic criteria, 56 of the occlu-sions were judged to be due to spontaneous in situ thrombosis within either grafts (30) or native arteries (26). The 16 occlusions that were judged to be due to embolism from a proximal source were usually in patients with a previous myocardial infarction and residual hypokinesia of a portion of the left ventricle. Only a few of the embolic occlusions were associated with atrial fibrillation.

Table 17-3 demonstrates the correlation between 30-day outcome of PIAT and the etiology (embolus versus thrombus), loci (supra- versus infrainguinal), and type of conduit (graft versus native artery) occlusion. Comparison of these tables demonstrates that the strongest correlation was between the angiographic pattern/clinical degree of ischemia and outcome.

These findings have led us to believe that the patient with intact sensorimotor function (viable), single-segmental occlusion, patent collaterals, and open distal vessels (category I) is an excellent candidate for thrombolysis with an expectation of 100% success. Unfortunately, in our experience, these represent a minority of the patients (20%).

The vast majority of patients with ALLI, 71% in our experience, present with more than one segment of occlusion (angiographic category II) and associated sensorimotor impairment ("threatened" clinical classification). Nonethe-

TABLE 17-2. Correlation Between the Initial Angiographic Category of Acute Occlusion and Outcome of PIAT

Occlusions		Outcome at 30 Days		
Angiographic Category	No.	% Patent	% Amputation	% Mortality
I	13	100	0	0
II	51	85	7.8	0
III	8	63	25	12.5

TABLE 17-3. Correlation Between Outcome of PIAT and Etiology, Loci, and Type of Occluded Conduit

Occlusions		30-Day Outcome of PIAT		
Characteristic	No.	% Patency	% Mortality	% Amputation
Etiology				
Embolus	16	94	0	0
Thrombosis	56	86	12	11
Loci				
Suprainguinal	25	84	4	8
Infrainguinal	47	85	0	8.5
Conduit				
Artery	42	88	2	7
Graft	30	80	0	10
OVERALL	72	85.9	1.6	8.5

less, these patients had patent collaterals and distal vessels. This persistence of some blood flow is felt to best account for the absence of mortality and the relatively low amputation rate of 7.8% in this group. We postulate that the ability of skeletal muscle to survive with very low blood flow, when at rest, prevents muscle necrosis while the branch and distal vessels remain open. Heparin can maintain the patency of the distal vessels while the thrombolytic agent clears the main occlusion. Furthermore, the main occlusion can be expected to be fresh clot, which should lyse promptly and completely.

The least frequent presentation (11%) was that of multiple segmental occlusions with absence of angiographic demonstration of patency of the distal vessels due either to thrombosis of those vessels or to occlusion of all the collaterals as well as the main channel (angiographic category III). These patients had anesthesia and paralysis ("irreversible" clinical classification). We were somewhat surprised that PIAT yielded a patency rate of 63% at 30 days in this group. This group, as expected, had the highest amputation rate (25%) and mortality rate (12.5%). In this group, we must fear that there is virtually no blood flow to the muscle and that necrosis will be present.

It is also noteworthy that there was a relatively strong correlation between the etiology of the occlusion and the outcome of PIAT. Specifically, the results of treating embolic occlusions were significantly better than those achieved when treating spontaneous thrombotic occlusions. Treatment of embolic occlusions yielded a 30-day patency rate of 94%, 0% amputations, and 0% mortality versus the 30-day patency of 82%, 11% amputations, and 2% mortality experienced with treating spontaneous thrombotic occlusions.

A trend toward better results was noted with treatment of arterial occlusions versus graft occlusions with respective 30-day patencies of 88% versus 80%, amputation rates of 7% versus 10%, and mortality rates of 2% versus 0%. Comparison of suprainguinal versus infrainguinal occlusions demonstrated a trend toward higher mortality in the more proximal occlusions.

Our interpretation of these analyses is that it

is the degree to which the occlusive process reduces collateral and distal flow that has the greatest effect on the presenting degree of clinical ischemia and the outcome. In the presence of open collaterals which are seen to fill the patent distal vessels, the patient and the limb appear to be able to tolerate the time required for PIAT to restore blood flow. These angiographic findings are present in categories I and II. Combining the results of PIAT for both categories I and II yielded a respectable 30-day patency of 88%, an amputation rate of 6%, and a 0% mortality rate.

These patterns of occlusion and clinical degrees of ischemia correlate with the underlying preocclusive state of the vascular tree. This is thought to account for the markedly better results of 30-day patency of 94% without associated amputations or mortality in the embolic occlusion group versus 82% 30-day patency, 11% amputation rate, and 2% mortality rate in the patients with spontaneous thrombotic occlusions. The latter are superimposed on much more extensive underlying vascular disease than the former.

Similarly, spontaneous arterial occlusions are often associated with a less extensive occlusive process (clot propagation) than is associated with occlusion of synthetic grafts. In the latter group, the graft often occludes due to the interval development of more distal disease such that when the graft clots, the thrombotic process is more likely to propagate distally through the next low-flow segment than when a diseased arterial segment occludes. In the synthetic graft situation, the main low-flow segment may well be the distal contiguous artery, but with the lack of side branches, the graft cannot form collaterals to help it maintain flow and patency despite progressive slowing of flow with progression of distal disease. Thus it thromboses simultaneously with occlusion of the distal contiguous vascular segment. However, in the case of an in situ arterial thrombosis, the occlusion occurs at the site of the low-flow lesion, and collateral blood flow protects the distal contiguous arterial segment from thrombosis unless it also contains a preocclusive lesion.

In all these instances, documentation of the extent of the occlusion and the presence of patent collaterals and distal vessels can be very useful in predicting the outcome of PIAT for ALLI. The six amputations were all in patients who had at least tandem lesions, and a higher proportion was noted in those in whom distal vessels could not be demonstrated than in those in whom they were seen to fill via collaterals (25% versus 7.8%).

In the absence of anesthesia, paralysis, occlusion of collaterals, and obliteration of distal vessels, the risk of mortality with PIAT for ALLI appears to be minimal, 0% in our experience. The presence of these findings increases the risk of both amputation and mortality. However, mortality due to systemic reperfusion syndrome is minimal in the absence of prolonged total occlusion of blood supply to a large muscle mass. Our experience matches that of Stallone et al.[44,48] in that we believe that the risk of life-threatening reperfusion complications is minimal if the ischemia is limited to the arm or to below the knee.

Both local (compartment syndrome) and systemic reperfusion complications are more likely to occur the more completely blood flow has been occluded. This statement is based on our own angiographic correlation with outcomes, as well as on clinical and experimental studies of complete vascular occlusion and limb reimplantation.[49–51] Simply put, the more completely the clotting process has occluded blood flow, the more likely and rapid is the development of lethal biochemical and coagulation products. We experienced a low incidence of compartment syndrome (4%) in our series of 72 infusions. This lower than expected incidence may have been due to the protective effect of the gradual reperfusion inherent in current PIAT methods. There is animal and clinical evidence that the slow restoration of flow over a period of hours may significantly reduce the risk of severe swelling that occurs following sudden restoration of flow at normal arterial pressure following surgical reperfusion of ischemic, skeletal, and cardiac muscle.[52–55]

An elegant animal experiment that was designed to answer the question of when distal spontaneous thrombi begin to develop in small branch and skin arteries supports our findings that these are unlikely to develop in the presence of patent collaterals and distal vessels. In 1973, Dunant and Edwards[49] performed a classic experiment to evaluate this question. They found that although small distal clots began to form after 6 h of occlusion of the canine common femoral artery and all the collateral vessels, none of these changes was noted if either the collateral or the main channel was left open despite occlusion of the other vessel for up to 24 h. Virtually every animal experiment to study local reperfusion phenomena has required that the limb or muscle group be totally devascularized.[52,56–59] The combination of these clinical and experimental findings leads us to believe that in the absence of anesthesia and paralysis, arteriography should be performed. If this demonstrates patency of collateral and distal vessels, then PIAT is an efficacious alternative therapy. Our experience suggests that it may be associated with a lower mortality rate without an associated higher amputation rate than experienced with thromboembolectomy or reconstructive surgery. Progression to either more extensive or complete occlusion can be reasonably expected to be prevented by appropriate dosages of intravenous heparin.

Prompt surgical treatment can be performed following PIAT without the expectation of untoward bleeding. Following our 72 infusions, 12 patients went on to have surgery within 24 h of cessation of thrombolytic therapy. No untoward bleeding was noted in any of them. Furthermore, successful thrombolysis promotes a successful outcome from any subsequent surgical procedure, as demonstrated by a 100% incidence of successful surgery following successful thrombolysis versus 50% successful surgical outcome following an unsuccessful PIAT.[45]

PIAT for ALLI due to spontaneous thromboses of native arteries and bypass grafts usually can be followed by one or another endovascular technique to treat the underlying flow-limiting lesion. In the event that these are not deemed appropriate, the patients can be medically stabilized and evaluated in preparation for elective surgery. Successful PIAT allows for optimal arteriographic definition of the inflow vessel, the recanalized segment, and the outflow vessels. Although arteriography can be performed in the operating room following thrombectomy, it is more optimally performed in angiographic suites. PIAT provides an alternative for the group of patients with ALLI who have consistently had the poorest results from surgical treatment. Specifically, these are patients with spontaneous in situ arterial occlusions. They have had the lowest incidences of limb salvage and the highest incidences of mortality when treated with emergency surgery.[3,4,26-28,32] Fogarty has advised against the use of his procedure/catheter for these patients, and Blaisdell and McPhail have endorsed delayed primary reconstruction. Recently, Yeager et al.[1] have recommended urgent, but not emergency, reconstructive surgery for spontaneous in situ thrombosis of arteries and grafts, but their 30-day mortality and amputation rates have been substantial (15% and 30%, respectively).

In our experience, PIAT for thrombotic ALLI has yielded better results than reported in the preceding series utilizing either restorative (thrombectomy) or reconstructive surgery. It has not proven to be a panacea, but in our treatment of 56 thrombotic occlusions, we experienced a 30-day patency of 82%, mortality of 1.8%, and amputation rate of 10.7%. The 30-day patency results were somewhat better in the native arteries (88%) as opposed to graft occlusions (80%).

In surgical series, advanced age[2,60] and/or recent myocardial infarction (RMI)[1,2,40,60] have been associated with a marked increase in mortality. Our series included 5 patients with RMI and 20 patients 75 years of age or older. None of these patients experienced myocardial infarction or death. The only death was in a patient in whom the occlusion originated at the origin of the external iliac artery and continued through the leg with obliteration of main, collateral, and all distal vessels (category III). That arteriographic pattern was associated, as expected, with anesthesia and paralysis (irreversible ischemia). Furthermore, the patient had been in that clinical status for approximately 4 days. The limb was reperfused with PIAT, but the patient died of the systemic reperfusion syndrome.[45,46]

In contrast, the mortality in surgical series is most often due to myocardial infarction rather than to systemic reperfusion. Our lower incidence of mortality is apparently due to the absence of myocardial infarctions, pulmonary embolism,

and congestive heart failure. This difference could be explained on the basis of less stress with PIAT than with surgery and attendant anesthesia. An additional factor could be the decrease in serum fibrinogen levels associated with PIAT versus the expected rise following surgery. Fibrinogen has been demonstrated to have a strong correlation with the incidence of myocardial infarction.[61] Some have suggested that elevated fibrinogen levels represent a significant independent risk factor that should be lowered in those patients who are at higher than normal risk of myocardial infarction. Patients with ALLI are at increased risk of myocardial infarction, particularly those who are elderly and those with RMI.[1,2,40,60] Thus the lowering of fibrinogen levels associated with the so-called high-dose urokinase (UK) infusion that we utilize for PIAT may have had the unexpected benefit of reducing the risk of myocardial infarction.[45] In a prospective, randomized trial contrasting thrombolysis with surgery as the initial treatment for ALLI, Ouriel et al.[62] demonstrated a lower incidence of cardiopulmonary events in the thrombolysis-treated group. They documented a lowering of fibrinogen concentration levels in the thrombolysis-treated group versus a rise in fibrinogen levels in the surgically treated group. The latter was explained as an acute phase reaction. They demonstrated a statistically significant reduction in deaths during the first year following treatment in the thrombolysis-treated group. They attribute this difference to the initial lower incidence of cardiopulmonary events in the thrombolysis group. These data support our results and hypothesis.

TECHNIQUE

The initial agent used for PIAT was streptokinase (SK). This was introduced by Dotter et al. in 1974.[63] They introduced the concept of administering 5000 U/h, which represented 1/20 of a systemic dose. They reasoned that the direct intrathrombus deposition of the agent would produce clot lysis as effectively as systemic administration, but with a lower incidence of complications. Considerable subsequent experience has determined that intrathrombus administration is more effective than intravenous administration but that the preferred agent is urokinase (UK). Despite the early experience of Katzen and van Breda,[64] in which they experienced a 92% success rate within 7 h with a 17% incidence of significant bleeding in 12 patients, we and others were unable to duplicate these excellent results.[65,66] We and others were experiencing a success rate of 45%, requiring 41 h of infusion, with an associated significant bleeding complication rate of 13% utilizing the so-called low-dose streptokinase regimen.[65,66]

We were discouraged by these results, but before abandoning thrombolysis, we felt that investigation of the use of UK should be tried. At that time, the literature stated that low-dose SK and low-dose UK effected the same results, with SK being favored due to lower cost.[64,65] Thus our early investigations with UK utilized what we called a high-dose regimen. This consisted of 4000 IU/min with repositioning of the catheter at 2-h intervals until antegrade flow had been reestablished.[66] Many of our applications were in patients with ALLI, and we adhered to the hard-won lessons learned by our surgical colleagues and utilized concomitant heparin to protect the patients from the formation of more clot while their low-flow or no-flow state existed.

We were gratified to note that use of UK effected a significantly higher clinical success rate of 81% and complete clot lysis incidence of 75% in a shorter time period of 18 h. These results could be due to the use of an initially higher dose, which was approximately 80% of a systemic dose, as opposed to the 5% of a systemic dose recommended for SK. It should be noted that the higher dose of UK was utilized only until reestablishment of flow. Following that, a dosage of 1000 U/min was used. This represents approximately 20% of a systemic dose in a 70-kg patient, in that the recommended systemic dose is 4400 U/kg. In a patient who had an average duration of infusion of 18 h, only 4 h would have been at the higher dose and 14 h at the lower dose. Thus the dosages were dramatically different only until flow had been reestablished.

Although the difference in initial dosage

could account for the higher success rate and shorter duration of infusion, this same explanation would not seem to cover the lower bleeding rate experienced with UK versus SK. This difference is particularly striking when one recalls that the so-called high-dose UK regimen included concomitant heparinization with efforts to maintain the PTT at approximately 100 s versus absence of concomitant heparinization with the low-dose SK regimen because of the common experience of increased bleeding when treating patients with both SK and heparin.[67] The exact explanation for those differences in bleeding is not known. These differences have not been apparent when the drugs have been given intravenously. In the patient undergoing PIAT with these agents, there is, of course, a hole in the artery. This is the source of almost all the bleeding complications. The duration of the infusion appears to have more to do with the likelihood of puncture-site bleeding than does the dose of the agent.[68] However, in this author's experience, puncture-site bleeding was noted at a much earlier point in time during infusions of SK than with UK.

Several methods and dosages of UK for PIAT have been developed. We continue to utilize 4000 U/min until antegrade flow has been reestablished. When utilizing an endhole catheter, reexamination and repositioning are performed at 1- to 2-h intervals. The use of a coaxial or multisidehole system often enables the drug to be in contact with the entire extent of the clot.[69] In this instance, the catheter does not need to be advanced, and reexamination is performed at 4-h intervals for the purpose of altering the dose. During these intervals, the patient is returned to the ward so as to provide maximum patient comfort and to allow for use of the angiography suite. With either the endhole or multisidehole systems, flow is usually reestablished within 2 to 4 h.[45,46,66,69]

Once flow has been reestablished, the infusion catheter is withdrawn until the tip is just within the origin of the vessel/graft. This helps to maximize flow through the segment, which aids in further thrombolysis and also helps to reduce the risk of pericatheter thrombus formation. At this time, the requirements for systemic heparinization are less, and the dose is reduced so as to maintain the PTT in the usual therapeutic range of 45 to 60 s rather than the 100 s that is recommended during the time that the limb is at risk of further clot propagation.

Following reestablishment of flow, the dose is reduced to 1000 to 2000 IU/min to effect complete lysis of the small volume of residual clot. We arrived at this lower dose of 1000 IU/min on the basis of our empirical observation that the rate of clot lysis diminished after reestablishment of flow despite the continued use of 4000 IU/min. We found it to be quite effective to rely more on time, flow, and the low dose to minimize cost and bleeding.[66] This empirical observation has been confirmed experimentally.[70] It has been suggested that as the volume of clot decreases and as flow is present, the chance interactions between the thrombolytic agent and plasminogen and then between plasmin and fibrin occur less frequently. Thus we stretch out the time intervals between reexaminations so as not to mistake the lack of decrease in volume of residual clot as evidence that it represents an atherosclerotic plaque. In our experience, the treatment of residual clot with angioplasty can induce distal embolization, which can be difficult to clear and can make the patient more ischemic.

Although we invariably utilize 4000 IU/min to reestablish flow in patients with either threatened (category II) or irreversible (category III) ischemia, we will occasionally utilize only 1000 IU/min in patients who are judged to be in the viable clinical class of ischemia and whose angiogram demonstrates category I findings of a simple segmental occlusion with open collateral and distal vessels. Concomitant heparinization should prevent these patients from progressing to a more advanced state of occlusion and worsened ischemia. The lower dose rate is used in these patients (viable, category I) when prompt reexamination within 2 to 4 h is not possible. Thus, to keep both cost and risk to a minimum, the lower dose is utilized with the anticipated reexamination time somewhere between 6 and 12 h.

We have occasionally used doses of 6000 to 8000 IU/min in patients with particularly severe ischemia. It is our impression that these higher doses have effected clot lysis more quickly, but with a much more rapid fall in serum fibrinogen and more instances of significant bleeding. Therefore, we do not routinely use these higher dosages.

Other regimens include 4000 IU/min after deposition of a loading dose throughout the clot (lacing)[68] versus continuous infusion with a higher dose of 6000 IU/min (R. A. Graor, personal communication, 1992) without a loading dose. A dose of 10,000 IU/min is delivered in two different methods. In one, it is delivered as a pulsed jet of 0.2 mL containing 5000 IU every 30 s through multisidehole or multislit catheters.[71,72] The other variation is utilized in Japan. This consists of the delivery of an average dose of 10,000 IU/min delivered in a 2- to 3-ml bolus every few minutes.[73] Advocates of the pulse-spray technique propose that lysis is hastened by better dispersion of the drug through the clot, as well as by mechanical disruption of the clot. We have been somewhat concerned that this fragmentation might lead to more frequent embolization of small emboli. The smaller the emboli, the more difficult they would be to clear. The advocates of the pulse-spray state that this has not been a frequent complication. The experience in Japan has included a few instances of significant embolization. This author remains somewhat concerned that these methods may cause a higher incidence of significant embolizations, which would offset their theoretical advantages.

The pulse-spray technique utilizes 10,000 IU/min, frequent forceful boluses, admixture of heparin with the thrombolytic agent in the infusate, and significant but not complete clot lysis as the endpoint. Thus it is difficult to determine which of these differences in technique accounts for the reported shorter duration of infusion with this regimen than with the continuous-infusion method utilizing 4000 IU/min without admixture of the heparin and lytic agent and with complete clot lysis as the endpoint. An attempt to clarify this question was undertaken by Kandarpa et al.[74] They examined femoropopliteal grafts in which UK was administered. They controlled for dose, endpoint (complete clot lysis), and heparin (no admixture), with the groups differing only in whether the lytic agent was administered continuously versus pulsed following initial lacing of the clot. They did not demonstrate a significant difference in time to initial reestablishment of flow, time to 95% clot lysis, or overall success rate. Thus the difference in duration with pulse-spray versus continuous-infusion techniques may relate more to differences in dosage (4000 IU/min versus 10,000 IU/min) and the utilization of complete clot lysis as the endpoint versus accepting reestablishment of flow with a small volume of residual clot as the endpoint. The lack of a significant difference in embolization between the two study groups may be due to both groups being initially treated with "lacing," which may yield a higher incidence than encountered with only continuous infusion.

Still others use continuous infusions of 1000 to 1500 IU/min to avoid a systemic fibrinolytic effect. They also avoid the use of heparinization so as to minimize the incidence of bleeding.[75,76]

All investigators report approximately the same incidences of success. In general, those utilizing higher dosages reexamine the patient at shorter time intervals and report earlier reestablishment of flow. This would be in accord with experimental work (in vitro and in vivo) demonstrating more rapid lysis of fresh clot with higher dosages of plasminogen activator.[77–80] Definitive prospective, randomized clinical trials comparing the various doses, techniques, and delivery systems do not exist at this time. Most practitioners develop experience and skill with one regimen and apply it to all instances of ALLI that they encounter. This practice may be prudent in that these patients have a serious problem that threatens both life and limb, and the practitioner can most likely deliver the best care by utilizing the regimen and infusion system with which he or she is most familiar. Developing skill and expertise with another regimen is made difficult by the fact that one does not have an opportunity to treat ALLI on a daily basis.

In summary, ALLI can be treated effectively with PIAT as the initial therapy. This author recommends it for those presenting with clinical degrees of ischemia that would be classified as either viable or threatened.[47] These patients should have confirming angiographic demonstration of pa-

tency of the collateral and distal vessels (angiographic categories I and II).[45,46] This approach can be expected to yield a lower mortality rate without an accompanying higher amputation rate.[45,62] The improvement in mortality rates can be expected to be greatest in the elderly (>75), frail, and those with significant coronary artery disease or with RMI (<2 weeks). In this author's opinion, the maximum reduction in mortality rate will probably be achieved by the practice of following successful thrombolysis with PTA such that any surgical treatment could be delayed until the patient has fully recovered from the stress of ALLI. It is also noteworthy that PIAT can be definitive therapy for approximately 30% of the patients who present with ALLI.[45,62] Thus we are entering a new era in which PIAT may become the "gold standard" for many patients with ALLI. The correlations we have demonstrated between angiographic patterns of acute occlusions and outcome of PIAT should prove very useful in patient selection.

REFERENCES

1. Yeager RA, Moneto GL, Taylor LM, Porter J. Surgical management of severe acute lower extremity ischemia. J Vasc Surg 1992;15:385.
2. Jivegard L, Holm J, Scherstén T. Acute limb ischemia due to arterial embolism or thrombosis: influence of limb ischemia vs. pre-existing cardiac disease on postoperative mortality rate. J Cardiovasc Surg 1988;29:32.
3. Jivegard L, Holm J, Scherstén T. The outcome in arterial thrombosis misdiagnosed as arterial embolism. Acta Chir Scand 1986;152:251.
4. Blaisdell FW, Steele M, Allen RE. Management of acute lower extremity arterial ischemia due to embolism and thrombosis. Surgery 1978;84:822.
5. Labey G, cited by Mosny M, Dumont MJ. Embolie fémorale au cours d'un rétrécissment mitral pur artériotomie. Guérison Bull Acad Med (Paris) 1911;66:358.
6. Lerman J, Miller FR, Lund CC. Arterial embolism and embolectomy. JAMA 1930;94:1128.
7. Keeley JL, Rooney JA. Retrograde milking: an adjunct in embolectomy. Ann Surg 1951;184:1022.
8. Shaw RS. A method for the removal of the adherent distal thrombus. Surg Gynecol Obstet 1960;110:255.
9. Oeconomus N. L'embolectomie retrograde; tech-

nique simplifié et résultats. J Chir Paris 1961; 81:185.

10. Fogarty TJ, Cranley JJ, Krause RJ, et al. A method for extraction of arterial emboli and thrombi. Surg Gynecol Obstet 1963;116:241.

11. Fogarty TJ. Catheter technique for arterial embolectomy. J Cardiovasc Surg 1967;8:22.

12. Fogarty TJ, Dailey PO, Shumway NE, Krippaehne H. Experience with balloon catheter technique for arterial embolectomy. Am J Surg 1971;122:231.

13. Thompson JE. Acute arterial occlusions. N Engl J Med 1974;290:950.

14. Abbott WM, Maloney RD, McCabe CC. Arterial embolism: a 44-year perspective. Am J Surg 1982; 143:460.

15. Eriksson J, Holmberg JT. Analysis of factors affecting limb salvage and mortality after embolectomy. Acta Chir Scand 1977;143:237.

16. Haimovici H. Myopathic-nephrotic-metabolic syndrome associated with massive acute arterial occlusions. J Cardiovasc Surg (Torino) 1973;14: 589.

17. Abbott WM, McCabe C, Maloney RD, Wirthlin RS. Embolism of the popliteal artery. Surg Gynecol Obstet 1984;159:533.

18. Volmar J. Rekonstruktive Chirurgie der Arterien. Stuttgart: Thieme, 1982:263.

19. Balas P, Bonatsos G, Xeromeritis N, et al. Early surgical results on acute arterial occlusions of the extremities. J Cardiovasc Surg (Torino) 1985;26: 262.

20. Larean A, Mathieu P, Hellmer J, Fieve G. Severe metabolic changes following delayed revascularization: Legrain-Cormier syndrome. J Cardiovasc Surg (Torino) 1973;14:609.

21. Littoy FN, Baker WH. Acute aortic occlusion: a multi-faceted catastrophe. J Vasc Surg 1986;4:211.

22. Baetz W, Bruckner R. Symptomatik und therapie der aortenbifurkationsembolie. Chirurgie 1985; 56:166.

23. Couch NP, Wheeler HB, Hyatt DF, et al. Factors influencing limb survival after femoropopliteal reconstruction. Arch Surg 1967;95:163.

24. Fogarty TJ. Management of arterial emboli. Surg Clin North Am 1979;59:749.

25. Fogarty TJ. Complications of arterial embolectomy. In: Beebe HG, ed. Complications in vascular surgery. Vol. 4. Philadelphia: JB Lippincott, 1973:95.

26. Gordon D, Fogarty TJ. Peripheral arterial embolism. In: Rutherford RB, ed. Vascular surgery. 2nd ed. Philadelphia: WB Saunders, 1984:449.

27. McPhail MV, Fratesi SJ, Barber GG, Scobie TK. Management of acute thromboembolic limb ischemia. Surgery 1983;93:381.

28. Cambria RP, Abbott WM. Acute arterial thrombosis of the lower extremity. Arch Surg 1984; 119:784.

29. Haimovici H, Moss CM, Veith FJ. Arterial embolectomy revisited. Surgery 1975;78:409.

30. Freund U, Romanoff H, Flomen Y. Mortality rate following lower limb embolectomy: causative factors. Surgery 1975;77:201.

31. Fogarty TJ. Sudden arterial occlusion: surgical aspects. Cardiovasc Clin 1971;3:173.

32. Field T, Littoy FN, Baker WH. Immediate and long-term outcome of acute arterial occlusion of the extremities: the effect of added vascular reconstruction. Arch Surg 1982;117:1156.

33. Pearse HE Jr. Embolectomy for arterial embolism of the extremities. Ann Surg 1933;98:17.

34. Danzis M. Arterial embolectomy. Ann Surg 1933; 98:249.

35. Key E. Embolectomy in circulatory disturbances in the extremities. Surg Gynecol Obstet 1923;36: 309.

36. Petitpierre M. Ueber embolektomie der extremitate narterien. Dtsch Z Chir 1928;210:184.

37. Dschanelidze JJ. Embolektomie. Arch Klin Chir 1927;149:55.

38. Linton RR. Peripheral arterial embolism: a discussion of the post-embolic vascular changes and their relation to the restoration of circulation in peripheral embolism. N Engl J Med 1941;224:189.

39. Sterling, GR, Morris KN, Officer Brown CJ, Barnett AJ. Arterial embolectomy. Med J Aust 1963; 2:255.

40. Gregg RO, Chamberlain BE, Myers JK, Tyler DB. Embolectomy or heparin therapy for arterial emboli? Surgery 1983;93:377.

41. Spencer FC, Eisman B. Delayed arterial embolectomy—a new concept. Surgery 1964;55:64.

42. Fisher RD, Fogarty TJ, Morrow AG. Clinical and biochemical observations of the effect of transient femoral artery occlusion in man. Surgery 1970; 68:323.

43. Haimovici H. Arterial embolism, myoglobinuria and renal tubular necrosis. Arch Surg 1970;100: 639.

44. Stallone J, Lim C, Blaisdell FW. Pathogenesis of pulmonary changes following ischemia of the lower extremities. Ann Thorac Surg 1969;7:539.

45. McNamara TO, Bomberger RA, Merchant RF. Intra-arterial urokinase as the initial therapy for acutely ischemic lower limbs. Circulation 1991; 83(suppl I):I–106.

46. McNamara TO. The correlation of the initial arteriographic pattern with clinical degree of ischemia and outcome in acute lower limb ischemia. Presented at the 75th Annual Meeting of the Radiological Society of North America, Chicago, Dec. 1989.

47. Rutherford RB, Flanigan DP, Gupta SK, et al. Suggested standards for reports dealing with lower extremity ischemia. J Vasc Surg 1986;4:80.

48. Stallone RJ, Blaisdell FW, Cafferata HT, Levin SM.

Analysis of morbidity and mortality from arterial embolectomy. Surgery 1969;65:207.

49. Dunant JH, Edwards WS. Small vessel occlusion in the extremity after various periods of arterial obstruction: an experimental study. Surgery 1973;73:240.

50. Mehl RL, Paul HA, Shorey W, et al. Treatment of "toxemia" after extremity replantation. Arch Surg 1964;89:871.

51. Malette WG, Armstrong RG, Criscuolo D. A second mechanism in hypotension following release of abdominal aortic clamps. Surg Forum 1964; 14:292.

52. Beyersdorf F, Matheis G, Kruger S, et al. Avoiding reperfusion injury after limb revascularization: experimental observations and recommendations for clinical application. J Vasc Surg 1989;9:757.

53. Rosencranz ER, Buckberg GD. Myocardial protection during surgical coronary reperfusion. J Am Coll Cardiol 1983;1:1235.

54. Buckberg GD. Studies of controlled reperfusion after ischemia: I. When is cardiac muscle damaged irreversibly? J Thorac Cardiovasc Surg 1986;92: 483.

55. Allen BS, Okamoto F, Buckberg GD. Studies of controlled reperfusion after ischemia: XV. Immediate functional recovery after six hours of regional ischemia by careful control of conditions of reperfusion and composition of reperfusate. J Thorac Cardiovasc Surg 1986;92:621.

56. Randle PJ, Smith GH. Regulation of glucose uptake by muscle: the effect of insulin, anaerobiosis, and cell poisons on the uptake of glucose and release of potassium by isolated rat diaphragm. Biochem J 1958;70:490.

57. Newsholme EA, Randle PJ. Regulation of glucose uptake by muscle: V. Effects of anoxia, insulin, adrenalin, and prolonged starving on concentrations of hexosphosphates and isolated rat diaphragm and perfused isolated hearts. Biochem J 1961;80:655.

58. Falholt K, Falholt W. Metabolism in ischemic muscle before and after treatment with glucose-insulin-potassium infusions. Acta Med Scand Suppl 1984;687:77.

59. McKay DG. Disseminated intravascular coagulation. New York: Harper & Row, 1965:103.

60. Allermand H, Westergaard-Nielsen J, Nielsen OS. Lower limb embolectomy in old age. J Cardiovasc Surg 1986;27:440.

61. Wilhelmsen L, Svardsudd K, Korsan-Bengsten K, et al. Fibrinogen as a risk factor for stroke and myocardial infarction. N Engl J Med 1984;311:501.

62. Ouriel K. Comparison of initial thrombolysis versus surgery for acute limb ischemia: randomized, prospective trial. Presented at the Western AngioInterventional Society Annual Meeting, Portland, Oregon, October 3, 1993.

63. Dotter CT, Rosch J, Seaman AJ. Selective clot lysis with low-dose streptokinase. Radiology 1974;111: 31.

64. Katzen BT, van Breda A. Low dose streptokinase in the treatment of arterial occlusions. AJR 1981;136: 1171.

65. Totty WG, Gilula LA, McClellan BL, et al. Low dose intravascular fibrinolytic therapy. Radiology 1982;143:59.

66. McNamara TO, Fischer JR. Thrombolysis of peripheral arterial and graft occlusions: improved results using high-dose urokinase. AJR 1985;144: 769.

67. Mori KW, Bookstein JJ, Heeney DJ, et al. Selective streptokinase infusion: clinical and laboratory correlates. Radiology 1983;148:677.

68. Sullivan KL, Gardiner GA, Shapiro MJ, Levin D. Acceleration of thrombolysis with a high-dose transthrombus bolus technique. Radiology 1989; 173:805.

69. McNamara TO, Gardner K. Coaxial system improves thrombolysis of ischemia. Diagn Imaging 1991;8:122.

70. DeMunk GAW, Groeneveld E, Rijken DC. Comparison of the in vitro fibrinolytic activities of low and high molecular weight single chain urokinase type plasminogen activator. Thromb Haemost 1993;70:481.

71. Valji K, Roberts AC, Davis GB, Bookstein JJ. Pulsed-spray thrombolysis of arterial and bypass graft occlusions. AJR 1991;156:617.

72. Mewissen MW, Minor PL, Beyer GA, Lipchik EO. Symptomatic native arterial occlusions: early experience with "over-the-wire" thrombolysis. JVIR 1990;1:43.

73. Sato M, Yamada R. Ultra high-dose urokinase for arterial occlusions. Presented at the Western AngioInterventional Society Meeting, Portland, Oregon, October 3, 1993.

74. Kandarpa K, Chopra PS, Aruny JE, et al. Intraarterial thrombolysis of lower extremity occlusions: prospective, randomized comparison of forced periodic infusion and conventional slow continuous infusion. Radiology 1993;188:861.

75. van Breda A, Katzen BT, Deutsch AS. Urokinase versus streptokinase in local thrombolysis. Radiology 1987;165:109.

76. LeBlang SD, Becker GJ, Benenati JF, et al. Low-dose urokinase regimen for the treatment of lower extremity arterial and graft occlusions: experience in 132 cases. JVIR 1992;3:475.

77. Collen D, Stassen JM, Verstraete M. Thrombolysis with human extrinsic (tissue-type) plasminogen activator in rabbits with experimental jugular vein thrombosis: effect of molecular form and dose of activator, age of the thrombus, and route of administration. J Clin Invest 1983;71:368.

78. Korninger C, Matsuo O, Suy R, et al. Thrombolysis

with human extrinsic (tissue-type) plasminogen activator in dogs with femoral vein thrombosis. J Clin Invest 1982;69:573.

79. Matsuo O, Rijken DC, Collen D. Comparison of the relative fibrinogenolytic, fibrinolytic, and thrombolytic properties of tissue plasminogen ac-tivator and urokinase in vitro. Thromb Haemost 1981;45:225.

80. Walker JE, Flook V, Ogston D. An artificial circu-lation for the study of thrombolysis. Acta Haema-tol 1983;69:41.

18

Thrombolytic Therapy in the Management of Chronic Arterial Occlusions

William R. Flinn

Walter J. McCarthy

Michael B. Silva, Jr.

Suresh Amble

It is well documented that the natural history of mild to moderate lower extremity ischemia due to atherosclerotic occlusive disease is benign. Progression to more severe symptoms occur in no more than 15% to 20% of patients, and fewer than 10% of patients will be threatened with eventual limb loss. In the past, when the only effective therapy was surgical repair or bypass, surgeons were understandably conservative in their recommendations to patients with symptoms of uncomplicated claudication when no limb jeopardy was evident. Nevertheless, the pleasure and freedom of movement provided by unencumbered walking may be one of the last remaining degrees of freedom for our elderly patients. The loss of this independence may be far more important to these patients than those of us in good health would estimate. If a treatment strategy can be developed that provides gratifying relief of ambulatory ischemic symptoms with an acceptable treatment risk, a reasonable treatment cost, a reduced hospital stay, and a shortened recovery period compared with that required after surgical treatment, then we must logically reexamine the more conservative patient-selection criteria employed in the past when considering surgical options alone.

The therapeutic options for treatment of chronic atherosclerotic arterial occlusive lesions of the lower extremities have been expanded significantly during the last decade by the evolution of invasive nonsurgical or "endovascular" techniques such as percutaneous transluminal ("balloon") angioplasty (PTA), laser-assisted angioplasty, intraarterial stents, and a variety of atherectomy devices. Understandably, there was great initial enthusiasm for techniques that might disobliterate arterial occlusive lesions without surgery. However, the early reocclusion and restenosis rates after many of these procedures have led to a critical reevaluation of their utility in many patients. This is coupled with a logical and essential concern about the costs of these various technologies—not only the initial outlay but also the cumulative costs of repetitive treatments when required.

It was initially recognized that PTA provided very successful treatment for isolated short segmental arterial stenoses, especially in larger, higher-flow vessels such as the iliac arteries. As PTA and other endovascular procedures were used to treat lesions below the inguinal ligament, however, their efficacy and durability were observed to be compromised. This seemed to be particularly true when treating longer segmental femoral-popliteal arterial *occlusions*.[1,2] Since femoral-popliteal occlusion is by far the most prevalent lower extremity arterial occlusive lesion producing ischemic symptoms in our population, initial enthusiasm for endovascular procedures in these patients waned. It was then hoped and assumed that laser systems would have a most dramatic effect on these longer femoral arterial occlusions, allowing subsequent PTA once a "channel" through the occluding lesion was forged with the laser. The early experience with virtually every laser system, however, has led to a recognition that the guidance systems and strategies for plaque ablation using laser systems need to be significantly modified before this technology will achieve any permanent role in this therapy, as will be evident from later discussion.

The more aggressive investigation of thrombolytic agents in the management of acute myocardial infarction and the development of newer and more effective thrombolytic agents such as urokinase (UK) and recombinant tissue-type plasminogen activator (rt-PA) led to the logical question of whether these agents would be useful in the treatment of a wider variety of lower extremity arterial occlusions. The adjuvant use of thrombolytic therapy with the more contemporary endovascular treatment modalities such as PTA or atherectomy has not been well documented in the past, but when one considers the underlying pathophysiologic events that contribute to the progression of arterial occlusive lesions or failure of endovascular manipulations, it seems reasonable to consider this as a logical addition to the overall therapeutic strategy in these patients. The basic underlying cause of arterial occlusions in the vast majority of patients is progressive obliteration of the arterial lumen by the atherosclerotic plaque. However, it has long been recognized that the terminal event in all cases is *thrombosis* and that propagation of this thrombus within the arterial lumen may occur for an unpre-

dictable distance proximal or even distal to the actual atherosclerotic occlusive lesion. The difficulty that exists at present is determining the presence and extent of the thrombotic component of the occlusion. The arteriographic appearance of a femoral-popliteal arterial occlusion offers absolutely no insight into the composition of the lesion (Fig. 18-1). Indeed, no presently available invasive or noninvasive technique can reliably characterize the precise morphology of an arterial occlusive lesion to tell whether the bulk of the lesion is plaque or thrombus. Several other important clinical observations have been made in the early experience with thrombolytic therapy for chronic arterial occlusions. First, there appears to be little relationship between the arteriographic appearance of a lesion or the duration of the ischemic symptoms and the possibility of achieving some identifiable thrombolysis in chronic lesions. Thus "dating" the thrombus by historical association with the onset of or worsening of the patient's symptoms appears less important than once assumed in predicting a successful response to lytic therapy. Additionally, it has been observed that

FIGURE 18-1. *In this schematic representation of two arterial occlusions, it is evident that the arteriographic appearance of the two lesions would be identical. However, the morphologic composition of each is quite different. The thrombus-dominant occlusion would be expected to have a favorable response to thrombolytic therapy, thus allowing identification and more effective treatment of the residual short segmental stenosis.*

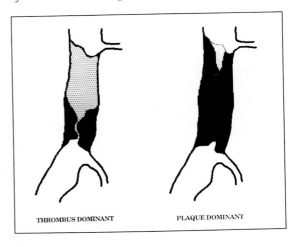

THROMBUS DOMINANT   PLAQUE DOMINANT

when a radiographic guidewire passes across an occlusive lesion without difficulty, a substantial portion of that lesion may be thrombus and thus subject to potential successful thrombolysis.

Recognizing that an unpredictable component of many femoral-popliteal arterial occlusions may be chronic thrombus, and noting that the initial efficacy and durability of present endovascular technology have been significantly compromised in these lesions, it is logical to investigate the impact of thrombolytic therapy in such clinical situations. Technologies such as PTA, laser, and atherectomy are designed as *plaque-specific* techniques, and their application to chronic thrombus logically would be ineffective. Similarly, residual thrombus within the arterial lumen after any form of therapy, regardless of the immediate therapeutic effect, would remain as a nidus for further thrombus deposition and would be expected to compromise the durability of whatever had been done. Successful initial thrombolysis in such cases might allow the more efficient application of plaque-specific technologies and might ultimately improve both the efficacy and durability of all such procedures.

When embarking on the investigation of new therapeutic strategies, it is critical to use standardized, objective techniques for assessment of the outcome. The failure to provide this objective documentation of measurable improvement in some reports describing the efficacy of endovascular techniques has led to justifiable criticism as well as an uncertainty about the true durability of these procedures. Vascular surgeons have scrutinized the results of their own surgical procedures more rigorously than perhaps any other surgical specialty. They have been actively involved in the development of noninvasive vascular testing that allows objective assessment of the hemodynamic efficacy of any therapeutic modality, surgical or nonsurgical, and provides a risk-free means for long-term follow-up. The early success rates and long-term patency of the time-honored surgical procedures such as femoral-popliteal or femoral-tibial bypass have been rigorously studied and well documented.[3] Clearly, any new therapeutic strategies must be similarly scrutinized using the same definitions[2] employed in

the past for assessment of the efficacy and durability of surgical revascularization for comparable groups of patients.

The critical questions that must therefore be answered about any newer therapeutic strategies for the treatment of chronic atherosclerotic arterial occlusive lesions of the lower extremities, before they will be accepted in comparison with available surgical procedures (whose risks and results are historically well documented), are basically threefold:

- *Is it effective?* The procedure must produce acceptable short-term success determined not solely by the arteriographic appearance of the lesion treated but also by a significant measurable hemodynamic improvement in lower limb arterial perfusion. This also must be achieved at an early risk and recovery rate that is measurably superior to standard surgical treatment of similar lesions.

- *Is it durable?* Interval noninvasive hemodynamic monitoring must be conducted prospectively in all treated patients to objectively document the intermediate and long-term efficacy of the procedure in comparison with known surgical alternatives. The durability of these procedures must be analyzed carefully in light of the initial expense of the technology employed (e.g., laser systems), as well as the expense and risks of repetitive treatments for recurrent or adjacent lesions when required.

- *Is it safe?* Newer treatment modalities must provide hemodynamic improvement with an acceptable periprocedural morbidity, an especially critical issue when thrombolytic therapy is employed. Additionally, failure to technically modify the lesion or early reocclusion after treatment should (ideally) not produce a *worsening* of ischemia over preprocedural levels with limb jeopardy that necessitates urgent or emergent surgical intervention. This latter criterion is especially critical if we are to liberalize the indications for treatment to include substantial numbers of patients with less severe, non-limb-threatening degrees of ischemia.

Endovascular technology that successfully answers these three generic questions will clearly be welcomed by all physicians caring for patients with lower extremity arterial occlusive disease. Unfortunately, to date, most of this technology has not achieved universal success. At the Northwestern University McGaw Medical Center–affiliated hospitals, we have performed preliminary investigations of several contemporary endovascular treatment strategies for the management of femoral artery occlusions. This has included excimer laser-assisted angioplasty and the adjuvant use of thrombolytic therapy with PTA or atherectomy. As will be discussed below, the use of one or another treatment modality was not based on a rigorous scientific protocol. However, a retrospective review of some of the initial experience provided some useful insight into the application of these rapidly evolving technologies.

EXPERIENCE WITH LASER-ASSISTED ANGIOPLASTY

Interest in the aggressive application of endovascular therapy to infrainguinal arterial occlusions led to our initial investigation of an excimer laser system.[5] As noted earlier, it was hoped that laser systems would significantly expand and improve the application of PTA, especially to longer segmental femoral artery occlusions. Virtually all conventionally available wavelengths have been applied experimentally or clinically to the ablation of atheromatous lesions. The ultraviolet excimer laser systems (308 nm, pulsed wave) had the theoretical advantages of producing tissue vaporization at the point of application without significant adjacent thermal injury. They also were effective even in the presence of plaque calcification, which was a significant limitation of thermal laser systems such as the familiar argon "hot-tip" laser. Additionally, the excimer laser was adaptable to available fiberoptic delivery systems.

One of the disadvantages of the excimer laser and other commercially available laser systems for atherolysis is catheter guidance. If a standard 0.018-in guidewire can be passed across the occlusive lesion, a 1.6- to 2.2-mm "over the wire"

laser catheter can be used. When guidewire passage is not possible, a no. 7 French balloon catheter with a 1.1-mm laser fiberoptic tip is used. Balloon inflation within the patent segment of the arterial lumen is thus used to stabilize and centrally locate (ideally) the laser fiber for passage into the plaque. Obviously, this latter, relatively blind, end-on approach has a higher risk of arterial wall perforation. Additionally, even after successful passage of the laser across the occlusive lesion, the maximum luminal diameter of the laser-treated lesion is only 2.2 mm, and thus all procedures require adjuvant PTA to achieve effective hemodynamic improvement.

A total of 26 superficial femoral artery (SFA) lesions in 23 patients were treated with excimer laser–assisted PTA. Patients were treated for claudication alone in 18 limbs (78%), for ischemic rest pain in 1 limb, and for ulceration or gangrene in 7 limbs. This group of patients included 13 women and 10 men with a mean age of 67 years. Segmental SFA occlusion was present on pretreatment arteriograms in 21 limbs (81%), and long segments of arterial stenoses were noted in the remaining 5 limbs. The mean pretreatment Doppler-derived ankle/brachial index was 0.49 for this group of limbs.

Results

Initial results of excimer laser–assisted PTA were classified as successful in 15 of 26 limbs (58%), as defined by arteriographic patency of the treated segment and a significant improvement in Doppler-derived ankle/brachial index. Arterial wall perforation necessitated termination of the procedure in 6 limbs, and technical failure occurred in the remaining 5 limbs. Short-segment lesions (<5 cm) were treated successfully in 83% of patients, while longer segments (>10 cm) were successful in only 22% of patients.

The initial follow-up for these patients extended from 2 to 14 months. During this first year, 8 of the 15 limbs treated successfully with excimer laser–assisted PTA experienced reocclusion. Thus early hemodynamic success was *sustained* in only 47% of patients, representing 27% of limbs selected for initial treatment.

Complications

As noted earlier, arterial wall perforation was recognized during laser treatment in 6 limbs, and 3 of these had arteriovenous communications demonstrated arteriographically. Arterial perforation necessitated termination of the therapeutic intervention and thus was clearly a major source of early technical failure. However, none of these cases of perforation or arteriovenous communication required surgical intervention; all closed spontaneously without identifiable patient morbidity.

Distal embolization of atherothrombotic material was seen in 3 patients. One patient required urgent surgical revascularization, and one was treated successfully with UK infusion. The third patient was medically unsuitable for surgical revascularization and underwent elective amputation. Two patients developed bleeding from the femoral artery at the site of catheterization which required surgical treatment.

Conclusions

Our experience and that of others[6] suggest that the excimer laser may be ideal for atherolysis; however, guidance problems significantly compromise early technical results, especially in longer lesions. Immediate efficacy of excimer laser–assisted angioplasty (53% in this experience) was compromised, but obviously, this cannot be solely attributed to the laser treatment alone, since adjuvant therapy (PTA in this series) was required in every case. These observations may simply represent confirmation of the compromised durability of PTA in more complex, longer femoral artery occlusive lesions. This also might suggest that the application of one, two, or more plaque-specific mechanisms to unpredictable segments of thrombus within the vessel will have a predetermined higher failure rate.

This initial experience with excimer laser–assisted PTA would suggest that the impact of this technology on the management SFA occlusive lesions is insufficient at present to justify the complexity and expense of existing laser systems. Rather than discard this technology, however, we

must look for methods to improve its efficacy. These would include improved guidance systems and development of larger laser catheters capable of producing extended plaque ablation and a larger resultant arterial lumen. Additionally, pretreatment or adjuvant thrombolysis may allow more direct application of this plaque-specific technology to residual atheromatous lesions.

EXPERIENCE WITH ADJUVANT THROMBOLYTIC THERAPY

During a similar time period, we undertook a preliminary investigation of the regular use of adjuvant thrombolytic therapy with endovascular treatment in patients with chronic infrainguinal arterial occlusions that were arteriographically and symptomatically similar to those treated with excimer laser–assisted angioplasty. These investigations were temporally parallel, but neither was consecutive, nor were patients randomized to one or the other of the two strategies. The treatment of patients was based on both specific selection criteria (outlined below) and available institutional resources at two separate affiliated institutions. The fundamental difference in these two experiences, however, was that this latter study involved the routine pre- and periprocedural infusion of thrombolytic therapy with UK.

Patients treated with adjuvant thrombolytic therapy were selected for this form of treatment based on characteristics of their arteriographic anatomy. These were not arteriograms that clearly demonstrated thrombi or emboli within the arterial lumen but rather those which had the familiar arteriographic appearance of "classic" atherosclerotic femoral-popliteal occlusions. Segmental superficial femoral or popliteal arterial occlusions were selected that were accessible by uncomplicated *antegrade* arterial catheterization. Rapid and successful thrombolysis is facilitated by infusion of the thrombolytic agent directly into the thrombus, and ipsilateral antegrade catheter placement is desirable. Patients with previous aortic or femoral grafts in the groin were excluded from this initial study to avoid potential complications unrelated to the treated lesions. Additionally, limbs were selected for infusion of thrombolytic therapy *only* if the arteriographic guidewire passed through or for a significant distance into the lesion initially. These characteristics were chosen to maximize the safety of this intervention but also to help intuitively identify those lesions which were likely to have some significant component of thrombus.

A total of 36 limbs in 29 patients with chronic femoral-popliteal arterial occlusions underwent treatment with thrombolytic therapy and adjuvant endovascular treatment. Intervention was performed for claudication in 17 limbs (47%) and for rest pain or ischemic ulceration in the remaining 19 limbs (53%). All limbs had preprocedural Doppler arterial examinations, and the mean preoperative ankle/brachial index was 0.42 for these 37 limbs. It is clear that this was a group of patients clinically similar to that treated with the excimer laser.

An initial high-dose infusion of 250,000 IU/h of UK as described by McNamara and Fischer[7] was begun directly into the lesion while the patient remained under observation in the arteriographic suite. During this initial infusion, additional arteriographic studies of the area of involvement were performed, and an attempt was made to differentiate ongoing lysis of thrombus from underlying residual plaque. If there was no evident lysis or change in the morphologic appearance of the occlusive lesion after a period of 3 to 4 h of this initial high-dose infusion, the procedure was terminated and the catheter removed. If lysis was evident but incomplete on the repeat arteriogram (Fig. 18-2), the UK infusion was continued at the original rate for an additional 3 to 4 h or until lysis was felt to be complete or the apparent underlying atheromatous lesion was identified. Adjuvant endovascular therapy was then undertaken and included standard PTA in 22 limbs and atherectomy in 11 limbs in this series. If residual thrombus was suspected by arteriogram during or after adjuvant endovascular treatment, the patient was maintained on a lower-dose UK infusion at 60,000 IU/h overnight in the intensive care unit, and repeat arteriography was performed the following morning prior to removal of the infusion catheter system. Addition-

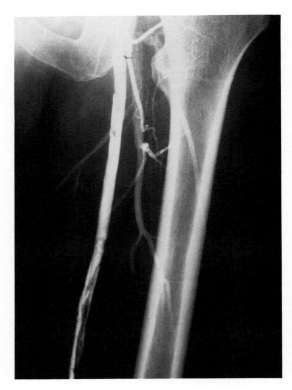

FIGURE 18-2. *Repeat arteriography reveals patency of almost the entire superficial femoral artery after the initial high-dose infusion of UK in a patient treated for a femoral-popliteal occlusion. Residual thrombus in the lumen identifies the need for continuing intraarterial infusion of UK.*

ally, all patients were maintained on systemic heparin therapy during treatment to prevent pericatheter thrombus formation. This overall therapeutic strategy was designed to promote rapid thrombolysis requiring a shorter infusion period to reduce hemorrhagic complications, most of which have been related to the indwelling catheter.

Significant initial thrombolysis (as determined by identifiable morphologic changes in the arteriographic appearance of the original occlusive lesion) was observed in 33 of these 36 limbs (91%). Early rethrombosis of treated lesions (<24 h) occurred in 6 limbs, and in 3 others no improvement in distal arterial perfusion was measurable despite arteriographically patent segments. None of the 6 patients who experienced early rethrombosis of treated lesions developed worsening of their previously stable ischemia, and none required urgent surgical intervention. Thus, after initial significant thrombolysis and adjuvant endovascular therapy, sustained, measurable hemodynamic improvement was observed in 24 limbs (73%) (Fig. 18-3). The mean postprocedural ankle/brachial index was 0.91 in these 24 limbs. Over a mean follow-up of 24 months, there have been 5 recurrent occlusions. No patients from this group have died during this period of observation, and none has required amputation;

thus the 2-year life-table patency rate was 79% for limbs that had initial successful treatment.

There were three major complications in this patient group. Two patients developed retroperitoneal hematomas while on heparin after the UK infusion. These both resolved spontaneously after cessation of heparin and required no surgical intervention. A third patient developed a hematoma in the rectus abdominis muscle during infusion of UK which appeared to be the result of dissection of blood upward from the femoral artery catheter insertion site. This did not require surgical intervention but necessitated cessation of the therapy and resulted in a technically unsuccessful

FIGURE 18-3. (A) Occlusion of the SFA near the adductor hiatus with large collateral (arrow) characteristic of chronic arterial occlusion. (B) The entire SFA and popliteal arteries are patent below the collateral (arrow) after thrombolytic therapy and adjuvant PTA.

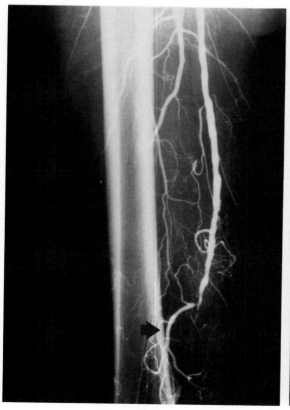
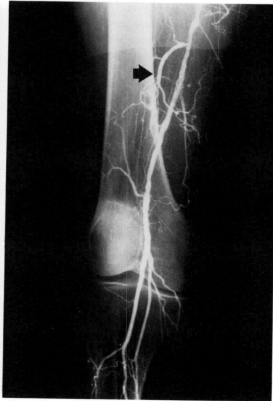

A
B

treatment of the arterial occlusive lesion in that patient.

Conclusions

Is it Effective? In this selected group of patients with the symptoms and arteriographic findings of "classic" chronic atherosclerotic occlusive lesions, arteriographic evidence of some thrombolysis, as evidenced by morphologic changes in the appearance of the lesion after UK infusion, was observed in over 80%. This response would surely not have been predicted based on our historic assumptions about the composition of femoral arterial occlusive lesions. The overall strategy of employing thrombolytic therapy with adjuvant endovascular treatment was hemodynamically successful in more than 70% of patients. While this is not strikingly different from the very best early success rates for PTA alone, the lesions ultimately undergoing plaque-specific treatment in this series were invariably shorter, more localized, and thus presumably more favorable lesions for standard endovascular therapy *after* UK infusion. This initial experience also would seem to confirm earlier observations that neither the nature of the patients symptoms nor the arteriographic appearance of the occlusive lesion at the outset of treatment can be used to accurately predict the response to thrombolytic therapy.

Is it Durable? Thrombolytic agents only lyse thrombus and have no impact on the underlying atherosclerotic occlusive lesion(s). The durability of these therapeutic interventions is primarily determined by the adjuvant technique employed, and significant debate and investigation continue concerning PTA, lasers, atherectomy devices, and arterial stents. Intuitively, however, the durability of any of these endovascular therapies will be improved by elimination of residual thrombus, allowing plaque-specific technologies to be directed more reliably at underlying atherosclerotic lesions. The patients treated in this series were carefully selected, and the number treated was small, which increases the risk of a type II error. Nevertheless, the follow-up period has been respectable, and successes to date have been encouraging enough to justify further investigation. This treatment strategy appeared to be more successful and less complex than the experience with excimer laser–assisted angioplasty.

Is it Safe? The major complications in this small series were self-limited. Additionally, no patients required urgent or emergent surgical treatment for complications or failure of therapy. It should be remembered that all thrombolytic agents produce *systemic* fibrinolysis, and if associated medical conditions in any patient make this an unacceptable or undesirable effect, then fibrinolytic agents should not be employed. Similarly, it should be remembered that the half-life of drugs such as UK or rt-PA is less than 30 minutes, and the initial decision to employ thrombolytic therapy does not justify that every subsequent complication be irrevocably associated with the decision to use the thrombolytic agent.

The improved safety of modern thrombolytic agents has led to an increasing recognition of their usefulness in the complex strategies for management of lower extremity arterial occlusive disease. It seems evident from this preliminary experience that many femoral-popliteal occlusive lesions have a component of thrombus which may respond to treatment by thrombolysis. The use of thrombolytic agents in these lesions may thereby improve the efficacy and durability of other mechanical endovascular devices. The issue of the relative cost of each of these strategies still remains to be carefully studied, but it has become increasingly evident that the costs of existing laser systems is probably unjustifiable. Expanded and extended clinical study will, of course, be necessary to more clearly define their precise role of thrombolytic therapy in the treatment of these difficult patients.

References

1. Jeans WD, Armstrong S, Cole SE, et al. Fate of patients undergoing transluminal angioplasty for lower limb ischemia. Radiology 1990;177(2):559.
2. Krepel VM, Andel GJ, van Erp WRM, et al. Percutaneous transluminal angioplasty of the femoropopliteal artery: Initial and long term results. Radiology 1985;156:325.
3. Veith FJ, Gupta SK, Ascer E, et al. Six-year

prospective multicenter randomized comparison of autogenous saphenous vein and expanded poly-tetrafluoroethylene grafts in infrainguinal arterial reconstruction. J Vasc Surg 1986;3:104.

4. Rutherford RB. Standards for evaluating results of interventional therapy for peripheral vascular disease. Circulation 1991;83(suppl I):I-6.

5. McCarthy WJ, Vogelzang RL, Nemcek AA Jr, et al. Excimer laser–assisted femoral angioplasty: early results. J Vasc Surg 1991;13:607.

6. Litvack F, Grundfest WS, Adler L, et al. Percutaneous excimer-laser and excimer-laser–assisted angioplasty of the lower extremities: results of initial clinical trial. Radiology 1989;172:231.

7. McNamara TO, Fischer JR. Thrombolysis of peripheral arterial and graft occlusions: improved results using high-dose urokinase. AJR 1985;144:769.

Anthony J. Comerota (Ed.). *Thrombolytic Therapy for Peripheral Vascular Disease.* Copyright © 1995 J. B. Lippincott Company.

19

REGIONAL THROMBOLYSIS FOR FAILED LOWER EXTREMITY ARTERIAL BYPASS GRAFTS

Geoffrey A. Gardiner, Jr.

The use of thrombolytic agents to recanalize occluded arterial bypass grafts remains somewhat controversial. Despite the diversity of opinion about the efficacy of graft thrombolysis, however, there continues to be great interest in this procedure. A major reason for this is the relatively poor results often encountered using surgical techniques alone to salvage occluded bypass grafts.[1-3] Although total graft replacement remains a viable alternative in some patients, others who have had multiple previous graft placements or revisions or who represent high operative risk may benefit from a nonoperative approach. Although successful lysis of an occluded graft does not always eliminate the need for a surgical procedure, it can at least provide information regarding the cause of graft failure, allowing for optimal surgical planning and a more limited or focused surgical procedure.

The theoretical advantages of successful thrombolysis for thrombosed arterial bypass grafts include angiographic demonstration of the underlying stenoses and the removal of clot from distal runoff vessels and from side branches or collateral beds which are inaccessible to balloon thrombectomy. This may have important implications for long-term patency, even in cases of graft replacement.[3] In addition, thrombolysis may be less damaging to arterial or vein graft walls compared with mechanical removal using a balloon catheter.

TECHNIQUE

Direct transcatheter intraarterial (regional) infusion is the method of choice for recanalizing thrombosed grafts using thrombolysis. The infusion catheters and infusion rates used for regional thrombolysis of grafts are the same as for occluded native arteries. Many special-purpose catheters and guidewires have been developed for use in regional thrombolysis. These wires or catheters have sideholes or slits which permit injection of the thrombolytic agent over various lengths rather than only at the endhole.

Placement of the infusion catheter into the occluded graft is mandatory for efficient clot lysis.

Blood flow through collateral vessels will divert most of the thrombolytic agent away from the occluding thrombus if the infusion is made above the graft origin. Direct injection of the plasminogen activator into the thrombus allows exposure of the clot to high concentrations of the lytic agent while minimizing systemic activation of the fibrinolytic system, since lower dosages can be used. Selective catheterization of the occluded graft may be technically challenging if the origin of the graft is not evident on preliminary angiograms or if the graft origin lies at an awkward angle. Also, advanced vascular disease or tortuous vessels proximal to the graft may make catheterization difficult. Finding the graft origin and entering the graft with the infusion catheter are sometimes prevented by severe stenosis at the proximal anastomosis, usually produced by intimal hyperplasia.

Once selective catheterization has been accomplished, a number of infusion methods have been described. Technical variables include the type of plasminogen activating agent used, the infusion rate, and the injection technique. The choice of thrombolytic agent seems to play an important role in determining initial success. Primary success rates for graft thrombolysis have been consistently lower using streptokinase (SK) than with the use of urokinase (UK) or recombinant tissue-type plasminogen activator (rt-PA). Reported success rates have varied from 27% to 72% in series using SK,[4-7] compared with 66% to 97% with UK or rt-PA.[6-11] Similar results have been demonstrated with these agents when used for native artery thrombolysis.[12]

The rate of infusion also has been studied as a possible determinant of success. In a randomized comparison of two different infusion rates of UK, Cragg et al.[10] found no difference in the initial success rate between a high- and a low-dose infusion. In addition, no significant advantages have been demonstrated in studies using rapid (high-dose) infusions[8,13] compared with slow (low-dose) infusions.[14]

However, more aggressive infusion techniques may reduce the time necessary for complete thrombolysis to occur. Slow injection of a concentrated bolus of thrombolytic agent throughout the thrombus prior to infusion has been demonstrated to shorten the duration of infusion, although it does not seem to affect the overall success rate.[15] Hess et al.[16] have shown in native arteries that frequent low-dose bolus injections associated with rapid advancement of the catheter tip as thrombolysis occurs are an effective method of rapid clot lysis. The pulse-spray technique[17,18] also seems to have the potential of significantly reducing the time necessary for complete clot lysis, but no conclusions can yet be made. The objective of all these techniques is to increase the surface area of the thrombus exposed to the lytic agent and thereby increase the speed at which lysis occurs.

Rapid return of antegrade blood flow through a thrombosed graft or artery is key to successful thrombolysis. In the absence of blood flow, new clot formation may occur, even with ongoing infusion of a lytic agent and adequate anticoagulation. Advanced vascular disease in the distal runoff vessels may prevent restoration of adequate blood flow despite effective thrombolysis. In practice, it is often difficult to distinguish atherosclerotic from thrombotic occlusion in the distal arteries. This uncertainty makes decisions regarding continuation of lytic infusions difficult in some cases where thrombolysis is not progressing rapidly and the status of the distal runoff vessels is unknown. Flow-limiting stenoses proximal to an occluded graft must be treated effectively before beginning thrombolytic infusion.

The duration of infusion is an important limitation of thrombolysis. Most studies report infusions of approximately 24 h in successful cases of graft thrombolysis. Although this in itself may not be a problem, it does require patient monitoring, usually in an intensive care setting, and multiple repeat angiograms. This may add significantly to the cost and risk of the procedure. There is some indication that the complication rate increases as the infusion time increases.[15] In addition, patients with critical ischemia may not be able to tolerate a period of 2 to 6 h before blood flow is restored. These and other factors have stimulated the continuing search for techniques and agents that will reduce the time necessary for effective thrombolysis.

RESULTS

Successful recanalization of thrombosed grafts depends on several key factors. The age of the thrombus is one potential factor affecting initial success. However, the duration of graft occlusion is a difficult variable to assess clinically. Most patients present acutely, since limb viability depends on graft patency; therefore, few chronically occluded grafts are treated. For this same reason, however, occlusion age is generally not an important issue in graft thrombolysis. Graft location, graft material, and the etiology of graft occlusion are other factors that may play an important role in the primary results of graft thrombolysis.

Thrombosed lower extremity grafts as a group have been treated successfully by regional thrombolysis in 53% to 97% of reported cases,[9–11,13,14,20] depending on the thrombolytic agent used and the criteria used to define success. Technical success, defined as complete or near-complete resolution of thrombus within the occluded graft, has been reported in 58% to 97% of procedures using UK.[8–11,13,14,20] Clinical success generally requires complete thrombolysis with restoration of antegrade blood flow and resolution of ischemic symptoms. This definition of success also includes all adjunctive surgical or interventional procedures used to treat underlying vascular lesions in or adjacent to the graft. Clinical success has been reported in 66% to 87% of procedures.[8–10,13,14] Combining reported series, adjunctive surgical or interventional procedures were required in 64% of patients (151 of 235).

Most of the important determinants of long-term graft patency are unrelated to the thrombolysis procedure itself. A critical aspect of graft thrombolysis which is often overlooked in the analysis of results is the influence various clinical factors have on long-term patency. Factors such as patient selection criteria used for the original graft placement, the severity of associated vascular disease, cardiac status, hypercoagulable states, the technical skill and judgment of the operating surgeon, and patient compliance all affect primary graft patency and will undoubtedly affect the durability of secondary graft patency once recanalization has been achieved.

The overall outcome of patients submitted to graft thrombolysis is dependent on a complex combination of both clinical and technical factors. The wide range of clinical variables encountered in these patients, the continually changing techniques, and the poor application of standard definitions and criteria for determining outcome probably account for much of the variation in reported results and have contributed to the difficulty in determining the precise indications for graft recanalization using regional thrombolysis.

Infrainguinal Grafts

The infrainguinal location is the most frequent site for graft thrombolysis. Grafts in this location also have the widest variation in materials, clinical presentations, and underlying causes for graft thrombosis. Successful recanalization of thrombosed infrainguinal grafts has been reported in 57% to 91% of cases.[7–9,13,15,30,31] The 1-year patency for infrainguinal grafts using regional thrombolysis in unselected patient populations ranges from 20% to 56% using life-table analysis.[15,30–32] These results vary depending in part on whether initial failures were included in the analysis.

One of the most important factors influencing short- and long-term results of infrainguinal graft thrombolysis is graft material. To some extent, this is related to differences in the etiologies of vein and prosthetic graft failure. During the first few weeks after graft placement, technical errors and inadequate blood flow are the major causes of graft thrombosis. After this period, the most common identifiable cause of polytetrafluoroethylene (PTFE) graft thrombosis is progression of atherosclerotic vascular disease. This is the reported etiology of PTFE graft failure in 30% to 81% of cases.[21–25] In the large majority of these cases, disease progression occurs in the distal vessels. Intimal hyperplasia involving the distal or proximal anastomosis is the second most common identifiable cause, responsible for about 20% of graft failures.

By comparison, the most frequent cause of vein graft thrombosis is intrinsic graft abnormalities such as focal strictures, fibrotic valves, intimal hyperplasia occurring at a clamp site, or diffuse luminal narrowing possibly related to chronic ischemia. Such lesions account for about half of vein graft failures.[26–29] Intimal hyperplasia at the proximal or distal anastomosis and progression of atherosclerotic vascular disease are also important but less frequent etiologies of vein graft failure.

The initial success rates are generally higher with prosthetic compared with vein grafts.[9,19] This trend is related in part to the intrinsic abnormalities that are a frequent cause of vein graft failure. Such lesions may severely compromise the graft lumen, making it difficult to effectively restore blood flow. Even when thrombus is resolved successfully, the graft may be so severely diseased that it is an unusable conduit (Fig. 19-1). These types of lesions do not occur in prosthetic grafts.

However, once successfully recanalized with restoration of good antegrade blood flow, vein grafts seem to have a better long-term patency rate (Fig. 19-2). A 1-year patency rate as high as

70% can be expected when successful lysis plus any required adjunctive treatment results in a reasonably normal appearing vein graft.[19,30] The progressive distal vascular disease more commonly encountered with PTFE graft occlusions is more difficult to treat, which could partially explain the poorer long-term patency with PTFE grafts.

Another possible difference between autogenous and prosthetic grafts is the tendency for thrombosis of the outflow arteries to occur in association with PTFE graft thrombosis. The presence of thrombus in the distal runoff vessels has a deleterious effect on outcome after graft recanalization or replacement.[3] This complicating feature of PTFE graft thrombosis is not seen with vein grafts. Thrombus in the distal vessels often responds well to thrombolysis and should be considered a specific indication for lytic therapy before attempted graft salvage or replacement. However, as previously noted, thrombosis of the distal runoff vessels is sometimes difficult to distinguish angiographi-

FIGURE 19-1. (A,B) *Intraoperative angiograms demonstrating distal in situ saphenous femoral–anterior tibial bypass graft (with patent perforating branches).* (C) *Repeat angiogram at 8 months shows occluded graft.* (D) *Recanalization using regional thrombolysis demonstrates diffuse narrowing of graft. Reocclusion occurred within 30 days resulting in above-knee amputation.*

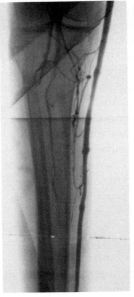
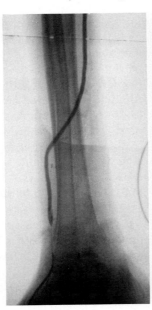
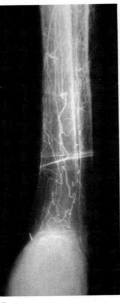
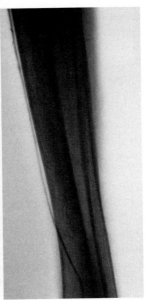

A   B   C   D

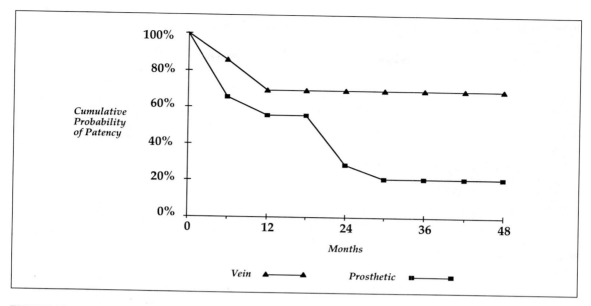

FIGURE 19-2. *Comparison of cumulative patency of vein and prosthetic grafts by means of Kaplan-Meier survival curves. (Reprinted with permission from Gardiner GA Jr, Kandarpa K, et al. Efficacy of thrombolysis in infrainguinal bypass grafts. Circulation 83(suppl I):I-99, 1991.)*

cally from progression of atherosclerotic vascular disease.

The most important determinant of long-term patency is the presence of a discrete lesion or lesions in or adjacent to the occluded graft thought to be responsible for graft failure (Fig. 19-3). Such lesions are found in 49% to 91% of successfully recanalized grafts[15,30-32] and are found more commonly in vein than in PTFE graft occlusions. Successful treatment of these lesions by balloon angioplasty or surgery can result in 2-year patency rates as high as 79%, compared with 10% in grafts without a demonstrable cause for graft failure (Fig. 19-4). The majority of patients with detectable lesions as a cause for graft thrombosis require limited surgical procedures, usually graft revision or short "jump" grafts. Some lesions are amenable to transluminal angioplasty or other interventional technique. No difference in long-term outcome has been documented between interventional or surgical therapies; however, they probably do not represent comparable groups. Recanalized grafts without an obvious cause for graft occlusion may benefit from long-term anticoagulation.

Suprainguinal Grafts

Most experience with regional thrombolysis for occluded grafts has been accumulated with infrainguinal grafts. Limited experience with thrombolysis of aortofemoral graft limbs suggests that higher initial success rates can be expected in these grafts. McNamara and Bomberger[8] achieved a 91% success rate in aortobifemoral grafts compared with 68% success in infrainguinal grafts. Durham et al.[9] reported an 88% success rate for suprainguinal grafts compared with a 59% infrainguinal graft success rate. In our own experience, 85% of suprainguinal grafts have been recanalized successfully versus 66% of infrainguinal grafts.[20] Although the significance of these differences is limited by the small numbers of patients in each study, this appears to be a consistent finding in most series.

Higher initial success rates in suprainguinal grafts may be related to the graft material used for these grafts. Prosthetic infrainguinal grafts also tend to have higher initial success rates compared with autogenous vein infrainguinal grafts.[9,19] In addition, thrombolytic recanalization is often

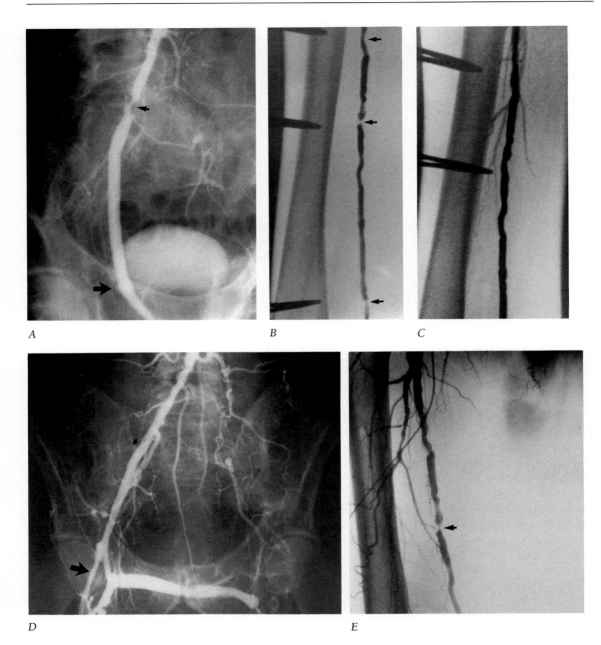

FIGURE 19-3. (**A**) *Initial angiogram demonstrates stenotic lesion in right iliac artery (small arrow) and chronic occlusion of left iliac artery. Right-sided reversed saphenous vein femoral-popliteal (large arrow) and femoral-femoral (not shown) grafts are occluded.* (**B**) *Following successful balloon angioplasty of right iliac lesion and successful thrombolysis of femoral-femoral and RSV femoral-popliteal grafts, three stenotic lesions demonstrated in femoral-popliteal graft (arrows).* (**C**) *Widely patent femoral-popliteal graft following successful thrombolysis and balloon angioplasty.* (**D**) *Three years later, repeat angiogram shows patent iliac angioplasty site (small arrow), femoral-femoral graft (large arrow), and femoral-popliteal graft.* (**E**) *New stenotic lesion in RSV femoral-popliteal graft (arrow).*

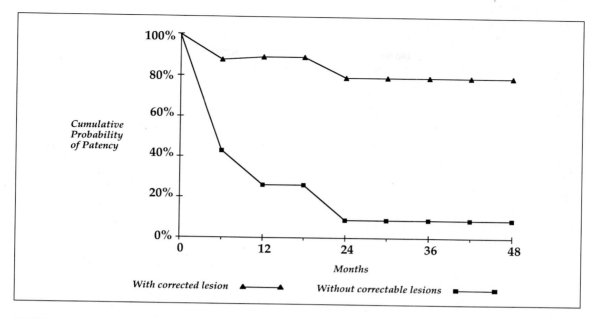

FIGURE 19-4. *Comparison of cumulative patency of grafts with and without corrected lesions by means of Kaplan-Meier survival curves. (Reprinted with permission from Gardiner GA Jr, Kandarpa K, et al. Efficacy of thrombolysis in infrainguinal bypass grafts. Circulation 83(suppl I):I-99, 1991.)*

technically easier for occluded aortobifemoral graft limbs compared with infrainguinal grafts. Access to the occluded limb from the arm or the contralateral femoral limb is generally much simpler than for infrainguinal grafts, partly because of the larger size and more proximal location of these grafts.

The large majority of lesions responsible for aortobifemoral limb thrombosis are located at the femoral anastomosis.[13] Most frequently, a stenotic lesion, often produced by intimal hyperplasia, is present. Less commonly, a pseudoaneurysm at the distal anastomosis or progressive atherosclerotic occlusive disease of the superficial femoral artery is responsible.

No significant difference in long-term graft patency has been demonstrated between suprainguinal and infrainguinal grafts,[13,19] although McNamara found that suprainguinal grafts had better long-term patency than infrainguinal grafts.[8] All these studies, however, are limited by the small numbers of cases in each series.

Extraanatomic Grafts

Little has been reported about the results of thrombolytic therapy for occluded axillofemoral or femorofemoral bypass grafts. In a compilation of published series representing thrombolysis of 374 lower extremity grafts,[4,8–11,13,14,20] only 25 extraanatomic grafts were reported. Results of lytic therapy in these grafts were not always distinguished from the other lower extremity grafts, but in 19 documented cases, 14 (74%) were recanalized successfully. Virtually nothing is known about long-term patency.

FAILURE OF THROMBOLYSIS

Clinical failure of thrombolysis is associated with varying degrees of thrombus resolution. Durham et al.[9] reported 24 graft thrombolysis failures with complete thrombolysis occurring in 8, partial thrombolysis in 11, and no lysis in 5 procedures.

Failed procedures are related to one of two causes in the large majority of cases. Premature discontinuation of lytic infusions due to a complication is one of the most frequent causes. Bleeding is the usual complication responsible for this circumstance. The inability to restore blood flow, associated with partial or even complete thrombolysis, is the other major cause of failed procedures. This is usually related to a severe stenotic lesion, most often in the graft or at the distal anastomosis, or to advanced peripheral vascular disease involving the outflow arteries. Occasionally, intimal hyperplasia at the proximal anastomosis causes complete or near-complete luminal occlusion and prevents passage of a guidewire or catheter selectively into the graft. Under such circumstances, proximal infusion of lytic agents will be futile. Rarely, the obstructing thrombus is unresponsive to lytic infusion, and no lysis occurs. This is sometimes related to chronically organized thrombus.

The effect of failed graft thrombolysis procedures on subsequent surgical management has not been well evaluated. Although distal embolization resulting in amputation has been reported occasionally, such instances appear to be rare. Delayed recanalization may increase the risk of reperfusion syndrome in severely ischemic patients, and progressive ischemia in some patients may complicate surgical treatment. However, proper patient selection and monitoring should minimize this risk. In general, failed procedures seem to have few adverse consequences for subsequent surgical management[19] and may have some benefit if partial lysis occurs or if the etiology for graft thrombosis can be identified.

COMPLICATIONS

Complications occurring during lytic infusions of thrombosed grafts have been reported in 17% to 30% of procedures.[9,11,19,20,30,32] Bleeding remains the most frequent complication. Bleeding complications have been reported in 7% to 17% of attempted graft thrombolysis. Fortunately, the large majority of these occur locally at the arterial puncture site or in the extremity being treated, often at the site of a recent or faulty anastomosis. These cases usually can be controlled by local compression but will frequently require the discontinuation of the lytic infusion and may result in a failed procedure. Bleeding also commonly occurs at skin puncture sites such as injection sites for intramuscular medications. It is important to avoid such injections during lytic therapy. Transgraft extravasation has been reported through both Dacron and polytetrafluoroethylene (PTFE) grafts[33–36] and, although it may be life-threatening if undetected, is rarely a significant problem.

Remote bleeding sites most often involve the retroperitoneum and less often the gastrointestinal or urinary tracts. Retroperitoneal bleeding should be suspected immediately in patients who complain of vague back or flank pain. Since thrombolytic infusions require patients to lie supine for many hours, symptoms of back discomfort are relatively common. The etiology of these symptoms may be difficult to determine clinically, and in suspicious cases, computed tomography or ultrasound may be helpful. Intracranial bleeding is one of the most serious complications of lytic therapy and is reported in 0.5% of regional thrombolytic infusions.[37] To date, no laboratory study or clinical criteria are able to predict with reliability the occurrence of this complication. Fortunately, it is a rare event using regional low-dose infusions.

Other complications such as distal embolization, sepsis, and reperfusion syndrome are well recognized risks associated with lytic therapy and are not unique to graft thrombolysis. Rethrombosis is a constant threat while a foreign body (catheter) remains in a vessel with little or no blood flow. Adequate anticoagulation using heparin (if UK or rt-PA is used as the plasminogen activator) and rapid restoration of antegrade flow are the keys to avoiding this problem. Distal embolization can produce increased ischemia during thrombolytic infusions. However, this is almost always temporary and will resolve with continued infusion. It may be necessary to advance the infusion catheter into the distal vessel for direct bolus injection or infusion of the thrombolytic agent to resolve this problem in some patients. Although amputation as a result of distal embolization has been reported, it is rare.

The probability of complications appears to increase with the duration of the thrombolytic infusion.[5] This may be related to the increasing likelihood of developing a systemic lytic state leading to bleeding complications. Also, prolonged catheterization can lead to sepsis. The choice of thrombolytic agent is another factor that may affect complication rates. Complications have been reported less often with UK compared with SK or rt-PA.[6] Finally, contrast-induced renal failure can result from repeated angiograms during a short time interval.

Careful patient selection remains the most crucial factor for safe procedures. In addition to standard exclusion criteria used for all forms of lytic therapy, a relative contraindication to graft thrombolysis is patients with thrombosis of a recently placed graft. Bleeding from the graft anastomosis is fairly common in such patients, and although usually easily detected and potentially controllable by local compression, the poor results of lytic therapy in this group do not seem to justify the risk.[19] Profound ischemia of the limb with loss of motor and sensory function is an absolute contraindication. The threat of reperfusion syndrome should be kept in mind whenever lysis of an occluded graft in a severely ischemic extremity is considered.

CURRENT ROLE OF GRAFT THROMBOLYSIS

Conclusive statements regarding the value of regional thrombolysis in patients with occluded grafts are difficult to make at present. This is a relatively new procedure that has undergone and continues to undergo rapid changes as new and innovative techniques and better thrombolytic agents are developed. Also, since a key aspect of graft thrombolysis is the durability of graft patency following successful procedures, and since the underlying cause of graft thrombosis is a major determinant of long-term outcome, the value of this procedure does not depend on the effectiveness of thrombolysis alone.

Although the ultimate role of regional throm-bolysis in patients with occluded grafts remains to be established, the potential value of this technique has been documented in many small series and individual patients. Regional thrombolysis has been demonstrated to be an effective means of removing thrombus from occluded grafts and distal vessels.

The issue of salvage versus replacement of grafts once thrombosis has occurred remains controversial. There is little doubt that replacement of a thrombosed graft by a new autogenous vein graft will result in the best long-term outcome. Therefore, regional thrombolysis should be considered only in situations where salvage of an existing graft is thought to be advantageous. The goal of graft thrombolysis should be considered not only therapeutic but also (and perhaps primarily) diagnostic. It should provide the surgeon with enough information about the cause of graft thrombosis to allow for a more informed decision about which grafts are potentially salvageable and which would be better treated by replacement. Consequently, successful graft thrombolysis allows for better surgical management.

Successful thrombolysis potentially offers both therapeutic and diagnostic advantages compared to surgical management alone. The clinical benefits of this will depend on the degree of associated vascular disease and the effectiveness of adjunctive surgical or interventional procedures in treating the underlying cause of graft thrombosis. In successful cases, good long-term results can be expected. The current challenge is to determine the appropriate indications for graft thrombolysis and to establish criteria for the selection of patients who are most likely to benefit from this procedure. Anticipation of further refinements of infusion technique and continued development of better thrombolytic agents should allow successful procedures in a high percentage of patients with minimal risk.

REFERENCES

1. Bandyk DF, Bergamini TM, Towne JB, et al. Durability of vein graft revision: the outcome of secondary procedures. J Vasc Surg 1991; 13:200.
2. Whittemore AD, Clowes AW, Couch NP, et al.

Secondary femoropopliteal reconstruction. Ann Surg 1981;193:35.

3. Green RM, Ouriel K, Ricotta JJ, et al. Revision of failed infrainguinal bypass graft: principles of management. Surgery 1986;100:646.

4. van Breda A, Robison JC, Feldman L, et al. Local thrombolysis in the treatment of arterial graft occlusions. J Vasc Surg 1984;1:103.

5. LeBolt SA, Tisnado J, Shao-Ru C. Treatment of peripheral arterial obstruction with streptokinase: results in arterial vs graft occlusions. AJR 1988; 151:589.

6. Graor RA, Olin J, Bartholomew JR, et al. Efficacy and safety of intraarterial local infusion of streptokinase, urokinase, or tissue plasminogen activator for peripheral arterial occlusion: a retrospective review. J Vasc Med Biol 1990;2:310.

7. Gardiner GA Jr, Koltun W, Kandarpa K, et al. Thrombolysis of occluded femoropopliteal grafts. AJR 1986;147:621.

8. McNamara TO, Bomberger RA. Factors affecting initial and 6-month patency rates after intraarterial thrombolysis with high dose urokinase. Am J Surg 1986;152:709.

9. Durham JD, Gellar SC, Abbott WM, et al. Regional infusion of urokinase into occluded lower-extremity bypass grafts long-term clinical results. Radiology 1989;172:83.

10. Cragg AH, Smith TP, Corson JD, et al. Two urokinase dose regimens in native arterial and graft occlusions: initial results of a prospective randomized clinical trial. Radiology 1991;178:681.

11. Seabrook GR, Mewissen MW, Schmitt DD, et al. Percutaneous intraarterial thrombolysis in the treatment of thrombosis of lower extremity arterial reconstructions. J Vasc Surg 1991;13:646.

12. van Breda A, Katzen BT, Deutsch AS. Urokinase versus streptokinase in local thrombolysis. Radiology 1987;165:109.

13. DeMaioribus CA, Mills JL, Fugitani RM, et al. A reevaluation of intraarterial thrombolytic therapy for acute lower extremity ischemia. J Vasc Surg 1993;17:888.

14. LeBlang SD, Becker GJ, Benenati JF, et al. Low-dose urokinase regimen for the treatment of lower extremity arterial and graft occlusions: experience in 132 cases. JVIR 1992;3:475.

15. Sullivan KL, Gardiner GA Jr, Shapiro MJ, et al. Acceleration of thrombolysis with a high-dose transthrombus bolus technique. Radiology 1989; 173:805.

16. Hess H, Mietaschk A, Bruckl R. Peripheral arterial occlusions: a 6-year experience with local low-dose thrombolytic therapy. Radiology 1987;163: 753.

17. Kandarpa K, Drinker PA, Singer SJ, et al. Forceful pulsatile local infusion of enzyme accelerates thrombolysis: in vivo evaluation of a new delivery system. Radiology 1988;168:739.

18. Valji K, Roberts AC, Davis GB, et al. Pulsed-spray thrombolysis of arterial and bypass graft occlusions. AJR 1991;156:617.

19. Sullivan KL, Gardiner GA Jr, Kandarpa K, et al. Efficacy of thrombolysis in infrainguinal bypass grafts. Circulation 1991;83(suppl I):I-99.

20. Gardiner GA Jr, Harrington DP, Koltun W, et al. Salvage of occluded arterial bypass grafts by means of thrombolysis. J Vasc Surg 1989;9:426.

21. Taylor RS, McFarland RJ, Cox MI. An investigation into the causes of failure of PTFE grafts. Eur J Vasc Surg 1987;1:335.

22. O'Donnell TF, Mackey W, McCullough JL, et al. Correlation of operative findings with angiographic and non-invasive hemodynamic factors associated with failure of polytrafluoroethylene grafts. J Vasc Surg 1984;1:136.

23. Veith FJ, Gupta SK, Daly V. Management of early and late thrombosis of expanded polytetrafluoroethylene (PTFE) femoropopliteal bypass grafts: favorable prognosis with appropriate reoperation. Surgery 1980;87:581.

24. Sterpath AV, Schultz RD, Feldhaus RJ, Peetz DJ. Seven-year experience with polytetrafluoroethylene as above-knee femoropopliteal by-pass graft. J Vasc Surg 1985;2:907.

25. Ascer E, Collier P, Gupta SK, Veith FJ. Reoperation for polytetrafluoroethylene bypass failure: the importance of distal outflow site and operative technique in determining outcome. J Vasc Surg 1987;5:298.

26. Mills JL, Fujitani RM, Taylor SM. The characteristics and anatomic distribution of lesions that cause reversed vein graft failure: a five-year prospective study. J Vasc Surg 1993;17:195.

27. Donaldson MC, Mannick JA, Whittemore AD. Causes of primary graft failure after in situ saphenous vein bypass grafting. J Vasc Surg 1992; 15:113.

28. Bandyk DF, Bergamini TM, Towne JB, et al. Durability of vein graft revision: the outcome of secondary procedures. J Vasc Surg 1991;13:200.

29. Berkowitz HD, Greenstein S, Barker CF, Perloff LJ. Late failure of reversed vein bypass grafts. Ann Surg 1989;210(6):782.

30. Miller BV, Sharp WJ, Hoballah JJ, et al. Management of infrainguinal occluded vein bypasses with a combined approach of thrombolysis and surveillance. Arch Surg 1992;127:986.

31. Belkin M, Donaldson MC, Whittemore AD, et al. Observations on the use of thrombolytic agents for thrombotic occlusion of infrainguinal vein grafts. J Vasc Surg 1990;11:289.

32. Graor Ra, Risius B, Young JR, et al. Thrombolysis of peripheral arterial bypass grafts: surgical thrombectomy compared with thrombolysis. J Vasc Surg 1988;7:347.

33. Perler BA, Kinnison M, Halden WJ. Transgraft hemorrhage: a serious complication of low-dose thrombolytic therapy. J Vasc Surg 1986;3:936.

34. Rabe FE, Becker GJ, Richmond BD, et al. Contrast extravasation through Dacron grafts: a sequela of low-dose streptokinase therapy. AJR 1982;138: 917.

35. Becker GJ, Holden RW, Rabe FE. Contrast extravasation from a Gore-Tex graft: a complication of thrombolytic therapy. AJR 1984;142:573.

36. Rosner NH, Doris PE. Contrast extravasation through a Gore-Tex graft: a sequela of low-dose streptokinase therapy. AJR 1984;143:633.

37. Gardiner GA Jr, Sullivan KL. Complications of regional thrombolytic therapy. In: Kadir S, ed. Current practice of interventional radiology. Philadelphia: BC Decker, 1991:87.

20

Devices for Delivery of Thrombolytic Agents

Barry T. Katzen

In the past decade, catheter-directed thrombolysis has become an accepted alternative in the treatment of occlusive vascular disease, despite a slow acceptance during the first years following initial description by Dotter et al.[1] and confirmation by others[2] in subsequent years. There have been increasing reports of clinical application, with attempts to analyze the variables involved in success, including patient selection, agent, dosage, concentration, delivery systems, and effects of mechanical intervention on the occluded segment.

The technical aspects of catheter-directed lysis are varied, but in recent years, individual centers have settled on techniques, systems, and dosages that have produced predictable results. None the less, technique, setup, and decision making remain the areas of greatest question among visiting fellows at the Miami Vascular Institute.

Successful lysis with low morbidity depends on many factors, but it is important that each institution establish standard and predictable protocols for patient selection and drug delivery, provide optimal patient care facilities and observation, and have an interventionist capable of making the on-line decisions regarding continuation or termination of infusion, repeat angiography, etc.

While many investigators with great experience have developed preferences for technique and protocols, at this time there is no clearly defined "right way to do it." In general, the catheter delivery systems preferred in an institution will reflect the overall technical approach that has evolved, i.e., single-lumen versus coaxial versus pulse-spray. Drug delivery systems of a variety of types and designs are available from most manufacturers of interventional products, each having design benefits and limitations. A review of all products currently available is beyond the scope of this chapter, but a review of general types of systems is presented. The following discussion reflects the author's approach to techniques and other variables in thrombolysis. They represent guidelines and are intended to give the reader an understanding of how I choose delivery systems.

BASIC CONCEPTS

The most fundamental concept of catheter-delivered thrombolysis is that effective lysis can be achieved at significantly lower doses when the agent is delivered directly *into* the thrombus. Intuitively, it seems,that further enhancement in efficacy and possible reduction in time of lysis might be achieved by *even distribution* of the agent throughout the occlusion. Although no studies have proven that more even delivery is beneficial, it is intuitive and has been my clinical experience over many years with simple endhole delivery catheters that better distribution of the agent produces improved and more predictable outcomes. The work of Bookstein[2,3] and others has demonstrated the potential benefit of high-pressure delivery (pulsed spray) of high concentration of the agent into occlusions. While clearly of value, at the time of this writing, this technical approach has not replaced more conventional continuous-infusion techniques in native arteries. It has, however, prompted the development of delivery devices that can function for both traditional infusion and spray modes and has seen increased use in the treatment of thrombosed dialysis access grafts.

Regardless of the system employed, I am guided by certain concepts when selecting catheters, guidewires, and sheaths for thrombolytic infusions which have served me well in clinical experience.

First, it is important that the devices be sized optimally to prevent limitation of flow *proximal* to the access and infusion sites. One French size may be critical in leading to pericatheter retrograde thrombosis. Careful attention to the puncture site arterial size should be paid when infrainguinal infusions are performed from the ipsilateral side. Approaching infrainguinal lesions from the contralateral side eliminates this potential problem but adds other technical problems depending on the aortic bifurcation and the extent of disease in the iliac circulation.

The second important concept is to select a device that will offer distribution of the thrombolytic agent throughout the entire length or greatest portion of the occluded segment. This may require several coaxial catheters and wires and generally two infusion pumps. On rare occasions it may be necessary to utilize three pumps.

While most investigators employ concomitant systemic heparinization, it is my practice to be selective in the use of high doses of heparin. At my institution, experience has shown no significant incidence of pericatheter thrombosis, either with or without the use of anticoagulation. It should be noted, however, that careful assessment of flow proximal to and around the occluded segment is made fluoroscopically, and these observations help to determine whether to use anticoagulation or not. In antegrade punctures, sheaths are used universally, and low doses of urokinase (20,000 IU/h) or heparin (100 IU/h) are administered through the sheath.

DEVICES FOR INFUSION

Endhole Infusion Catheters

The simplest device for infusion of thrombolytic agents is a small diagnostic catheter (Fig. 20-1). Original descriptions by Dotter et al.,[1] this author,[4] and others showed the ability to lyse thrombus successfully simply by embedding a single-lumen catheter into the proximal portion of the occluded segment. While effective, newer devices offer potential benefits, and this type of infusion is limited to the distal portion of coaxial infusions or small arteries such as the infrapopliteal vessels of the lower extremity or the vessels of the forearm. These infusions may be made through no. 3 French catheters passed through proximal no. 5 French catheters (Fig. 20-2) or may be smaller open-ended infusion wires such as the SOS,[5] Cragg,[6] or tracker wires.

Endhole infusion catheters are characterized by their simplicity of use and setup but are associated with less positional stability.[6] If the catheter tip is embedded in the proximal 1 cm of the occlusion, relatively little patient motion or leg bending could dislodge the tip from the occlusion, negating any benefit of thrombolysis. Attention to detail and periodic angiographic assessment are necessary to ensure proper catheter

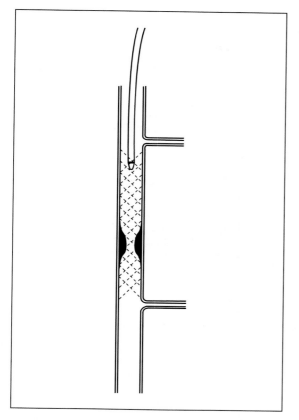

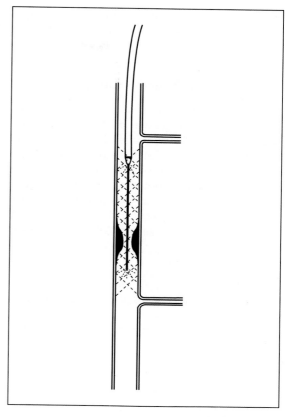

FIGURE 20-1. *Single-lumen endhole catheter. Originally used diagnostically, it was the first catheter used to deliver thrombolytic agents intraarterially by placing its tip into the proximal portion of the occluded vessel.*

FIGURE 20-2. *Smaller catheter (3–5F) advanced through a larger catheter (5–6F) allows better penetration of thrombus, resulting in improved stability during infusion and more effective drug delivery.*

position and occasionally to advance the catheter as lysis progresses.

Coaxial Endhole Infusion Systems

Because of the limitations of the simple systems, alternative devices for delivery of thrombolytic agents began to develop. The goals of these systems were to achieve predictable results by allowing more even distribution of the agent throughout the maximum length possible. The first attempts were the use of coaxial systems (see Fig. 20-2) of larger and smaller catheters or open-ended guidewires (SOS wire, Bard, Inc.). By using a no. 5 or 6 French catheter proximally with a no.

3 or 5 French catheter distally, multiple sites of infusion could be established within the occluded segment. This "catheter within a catheter" approach offered greater stability and produced considerably more certainty that the catheters would remain properly positioned throughout the length of infusion. A gradual elimination of the need for periodic angiographic evaluation during infusions also occurred. It did, however, add to the complexity of setup, since there were now sheaths, a catheter, and a smaller catheter within, requiring multiple infusion pumps, Tuehy-Borst (Y) adapters, and more critical monitoring of infusion pumps by nursing staff. Nonetheless, attentive consensus[8] developed that these methods

produced superior results, and the use of simple endhole catheter infusions has diminished in my experience.

Multisidehole Infusion Catheters

One of the earliest modifications in delivery devices was the development of infusion catheters with multiple sideholes (Fig. 20-3). Because of fluid mechanics, this became a more difficult engineering problem. While the characteristics of fluid injected at high pressures and volumes have been studied in detail, information about the distribution of fluid injected at low pressures and volumes is relatively scarce. Placing additional

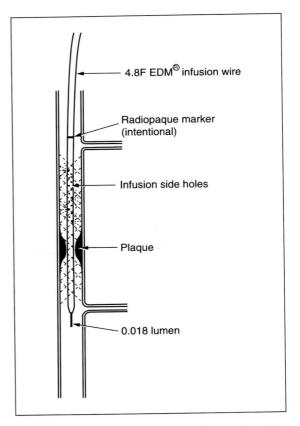

FIGURE 20-4. Multilumen infusion catheter with multiple sideholes, allowing even infusion over long lengths of occlusion.

FIGURE 20-3. Catheter with an infusion wire which has a single lumen with multiple sideholes added. This did not ensure even infusion of drug due to variable outflow resistance.

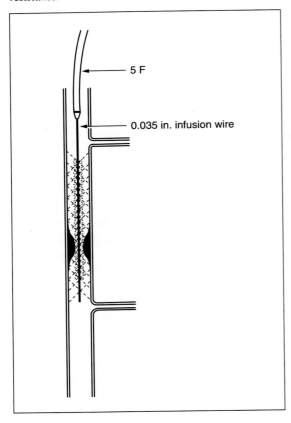

sideholes did not produce the desired effect of even infusion of the agent across the entire length of the sideholes but resulted in uneven infusion and no infusion through many of the holes, depending on design and variability of outflow resistance. It was apparent that design modification would be required to achieve the intended goal of symmetrical extrusion of fluid from the catheter.

One of the first catheters developed was a multilumen no. 4.8 French catheter with a 0.018-in central lumen (EDM catheter, Peripheral Systems Group, Mountain View, CA). This catheter allowed even infusion over long lengths of occlusion and was particularly suited for occluded femoropopliteal bypass grafts and upper extremity venous occlusions. While quite effective, it is more expensive, and smaller guide wires must be used. A similar device is the Cook multisideport infusion catheter (Cook, Inc., Bloomington, IN). These devices are more expensive than conventional catheters but may offer some cost savings by requiring only one infusion pump for long segments of disease.[9] Other multisidehole devices include the Mewissen catheter and Katzen infusion wire (Boston Scientific Corp., Watertown, MA) (Fig. 20-4), which can be used in combined fashion.[10] These devices also provide even distribution of the infusate throughout long segments and can be used with single infusion pumps when used alone. When used in combination with each other or other catheter/wire combinations, additional

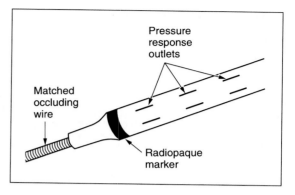

FIGURE 20-6. *Coaxial infusion catheter system using "slits" instead of sideholes. There are four pressure response outlets located at 90° every 5mm.*

infusion pumps are required. The McNamara coaxial catheter (Cook, Inc.) (Fig. 20-5) offers the advantage of variable length of infusion with the same device. More recently, an infusion catheter with slits (Fig. 20-6) instead of holes (Angiodynamics, Glen Falls, NY) has been added to the marketplace and has been clinically effective.

At present, a variety of multisidehole infusion systems are available, with varying physical characteristics and limitations (Table 20-1). There has been no scientific evidence to show superiority of one system over the other, although some have investigated the flow characteristics of different devices. McNamara[11] has found that when sideholes are placed 0.5 cm apart, a larger percentage of fluid will pass through the proximal holes and that as sideholes become closer, the catheter behaves like a "single" sidehole catheter. Use at a specific institution may be more dependent on personal preferences and intuitive analyses of performance differences. Most of the newer devices are suitable for both slow infusion and pulse-spray techniques.

FIGURE 20-5. *A coaxial multisidehole infusion catheter (5F). This system permits variable-length infusion with a single device.*

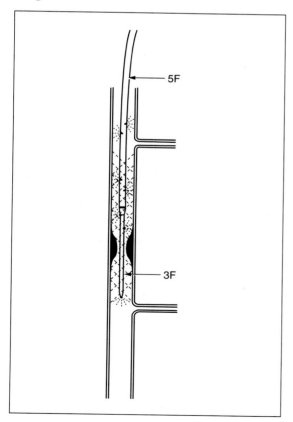

CONCLUSION

A number of devices have been developed for the infusion of thrombolytic agents using both traditional infusion and pulsed-spray techniques. Many devices have been developed to perform

TABLE 20-1. *Characteristics of Some Currently Available Multidisciplinary Catheters*

Type	Advantages	Disadvantages
EDM	Separate infusion lumens Even distribution of drug Only one infusion pump required Preassembled	Required two pumps Requires obturating wire Production of "hot spots" during infusion (from overlapping catheters)
Mewissen catheter	Accommodates 0.038-in guidewire Easier to inject contrast Pulse-spray capable Can be used with Katzen wire (coaxial)	Requires obturating wire Requires sidearm adapter Requires two pumps, and costs are relatively high if used with Katzen wire Less even distribution (infusion lumen is also guidewire lumen)
Cook multisideport catheter	Accommodates 0.038-in guidewire Advantages are same as Mewissen catheter	Requires tip occluder for infusion Other disadvantages same as Mewissen catheter
Katzen wire	0.035-in size is less occlusive Coaxial with Mewissen or Cook catheter Pulse-spray capable Guidewire "trackability"	Low flow rate for angiography Requires directional catheter if subselection necessary Production of "hot spots" with coaxial infusions secondary to uneven dispersion
McNamara coaxial catheter (Cook, Inc.)	Length can be tailored to occlusion Outer catheter used for angiography Both catheters are pulse-spray capable	Requires two pumps Requires obturating wire Production of "hot spots" during infusion (from overlapping catheters)
Pro infusion catheter (AngioDynamics)	Homogeneous distribution of fluid Pulse-spray or infusion capable Single pump	Requires obturating wire Size

both. It is my impression, and general clinical acceptance, that these devices produce more predictable and effective outcomes, but this has not been documented scientifically. Nonetheless, industry has developed relatively sophisticated devices with precise physical characteristics. There is no "best" delivery system, but rather an assortment of devices with inherent advantages and limitations from which the interventionist can choose depending on the anatomic area of thrombosis, length of occlusion, and type of infusion to be conducted. Clearly, these devices have improved the quality of therapy by offering predictable performance, stability of placement, and reduction in the need for frequent angiographic checks. The interventionist should review the available devices and make individual preference based on performance, cost, and general fit with the techniques and approaches used in his or her institution.

References

1. Dotter CT, Rosch J, Seaman AJ. Selective clot lysis with low-dose streptokinase. Radiology 1974; 111(1):31.

2. Bookstein JJ, Saldingere E. Accelerated thrombolysis: in vitro evaluation of agents and methods of administration. Invest Radiol 1985;20(7):731.

3. Bookstein JJ, Valji K. Pulse-spray pharmacomechanical thrombolysis. Cardiovasc Intervent Radiol 1992;15(4):228.

4. Katzen BT, van Breda A. Low dose streptokinase in the treatment of arterial occlusions. AJR 1981; 136(6):1171.

5. Sos TA, Cohn DJ, Srur M, et al. A new open-ended guidewire/catheter. Radiology 1985;454:817.

6. Barnhart W, Snidow JJ, Smith TP, et al. New guidewire for high-flow infusion. Radiology 1990; 174:1058.

7. Hicks ME. Delivery systems for various clinical applications in peripheral arterial thrombolysis: a practical approach. Semin Intervent Radiol 1992; 9:211.

8. McNamara TO, Gardiner K. Results of thrombolytic infusions with single catheter versus coaxial catheter systems (abstract). RSNA Sci Prog 1990;177:126.

9. Hicks ME, Picus D, Darcy MD, Kleinhoffer MA. Multilevel infusion catheter for use with thrombolytic agents. JVIR 1990;1:43.

10. Mewissen MW, Minor PL, Beyer GA, Lipchik EO. Symptomatic native arterial occlusions: early experience with "over-the-wire" thrombolysis. JVIR 1990;1:43.

11. McNamara TO. Personal communication, March 1994.

Anthony J. Comerota (Ed.). *Thrombolytic Therapy for Peripheral Vascular Disease.* Copyright © 1995 J. B. Lippincott Company.

21

Pharmaco-
mechanical
Thrombolysis
in the Peripheral
Vasculature
(Pulse-Spray
Technique)

Joseph J. Bookstein

Karim Valji

Anne C. Roberts

Principles

Pulse-spray pharmacomechanical thrombolysis (PSPMT) is a method for selective thrombolysis consisting of brief high-pressure pulsed injections of a concentrated fibrinolytic agent throughout clot via a multisideslit catheter. The method was designed to more fully exploit the potentials of the selective catheter in increasing the speed, consistency, and safety of thrombolysis. Its rationale was originally based on laboratory experiments that demonstrated quantifiable advantages of (1) intrathrombic rather than suprathrombic injection, (2) high concentrations of urokinase (UK) or tissue-type plasminogen activator (but not streptokinase), and (3) clot maceration during thrombolysis.[1–3] Further experiments also provided rationale for (4) admixture of the fibrinolytic agent with heparin[4] and (5) simultaneous administration of aspirin or other platelet-inhibiting agents.[5]

With current methodology, PSPMT usually achieves thrombolysis adequate for transluminal angioplasty within 20 to 35 minutes in dialysis grafts and within 60 to 150 minutes in native arteries (Fig. 21-1) or arterial bypass grafts (Fig. 21-2).[6–11] Lysis can almost always be achieved when thrombi can be penetrated by guidewire or catheter, regardless of clot age. The high efficiency of the method enables marked reduction in the usual required dose of thrombolytic agent (mean dose for arterial thrombolysis 500,000 units UK). Possibly related to the low dose of thrombolytic agent, the brevity of the procedure, and the fact that the patient is under continuous observation, hemorrhagic complications are rare.

As the name implies, mechanical adjuncts are an inherent part of the pharmacomechanical method. Initially, the mechanical effect of the high-pressure pulses helps macerate clot and more effectively admix clot and fibrinolytic agent. In addition, a balloon catheter can be used to macerate small amounts of resistant clot that may become apparent late in the lytic process (see below). Finally, in order to inhibit rethrombosis and augment and maintain flow, underlying stenoses responsible for thrombosis are usually treated by balloon angioplasty, atherectomy, and/or stenting upon completion of lysis (Fig. 21-3). Recognition

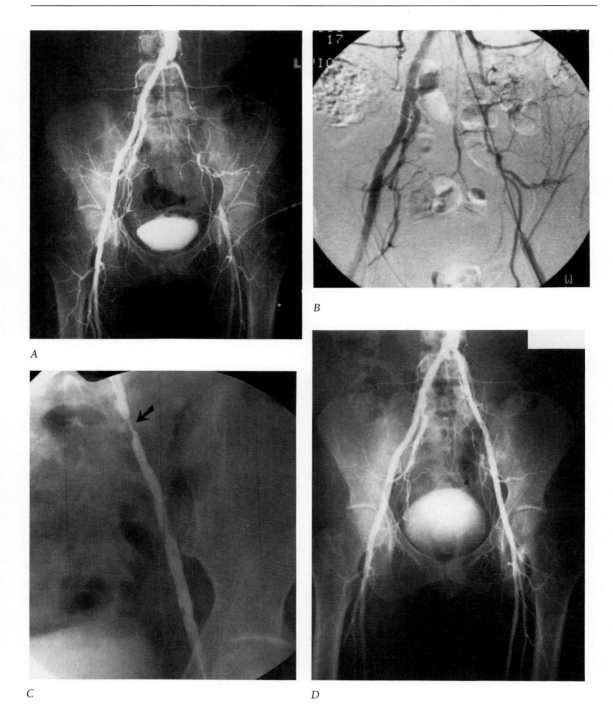

FIGURE 21-1. *Example of favorable responses of thrombus, embolus, and atherosclerosis to PSPMT and angioplasty. A 58-year-old woman with sudden onset of mild claudication of the left lower extremity 30 days earlier and marked sudden worsening of left calf claudication 6 days earlier. (A) Abdominal aortogram shows occlusion of the left common and external iliac artery. The films of*

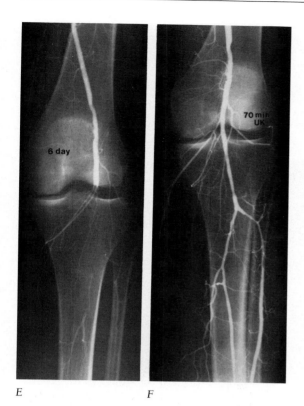

E *F*

FIGURE 21-1. (Continued).

cluding devices for rotational maceration, aspiration, and ultrasonic dissolution.[12–17] While most of these devices also can be used in conjunction with pharmacologic methods, PSPMT enables the most convenient marriage of pharmacologic and mechanical adjuncts, using relatively simple, inexpensive, and readily available equipment. The basic instrument for PSPMT is the catheter, modified for sideslit injection. Pulsed injections are currently given manually via tuberculin-like syringes, although a pulse injector is under development. The balloon catheter is the basic supplemental mechanical tool. Of the several currently available methods for pharmacomechanical thrombolysis, clinical experience sufficient for evaluation has been accumulated only with the pulse-spray method.[7–11]

Also contributing to advances in thrombolysis is greater understanding of the behavior of thrombi. Within the last decade, many accepted teachings have undergone significant modification. For example, it has become apparent that thrombi may be lysed in minutes rather than many hours or even several days; that thrombi contain sufficient plasminogen for lysis, obviating the need for additional plasminogen via inflow of blood; that chronic thrombi often fail to organize and may remain lyseable for months or even years; that long occlusions often consist of thrombus situated above a short atherosclerotic stenosis, rendering such long lesions amenable to a combination of thrombolysis and angioplasty; that thrombi often consist of platelet-rich and

and exploitation of the synergistic potentials of mechanical adjuncts represent a significant advance in thrombolytic methodology.

Many new devices for mechanical thrombolysis are undergoing preliminary evaluation, in-

---

the legs showed abrupt occlusion of the left popliteal artery suggesting embolus (see Fig. 21-1E). **(B)** After ipsilateral puncture, pharmacomechanical thrombolysis (PSPMT) with 400,000 units of UK was performed for 40 minutes, but the pulse had not returned and there was no direct flow in the common or external iliac artery on digital arteriography. It was considered likely that the catheter was obstructing an underlying atherosclerotic stenosis. **(C)** The catheter was partially withdrawn, and flow became immediately apparent fluoroscopically. A 105-mm spot film demonstrates the underlying atherosclerotic stenosis (arrow) which presumably caused thrombosis. Note small amounts of residual thrombotic material. Angioplasty in the presence of this small amount of thrombus may be performed without concern regarding excessive risk of thromboembolism. **(D)** After angioplasty with a 7-mm balloon catheter, there is good recanalization. Patency has persisted to the present, 24 months after treatment. **(E)** The next day the popliteal embolus was approached. Arteriography showed no change from the original arteriogram. **(F)** After 450,000 units of UK was pulse sprayed over 70 minutes, the embolus is completely lysed. The left ankle pulses remain normal 2 years later. (Used with permission from Bookstein JJ, Valji K: Pulse-spray pharmacomechanical thrombolysis: Updated clinical and laboratory observations. Semin Intervent Radiol 9:174, 1992.)

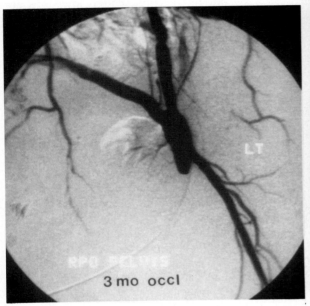

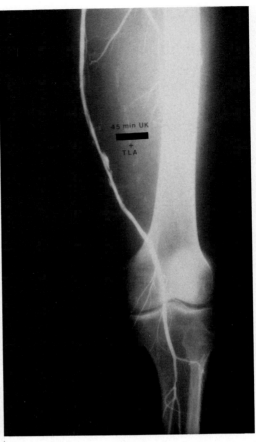

A   B

FIGURE 21-2. PSPMT of thrombosed PTFE graft. A 70-year-old man with femoral-femoral and femoral-popliteal bypass grafts. The history and physical examination suggested left femoral-popliteal graft occlusion of 90 days' duration. (A) Arteriography via a femoral-femoral graft demonstrates occlusion of the origin of the left femoral-popliteal graft. (B) A catheter with 15-cm sideholes was passed sequentially into the graft. After pulsed injection of 750,000 units of UK in 45 min, the graft is adequately patent.

platelet-poor segments, with the platelet-rich segment being relatively thrombolysis resistant; that thrombolysis is a process in dynamic equilibrium with rethrombosis; and that ongoing rethrombosis is a factor that limits the rate and extent of thrombolysis (see below).

The PSPMT method manipulates the intrathrombic microenvironment to maximize thrombolysis and inhibit rethrombosis. The cardinal pharmacomechanical principles and rationale of PSPMT may be outlined as follows:

1. Penetrating intrathrombic injections of fibrinolytic spray, thus macerating clot and augmenting interactive surface area
2. Intrathrombic containment of thrombolytic agents, minimizing dilution, inhibition of fibrinolysis by plasmin inhibitors, and systemic effects
3. Simultaneous treatment of the entire thrombus, increasing the rate of lysis
4. Concentrated agent, usually UK, increasing the rate of lysis

5. Intrathrombic heparin and systemic aspirin, significantly inhibiting rethrombosis
6. Small pulse volumes and briefly delayed treatment of a small distal plug of thrombus in order to minimize embolization
7. Balloon maceration of resistant thrombic foci after lytic stagnation (see below)
8. Transluminal angioplasty or atherectomy upon completion, as indicated

INDICATIONS

Indications for thrombolysis of peripheral thromboembolic disease remain individualized and not yet precisely defined at our institution. In general, however, acceptance of thrombolysis increases with increasing recognition of the speed and safety of the PSPMT method. The following conditions serve as relative indications for thrombolysis of the peripheral vasculature:

1. Acute arterial or bypass graft occlusions of any length, with demonstrable distal runoff
2. Chronic iliac occlusions, particularly unilateral
3. Chronic, relatively short, infrainguinal occlusions, often before PTA
4. Sudden worsening of chronic ischemic symptoms with angiographic appearance compatible with superimposed acute thrombus
5. Thrombi that develop during PTA

When thrombolysis is performed, PSPMT is almost always the thrombolytic method employed. In exceptional cases (e.g., multiple very distal emboli), the selective infusion method may be performed from above the thrombi. PSPMT has been used rarely for thrombosis of subclavian and portal veins or for thrombosed transjugular intrahepatic portosystemic stent-shunts (TIPS). Because PSPMT is so rapid and successful, distinction between thrombosis and embolism becomes less of an important factor in deciding on thrombolysis. Likewise, the clinical degree of ischemia is not usually a determining factor, although irreversible muscle injury remains a contraindication. Clot age is relatively irrelevant as long as

the obstruction is at least partially penetrable by catheter or guidewire, thus avoiding futile attempts at lysing organized thromboemboli or pure atherosclerosis.[18]

The usual relative contraindications to thrombolysis also apply to PSPMT. These include

1. Major abdominal, thoracic, or intracranial surgery within 2 to 3 weeks
2. Major trauma within 2 to 3 weeks
3. Stroke within the past 12 months
4. Severe hypertension
5. History of gastrointestinal bleeding within the past 12 to 24 months
6. Hemorrhagic diathesis
7. Pregnancy

However, because PSPMT is performed so rapidly with the patient under direct observation, and because the total doses of thrombolytic agent are relatively low, we have performed PSPMT despite recent vascular or abdominal surgery in several patients without significant complication.

RATIONALE OF EQUIPMENT DESIGN

In order to exploit the maceration effect of pulsed injections, to inject the fibrinolytic agent simultaneously and homogeneously throughout thrombus, and to minimize embolization, it is advantageous to use

1. An end-occluded noncompliant catheter with multiple tiny sideslits or extremely fine holes over an active length equal to the clot length but not to exceed 20 to 30 cm
2. An end-hole occluding system constructed with a fine-wire shaft to minimize impairment of pulse transmission through the catheter
3. Small pulse volumes of injectate (~0.2 to 0.4 mL) to minimize embolization
4. Brief pulse duration and steep pressure ascent and descent to maximize penetrance by a given pulse volume

Our currently preferred catheter system (Angiodynamics, Inc., Glens Falls, N.Y.) is designed

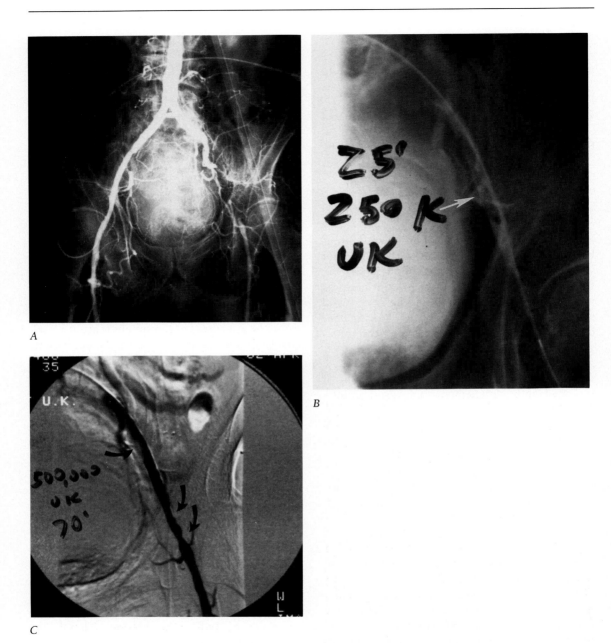

A

B

C

FIGURE 21-3. *The use of the principle of lytic stagnation to determine a thrombolytic endpoint. A 68-year-old man with a history suggesting left iliac occlusion of 30 days' duration. (**A**) Abdominal aortogram shows occlusion of the left external iliac artery. (**B**) A sideslit catheter was passed around the aortic bifurcation into the thrombus. After pulsed injections of 250,000 units of UK, there is considerable lysis and some flow, but a large residual thrombus is evident (arrow). The amount of residual thrombus obviated angioplasty at that time. (**C**) After pulsed injections of 500,000 units of UK in 70 min, there is marked further lysis, but minor mural irregularity persists (arrows). (**D**) After additional pulsed injections of another 250,000 units in 20 min, lytic stagnation is observed, characterized by absence of further resolution of the residual mural defects. Transluminal angioplasty was performed immediately thereafter. (**E**) Slight further resolution of the mural protuberances is noted after angioplasty. The irregularities most likely represent organized thrombus or atherosclerosis.*

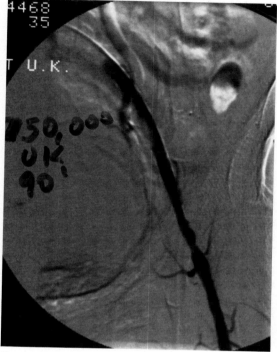

D

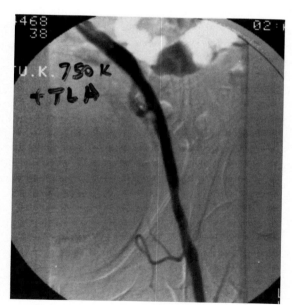

E

FIGURE 21-3. (Continued).

specifically to meet these objectives. The catheter has multiple, extremely fine sideslits so that intra-catheter pressure is maintained during pulsing, tending to equalize the volume ejected through each sideslit. When 0.2 to 0.4 mL of fluid is force-fully injected by a small syringe, a penetrating jet is emitted from each slit. In laboratory tests, the volumes ejected through each of the sideslits did not differ by a factor of more than 2 (Bookstein JJ, unpublished data). Other tests demonstrated no significant difference in the volume of ejectate through slits that were situated above clot as com-pared with slits that were within clot.[19] Other catheter systems that may be used with pulse-spray methodology are currently marketed by Cook, Inc., Meditech, Inc., and PSG, Inc.

METHODOLOGIC DETAILS

In addition to understanding the general princi-ples of PSPMT discussed above, exact knowledge of technical details is important in maximizing ef-ficacy and safety (modified from ref. 8, with per-mission). *It must be emphasized that the following methods relate to the pulse-spray method only and may be inappropriate or contraindicated for other thrombolytic methods.*

1. *Catheter placement.* When preparing for thrombolysis of bypass grafts or native arteries, the tip of the multislit catheter is initially placed approximately 2 cm proximal to the distal end of clot. The distal untreated clot then acts as a plug to delay washout of fibrinolytic agent and early downstream clot embolization. After about 15 minutes, the catheter is advanced so that the plug is also treated.

2. *Thrombolytic mixture, anticoagulation, and antiplatelet regimens.* At present, we usually use concentrated UK as the fibrinolytic agent, but concentrated tissue-type plasminogen activator (t-PA) also has been effective.[20] Unless the patient is already well heparinized, the first 250,000 units of UK is diluted in 9 mL of sterile water, to which is added 1 mL of heparin solution containing 5000 units/mL. Additional ampules of UK, if nec-essary, are dissolved in 10 mL of sterile water *without heparin.* An additional 2000 units of hep-

arin is often given systemically with onset of treatment. Aspirin (325 mg) is given, preferably several hours before thrombolysis. Maximum dose of UK for pulse-spray methods is about 1.25 million units.

Applying similar principles, we have used t-PA in 26 patients. The concentration of t-PA has been 295,000 units/mL (0.5 mg/mL). As with UK, heparin, in concentrations indicated above, has been diluted into the first 10 mL. Mean total dose of t-PA has been ~7 mg, with maximal required dose in one patient of 14 mg and absolute limit imposed by protocol of 20 mg.

The degree of anticoagulation can be conveniently monitored within the angiography suite by determination of the activated clotting time (ACT) using an automated device (Hemotec, Englewood, Colo.). Additional heparin may then be given systemically during the procedure, and particularly before angioplasty, to prolong the ACT to at least 250 to 300 s (control usually near 120 ss). Adequate prolongation of clotting times is essential for rapid thrombolysis by the PSPMT method. When thrombolysis is proceeding more slowly than expected or rethrombosis becomes a problem, we usually find insufficient prolongation of the ACT, and additional heparin usually accelerates thrombolysis.

3. *Lacing.* The entire system (catheter, reservoir and tuberculin syringes, and adapters) must first be carefully flushed of all air in order to minimize compliance so that pulses can be brief and forceful. The injection pulses should be as sudden and powerful as possible, and "lackadaisical pulsing" is one pitfall of the method. In native arteries or bypass grafts, the entire thrombus is initially laced with pulses of 0.2 to 0.3 mL, except for a 2-cm plug that is left unlaced for the first 15 minutes. (*Caveat:* Pulses larger than 0.3 to 0.4 mL may increase the incidence of distal embolization.) If the thrombus is longer than the active length, lacing is begun within the distal portion of the thrombus (except for the 2-cm distal plug); the catheter is then withdrawn sequentially into unlaced thrombus at 5- to 10-minute intervals and then is periodically advanced and withdrawn during lacing to repeatedly expose the entire thrombus to the thrombolytic agent. The initial pulse rate is two to three pulses per minute. After

100,000 to 150,000 units has been delivered to each 20-cm length of clot, the pulse rate is usually slowed to one per minute.

4. *Duration of treatment.* In arteries and bypass grafts, pulse-spray pharmacomechanical thrombolysis may be continued until luminal caliber is fully restored, until further lysis fails to occur on 20- to 30-minute interval angiograms, or until 1.25 million units of UK has been administered, whichever occurs first. If lysis appears unsatisfactory after 1.25 million units has been delivered by PSPMT, chances for complete recanalization are small, and thrombolysis may be terminated. Residual luminal narrowing at this time likely represents atheroma, organized thrombus, neo-intimal hyperplasia, arterial atrophy, or thrombolysis-resistant white (high-platelet) thrombus. Some investigators, however, prefer to continue thrombolysis via a prolonged low-dose infusion at 60,000 to 100,000 units/h for up to 24 h or more while the partial thromboplastin time (PTT) is monitored and maintained at 1.5 to 2 times control. From our limited experience with this practice, we suspect an increased incidence of hemorrhagic complications when infusion time is extended.

Some users of pulse-spray methods have preferred to begin thrombolysis by pulse spray and then, for logistic reasons, to transfer the patient from the angiography suite to an intensive-care unit (ICU) to complete the procedure by local infusion. This practice does succeed in achieving rapid initial vascular patency, and we too have used this method on occasion. Nevertheless, this terminal infusion modification does compromise other advantages of the PSPMT method and incurs the added expense of the ICU.

5. *Dialysis grafts.* The technique is modified significantly for dialysis grafts as follows: First, two catheters are used in crisscross fashion, and two hand injection systems are recommended.[6] Second, the entire clot is treated simultaneously, and distal plugs are not initially spared. Third, a high-platelet thrombolysis-resistant clot segment is often present near the arterial anastomosis which is pulled into the graft and mechanically disrupted early (after ~10 minutes) in the lytic process. Finally, angioplasty in dialysis grafts can be performed after most thrombus has lysed and

despite persistence of small to moderate amounts of remaining thrombus (see below).

6. *Mechanical thrombolysis.* Small lysis-resistant portions of clot are frequently present at the arterial anastomosis of dialysis or bypass grafts. These portions of thrombus can be broken mechanically by balloon catheter (occlusion or angioplasty types) after most other thrombus has lysed. In dialysis grafts, we tend to lyse these segments relatively early, often after about 10 minutes of lysis. The segment is pulled from near the arterial anastomosis, preferably with an occlusion balloon to prevent distal embolization, and then is crushed. In bypass grafts or native arteries, mechanical manipulation of the resistant segment is delayed longer, for perhaps 60 to 90 minutes.

To monitor lysis, we perform arteriography at 20- to 30-minute intervals. When progressive lysis is no longer demonstrated on interval films obtained during PSPMT (so-called lytic stagnation), we are reasonably confident that most thrombus has been lysed and that angioplasty can be performed without undue risk of significant embolization.[21] Residual luminal compromise at this time sometimes represents small foci of resistant (high-platelet) thrombus but more frequently organized thrombus, atherosclerosis, neointima, or (possibly) arterial atrophy.

7. *Catheter removal.* Upon completion of lysis, the catheter is removed when the ACT is under 200 s. Up to 20 mg (2 mL) of protamine sulfate may be given in 10-mg increments if hemostasis is not achieved after 20 to 30 minutes of compression. After arterial thrombolysis, a compression dressing is recommended. In view of the brevity of the procedure and usual absence of hemorrhagic problems, fibrinogen, PTT, and other coagulation parameters are not usually monitored.

PSPMT RESULTS WITH UK

As of October 1992, 202 PSPMT procedures had been attempted with UK at UCSD or the affiliated VA hospital. Lysis was considered complete or adequate for angioplasty in 196 cases. The thrombolysis times and dose requirements are presented in Table 21-1. Complications are presented in Table 21-2. Analyses of immediate and long-term results of portions of these data have been published previously.[10,11]

PSPMT WITH T-PA

We evaluated t-PA as an alternative to UK for PSPMT in a series of 27 patients. t-PA was used in a concentration of approximately 0.5 mg/mL, and as with UK, heparin was admixed with the first 5 mg to a concentration of 500 units/mL.

The single failure (Table 21-3) was due to hypercoagulability associated with metastatic hypernephroma.

In general, the speed and efficacy of PSPMT with t-PA approximated that of UK. No acceleration of lysis by t-PA was observed in dialysis grafts. It must be noted, however, that mechanical methods are applied early in dialysis grafts, tending to obscure possible acceleration of pharmacologic thrombolysis. There was a suggestion of acceleration in occlusions of native arteries or arterial bypass grafts, but the number of cases was small and differences were of marginal statistical significance. There also was a suggestion of increased early rethrombosis of dialysis grafts after therapy with t-PA when the t-PA series was compared with a cotemporal but nonrandomized series of thrombosed dialysis grafts treated with UK PSPMT. Others investigators also have suggested

TABLE 21-1. *Pulse-Spray Pharmacomechanical Thrombolysis with UK: 196 Successful Lyses/ 202 Attempts (97%)*

Classification	n	Total Lysis Time (min)	Units UK (000)
Successful lysis	196	56 ± 47	396 ± 211
Dialysis graft	133	36 ± 20	327 ± 141
Native artery	38	89 ± 47	540 ± 235
Bypass graft	25	109 ± 72	576 ± 262
Artery or bypass ≤2 days old	25	100 ± 78	571 ± 256
Artery or bypass >2 days old	38	93 ± 44	584 ± 239

Note: The six failures were all explainable. In arterial or bypass thromboses, there was one intramural catheter passage, one instance where the thrombus was probably organized thrombus, and one instance of diffuse spasm of a venous bypass graft. In dialysis grafts, there was an inability to access the entire thrombus in two and hypercoagulability in one.

TABLE 21-2. Complications in 202 Attempts at UK
Pulse-Spray Pharmacomechanical Thrombolysis

Complications   19 (9%)
Additional therapy required in 7 (3%)
0   Intracranial hemorrhages
7   Hemorrhages
   0   Requiring transfusion
   4   Moderate-sized groin hematomas, no Rx
   1   Large flank hematoma, prolonging hospitalization
   1   Large groin hematoma, requiring evacuation
   1   Gl hemorrhage, not requiring transfusion
8   Distal emboli (7 in arterial or bypass grafts, 1 dialysis
    graft)
   3   Lysed
   2   Removed optionally during bypass for other reasons
   1   Embolectomy dorsalis pedis artery
   1   Embolectomy posterior tibial artery
   1   No treatment
2   Perforation or dissection
2   Sepsis from lysis of infected graft

an increased incidence of rethrombosis after t-PA
(in coronary thrombolysis).[22–24]

COMPARISON OF PSPMT AND SELECTIVE INFUSION METHODS

Comparison of the results of PSPMT with those of
selective infusion is difficult for a number of reasons. In arterial or bypass occlusions, we consider
PSPMT to be successful when flow has been reconstituted, virtually all thrombus has lysed, and
lysis is sufficient for performance of angioplasty
or decisions regarding operation. Others[25] require
a favorable clinical outcome at up to 30 days for
classification of success. It must be emphasized,
however, that clinical outcome involves many
variables besides lysis, particularly underlying
disease process and adjunctive use of surgery or
angioplasty. Thus 30-day outcome includes confounding variables, while immediate angiography
enables more accurate assessment of thrombolysis itself.

The method against which thrombolytic results are commonly compared was published by
McNamara and Fisher[25] in 1985. This article presented results in 93 thromboembolic occlusions
of peripheral arteries or grafts in 85 patients.
Urokinase was infused at 4000 IU/min until antegrade blood flow was reestablished and then at
1000 to 2000 IU/min until clot lysis was complete. Thrombolysis was interrupted for a variety
of reasons in 9 patients. In the 84 completed procedures, mean duration of lysis was 18 ± 20 h,
and the incidence of complete clot lysis was 83%.
Average dose of UK, as estimated from data presented in the paper, was about 2 million units.
The incidence of complications was 15%, including 4 cases of hemorrhage requiring transfusion.
Succeeding articles from this group report comparable results.[26,27]

Relative to the McNamara and Fisher
method, PSPMT enables approximately 10-fold
reduction in thrombolysis times, a higher usual
rate of successful thrombolysis (83% versus 95%),
fourfold reduction in required dose of UK, reduced incidence of significant hemorrhage (Table
21-4), and significant cost savings attributable to
decreased dose of UK and avoidance of ICU
admission.

A major advantage of PSPMT is the high rate
of successful thrombolysis. Our overall success

TABLE 21-3. Pulse-Spray Pharmacomechanical
Thrombolysis with t-PA: 26 Successful Lyses/
27 Attempts (96%)

Classification	n	Total Lysis Time (min)	t-PA (mg)
Successful lysis	26	39 ± 22	
Dialysis graft	21	32 ± 16	7.0 ± 4.0
Native artery	2	73 ± 8	9.0 ± 1.0
Bypass graft	3	67 ± 29	5.8 ± 0.8
Thrombi 1–2 days	18	33 ± 18	7.0 ± 4.0
Thrombi 3–75 day	8	53 ± 26	7.4 ± 2.0

TABLE 21-4. Comparison of PSPMT and McNamara[25]
Infusion Method for Thrombolysis in Arteries
and Bypass Grafts

	PSPMT	Selective Infusion
Mean lysis time (min)	96 ± 59	1080 ± 1200
Successful lysis	95%	83%
Units urokinase (× 1000)	554 ± 246	~2000
Transfusion required for hemorrhage	0%	4%

rate, judged by complete lysis or lysis adequate for transluminal angioplasty, was 97%. In peripheral arterial or bypass occlusions, PSPMT produced thrombolysis in 63 of 66 cases (95%), compared with 83% to 88% in most other infusion studies;[25,28] a recent infusion study,[29] however, obtained a 95% success rate.

In dialysis grafts, comparison of PSPMT and infusion methods is difficult because of varying methods of infusion, use of either UK or streptokinase (SK) as the fibrinolytic agent, and various criteria for success. Bearing these limitations in mind, tabulation of results of 6 reported series[30–35] totaling 228 thrombolytic attempts in clotted dialysis grafts indicated success rates of from 59% to 100% (weighted average 66%). This compares with successful lysis in 133 of 136 patients (98%) treated by PSPMT, with continued patency allowing at least one successful dialysis in 129 patients (95%). Very much to the point is the paper by Kumpe and Cohen,[36] in which the rate of successful lysis of dialysis grafts was increased from 64% to 89% with adoption of the cross-catheter technique, a cardinal component of PSPMT in dialysis grafts.[6]

Another major advantage of PSPMT is the rapidity of lysis, a feature of particular value in patients with thrombosed hemodialysis access grafts. Typically, thrombosis is discovered at the time the patient presents for dialysis. The patient usually can be worked into that days angiography schedule; thrombolysis plus the usually required angioplasty is performed in about 90 minutes on an outpatient basis. The patient can then be dialyzed that same day, without interruption of the dialysis schedule.

Speed is also important in treating peripheral arterial occlusions. The rapidity of PSPMT enables performance of both lysis and angioplasty at a single sitting, increasing comfort and convenience for the patient and avoiding the costs and logistic difficulties involved in using the ICU. Speed is also important in the patient with an acutely ischemic, marginally viable limb, in whom prompt reestablishment of flow should minimize tissue necrosis, compartment syndrome, and renal toxicity of reperfusion.[37] When the angiographic catheter is already in place for diagnostic arteriography, subsequent revascularization by PSPMT and angioplasty is usually faster than is logistically feasible by surgery. While McNamara and Gardner[38] report moderate acceleration of thrombolysis (mean times 10 h) by infusing through a multisidehole catheter, others have not confirmed this advantage.[39] Our experimental work (unreported) indicates that a multisidehole catheter offers only modest improvement in homogeneity of distribution of thrombolytic agent unless combined with abrupt pulsing and extremely fine sideholes, inherent attributes of PSPMT methodology.

One significant concern regarding PSPMT is the incidence of distal embolization after lysis of arteries or bypass grafts. The incidence of embolization in our arterial or bypass cases was 11% (7 of 61) (see Table 21-2); most emboli were asymptomatic and/or disappeared after further lysis. This incidence is roughly comparable with the 15% incidence of distal migration observed after high-dose UK infusion therapy[27] and marginally higher than the 7% incidence observed after low-dose infusion therapy.[29]

Data enabling direct comparison of long-term results of PSPMT and infusion methods are not available. There is, however, no evidence to suggest that patency reestablished by PSPMT is more or less durable than patency reestablished by other thrombolytic means. Indeed, our prior analysis of long-term dialysis graft patency after pulse-spray or another form of pharmacomechanical thrombolysis indicated 1-year primary and secondary patency rates of 26% and 51%, respectively,[10] rates that approach the 60% to 72% secondary rates reported after surgical revision[40–42] or the 59% 1-year patency rate (excluding initial failures) reported by Poulain et al.[35] in patients treated by lysis and clot aspiration.

In considering arterial and bypass graft occlusions, the long-term results of successful lysis appear to be more dependent on the underlying disease than on the thrombolytic method used. Our prior analysis of midterm results in thrombosed arteries or bypass grafts to the lower extremity indicated anatomically successful lysis in 47 of 48 obstructions.[11] Seventeen patients (36%) in this group then underwent operation (somewhat confounding interpretation of long-term results of the thrombolysis). Of 15 recanalized arterial obstructions that did not undergo operation, 7 (47%) remained patent at 3 to 28 months of follow-up. This figure seems roughly comparable with the patency rate of McNamara and Bomberger,[26] in which 45% of 100 thrombolytic infusions showed patency at 6 months (59% patency if technical failures are excluded).

PSPMT AND RETHROMBOSIS

A mounting body of evidence indicates that thrombolysis and rethrombosis are processes in dynamic equilibrium. In keeping with other thrombolytic methods, PSPMT is also susceptible to rethrombosis. Indeed, because the patient undergoes relatively frequent fluoroscopic angiography during PSPMT, transient rethrombosis is recognized frequently. The increased awareness of rethrombosis during thrombolysis has stimulated aggressive antithrombic and antiplatelet interventions during thrombolysis.

Rethrombosis seems largely attributable to phenomena inherent in the thrombolytic process itself. Thrombin, apparently active, is released during thrombolysis in a form bound to fibrin degradation products (i.e., thrombin-FDP).[43–45] The acceleration of thrombolysis by heparin[46–49] and other antithrombic agents probably reflects the prothrombotic effects of thrombin during lysis.

Thrombolysis also activates platelets, and platelet activation has been implicated in lysis resistance and rethrombosis.[50–54] High-platelet thrombi have been shown to be much more resistant to lysis than thrombi rich in red cells[55] and much more prone to rethrombosis.[56] Platelets release a number of products potentially capable of interfering with the activity of plasminogen activators: plasminogen activator inhibitor type 1 (PAI-1),[57] α_2-antiplasmin,[58] transforming growth factor β (a potent stimulus for endothelial release of PAI-1),[59] and platelet factor 4, which inactivates heparin.[60] More important, by providing cofactors that increase prothombinase activity as much as 300,000-fold,[51,61] platelet activation

markedly enhances conversion of prothrombin to thrombin. Platelets also promote fibrin cross-linkage and clot retraction, decreasing available binding sites for t-PA—additional mechanisms explaining impaired thrombolysis of high-platelet clots.[62] Penny and Ware[63] believe that the platelet activation is attributable to both thrombin and the direct action of plasmin on platelets, with ADP as an important cofactor.

Shear activation of platelets is a well-recognized phenomenon,[64,65] a factor of particular relevance to PSPMT. Platelet activation by fluid jet was nicely shown by Bernstein et al.,[64] suggesting that the pulse spray of PSPMT might be procoagulant via platelet activation or other effects. In a pilot series of in vitro experiments, we have shown significant procoagulant effects of a single pulse of saline (delivered via PSPMT equipment) into fresh human blood in vitro.[20] The pulse also produced hemolysis, presumably releasing ADP and other procoagulants from red blood cells.

As indicated above, we routinely admix heparin with the fibrinolytic agent. This practice was initially based on uncontrolled clinical observations that suggested an association between inadequate anticoagulation and thrombolytic failure. We also noted that when rethrombosis became problematic, the ACT was often near normal despite the administration of heparin, suggesting heparin resistance. Some experimental evidence, however, suggests adverse effects of heparin on thrombolysis,[66,67] prompting us to perform experiments to evaluate heparin with parameters specifically relevant to PSPMT. In an initial set of in vitro experiments, admixture of 500 units/mL heparin with UK augmented 1-h lysis by 9% ($p < 0.05$), while admixture with t-PA inhibited lysis by 12% ($p < 0.05$).[20]

In related in vivo experiments, we have used a rabbit inferior vena caval thrombosis model to evaluate the prothrombolytic effects of various antithrombotic or antiplatelet agents that may be incorporated into PSPMT. Our data indicated that PSPMT with t-PA admixed with heparin significantly augmented thrombolysis relative to PSPMT with t-PA and systemically administered heparin.[4] An analogous experiment comparing admixture of t-PA and the antiplatelet agent PGE_1

with t-PA plus systemic PGE_1 showed comparable advantage of the admixture.[5] This latter study provides supportive evidence for an ongoing clinical evaluation of admixture of PGE_1 in PSPMT.

SUMMARY

Further elucidation of the behavior of thrombi and the process of thrombolysis has been exploited clinically via the method of pulse-spray pharmacomechanical thrombolysis. This method has significantly increased the speed, consistency, safety, and efficacy of thrombolysis. Ongoing rethrombosis and lysis resistance are recognized as important limiting factors in thrombolysis and emphasize the need for more effective antithrombic and antiplatelet agents and regimens. The value of mechanical adjuncts is also increasingly recognized, as are the inherent mechanical attributes of the pulse-spray method. An important recent development in the practice of pulse-spray thrombolysis is the use of mechanical maceration and removal of foci of resistant thrombus by balloon catheter after lytic stagnation.

REFERENCES

1. Bookstein JJ, Saldinger E. Accelerated thrombolysis: in vitro evaluation of agents and methods of administration. Invest Radiol 1985;20:731.
2. Valji K, Bookstein JJ. Fibrinolysis with intrathrombic injection of urokinase and tissue-type plasminogen activator: results in a new model of subacute venous thrombosis. Invest Radiol 1987; 22:23.
3. Kandarpa K, Drinker PA, Singer SJ, Caramore D. Forceful pulsatile local infusion of enzyme accelerates thrombolysis: in vivo evaluation of a new delivery system. Radiology 1988;168:739.
4. Valji K, Bookstein JJ. Efficacy of adjunctive intrathrombic heparin with pulse spray thrombolysis in rabbit inferior vena cava thrombosis. Invest Radiol (accepted).
5. Valji K, Bookstein JJ. Intrathrombic prostaglandin E_1 promotes pulse spray thrombolysis with t-PA in experimental thrombosis. Radiology (accepted).
6. Davis GB, Dowd CF, Bookstein JJ, et al. Efficacy of intrathrombic deposition of concentrated urokinase, clot maceration and angioplasty. AJR 1987; 149:177.
7. Bookstein JJ, Fellmeth B, Roberts A, et al. Pulsed-spray pharmacomechanical thrombolysis: Preliminary clinical results. AJR 1989;152:1097.
8. Bookstein JJ, Valji K. "How I do it": pulse-spray pharmacomechanical thrombolysis. Cardiovasc Intervent Radiol 1992;15:228.
9. Mewissen MW, Minor PL, Beyer GA, Lipchik EO. Symptomatic native arterial occlusions: early experience with "over-the-wire" thrombolysis. J Vasc Intervent Radiol 1990;1:43.
10. Valji K, Bookstein JJ, Roberts AC, Davis GB. Pharmacomechanical thrombolysis and angioplasty in the management of clotted hemodialysis grafts: early and late results. Radiology 1991;178:243.
11. Valji K, Roberts AC, Davis GB, Bookstein JJ. Pulsed-spray thrombolysis of arterial and bypass graft occlusions. AJR 1991;156:617.
12. Yedlicka JW, Carlson JE, Hunter DW, et al. Thrombectomy with the transluminal endarterectomy catheter (TEC) system: experimental study and case report. J Vasc Intervent Radiol 1991; 2:343.
13. Schmitz-Rode T, Gunther RW, Muller-Leisse C. US-assisted aspiration thrombectomy: in vitro investigations. Radiology 1991;178:677.
14. Ponomar E, Carlson JE, Kindlund A, et al. Clot-trapper device for transjugular thrombectomy from the inferior vena cava. Radiology 1991; 179:279.
15. Bildsoe MC, Moradian GP, Hunter DW, et al. Mechanical clot dissolution: new concept. Radiology 1989;171:231.
16. Johnson CC, Dewhurst TA, Vracko R, et al. Thrombolysis by rotational thrombectomy followed by tissue plasminogen activator: evaluation by angioscopy. Cathet Cardiovasc Diagn 1991;24: 214.
17. Guenther RW, Vorwerk D: Aspiration catheter for percutaneous thrombectomy: clinical results. Radiology 1990;175:271.
18. Smith DC, McCormick MJ, Jensen DA, Westengard JC: Guide wire traversal test: retrospective study of results with fibrinolytic therapy. J Vasc Intervent Radiol 1991;2:339.
19. Cho KJ, Recinella DK, Bookstein JJ. Dispersal pattern for new catheter for pulse-spray delivery of thrombolytic agents: Design, theory, and results. Radiology 1991;181(suppl):219.
20. Bookstein JJ, Valji K. Pulse-spray pharmacomechanical thrombolysis: updated clinical and laboratory observations. Semin Intervent Radiol 1992; 9:174.
21. Valji K, Bookstein JJ, Roberts AC. Lytic stagnation as an endpoint for pulse-spray pharmacomechanical thrombolysis of occluded arteries and bypass grafts. In preparation.
22. Morris JA, Muller DWM, Topol EJ. Combination

thrombolytic therapy: a comparison of simultaneous and sequential regimens of tissue plasminogen
and urokinase. Am Heart J 1991;122:375.

23. Califf RM, Topol EJ, Stack RX, et al for the TAMI
Study Group. Evaluation of combination thrombolytic therapy and timing of cardiac catheterization in acute myocardial infarction: results of
thrombolysis and angioplasty in myocardial infarction phase 5 randomized trial. Circulation
1991;83:1543.

24. Neuhaus K-L, Tebber U, Gottwik M, et al for the
GAUS Group. Intravenous recombinant tissue
plasminogen activator (rtPA) and urokinase in
acute myocardial infarction: results of the German
Activator Urokinase Study (GAUS). J Am Coll
Cardiol 1988;12:581.

25. McNamara TO, Fischer JR. Thrombolysis of peripheral arterial and graft occlusions: Improved
results using high-dose urokinase. AJR 1985;144:
769.

26. McNamara TO, Bomberger RA. Factors affecting
initial and 6 month patency rates after intra-arterial thrombolysis with high dose urokinase. Am J
Surg 1986;152:709.

27. McNamara TO, Bomberger RA, Merchant RF.
Intra-arterial urokinase as the initial therapy for
acutely ischemic lower limbs. Circulation 1991;
83(suppl1):106.

28. Sullivan KL, Gardiner GA, Kandarpa K, et al. Efficacy of thrombolysis in infrainguinal bypass
grafts. Circulation 1991;83(suppl1):99.

29. LeBlang SD, Becker GJ, Benenati JF, et al. Low-
dose urokinase regimen for the treatment of lower
extremity arterial and graft occlusions: experience
in 132 cases. J Vasc Intervent Radiol 1992;8:475.

30. Mangiarotti G, Canavese C, Thea A, et al. Urokinase treatment for arteriovenous fistulae declotting in dialyzed patients. Nephron 1984;36:60.

31. Klimas VA, Denny KM, Paganini EP, et al. Low-
dose streptokinase therapy for thrombosed arteriovenous fistulas. Trans Am Soc Artif Intern
Organs 1984;30:511.

32. Docci D, Turci F, Baldrati L. Successful declotting
of arteriovenous grafts with local infusion of
urokinase in hemodialyzed patients. Artif Organs
1986;10:494.

33. Schilling JJ, Eiser AR, Slifkin RF, et al. The role of
thrombolysis in hemodialysis access occlusion.
Am J Kidney Dis 1987;10:92.

34. Zeit RM, Cope C. Failed hemodialysis shunts: one
year experience with aggressive treatment. Radiology 1985;154:353.

35. Poulain F, Raynaud A, Bourquelot P, et al. Local
thrombolysis and thromboaspiration in the treatment of acutely thrombosed arteriovenous hemodialysis fistulas. Cardiovasc Intervent Radiol
1991;14:98.

36. Kumpe DA, Cohen MAH. Angioplasty/throm-

bolytic treatment of failing and failed hemodialysis
access sites: comparison with surgical treatment.
Prog Cardiovasc Dis 1992;34:263.

37. Lang EK. Streptokinase therapy: complications of
intra-arterial use. Radiology 1985;154:75.

38. McNamara TO, Gardner K. Results of thrombolytic infusions with single catheter versus coaxial catheter systems. Radiology 1990;177(suppl):
126.

39. Gilarsky BP, Kaufman SL, Martin LG, et al. Urokinase thrombolysis with a multiple-side-hole infusion catheter. Radiology 1990;177(suppl):126.

40. Palder SB, Kirkman RL, Whittmore AD, et al. Vascular access for hemodialysis: patency rates and
results of revision. Ann Surg 1985;202:235.

41. Puckett JW, Lindsay SF. Midgraft curettage as a
routine adjunct to salvage operation for thrombosed polytetrafluorethylene hemodialysis access
grafts. Am J Surg 1988;156:139.

42. Etheridge EE, Haid SD, Maeser MN, et al. Salvage
operations for malfunctioning polytetrafluoroethylene hemodialysis access grafts. Surgery 1983;94:
464.

43. Mirshahi M, Soria J, Soria C, et al. Evaluation of
the inhibition by heparin and hirudin of coagulation activation during r-tPA-induced thrombolysis. Blood 1989;74:1025.

44. Francis CW, Markham RE, Barlow GH, et al.
Thrombin activity of fibrin thrombi and soluble
plasmic derivatives. J Lab Clin Med 1983;102:220.

45. Bloom AL. The release of thrombin from fibrin by
fibrinolysis. Br J Haematol 1962;8:129.

46. Gulba DC, Barthels M, Westhoff-Bleck M, et al. Increased thrombin levels during thrombolytic therapy in acute myocardial infarction: relevance for
the success of therapy. Circulation 1991;83:937.

47. Andrade-Gordon P, Strickland S. Interaction of
heparin with plasminogen activators and plasminogen: effects on the activation of plasminogen.
Biochemistry 1986;25:4033.

48. Fears R. Kinetic studies on the effect of heparin
and fibrin on plasminogen activators. Biochem J
1988;249:77.

49. Susawa T, Yui Y, Hattori R, et al. Heparin requirement in tissue-type plasminogen activator–
induced experimental coronary thrombolysis:
comparison with urokinase-induced coronary
thrombolysis. Jpn Cir J 1987;51:431.

50. Coller BS. Platelets and thrombolytic therapy. N
Engl J Med 1990;322:33.

51. Fitzgerald DJ, FitzGerald GA. Antiplatelet and anticoagulant therapy during coronary thrombolysis. Trends Cardiovasc Med 1991;1:29.

52. Fitzgerald DJ, Catella R, Roy L, Fitzgerald GA.
Marked platelet activation in vivo after intravenous streptokinase in patients with acute myocardial infarction. Circulation 1988;77:142.

53. Fitzgerald DJ, Roy L, Wright F, Fitzgerald GA.

Functional significance of platelet activation following coronary thrombolysis. Circulation 1987; 76(suppl 4):151.

54. Ohlstein EH, Shebuski RJ. Tissue-type plasminogen activator (t-PA) increases plasma thromboxane levels which is associated with platelet hyperaggregation. Circulation 1987;76(suppl 4):100.

55. Jang I-K, Gold HK, Ziskind AA, et al. Differential sensitivity of erythrocyte-rich and platelet-rich arterial thrombi to lysis with recombinant tissue-type plasminogen activator. Circulation 1989;79: 920.

56. Haskel EJ, Prager NA, Sobel BE, Abenschein DR. Relative efficacy of antithrombin compared with antiplatelet agents in accelerating coronary thrombolysis and preventing early reocclusion. Circulation 1991;83:1048.

57. Erickson LA, Ginsburg MH, Loskutoff DJ. Detection and partial characterization of an inhibitor of plasminogen activator in human platelets. J Clin Invest 1984;74:1465.

58. Plow EF, Collen D. The presence and release of alpha$_2$-antiplasmin from human platelets. Blood 1981;58:1069.

59. Loskutoff DJ. Type 1 plasminogen activator inhibitor and its potential influence on thrombolytic therapy. Semin Thromb Hemost 1988;14:100.

60. Bock PE, Luscombe M, Marshall SE, et al. The multiple complexes formed by the interaction of platelet factor 4 with heparin. Biochem J 1980; 191:769.

61. Miletich JP, Jackson CM, Majerus PW. Interaction of coagulation factor Xa with human platelets. Proc Natl Acad Sci USA 1977;74:4033.

62. Kunitada S, FitzGerald GA, Fitzgerald DJ. Inhibition of clot lysis and decreased binding of tissue-type plasminogen activator as a consequence of clot retraction. Blood 1992;79:1420.

63. Penny WF, Ware JA. Platelet activation and subsequent inhibition by plasmin and recombinant tissue-type plasminogen activator. Blood 1992; 79:91.

64. Bernstein EF, Marzec U, Johnston GG. Structural correlates of platelet functional damage by physical forces. Trans Am Soc Artif Intern Organs 1977;23:617.

65. Colantuoni G, Hellums JD, Moake JL, Alfrey CP. The response of human platelets to shear stress at short exposure times. Trans Am Soc Artif Intern Organs 1977;23:626.

66. Kawano K, Ikeda Y, Handa M, et al. Enhancing effect by heparin on shear-induced platelet aggregation. Semin Thromb Hemost 1990;16:60.

67. Gorog P, Ridler CD, Kovacs IB. Heparin inhibits spontaneous thrombolysis and the thrombolytic effect of both streptokinase and tissue-type plasminogen activator: an in vitro study of the dislodgment of platelet-rich thrombi formed from native blood. J Intern Med 1990;227:125.

Anthony J. Comerota (Ed.). *Thrombolytic Therapy for Peripheral Vascular Disease.* Copyright © 1995 J. B. Lippincott Company.

22

INTRAOPERATIVE INTRAARTERIAL THROMBOLYTIC THERAPY

Anthony J. Comerota

A. Koneti Rao

Intraarterial delivery of thrombolytic agents via catheter-directed techniques has become well established in the treatment of arterial and graft occlusion. Activation of fibrin-bound plasminogen is the basis for thrombolytic therapy, and the intraarterial delivery of high concentrations of lytic agents accelerates lysis of pathologic thrombi.

A recent operation is considered a contraindication to intravenously delivered fibrinolytic therapy. For this reason, most vascular surgeons were reluctant to infuse lytic agents intraarterially during the course of an operation.

This chapter reviews the clinical and laboratory rationale for use of thrombolytic agents intraoperatively and examines supporting laboratory data. The published clinical experience is reviewed, and the results of our clinical experience are updated. A recent prospective, randomized study evaluating the hematologic details of intraoperative urokinase (UK) infusion is presented.

RATIONALE

In 1981, two interesting patients were treated with catheter-directed infusion of streptokinase (SK) for acute embolic occlusion. The first patient suffered a massive pulmonary embolus to the right main pulmonary artery[1] (Fig. 22-1). After 90 minutes of direct intrapulmonary artery infusion of SK, reperfusion was observed to the right lower lobe, with a significant drop in pulmonary artery pressures (Fig. 22-1B). After 12 to 24 h, the patient had excellent reperfusion (Fig. 22-1C) but by this time demonstrated a systematically lytic state, as evidenced by his hematologic profile. However, the most pertinent observation relative to the present discussion was that early in the course of therapy, substantial lysis of the thrombus occurred, resulting in reperfusion of the lower lobe and a marked drop in pulmonary artery pressure without evidence of a systemic lytic effect.

A second patient presented in profound shock with a gunshot wound through his common femoral artery.[2] Resuscitation was achieved with intermittent digital occlusion of the injured artery. Primary repair was accomplished by resec-

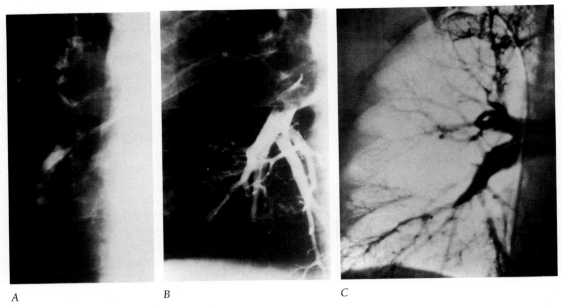

A   B   C

FIGURE 22-1. Rapid clot lysis during catheter-directed thrombolytic therapy of a massive pulmonary embolus. (A) Pulmonary arteriogram showing massive pulmonary embolus of right main pulmonary artery with significantly elevated pulmonary artery pressures. (B) Pulmonary angiogram following 1.5 h of intrapulmonary artery SK infusion at a rate of 50,000 IU/h. Reperfusion of the right lower lobe is observed with a significant drop in pulmonary artery pressures. (C) Following 12 to 24 h of infusion, the pulmonary angiogram shows excellent reperfusion of the right lung with normal resting pulmonary artery pressures. The important observation, however, is that clot lysis and reperfusion occurred early in the course of therapy without systemic fibrino(geno)lysis.

tion of the damaged vessel and end-to-end anastomosis following retroperitoneal mobilization of the entire external iliac artery. Postoperatively, the patient had a cold foot, and an arteriogram showed embolic occlusion of all three infrapopliteal arteries (Fig. 22-2A). Since the embolized thrombus was acute, and since all infrapopliteal arteries were occluded, it was decided to treat this patient with a limited dose of SK over a short period of time. With direct catheter infusion, the thrombus was lysed and normal perfusion restored (Fig. 22-2B) without laboratory evidence of a coagulopathy and without any evidence of bleeding. These clinical examples indicate that direct intraarterial infusion of lytic agents can dissolve blood clots within a short period of time without undue bleeding.

These observations were welcome in light of the uniform recognition that persistence of resid-

ual intraarterial thrombi was the rule following both clinical and experimental balloon catheter thromboembolectomy for acute arterial occlusion. Greep et al.[3] showed that almost all patients treated with the standard balloon catheter technique had additional thrombus removed with a modified wire basket catheter retrieval system. Plecha and Pories[4] performed an angiographic study and showed that 36% of patients had residual thrombus extracted following their best attempts at balloon catheter thromboembolectomy for acute arterial occlusion. These data were corroborated by Quinones-Baldrich et al.[5] in an experimental study where they demonstrated that 85% of dogs had angiographically demonstrable residual thrombi following balloon catheter thromboembolectomy. The existence of residual thrombi provides a strong rationale to administer thrombolytic agents. Moreover, in the intraopera-

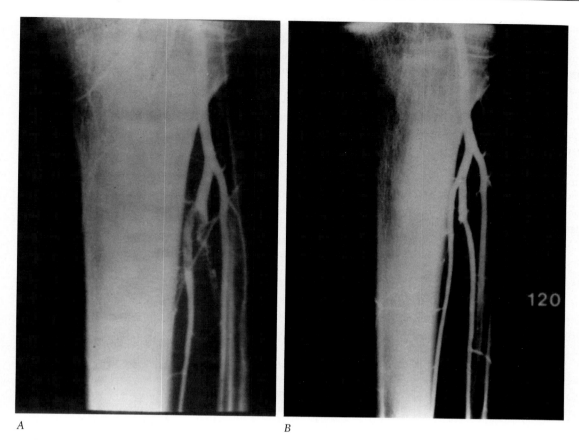

A   B

FIGURE 22-2. Early reperfusion with regional administration of thrombolytic therapy in a patient with acute arterial occlusion. (A) All infrapopliteal vessels are occluded in this patient following his resuscitation and subsequent repair of a gunshot wound of his common femoral artery. (The anterior tibial artery is occluded below the cut of this film.) A catheter was placed around the aortic bifurcation, through the repaired femoral artery, and into the distal popliteal and tibioperoneal trunk. (B) Following 2h of infusion of SK at 35,000 IU/h, all infrapopliteal thrombus is lysed (except for a small branch of the peroneal artery), with reperfusion of the foot and palpable distal pulses. The patient showed no systemic fibrinogenolysis, and there was no bleeding complication.

tive setting, the careful use of lytic agents with a short half-life may minimize or avoid a systemic lytic effect persisting after wound closure.

EXPERIMENTAL STUDIES

Dunnant and Edwards[6] demonstrated that experimental hindlimb ischemia produced arteriolar thrombosis following 6 h of inflow occlusion. The extensive degree of thrombosis indicated that simple mechanical thrombectomy would not restore perfusion to the nutrient vessels from the main arteries.

Quinones-Baldrich et al.,[5] in a controlled canine hindlimb perfusion study, showed that thrombolysis following the best attempts at balloon catheter thromboembolectomy produced significantly improved angiographic results and a marked trend (though not statistically significant) toward improved flow compared with control limbs. Belkin et al.,[7] in an isolated limb ischemic muscle preparation, demonstrated that UK infusion salvaged more ischemic muscle compared with a control group. Additionally, significantly less injury (as shown by reperfusion edema) was noted in the lytic group compared with control muscles. In this study there also was a trend toward improved blood flow. Therefore, experimental animal models confirm the clinical observations that balloon catheter thromboembolectomy frequently leaves residual thrombus. The data also demonstrate that arteriolar perfusion can be restored, tissue salvaged, and reperfusion injury reduced with the judicious use of intraarterial infusion of lytic agents.

CLINICAL EXPERIENCE

An early report on the use of intraoperative SK dampened the enthusiasm of many surgeons for intraoperative thrombolysis. Cohen et al.[8] treated 12 patients with SK in doses ranging from 25,000 to 250,000 IU using a repeated-bolus technique over 30 to 150 minutes of inflow occlusion. There was a 42% mortality, and 42% of the patients suffered a bleeding complication. It is likely that patient selection, choice of lytic agent, and method of infusion contributed to the high complication rate. Quinones-Baldrich et al.[9] reported 5 patients with angiographically documented residual thrombi following balloon catheter thrombectomy who were treated with intraarterial SK over a shorter period of time. All 5 had successful lysis without bleeding complications.

Norem et al.[10] demonstrated an alternative clinical benefit from intraoperative thrombolysis. They found that after balloon catheter throm-

boembolectomy, additional thrombus could be retrieved following intraoperative intraarterial infusion of SK. In 19 patients having thromboembolectomy for acute arterial ischemia, intraarterial SK was infused in the operating room. After a short waiting period, repeat balloon catheter thrombectomy retrieved additional thrombus, and all patients demonstrated angiographic improvement. Similar findings occurred with the use of intraoperative UK infusion.[11]

Parent et al.[12] treated 28 patients with acute ischemia and residual thrombus following balloon catheter thrombectomy. Seventeen patients had operative angiograms demonstrating thrombi. Of those 17, 15 had successful lysis when treated with intraoperative thrombolytic therapy. Both SK and UK were used and were shown to be equally effective (Table 22-1). However, hypofibrinogenemia and bleeding complications were significantly more frequent in those treated with SK compared with those treated with UK.

At Temple University Hospital, 53 patients who had impending limb loss and occlusions of their "runoff" vessels have been treated with intraoperative intraarterial lytic therapy over the past 10 years. Included are patients with extensive distal thrombosis in whom complete thrombectomy was difficult or impossible and for whom the attending surgeon believed that tissue loss was imminent (Table 22-2). SK, UK, or recombinant tissue-type plasminogen activator (rt-PA) were infused into the most distal vessel containing the thrombus with a short-duration infusion (either single- or double-bolus technique). Up to 50,000 IU of SK, 250,000 IU of UK, or 10 mg of rt-PA were used for routine intraoperative use (excluding patients having the isolated

TABLE 22-1. *Intraoperative Intraarterial Fibrinolytic Therapy: Overall Results*

Agent	No. of Patients	Success (%)	Bleed (%)	Fibrinogen (mg/dL)	Percent of Patients with Fibrinogen < 100 mg/dL
SK	7	6/7 (85%)	2/7 (29%)	−130	43
UK	21	19/21 (91%)	1/21 (5%)	−46	5
p Value		N.S.	< 0.05	=0.054	< 0.05

Created with data from ref. 12.

TABLE 22-2. *Results of Intraoperative Intraarterial Thrombolysis as an Adjunct to Revascularization for Patients with Distal Arterial Thrombosis*

Successful revascularization and limb salvage	70% (37/53)
Lysis	70% (26/37)*
Indeterminant	30% (11/37)*
Amputation	30% (16/53)
Mortality	9% (5/53)†
Bleeding complications	2% (1/53)‡

*Denominator refers to those patients treated successfully.
†None due to lytic agent.
‡Patient on heparin infusion postoperatively. Bleeding complication occurred on the third postoperative day.

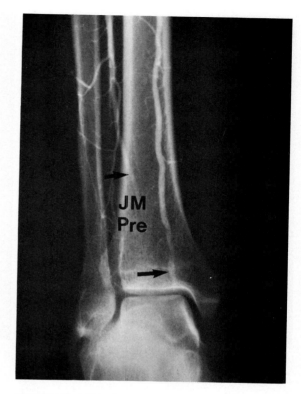

limb perfusion technique). Inflow was restored to the site of infusion in each instance by thrombectomy or bypass, whichever was necessary (Figs. 22-3 and 22-4). Limb salvage was achieved in 70%. In 47%, limb salvage was directly attributable to thrombolytic therapy. Since thrombectomy or bypass procedures also were performed in these patients, it often was difficult to determine precisely the predominant intervention contributing to the limb salvage. This occurred in 23%, and these were identified as indeterminate outcomes. Thirty percent ultimately had a major amputation. Although there was a 9% mortality, none of the deaths was thought to be due to the lytic therapy. One major bleeding complication occurred on the third postoperative day in a patient who was on heparin, and this was attributed to anticoagulation.

A promising new approach is "high-dose isolated limb perfusion."[13] This procedure is indicated in patients with multivessel occlusion in whom a single- or double-bolus infusion is likely to be inadequate and in patients in whom any degree of systemic fibrinolysis would pose significant risk. This technique includes full anticoagulation, exsanguination of venous blood from the limb with a rubber bandage, application of a tourniquet to achieve complete arterial and venous occlusion, direct arterial infusion into the affected vessels with a high dose of UK (1 million IU or more) or rt-PA (40 mg or more), and drainage of the venous effluent (Fig. 22-5). Infusion of a lytic agent in the limb for 45 to 60 min-

FIGURE 22-3. *Distal arteriogram of a 46-year-old woman presenting with acute arterial thrombosis of her right leg. Acute thrombus was present in the external iliac, common femoral, superficial femoral, and profunda femoris arteries. Additionally, arterial occlusion of the dorsalis pedis and posterior tibial arteries (arrows) is documented. The acute thrombus in large vessels was easily removed with balloon catheter thromboembolectomy. It was evident that without removal of the thrombus in the foot, the patient would require an amputation below the knee. One year earlier she had suffered an above-knee amputation on her opposite leg for an undefined coagulopathy resulting in massive arterial thrombosis. A cutdown on the dorsalis pedis and posterior tibial arteries was performed. A thrombectomy catheter could not be advanced distally; however, a small silicone catheter was placed and 50,000 IU of SK slowly infused into the foot. The arteriotomies were closed. This resulted in limb salvage with the loss of only one toe.*

utes has yielded impressive results in a small number of patients suffering from acute multivessel distal thrombi or emboli. Seven patients have been treated for severe ischemia with the isolated limb perfusion method. Four had a good response

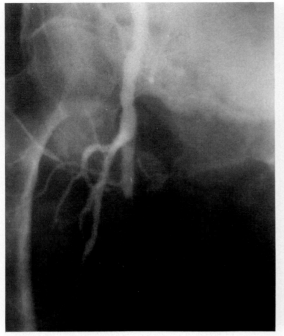

A

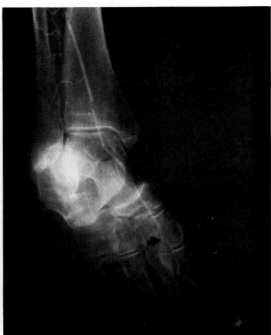

B

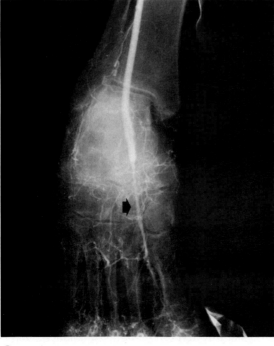

C

FIGURE 22-4. The use of intraoperative intraarterial thrombolysis to dissolve clots in the runoff bed before construction of a more proximal bypass. This patient presented with acute occlusion of her femoral–anterior tibial bypass graft. (A) All named arteries below the profunda femoris artery were occluded. The distal extent of the anterior tibial artery is visualized (B), showing progressive atherosclerotic disease in several areas. There was segmental occlusion of the dorsalis pedis artery (arrow) that appeared consistent with a thrombotic occlusion. UK (60,000 IU) was infused distally from an arteriotomy in the dorsalis pedis before thrombectomy of the femoral–anterior tibial artery bypass. Once thrombectomy was performed, the graft was extended to the dorsalis pedis with a 4-mm PTFE graft. A completion arteriogram (C) shows complete lysis of the thrombus in the distal dorsalis pedis artery. The patient was continued on low-dose warfarin, and her graft remained patent for 3.5 years.

with limb salvage, and three patients failed to improve. If distal vessel occlusion is due to atheromatous emboli or organized thrombus, treatment has not been successful. This novel approach deserves further evaluation.

PROSPECTIVE STUDY OF INTRAOPERATIVE UK

The preceding discussion reviewed the role of intraoperative intraarterial delivery of thrombolytic agents. They have been shown to be effective in dissolving distal thrombi in occluded arteries and grafts, clearing the distal circulation before or after lower extremity operative reconstruction, and assisting in more effective mechanical removal of the thrombus.[14] However, high rates of bleeding complications have been reported.[8] During the evolution of intraarterial catheter-directed lytic therapy for arterial and vascular graft occlusion, UK has become the preferred agent because of its safety and efficacy profile. Recombinant tissue-type plasminogen activator (rt-PA) has been used less frequently.

The goal of intraoperative intraarterial thrombolytic therapy is to deliver a plasminogen activator at a high concentration to the thrombus, thereby promoting regional thrombolysis with minimal effects on plasma fibrinogen or clotting factors and with a low risk of bleeding complications. However, little information is available about the regional effects compared with the systemic effects of intraoperatively administered plasminogen activators. Moreover, the dose-response relationship to the infused plasminogen activators has not been evaluated. A prospective, multicenter randomized, blinded, and placebo controlled study was performed[15] to address a number of basic issues regarding intraoperative delivery of UK.

The purposes of this study were to evaluate

1. The regional and systemic effects on plasma fibrinogen and the fibrinolytic system of intraoperative intraarterial urokinase infusion.
2. Whether there is a dose-response relationship.

3. Whether there is breakdown of cross-linked fibrin in a limb undergoing routine lower extremity revascularization (chronic limb ischemia) following a bolus dose of UK.
4. Whether there is an increased risk of excessive bleeding, operative blood loss, or wound hematomas.

Materials and Methods

One-hundred and thirty-four patients were prospectively randomized to receive one of three doses of UK or a saline placebo infusion in a blinded fashion into the distal arterial circulation during routine infrainguinal lower extremity revascularization for chronic limb ischemia. The endpoints to be analyzed were the degree of plasminogen activation, the regional and systemic breakdown of fibrinogen and fibrin, the degree to which a dose-response relationship could be established, and the safety of intraoperative intraarterially infused urokinase. One of three doses of study drug or placebo was infused in a 30-cc volume as a bolus through the distal arteriotomy at the time of vascular reconstruction. Patient groups included (1) placebo (saline), (2) UK125 (urokinase, 125,000 IU), (3) UK250 (urokinase, 250,000 IU), and (4) UK500 (urokinase, 500,000 IU).

Blood samples (20 cc) were drawn simultaneously from the ipsilateral femoral vein to evaluate regional effects and the arm to evaluate the systemic effects at four time points: (1) preinfusion (pre)—following heparinization but prior to vascular clamping; (2) prereperfusion (prere)—after vascular reconstruction was completed but before vascular clamps were removed; (3) postreperfusion (postre)—approximately 1 minute after vascular clamps were removed and reperfusion restored; and (4) 2 hours (2 h) after the study drug was infused. The 2-h sample was a systemic sample only because by this time most patients were in the recovery room. A standardized dose of heparin was given intravenously (75 IU/kg) before vascular clamping, and subsequent anticoagulation or dextran was withheld until after the 2-h blood sample was drawn.

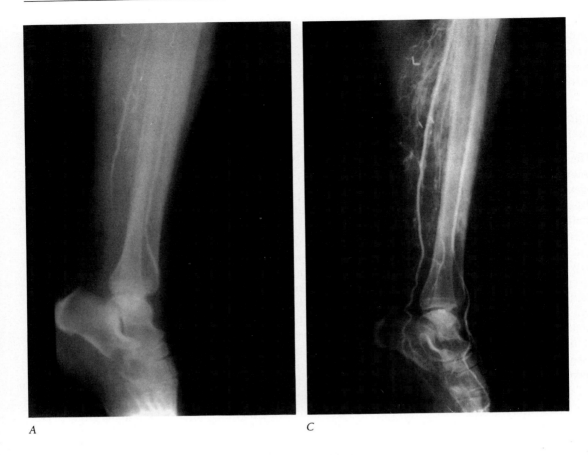

A

C

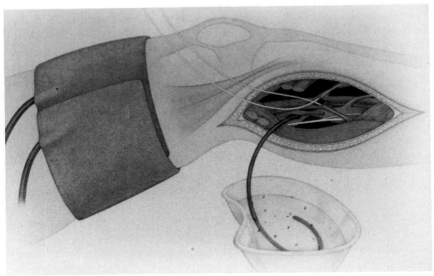

B

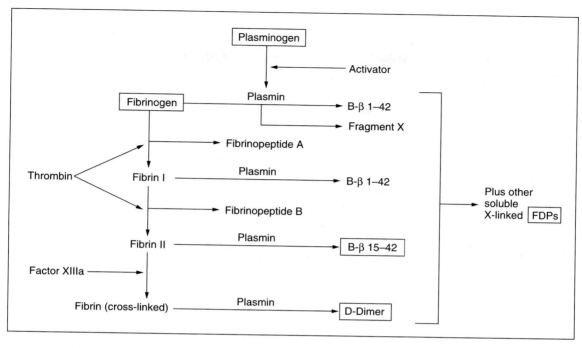

FIGURE 22-6. Schematic diagram of the markers of thrombin and plasmin-mediated proteolysis of fibrinogen and fibrin. ▭ = analyzed as endpoints of study.

Blood samples were analyzed at a central core laboratory at the Sol Sherry Thrombosis Research Center (Temple University School of Medicine, Philadelphia, PA) for (1) plasminogen activity, (2) fibrinogen, (3) fibrin(ogen) degradation products (FDPs), (4) D-dimer, and (5) fibrinopeptide

$B-\beta_{15-42}$ breakdown product. When thrombin interacts with fibrinogen, fibrin I and fibrin II are formed by the sequential release of fibrinopeptides A and B. Fibrin II is subsequently cross-linked by activated factor XIII (Fig. 22-6). Activation of plasminogen results in the formation of

FIGURE 22-5. The technique of high-dose isolated limb perfusion of a thrombolytic agent in a patient who could not have any degree of systemic fibrinolysis (having had a coronary artery bypass 2 days earlier) and who had acute multivessel distal occlusion that was unlikely to resolve with a single bolus of a fibrinolytic agent. The patient had an acute embolic/thrombotic arterial occlusion after percutaneous removal of an intraaortic balloon, which was required following her emergency coronary artery bypass. Shown is the intraoperative arteriogram after balloon catheter thrombectomy of her popliteal and tibial vessels. Additional thrombus could not be mechanically removed. Catheters were placed into the origin of the posterior tibial and anterior tibial arteries, and the arteriogram (A) was performed with this selective injection technique. There was no evidence of contrast material entering the foot. Since additional thrombus could not be retrieved, we believed the patient would suffer a major amputation. (B) The patient's limb was elevated and the venous blood exsanguinated with a rubber bandage. A sterile blood pressure cuff (tourniquet) was placed on the distal thigh and inflated to 250 mmHg. The popliteal vein was cannulated with a red rubber catheter and drained into a basin. One million units of UK was infused into the lower leg in a volume of 1 L of saline (500,000 IU in each of the anterior tibial and posterior tibial arteries) over 20 min. Following completion of the UK infusion, the limb was flushed with a heparin-saline solution. The venotomy was closed primarily, and the arteriotomy closed with a patch. (C) A postinfusion arteriogram documented significant improvement of perfusion to the foot. The patient had a palpable dorsalis pedis pulse and a pink foot following wound closure.

plasmin, which has proteolytic effects on fibrinogen, fibrin, and cross-linked fibrin. The assays used to measure degradation products (FDPs) do not distinguish between those from fibrinogen or fibrin. However, specific markers are available to detect plasmin-induced breakdown of fibrin and cross-linked fibrin. Action of plasmin on fibrin results in the formation of fragment B-β_{15-42}, and on cross-linked fibrin, production of D-dimer.

Statistical Analysis

For the laboratory data, the change from baseline (pre) values were calculated for each time point of prereperfusion, postreperfusion, and 2-h postreperfusion. Changes from baseline were compared between each dosage level and placebo using the maximum change from baseline in the expected direction assuming a treatment effect. Due to skewness of the data, median values were used for calculating the significance of maximum change. All comparisons between dosage levels and the placebo group were performed by Wilcoxon rank-sum analysis. Due to the number of comparisons being made, a more conservative level of significance of $p < 0.01$ was chosen for analysis of blood sample results.

Results

Patient characteristics were similar among treatment groups (Table 22-3), with the exception that

TABLE 22-3. Patient Characteristics According to Treatment Group

	Treatment Group				
	Placebo	UK125	UK250	UK500	Total
No.	33	32	34	35	134
Sex (%)					
Male	4.7	61.3	55.9	51.4	58.2
Female	35.3	38.7	44.1	48.6	41.8
Age (years)	63.0	69.4	69.6	67.1	67.2 ($p = 0.042$)*
Race (%)					
Caucasian	76.5	67.7	70.6	60.0	68.7
Black	14.7	25.8	23.5	31.4	23.9
Hispanic	2.9	3.2	2.9	8.6	4.5
Other	5.9	3.2	2.9	0.0	3.0
Diabetes (%)	41.2	48.4	47.1	51.4	47.0
CAD (%)	44.1	32.3	23.5	40.0	35.1
Hypertension (%)	32.4	51.6	44.1	54.3	45.5
Stroke (%)	2.9	9.7	11.8	11.4	9.0
Smokers (%)					
Yes	64.5	76.7	67.7	80.0	72.4
No	35.5	23.3	32.3	20.0	27.6
Signs/symptoms (%)					
Claudication	29.4	19.4	20.6	20.0	22.4
Rest pain	8.8	25.8	17.6	34.3	21.6
Tissue necrosis	58.8	51.6	58.8	45.7	53.7
None	2.9	3.2	2.9	0.0	2.3
Operative procedure (%)					
Saphenous vein	61.8	71.0	70.6	74.3	69.4
Prosthetic	26.5	22.6	11.8	14.3	18.7
Other	11.7	6.4	17.6	11.4	11.9
Anesthesia					
General	61.8	61.3	67.6	60.0	62.7
Epidural	32.4	29.0	32.4	34.3	32.1
Other	5.8	9.7	0.0	5.7	5.2

*By analysis of variance, only age was significantly different between placebo and treatment groups (UK125 and UK250). All other differences were not significant.

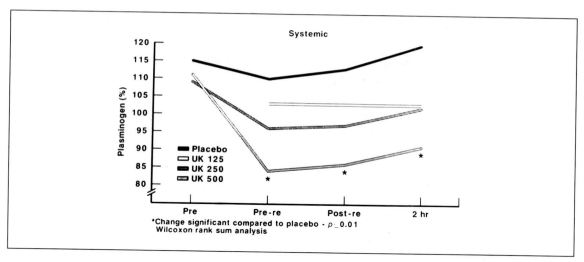

FIGURE 22-7. Mean plasma plasminogen levels in the systemic circulation by time period and dosage level. There appears to be a dose-related decline in plasminogen in the UK500 group which is significantly different from the placebo group (p < 0.001; normal = 112 ± 22%). *p < 0.001.

those in the placebo group were younger than patients receiving UK ($p = 0.042$). There were no significant differences across treatment groups with respect to the distribution of associated risk factors, degree of ischemia at presentation, type of operative procedure, or anesthesia administered.

Figures 22-7 to 22-11 show the plasma levels of the measured proteins by treatment group for each time point. Plasma plasminogen activity

(Fig. 22-7) was measured in the systemic circulation only. Compared with the placebo group, there was a dose-dependent decline in plasminogen activity which was significant ($p < 0.001$) only at the highest dose. Even at UK500, however, the mean values were still within the normal range. There was no significant decline in either the regional or systemic plasma fibrinogen following bolus UK infusion (Fig. 22-8). The plasma

FIGURE 22-8. Mean plasma fibrinogen levels in the regional and systemic circulations by time period and dosage level. There was no significant change in any of the UK treatment groups compared with placebo (normal = 294 ± 64 mg/dL).

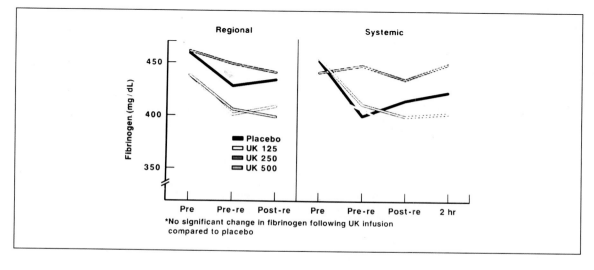

FDP levels (Fig. 22-9) were elevated in the treatment group in a dose-related fashion, with increases becoming significant ($p < 0.001$) relative to the placebo group at UK250 and UK500 in the regional circulation and at UK500 systemically ($p = 0.01$). There were significant elevations of D-dimer (Fig. 22-10) regionally at each UK dose ($p < 0.001$) which increased in a dose-response fashion. Systemic levels of D-dimer became significantly elevated at UK250 and UK500 ($p < 0.001$). Lastly, fragment B-β_{15-42} levels (Fig. 22-11) showed a trend toward elevation at the higher doses of UK but achieved significance only at UK500 ($p = 0.009$) at the prereperfusion time point in the systemic circulation.

Table 22-4 shows the maximal changes from baseline observed in the plasma measurements for each dosage level. Table 22-5 lists patient morbidity and mortality according to treatment groups. There was no difference in blood loss, the amount of blood replaced, or the assessment of excessive operative bleeding for any patient group. There was no difference in the frequency of wound hematomas comparing patients receiving UK with those receiving placebo. There is a trend toward a shorter length of stay in the

placebo group (10.8 days) compared with the treatment groups (15.6 to 22.7 days; $p = 0.06$). An unexpected finding was the increased mortality in the placebo group (12.1% in placebo compared with 2.0% in patients receiving UK; $p = 0.033$). There were no significant differences between the maximal changes noted in the systemic and regional circulations for any of the plasma measurements.

Discussion

An important observation of this multicenter, randomized study was the safety of intraoperatively infused UK in bolus doses up to 500,000 IU. No bleeding complications were identified. The increased mortality (12%) in the placebo group was an unexpected finding and cannot be easily explained. Interestingly, in another recent prospective, randomized study comparing catheter-directed thrombolysis with surgery in patients with acute limb ischemia, patients in the thrombolytic group had significantly better survival than patients randomized to surgery.[16] In our study, the postoperative length of stay appeared to be longer in the UK groups, although this was not

FIGURE 22-9. Mean levels of fibrin(ogen) degradation products (FDPs) in the regional and systemic circulations by time period and dosage level. The FDPs were significantly elevated regionally and systemically at all time periods in the UK500 group ($p < 0.001$). There was a significant systemic elevation after reperfusion in the UK250 group ($p < 0.001$).

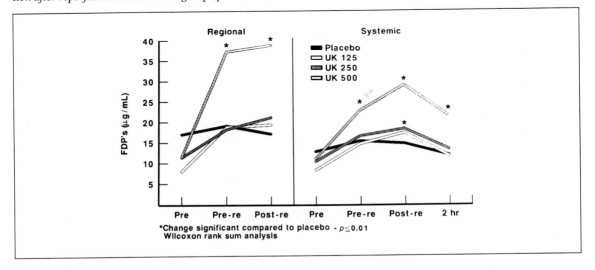

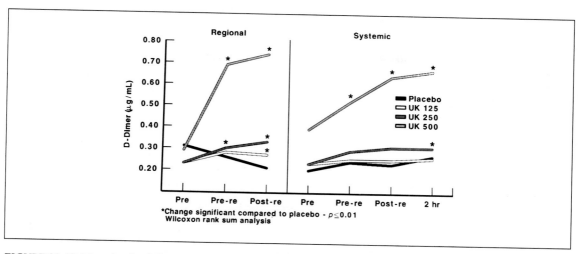

FIGURE 22-10. Mean levels of plasma D-dimer in the regional and systemic circulations by time period and dosage level (normal = 0.083 ± 0.014 μg/mL). Note the significant and dose-related elevations at all doses of UK regionally and at UK250 and UK500 systemically.

statistically significant (see Table 22-3). Since two deaths occurred by the second postoperative day and two deaths occurred 1 month postoperatively, the mortality in the placebo group was not a factor influencing length of stay. The longer mean length of stay in the UK-treated patients may be due to several outliers, some remaining hospitalized for more than 3 months. The fact that patients in the placebo group were significantly younger and more were treated for intermittent claudication also may have influenced postoperative length of stay. The median values for length of

FIGURE 22-11. Mean levels of B-β_{15-42} in the regional and systemic circulations by time period and dosage level (normal = 6.9 ± 1.1 pmol/mL). There appear to be dose-related increases in B-β_{15-42}; however, the only significant elevation occurred in the UK500-treated patients at the prereperfusion time point.

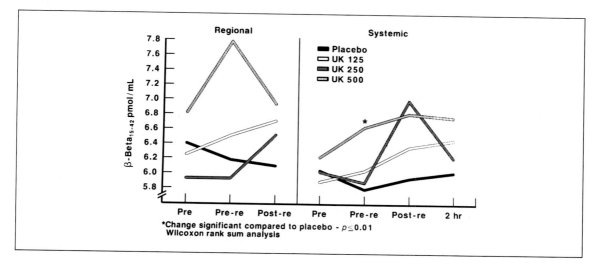

TABLE 22-4. *Maximal Changes from Baseline (values reported as mean/median)*

	Placebo ($n = 33$)	UK125 ($n = 32$)	UK250 ($n = 34$)	UK500 ($n = 35$)
Regional				
Plasminogen (%)	NA	NA	NA	NA
Fibrinogen (mg/dL)	−30.72/−27.00	−28.62/−28.0	−20.35/−22.00	−38.97/−41.00
FDPs (μg/mL)	2.75/0.00	11.25/0.00	9.65/0.00	27.20/18.00 ($p < 0.001$)
D-Dimer (μg/mL)	−0.106/−0.003	0.035/0.008 ($p < 0.001$)	0.100/0.029 ($p < 0.001$)	0.401/0.127 ($p < 0.001$)
B-β_{15-42} (pmol/mL)	−0.305/−0.226	0.461/0.143	0.595/0.136 ($p = 0.021$)	0.952/0.296 ($p = 0.017$)
Systemic				
Plasminogen (%)	−4.62/−6.50	−9.53/−10.50	−13.03/−15.00 ($p = 0.052$)	−27.46/−23.00 ($p < 0.001$)
Fibrinogen (mg/dL)	−43.78/−30.00	−30.52/−28.00	4.34/−10.00 ($p = 0.018$)	−50.91/−56.00
FDPs (μg/mL)	3.45/0.00	9.12/0.00	7.74/8.00 ($p = 0.005$)	18.00/10.00 ($p < 0.001$)
D-Dimer (μg/mL)	0.066/0.003	0.026/0.003	0.069/0.035 ($p = 0.005$)	0.288/0.111 ($p < 0.001$)
B-β_{15-42} (pmol/mL)	−0.249/−0.075	0.572/0.125	0.199/0.234 ($p = 0.025$)	0.552/0.301 ($p = 0.001$)

Note: p values refer to comparisons to placebo and were calculated using the Wilcoxon rank-sum analysis. $p < 0.05$ values are listed, but significance is assigned at $p \leq 0.01$.

stay, however, are relatively consistent for all treatment groups and placebo.

The goal of regionally delivered plasminogen activators is to achieve fibrinolysis with minimal breakdown of fibrinogen, clotting factors, and other plasma proteins. A major purpose of our study was to assess the impact of the intraoperative use of UK on plasminogen activation and lysis of fibrinogen and fibrin in the regional and systemic circulations. There was a dose-dependent decline in plasma plasminogen levels (see Fig. 22-7), indicating plasminogen activation, particularly at the highest dose. Although regional levels were not measured, it is reasonable to assume the same dose-response locally also, where the UK levels would be higher than peripherally. Activation of plasminogen results in the generation of plasmin, which induces lysis of fibrin clots as well as circulating fibrinogen with formation of degradation products. Of particular importance is the finding that even at the highest concentration of UK administered, there was no significant decline in plasma fibrinogen levels over those noted in the placebo group. The plasma levels of FDPs, which reflect the break-

down of both fibrin and fibrinogen, were significantly elevated (see Fig. 22-8). Overall, the changes in fibrinogen, plasminogen, and FDPs noted in our study are substantially lower than those noted in studies where thrombolytic agents have been administered to patients with acute myocardial infarction,[17,18] where much higher doses of thrombolytic agents are infused systemically over a longer duration. Our patients had relatively small doses of UK given intraarterially as a bolus into a relatively stagnant distal circulation.

Of particular interest to us was to determine if administration of UK would result in lysis of fibrin regionally and in the distal arterial bed, which would be a potentially beneficial effect. Because the FDP assay measures the sum of the breakdown products of fibrin and fibrinogen, additional markers of plasmin-mediated proteolysis were used to differentiate between the breakdown of fibrin and cross-linked fibrin (see Fig. 22-6). The action of plasmin on fibrin results in the release of fibrinopeptide B-β_{15-42}. Fragment D-dimer is derived from the action of plasmin on cross-linked fibrin. There was significant elevation in D-dimer levels regionally at all doses of UK and

TABLE 22-5. Patient Morbidity and Mortality According to Treatment Group

	Treatment Group					
	Placebo	UK125	UK250	UK500	Total	
Blood loss (mL)						
Mean	306.1	420.7	355.2	368.1	361.2	
Median	250.0	350.0	325.0	300.0	300.0	$(p = 0.12)$
Blood replaced (mL)						
Mean	146.9	150.0	140.9	187.6	156.8	
Median	0.0	0.0	0.0	0.0	0.0	$(p = 0.89)$
Excessive operative bleeding						
(% of patients)	5.9	9.7	2.9	2.9	5.2	$(p = 0.56)$
Wound hematoma (% of patients)						
None	91.2	86.7	87.5	94.1	90.0	
Mild	5.9	6.7	12.5	5.9	7.7	$(p = 0.71)$
Moderate–severe	2.9	6.6	0.0	0.0	2.3	
Death (%)	12.1	0.0	5.9	0.0	4.5	$(p = 0.034)$
Length of stay (postoperative days)						
Mean	10.8	22.7	15.7	16.2	16.3	
Median	9.5	16.0	9.0	11.0	10.0	$(p = 0.06)$

Significance: $p \leq 0.05$.

systemically at UK250 and UK500 (see Fig. 22-8). Levels of fragment B-β_{15-42} increased with increasing doses of UK but were significantly elevated in the systemic circulation at UK500. These findings suggest that there is degradation of fibrin by UK. The absence of such a rise in either B-β_{15-42} or D-dimer levels in the placebo group indicates that the observed elevations in the UK groups are not merely due to lysis by endogenous plasminogen activators of the clot formed during surgery to provide hemostasis. The elevated D-dimer levels suggest lysis of cross-linked fibrin in the regional circulation. It needs to be considered whether the observed high D-dimer levels are influenced by detection of other non-cross-linked FDPs in the assay, as reported by Lawler et al.[19] in subjects with extensive fibrinogen breakdown (>80% of baseline values) following administration of thrombolytic therapy. This is unlikely to be the case because in our patients the changes in plasma levels of plasminogen, FDPs, and D-dimer were substantially less than the levels observed by these authors, and more important, there was no significant decline in plasma fibrinogen levels. Moreover, no appreciable cross-reactivity with FDPs has been reported with the ELISA assay.[20,21]

Therefore, the elevated D-dimer levels suggest UK-induced dissolution of cross-linked fibrin in the extremity circulation. Whether such lysis of clinically silent fibrin deposits in the ischemic extremity translates into clinical benefit needs to be established.

Although the acutely ischemic limb with suspected distal thrombi is the most frequent indication for intraoperative fibrinolytic therapy, this study was designed to evaluate the effects of UK infusion in patients with chronic lower extremity ischemia with respect to its effects on activation of the fibrinolytic system and plasma fibrinogen. The significant dose-related elevation of D-dimer suggests that there is lysis of fibrin in the distal arterial circulation. If this is indeed the case, small distal vessel thrombosis may be part of the pathophysiology of chronic limb ischemia. Since no bleeding complications were observed, it seems reasonable to consider distal infusion of UK in patients undergoing operations for chronic severe limb ischemia. Although these results suggest that intraoperative UK infusion may be of value for patients undergoing revascularization for chronic limb ischemia, additional randomized studies are indicated to delineate clinical benefits.

Acknowledgments

Supported in part by NIH Grant K07 HL02658.

REFERENCES

1. Comerota AJ, Rubin R, Tyson R, et al. Intraarterial thrombolytic therapy in peripheral vascular disease. Surg Gynecol Obstet 1987;165:1.
2. Chaise LS, Comerota AJ, Soulen RL, et al. Selective intraarterial streptokinase therapy in the immediate postoperative period. JAMA 1982;247:2397.
3. Greep JM, Allman PJ, Janet F, et al. A combined technique for peripheral arterial embolectomy. Arch Surg 1972;105:869.
4. Plecha FR, Pories WJ. Intraoperative angiography in the immediate assessment of arterial reconstruction. Arch Surg 1972;105:902.
5. Quinones-Baldrich WJ, Ziomek S, Henderson TC, et al. Intraoperative fibrinolytic therapy: experimental evaluation. J Vasc Surg 1986;4:229.
6. Dunnant JR, Edwards WS. Small vessel occlusion in the extremity after periods of arterial obstruction: an experimental study. Surgery 1973;75:240.
7. Belkin M, Valeri R, Hobson RW. Intraarterial urokinase increases skeletal muscle viability after acute ischemia. J Vasc Surg 1989;9:161.
8. Cohen LJ, Kaplan M, Bernhard VM. Intraoperative fibrinolytic therapy: an adjunct to catheter thromboembolectomy. J Vasc Surg 1985;2:319.
9. Quinones-Baldrich WJ, Zierler RE, Hiatt JC. Intraoperative fibrinolytic therapy: an adjunct to catheter thromboembolectomy. J Vasc Surg 1985;2: 319.
10. Norem RF, Short DH, Kerstein MD. Role of intraoperative fibrinolytic therapy in acute arterial occlusion. Surg Gynecol Obstet 1988;167:87.
11. Garcia R, Saroyan RM, Senkowsky J, et al. Intraoperative, intraarterial urokinase infusion as an adjunct to Fogarty catheter embolectomy in acute arterial occlusion. Surg Gynecol Obstet 1990;171: 201.
12. Parent NE, Bernhard VM, Pabst TS, et al. Fibrinolytic treatment of residual thrombus after catheter embolectomy for severe lower limb ischemia. J Vasc Surg 1989;9:153.
13. Comerota AJ, White JV, Grosh JD. Intraoperative, intraarterial thrombolytic therapy for salvage of limbs in patients with distal arterial thrombosis. Surg Gynecol Obstet 1989;169:283.
14. Comerota AJ, White JV. Intraoperative, intraarterial thrombolytic therapy as an adjunct to revascularization in patients with residual distal arterial thrombus. Semin Vasc Surg 1992;5(2):110.
15. Comerota AJ, Rao AK, Throm RC, et al. A prospective, randomized, blinded, and placebo-controlled trial of intraoperative intraarterial urokinase infusion during lower extremity revascularization: regional and systemic effects. Ann Surg 1993;218 (4):534.
16. Ouriel K. Comparison of results: surgery or thrombolysis for acute limb ischemia. Symposium: thrombolytic therapy in the management of vascular disease. Satellite Symposium to the 11th UCLA Symposium: a comprehensive review and update of what's new in vascular surgery, Los Angeles, Oct 3–8, 1993.
17. Rao AK, Pratt C, Berke A, et al. Thrombolysis in myocardial infarction (TIMI) trial, phase I: hemorrhagic manifestations and changes in plasma plasminogen activator and streptokinase. J Am Coll Cardiol 1988;11:1.
18. Mueller HS, Rao AK, Forman SA, TIMI investigators. Thrombolysis in myocardial infarction (TIMI): comparative studies of coronary reperfusion and systemic fibrinogenolysis with two forms of recombinant tissue-type plasminogen activator. J Am Coll Cardiol 1987;10:479.
19. Lawler CM, Bovill EG, Stump DC, et al. Fibrin fragment D-dimer and fibrinogen Bβ peptides in plasma as markers of clot lysis during thrombolytic therapy in acute myocardial infarction. Blood 1990;76(7):1341.
20. Whitaker AN, Elms MJ, Masci PP, et al. Measurement of cross-linked fibrin derivatives in plasma: an immunoassay using monoclonal antibodies. J Clin Pathol 1984;37:882.
21. Elms MJ, Bundesen PG, Webber AJ, et al. Measurement of cross-linked fibrin degradation products: an immunoassay using monoclonal antibodies. Thromb Haemost 1983;50(2):591.

Anthony J. Comerota (Ed.). *Thrombolytic Therapy for Peripheral Vascular Disease.* Copyright © 1995 J. B. Lippincott Company.

23

THROMBOLYTIC THERAPY AND ANGIOPLASTY FOR TREATMENT OF CLOTTED AND FAILING HEMODIALYSIS ACCESS

Mark A. H. Cohen

David A. Kumpe

Janette D. Durham

There are at least 115,000 individuals in the United States with end-stage renal disease. In the absence of a successful renal transplantation, they require artificial dialysis for the rest of their lives. Eighty-five percent receive hemodialysis three times per week. Those undergoing hemodialysis require vascular access that is easily available and sustains a sufficiently high blood flow to allow uninterrupted shunting of at least 200 mL/min without thrombosis. Usually, the blood flow is 400 to 1500 mL/min.[1,2] The standard means of creating such an access is by surgically forming a subcutaneous arteriovenous conduit. The creation of a hemodialysis access site is now one of the most common vascular operations performed.[3]

These accesses have a high incidence of complications. Even the optimal access, an arteriovenous fistula (Brescia-Cimino fistula), has a high rate of failure. Complications associated with arteriovenous access are the most frequent cause of hospitalization for patients on chronic hemodialysis, who require, on average, approximately 1 month of hospitalization each year; half this time is for placement or revision of their arteriovenous communications.[4,5] Preservation of each access site is becoming more important as patients are being carried for longer periods on hemodialysis. In one series,[6] at 5-year follow-up, 73% of the surviving patients were still on hemodialysis (40% of the original cohort, while 40% had died and 16% had functioning renal allografts). Thus it is understandable that vascular access has been referred to as the "Achilles heel of the hemodialysis patient."[7,8]

The most common complication of the hemodialysis access is partial or complete obstruction of blood flow due to vascular stenosis or thrombosis. We will discuss the management and prevention of this complication. Management of less common complications, including aneurysm and pseudoaneurysm formation, steal syndrome, distal extremity edema, high-output congestive heart failure, and infection (particularly for prosthetic grafts), is beyond the intended scope of this chapter.

BACKGROUND

Types of Access for Hemodialysis

The types of accesses include external arteriovenous silicone cannula shunts (Quinton-Scribner), major venous cannulation with one or two catheters, native arteriovenous fistulas, and arteriovenous conduits created with prosthetic materials.

External Arteriovenous Shunts

Arteriovenous shunts[9] were the first method described for maintaining long-term access to the circulation among patients undergoing chronic hemodialysis. Now uncommonly used, the primary indication for their placement is patients who have acute, potentially reversible renal failure requiring repeated hemodialysis in whom major venous cannulation is contraindicated. Because of high rates of infection and thrombosis, these shunts are not satisfactory for chronic hemodialysis. The infection rate of these shunts is approximately 10 times higher, and their survival one-third as long, as that of arteriovenous fistulas.[10–12]

Venous Catheters

Major venous cannulation with polyurethane catheters is the principal means of obtaining immediate temporary access for hemodialysis. The catheters are used primarily in the setting of either chronic renal failure when the patient does not yet have a functional permanent access or acute renal failure if hemodialysis is needed. A double-lumen catheter is inserted into the superior or inferior vena cava, usually via a common femoral or subclavian vein route. The catheter is usually placed in the superior vena cava via a subclavian vein rather than an internal jugular vein because in this location the catheter can be easily covered with a sterile dressing. If the patient is bedridden, the catheter may be placed in a common iliac vein or inferior vena cava via a common femoral vein. These major venous access methods have supplanted the external arteriovenous silicone shunt in nearly all cases. However, subclavian insertion sites for these catheters are liable to develop stenoses[13] or thromboses[14,15] among chronic hemodialysis patients, particularly if the catheter is left in place for 4 weeks or more.[16–18]

Insertion of catheters in the internal jugular vein is also associated with a risk of central venous stenosis.[14] A prospective study before placement of a long-term dialysis graft demonstrated a 40% prevalence of moderate or severe subclavian vein stenosis in patients with prior or current ipsilateral subclavian temporary dialysis catheters.[19] Stenosis also has been reported in patients who have not had previous ipsilateral central venous cannulation.[20] Although stenoses in the innominate vein also are common, superior vena caval stenosis is relatively rare. The principal factor reported to be associated with an increased prevalence of central venous stenosis is prolonged central venous cannulation.[16,21] Female patients and those with a higher number of subclavian cannulations also have been reported to have an increased risk of stenosis.[21] The presence of a subclavian stenosis ipsilateral to an upper extremity vascular access often causes venous hypertension and marked upper extremity edema. Elevated venous pressure is a less specific presentation.[16] The reported intervals between the initial placement of the access and development of the edema has varied between 2 weeks and over 2 years.[16,17]

The stenosis may precipitate thrombosis of the access.[22] Because subclavian catheters can produce a subclavian stenosis, the use of large catheters in this location to "tide over" a hemodialysis patient whose access site has thrombosed is discouraged. Therefore, one goal in salvaging a thrombosed access is to have a technique that allows prompt use of the repaired access so that the interim placement of such subclavian catheters is not necessary. The frequency of use of subclavian catheters in the immediate posttreatment period after surgical revisions or lysis/angioplasty of thrombosed access sites, before dialysis is resumed, is seldom recorded by investigators.

Native Arteriovenous Fistulas

Since its description 27 years ago by Brescia et al.,[23] the optimal vascular access has been a native arteriovenous fistula (AVF) in an upper extremity. As a result of the formation of the fistula, there is dilation and arterialization (thickening of the vein wall) of the venous outflow. The fistula is usually created by anastomosis of the end or side of the cephalic vein to the side of the radial artery. Fistulas can be created between the basilic vein and the ulnar artery, but these are associated with a higher rate of thrombosis[24] and of finger ischemia, particularly in diabetics.[25,26] Other sites include more distal placement of the fistula in the snuff box,[27,28] fistulas between the brachial artery and cephalic vein of the upper arm,[29] and fistulas between the saphenous vein and the side of the femoral artery (saphenous loop).[30] AVFs are not commonly formed in the lower extremities because of a high infection rate[31,32] and poor accessibility. AVFs should be placed well in advance of their anticipated use to allow for maturation, since they usually require at least 3 to 8 weeks for sufficient venous dilation to allow for easy percutaneous access.[6] Patients who have very large veins can sometimes be dialyzed within several days of placement of the fistula. However, punctures performed when the veins are still thin-walled can result in early venous stenosis. The principal disadvantage of AVFs is that many patients do not have sufficiently large caliber superficial vessels in proximity to one another to allow formation of an adequate AVF. This may be because of small, atherosclerotic, or heavily calcified distal arteries in the wrist, particularly in diabetics; inadequately developed superficial veins in the forearm; deeply embedded forearm veins, usually in obese persons; or fibrosis of the forearm veins from previous intravenous lines, drug abuse, or external shunts. Early thrombosis is more common in AVFs than in prosthetic grafts and is due in part to adventitial bands, traumatized veins, twisted veins, and veins with proximal stenosis or sclerosis from previous phlebitis. These early failures cannot generally be corrected, and new accesses must be created as replacements.[31,33] On the other hand, AVFs, once functioning, have much lower long-term complication and failure rates than any other alternative long-term access. Table 23-1 shows published survival rates for AVFs. Although there is a relatively high failure rate during the first year, AVFs may survive more than 10 years.

Prosthetic Conduits

Since many hemodialysis patients initially do not have adequate native vessels to form an AVF or

TABLE 23-1. *Secondary Patency Rates of AVFs (percent)*

Author (No.)	1 Year	2 Years	3 Years
Kinnaert (202)	88	88	82
Rohr (126)	65	55	55
Silcott (78)	75	67	62
Kherlakian (100)	71	66	64
Palder (154)	60	53	45
Stevens (40)	95	87	

have failed AVFs, prosthetic conduits are commonly inserted as an alternative. In many medical centers, more prosthetic conduits are created than AVFs.[6,33] Prosthetic fistulas are now the most common type of vascular access in older patients, who now undergo dialysis with increasing frequency, because of the difficulty in finding satisfactory veins to create a new native fistula.[34] With the continued increase in the lifespan and average age of patients receiving hemodialysis, it is likely that the need for prosthetic accesses will increase.

There have been extensive studies to define the optimal prosthetic conduit. Autologous[30,35] and homologous[36-38] arteries and veins, human umbilical veins,[39,40] woven Dacron grafts,[41,42] and bovine arteries[35,43-46] have been used with some success. However, expanded polytetrafluoroethylene (ePTFE) grafts have proven to be superior to these and are now the standard prosthetic graft.[6,43,47-50] Expanded PTFE is easily inserted, is easily thrombectomized or recanalized with lytic agents with an acceptable patency, has moderate resistance to infection, and has a low incidence of aneurysm formation.[51-53] The ultrastructure of PTFE allows tissue ingrowth between fibrils, which results in transmural fibrous tissue and the formation of a neointima.[54] The fibrous tissue seals the opening in the prosthesis caused by each needle puncture. PTFE accesses are placed preferentially in the upper extremities because of the higher risk of infection for lower extremity grafts[55] and because, if arterial ligation is later necessary to treat a graft infection, limb-threatening ischemia can develop in the leg, whereas ischemia is rarely a problem in the upper extremity because of the richer collateral circulation in the arm.[3] Typically, PTFE grafts are placed as a straight segment or as a loop in either the forearm or arm. Although there have been no controlled studies, some retrospective investigations have suggested that forearm loop grafts have higher rates of patency than other grafts,[33,50,56,57] although other investigators favor straight grafts in the upper arm.[3] As the standard access sites fail in patients undergoing chronic hemodialysis, other sites in both the upper and lower extremities are utilized.[3,56] The usual graft diameter is 6 to 8 mm.[58]

PTFE grafts have a lower incidence of early thrombosis than AVFs because they are anastomosed to proximal vessels in the forearm, which are larger than the distal vessels typically used for AVFs. The placement of PTFE grafts is a technically less demanding operation, and the grafts have higher early postoperative flow rates than AVFs. For example, in Kherlakian's series,[6] early thrombosis (≤6 weeks after placement) occurred in 12% of the radial-cephalic arteriovenous fistula group and in 4% of the expanded PTFE graft group. Early thrombosis after placement of a PTFE graft is usually due to a technical error at the anastomosis, an anatomic problem such as an inadequate artery or vein, graft kinking, or graft compression due to a perigraft hematoma.[59] Nevertheless, PTFE grafts have higher rates of infection, pseudoaneurysm formation, venous hypertension, arterial steal and thrombosis than AVFs.[5,6,10,11,60–63] Despite aggressive treatment of access complications, with surgical revision if necessary, the 2-year patency rate for these accesses is usually 50% to 60%,[6,50,56,57,64–66] with a few reports in the 70% to 80% range[33,59,67] (Table 23-2). PTFE

grafts are therefore inserted only when native arteriovenous fistulas cannot be created.

FAILURE / THROMBOSIS

While the list of early and late complications of hemodialysis accesses, both native arteriovenous fistulas and prosthetics, is long, the most common problems are vascular stenosis and thrombosis, which account for over 80% of all complications of both AVFs and PTFE grafts.[6,33,50,64,66,68] We will confine our discussion to the management of these conditions.

Causes of Thrombosis

Stenosis at or near the venous anastomosis is the most common cause of late access thrombosis among both PTFE grafts and AVFs, being identified as the etiology in 58% to 81% of cases. Sites of stenosis among PTFE grafts are shown in Table 23-3.[50,53] Most stenoses in AVFs are located in the efferent limb, just distal to the anastomosis and near the site of arterial puncture.[69] The relative frequency of anatomic causes for AVF thromboses are discussed in a report by Romero et al.[70] They stated that 17% of thromboses were due to an arterial stenosis within a few millimeters of the anastomosis, 35% were due to venous stenosis within a few centimeters of the anastomosis, and 35% were due to both arterial and venous stenoses. In 13% of the thromboses, no anatomic cause was discerned. For clotted PTFE grafts, failure to identify a cause of thrombosis during surgical revision is a common problem; in series other than those cited in Table 23-3, no cause for the thrombosis was established in 42% to 52% of cases.[56,64,71,72] On the other hand, Valji et al.,[53] in a series of clotted PTFE grafts treated with interventional radiologic techniques (fibrinolysis and angioplasty), an anatomic cause for thrombosis was identified in 92% of cases. The discrepancy may be due to the better angiographic evaluation possible during lysis/angioplasty. Less common causes of access thrombosis are arterial and intragraft stenosis, subclavian vein stenosis, volume depletion, hypotension, heart failure, and external compression. Many dialysis nurses with whom we have

TABLE 23-2. Secondary Patency Rates
of PTFE Grafts (percent)

Author (No.)	1 Year	2 Years	3 Years	5 Years
Sterioff (203)	87	83	75	—
Munda (67)	67	50	—	—
Tordoir (100)	74	59	59	47
Kherlakian (100)	75	61	50	—
Rizzuti (189)	76	—	50	40
Puckett (127)	95	81	70	—
Sicard (185)	66	48	40	—
Palder (163)	80	68	68	—

TABLE 23-3. Etiology of Thrombosis of PTFE Grafts (percent)

Author (No.)	Venous Anastomosis Stenosis	Arterial Stenosis	Distal Venous Stenosis	None	Other
Munda (40)	58	7	0	35	0
Valji (117)	77	18	9	4	15

talked think that the incidence of access thrombosis has risen since the use of erythropoietin in dialysis patients was started several years ago. If this observation proves correct, the higher hematocrits presumably produce higher blood viscosity and a higher tendency for thrombosis.

Venous stenoses occur significantly more often with PTFE grafts than with Brescia-Cimino fistulas, and patients with Brescia-Cimino fistulas require fewer operative repair procedures. Swedberg et al.[5] found that failure due to venous stenosis occurred at 22.3 ± 13.1 months for Brescia-Cimino fistulas and at 16.0 ± 15.0 months ($p < 0.25$, NS) for PTFE grafts, although significant stenosis has been reported in PTFE grafts as early as 2 months.[50]

A detailed study of the histology of the intimal hyperplasia causing stenosis at hemodialysis access PTFE venous anastomosis sites has been published.[5] Immunocytochemical stains demonstrated that the intimal hyperplasia consists of a cellular and an extracellular component. The cellular element is almost exclusively composed of smooth-muscle cells. Smooth-muscle cells near the media contained more actin than those near the lumen, suggesting that the latter are younger, less well differentiated proliferating cells. Within the extracellular matrix, there are uniform gradients of collagen, elastin, and proteoglycan from the intima to the lumen, with collagen and elastin being most concentrated deep in the intima and proteoglycan most concentrated near the lumen. There was an absence of consistent signs of fibrin or hemosiderin within the intima and an absence of intimal macrophages and of intracellular or extracellular lipid deposits. The authors interpret these findings as suggesting that the intimal cellular proliferation is a steadily progressive rather than episodic process and that it is not due to subclinical thrombosis at the venous anastomosis or

to lipid accumulation. They postulated that the hyperplasia is due to two local factors—the release within the graft of platelet-derived growth factor due to platelet deposition at the puncture sites and localized intimal injury caused by highly turbulent blood flow at the anastomosis. The process is quite similar or identical to that causing stenoses near anastomoses in arterial bypass grafts and coronary artery bypass grafts.[73,74] The smooth-muscle nature of the stenosis accounts for its relatively poor long-term response to balloon dilation, since this is a different lesion from the atheromatous plaques that respond well to balloon dilation because of the known mechanism of dilation of atheromatous lesions, in which there is fracture of the stenosing plaque, separation of the plaque from the medial and adventitial layers of the artery, and stretching of the media and adventitia.[75] Intimal hyperplasia is more likely to undergo elastic recoil after being stretched by a balloon catheter.

Intragraft stenoses, occurring particularly at sites of repeated needle punctures, were reported in one study to be composed of stratified organizing thrombus rather than smooth-muscle-cell proliferation.[59] It is not clear whether the mechanism of intragraft stenosis formation is significantly different from that of anastomotic stenoses.

Clinical Presentation of a Failing Access Site

The best time to treat a failing hemodialysis access site is before it thromboses, although clinical evaluation can be difficult. Rising venous pressures and poor flow, sometimes accompanied by a decrease in the palpable anastomotic thrill or audible bruit or the presence of a palpable cord in the region of the venous anastomosis, characterize the clinical findings during this period. Poor flow during dialysis with collapse of the vein or graft ("arterial sucking") suggests an arterial anastomosis or arterial inflow problem. Failing Brescia-Cimino fistulas with an anastomosis near the wrist may have arterialization of the hand veins and localized edema of the hand and forearm or even localized edema of several fingers due to venous hypertension in the remaining patent veins in the hand.[76]

Hemodynamic and laboratory parameters are also helpful in evaluation of shunt function. Elevated venous pressures predicted venous stenosis with a sensitivity of 86% and a specificity of 93% in one recent study of patients undergoing dialysis at blood flow rates of 225 mL/min or less.[34] Whether measurement for elevated venous pressures is useful in all settings is not yet tested. High-efficiency hemodialysis is a new method in which blood is circulated at higher flow rates (350 to 450 mL/min instead of the traditional 150 to 250 mL/min) with resultant rapid dialysis and ultrafiltration. In this setting it is not known whether elevation of venous pressures is a useful means of detecting stenoses. Mixing of arterial and venous blood (recirculation) in the extracorporeal circulation also occurs with poor circulation through the fistula. In the setting of high-efficiency hemodialysis, detection of small amounts of recirculation through the dialyzer, calculated as an index of urea levels in the arterial line, venous line, and peripheral circulation, has been shown to be a specific method of detecting vascular stenoses in patients with PTFE grafts.[77] Eighty-two percent of patients with a recirculation fraction above 15% had significant stenoses (82% specificity), although the sensitivity of the method is not yet established.

The presence of low blood flow rates in grafts has been suggested as a means of identifying accesses at risk of thrombosis. Blood flow rates can be estimated from measurements of graft diameter and velocity with duplex ultrasound. Two studies suggest that accesses with a blood flow rate below 450 to 500 mL/min are at high risk for thrombosis within 9 weeks.[1,2] The utility of detecting a decrease in blood flow rate as a sign of vascular stenosis has not been directly demonstrated. Color Doppler sonography, which provides simultaneous information on vascular anatomy and flow, is potentially well suited to detect the presence of stenoses in vascular accesses. Preliminary results indicate that it reliably detects venous anastomotic stenoses noninvasively in PTFE grafts[78] but is less likely to be as useful in evaluating AVFs. Stenoses near the anastomosis in AVFs and complex perianastomotic venous collaterals may be difficult to interpret.[78,79]

In our own practice, we have found fistulography performed immediately after dialysis, before the dialysis needles are removed, to be the fastest and most accurate study to evaluate the need for intervention (see "Technique of Fistulography," below).

After thrombosis, the anastomotic bruit/thrill disappears entirely. The acutely thrombosed graft and draining vein are often tender. The diagnosis is often first made when puncture of the access yields no flow or only clots on aspiration of the dialysis needle. An important technical point, if thrombolytic treatment of the thrombosed site is planned, is for the dialysis nurses to leave the puncture needle in place. It may be that the needle can be used as a site for insertion of an infusion catheter, but even if not, the needle will tamponade potential hemorrhage from this site during lysis. If more than one needle is placed before the diagnosis of thrombosis is made, each needle should be left in place until after completion of lysis.

SURGICAL MANAGEMENT OF THROMBOSED ACCESS SITES

Thrombectomy

The traditional management of a thrombosed access has been a simple thrombectomy with an access revision if indicated. These procedures are usually performed under regional anesthesia within several days after the thrombosis is detected, although textbooks state that thrombectomies can be performed as late as 2 weeks after the thrombosis. If the access salvage procedure is uncomplicated, the patient is usually hospitalized overnight, although these procedures are also performed as an outpatient in some centers. In the absence of marked postoperative edema, the access can be used immediately, but care must be taken not to puncture the graft at the precise site of the revision. However, not infrequently, there is enough swelling around the graft after the revision that the graft cannot be used for several days. A simple thrombectomy is done via a small transverse incision, in the case of an autogenous AVF, near its anastomosis, in the case of a synthetic graft, near the venous anastomosis for straight forearm grafts, and at the nadir of the loop for loop grafts.[59,71] The clot is then removed with a Fogarty balloon-tipped catheter. The surgeon attempts to determine whether the thrombosis is due to a mechanical obstruction primarily by the resistance to passage of the catheter or of coronary dilators through the graft and its anastomoses. There are varied opinions about the utility of the estimate of stenosis obtained with the dilators.[71,80] Operative angiography[59] and angioscopy also may be used. An early reocclusion following a simple thrombectomy is often a sign of a residual untreated vascular stenosis. If a stenosis is present, then either a patch angioplasty, an interpositional graft, or less commonly, a venous endarterectomy is performed with the thrombectomy.

Surgical Revision

A patch angioplasty is usually performed to correct a local vascular narrowing due to a venous anastomosis stenosis. A longitudinal incision is made over the venous stenosis, and a small patch of native vein or prosthetic material is sutured in place, thereby widening the narrowed lumen. Placement of an interpositional graft involves cutting the distal end of the graft at or near the venous anastomosis, suturing an additional graft to the original graft, and anastomosing the other end of the new segment to normal vein above the stenosis. Interposition provides the most definitive surgical correction of anastomotic stenoses and can bypass stenoses which extend well beyond the immediate anastomosis. The relative efficacies of thrombectomy alone, patch angioplasty, and interposition are not well defined. In an uncontrolled, retrospective study comparing access patency following each of these three procedures, accesses treated by interpositional bypass had a statistically significant longer patency than the others.[33] On the other hand, surgical revision, especially interpositional bypass of outflow stenoses, has the major drawback of extending the vascular access graft further up the extremity; more proximal sites for potential future accesses may be permanently lost.

Surgical therapy of stenoses in the axillary and subclavian veins is technically difficult.[34] Thus there have been relatively few reports of surgical repair of stenosed or occluded subclavian veins.[81,82] Percutaneous angioplasty with and without stent placement has been the principal means of correcting central venous stenoses (see "Angioplasty for Maintenance of Access Patency," below).

Excluding reports before 1980, the initial success of thrombectomy/revision in reestablishing function of the dialysis access site is 70% to 100% for all patients with thrombosed access sites and 84% to 100% in patients who actually undergo the procedure.[33,52,64,65,83] The long-term patency rates following thrombectomy with or without a revision are not well defined, since most investigators have reported secondary patency results for all accesses rather than the results of the accesses requiring revision.[6,33,50,52,56,68,71] Only one report of which we are aware lists the unassisted patency after the first access site revision.[59] Most accesses remain patent for at least 1 month following a thrombectomy.[52,64,65,71] Puckett et al.[59] reported 12-month unassisted patencies following access revision of 15% and 36% among patients who had thrombosed PTFE grafts undergoing surgical revision with and without midgraft curretage. The other published data on surgical revisions of thrombosed access sites, however, are insufficient to estimate unassisted access patency rates more than 1 month after revision. There is general agreement that grafts or AVFs which require salvage because of thrombosis due to a flow-limiting stenosis will likely require further revisions and that patients who have "aggressive revision" (multiple revisions) will have long-term patencies near or equal to those untreated accesses of a similar type.[33,56,71]

Accesses can undergo repeated thrombectomies. Etheredge et al.[71] reported that 1-month patencies after first, second, and third revisions were 65%, 53%, and 44%. This group performed up to eight revisions to maintain functional patency of some of their accesses. In the experiences of Palder et al.[33] and Cada et al.,[84] approximately 60% of revised grafts required more than one secondary salvage procedure. The duration of patency after the initial thrombectomy does not predict the likelihood of a sustained patency following a subsequent thrombectomy. However, in comparison with accesses that have not needed a prior thrombectomy, accesses that have had multiple previous thrombectomies have a reduced probability of a 1-month survival following a subsequent thrombectomy.[71]

Only a minority of thrombosed AVFs can be salvaged surgically following a thrombosis.[70,85] For this reason, many surgeons recommend that the salvage procedures not be attempted on thrombosed AVFs.[6,31,33] If performed, the primary surgical means of salvaging the access are a simple thrombectomy or a thrombectomy followed by intraoperative angioplasty with a balloon catheter, a rigid dilator, or via a patch procedure. Alternatively, a new access may be created in the same region by anastomosis of the same vessels proximal to the original fistula to form an AVF or by interposition of a PTFE graft proximal to any stenoses. The patency of successfully revised AVFs approaches that of unrevised fistulas.[33,70,85]

INTERVENTIONAL RADIOLOGIC MANAGEMENT OF ACCESS-SITE STENOSES AND THROMBOSES

Thrombolysis

Thrombolysis and angioplasty play no significant role in the treatment of early thrombosis of either AVF or PTFE grafts. Early thrombosis of an AVF is most likely due to either a technical error or insufficient distal arteries or draining veins. Early thrombosis of a PTFE graft usually indicates a technical error. In the case of a PTFE graft, the best hope of salvage lies in surgical reexploration and revision of the problem, if possible. At the request of the surgical service, we have occasionally,

as a diagnostic maneuver, recanalized with fibrinolysis a thrombosed, freshly placed (≤3 weeks) PTFE access to define the underlying anatomic problem, although we make no attempt to repair any pathology with balloon angioplasty.

The principal alternative to surgical thrombectomy for an acute thrombosis of an established access site is thrombolysis. Performed under a variety of protocols, thrombolysis usually results in complete lysis of acute thrombosis (within less than 5 days) for PTFE grafts, with success rates of 58% to 90% (Table 23-4). The principal reason for the wide range of reported success rates for thrombolysis is probably the widely differing techniques, choice of lytic agent, and small number of cases in some instances. Earlier reports discussed administration of streptokinase (SK) at relatively low rates of infusion, about 10,000 IU/h.[86-88] Two of these reports had lysis rates in AVFs and PTFE grafts below 50%. Attempts in undefined types of thrombosed dialysis accesses to administer SK throughout the clot via multiple direct percutaneous injections with manual external massage of the access also have been reported, with a 68% to 77% success rate overall and a 52% success without surgical intervention.[89,90] More recently, urokinase (UK) has become the thrombolytic agent of choice. It offers the advantages over SK of having a shorter effective half-life and no antigenicity and thus the possibility of

TABLE 23-4. Results of Lytic Infusions for Thrombosed Accesses

Author	Number	Percent Clinical Success
Klimas	50	58
Mangiarotti	23	62
Ahmed	15	53
Docci	15	90
Valji*	121	90
Brunner*	14	79
UCHSC crossed-catheter technique*	73	85
UCHSC single-catheter technique	62	61

* Crossed catheter technique.

repeated administration in cases of recurrent thrombosis. UK is commonly administered in doses of 60,000 to more than 500,000 IU/h. Tissue-type plasminogen activator (t-PA) also has been used as a thrombolytic agent for thrombosed grafts, administered at 10- to 20-minute intervals with a maximal total dose of 30 mg. The reported success rates have been 92% and 67% in studies of, respectively, 14 and 15 thrombosed grafts.[91,92] There are insufficient published data to compare the complication rates associated the use of t-PA and UK as thrombolytic agents for treatment of thrombosed accesses. Contraindications to lysis of clotted hemodialysis access grafts include suspected graft infection, a contraindication to anticoagulation/fibrinolytic therapy, or severe allergy to contrast material.[53]

Thrombolysis has been used to treat central venous thrombosis ipsilateral to an access.[15,18,21,93–96] However, these reports have presented only a few cases of central venous thrombosis each, and often few details about management of the thrombus are given. Certainly central vein clot can be successfully lysed.[18,94,95] The most appropriate dose of the thrombolytic agent and the optimal technique to manage the underlying venous pathology, usually a stenosis at the site of a previous subclavian catheter, remain to be defined.

Technique of Fistulography

The patient comes to the radiology department immediately following dialysis with the dialysis needles still in place, heparin locked at the time the patient leaves the dialysis unit. If the dialysis unit is located away from the hospital (one of our main units is three blocks away from the radiology department), an elastic bandage is wrapped around both needles, and the patient either walks or is sent via motor transportation to the radiology department. Contrast material is injected through the proximal-most needle under fluoroscopy, and radiographic spot films are obtained in the most appropriate projection as determined fluoroscopically. The complex anatomy of the venous drainage from the access site may need to be depicted in multiple projections. The arterial anastomosis is evaluated by limiting arterial in-

flow. This is usually accomplished using a blood pressure cuff around the upper arm, which is inflated to a pressure (usually 250 to 300 mmHg) above systolic pressure, after which injected contrast material flows retrograde in the graft through the arterial anastomosis. Radiographic spot films are obtained, frequently in multiple projections, over 15 to 30 seconds. Dilute nonionic contrast material is used for studying the arterial anastomosis so that the patient experiences no discomfort while the contrast material is static in the artery adjacent to the anastomosis and the blood pressure cuff is expanded. The blood pressure cuff is deflated as soon as spot films are obtained. Cuff inflation time is 30 to 60 seconds.

Technique of Thrombolysis

The technique of administering the thrombolytic agent has a major effect on success rates. Lysis of a thrombosed PTFE graft is a more complex problem than intraarterial lytic therapy at other sites because of several factors: (1) the graft is punctured 300 times a year with large-bore needles, so recent puncture sites are present which may become points of hemorrhage, (2) an arterial anastomosis is present, which presents an alternative pathway for any thrombus pushed retrograde (arterial embolization), (3) one or multiple venous stenoses are present, which are more resistant to dilation than arterial stenoses, and (4) the venous outflow pattern is variable and must be delineated in each patient with careful fistulography. The placement of a single infusion catheter just within the thrombus, a technique used widely for intraarterial lysis of thromboses at other locations, has a lower success rate than two-catheter infusions. For example, we found that success rates increased from 61% to 85% after institution of a two-catheter lacing/infusion technique, described below, and preliminary lacing of the clot with 250,000 to 500,000 IU of UK.[95] These modifications in technique lessened the failure rate due to inability to lyse clot adjacent to the arterial anastomosis and to extravasation from recent puncture sites in the graft. The crossed-catheter technique appears to have a significantly higher success rate than a single-infusion-point technique.

Quick reestablishment of flow through a

thrombosed access helps decrease the frequency and severity of bleeding from puncture sites. To produce quick recanalization, concentrated UK (150,000 to 500,000 IU) is laced through the entire length of the clot via two catheters that have been placed in crossed fashion in the graft, one each directed toward the venous and arterial anastomoses.[97] Davis et al.[98] also rotated the catheters to mechanically disrupt the thrombus and increase the clot-agent interface. After the initial lacing of UK, the drug is infused through one or both catheters until lysis is complete or near complete, after which balloon angioplasty is performed on any arterial, midgraft, or venous outflow stenoses. Multiple-sidehole catheters used to deliver pulses of 0.2 mL of concentrated UK (25,000 IU/mL) and heparin (500 IU/mL) represent a further refinement of the crossed-catheter technique; this approach, combined with maceration of remaining clot with a balloon catheter, may obviate the need for an infusion after the initial lacing of the clot.[53] Figure 23-1 illustrates an example of lysis/angioplasty of a clotted access using the crossed-catheter technique and pulsed-spray thrombolysis. An alternative protocol has been proposed by Brunner et al.[99] Their approach is to continuously infuse concentrated UK (50,000 IU/mL) at 20,000 IU/minute via two crossed catheters with multiple sideholes without preliminary lacing of the drug through the clot. There has been no report of the administration of t-PA using the crossed-catheter technique. Following access recanalization with thrombolysis, there must be a correction of any associated hemodynamically significant vascular stenoses to prevent rethrombosis. Thorough fistulography after lysis is important to locate all potential stenoses for dilation, including the arterial anastomosis, venous anastomosis, midgraft region[56,59] and the venous outflow in the arm and subclavian region. Narrowings of 50% or greater undergo surgical repair or angioplasty.[53,86,87,95,98] Davis et al.[98] suggested that angioplasty of stenoses before complete thrombolysis with UK may result in a decreased time for complete lysis.

Results of Thrombolysis

The administration of high doses of UK via crossed-catheter technique to 41 thrombosed PTFE grafts resulted in a lysis rate of 90%.[98] This is the first series reported in which the crossed-catheter technique was used. The technique has now been adapted by many other interventional radiologists who treat thrombosed accesses. The same San Diego group has more recently reported a modified method of lacing the clot in PTFE grafts with UK[53] using a concentrated solution of UK (25,000 IU/mL) administered in pulsed boluses of 0.2 mL through crossed multiple-sidehole catheters. In 121 infusions in 73 patients, they achieved 90% success for all patients in whom treatment was attempted and a 93% rate of restoration of the access site using lysis and angioplasty among patients who had complete treatment. Lysis time using the pulsed-spray technique was 46 ± 21 minutes. Personal communication indicates that almost all these patients were treated as outpatients and without the need for placement of a subclavian catheter as a site for interim dialysis.[100] An alternative modification of the crossed-catheter technique has been introduced.[99] Highly concentrated UK (50,000 IU/mL) is administered at a rapid rate (20,000 IU/min.) via pediatric microdrip infusion pumps into the two catheters for 50 to 60 minutes, with an additional 250,000-IU infusion of UK if needed. The clots were not laced with the drug before starting the infusion. All patients were systemically anticoagulated with heparin. Patency was reestablished in 11 of 14 thrombosed accesses (AVF and PTFE grafts). The authors indicate that the continual infusion would reduce the manpower need in the angiography suite by obviating the need for someone to be present to manually perform the pulse injections. Also, they suggest that the risk of distal arterial embolization may be reduced. A larger study would be needed to compare the efficacy, safety, and efficiency of the pulsed and continuous administrations of UK.

A particular problem after otherwise complete lysis is the persistence of a rounded focal filling defect at the proximal end of the graft just distal to its arterial anastomosis in 18% of cases.[53] We have seen the identical phenomenon.[101,102] Similar plugs were reported by Etheredge and colleagues[71] during surgical thrombectomy. In that series, the plugs consisted of white clot, as opposed to red clot in the remainder of the graft. The white clot possibly represents platelet-rich thrombus, a composition that might explain its relative resistance to the thrombolytic agent. This focus of thrombus, when present after otherwise complete lysis, can be eliminated by prolonged infusion of UK or maceration with a balloon catheter.[53]

There are fewer reported attempts of thrombolysis of AVFs.[86,95,103,104] Gmelin et al.[103] treated occluded accesses with angioplasty without any thrombolysis or additional physical disruption of the thrombus. Of a group of 43 malfunctioning AVFs and 3 malfunctioning prosthetic shunts, this method led to salvage of only 13 of 28 thromboses (48%). We lysed 10 of 17 thrombosed AVFs (59%) using a single-catheter technique in almost all cases.[95] Poulain et al.[104] treated 14 thrombosed AVFs and 2 thrombosed autologous venous bypasses by a retrograde administration of UK and Lys-plasminogen into the thrombus, thromboaspiration via a no. 8 French catheter of thrombi resistant to thrombolysis, and angioplasty. This technique was successful in 12 (75%) cases. There are no studies of the efficacy of the crossed-catheter technique for lysis of thrombosed AVFs. The role of thrombolysis in the management of thrombosed AVFs has not yet been delineated.

There is also limited information about long-term access patency following thrombolysis. Some reports do not provide details of management after thrombolysis or patency rates.[86,105,106] Angioplasty immediately after thrombolysis has been reported to have a 79% to 93% success rate.[53,89,98] Following thrombolysis with angioplasty as necessary, the majority of accesses are patent after 3 months.[53,87,89,98,99] Again, there are insufficient data to determine whether patency rates after lysis and percutaneous transluminal angioplasty (PTA) differ between AVFs and PTFE grafts. Similar to surgical revisions, repeat treatment with PTA and thrombolysis/PTA will be necessary in over half of patients.[53,98] The highest rate of rethrombosis occurs in the first month after successful lysis/PTA. Shorter intervals between graft thrombosis predicted earlier subsequent graft failure. Unassisted patency of 26% and assisted patency of 51% at 1 year were reported by Valji et al.[53] This unassisted patency is comparable with the 12-month patency among a group of patients with PTFE grafts undergoing surgical thrombectomy, who had a 12-month primary patency of 36% without midgraft curettage and 15% with midgraft curettage.[59] The assisted patency of 51% at 12 months is comparable with the secondary patencies of Palder et al.[33] and Etheredge et al.[71] of 72% and 60% among patients receiving surgical thrombectomy/revision and was achieved without any surgical revision or loss of any further vessel which could later be used for construction of a new access site. In summary, intragraft thrombolysis with close patient follow-up, including angioplasty of any recurrent stenoses and repeated thrombolysis of additional thromboses, can maintain patency for at least 12 months in most patients following access thrombosis. We have found that the combination of fibrinolysis/PTA and surgical revision will lead to the longest patency of a single access site. When an access thromboses, fibrinolysis/PTA is used to reestablish its function; recurrent failure of the access is treated with repeat PTA, combined with lysis if thrombosis recurs; surgical revision of the same access is then performed when its anatomy has deteriorated to the extent that it cannot be treated adequately by percutaneous means; failure of the revised access is once again treated with PTA, with lysis as necessary, until both the interventional radiologic and surgical teams feel that the anatomy of the access has deteriorated to beyond repair.

Alternative Approaches

There has been a single report of attempted manual removal of access thrombosis with a guidewire and angioplasty in 5 accesses. This was successful in 4 cases, with no rethrombosis with a median follow-up of 18 weeks.[107] Another group has reported a 59% success rate with treating thrombosed fistulas and bovine and PTFE grafts with infusion of UK and Lys-plasminogen via a single catheter. If there is residual thrombus, this is followed by thromboaspiration of the residual clot by a no. 8 French catheter attached to a 50-mL syringe. Angioplasty is performed as indicated.[104]

Thrombolysis by direct graft puncture and infusion of the lytic agent without fluoroscopic guidance, with subsequent angiography and sur-

(Text continued on page 342)

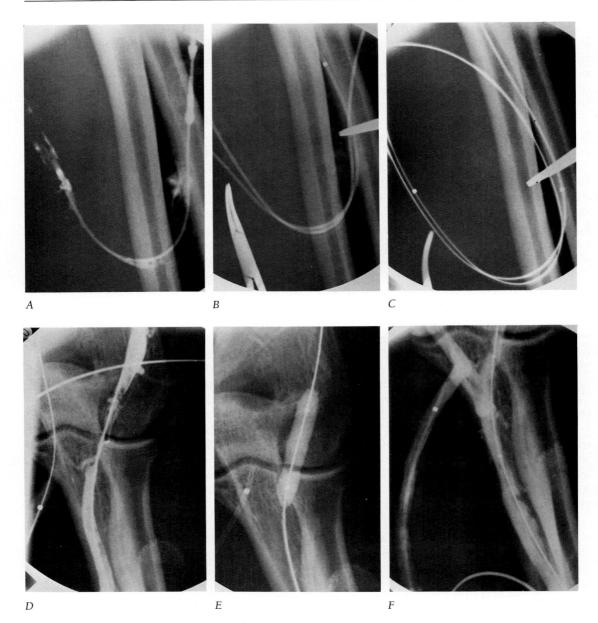

FIGURE 23-1. **(A)** *Clotted PTFE graft. Initial catheter placement toward the arterial anastomosis. Thrombus in the graft is outlined by contrast just distal to the tip of the catheter.* **(B)** *Crossed catheters have been inserted with their tips at the arterial and venous anastomoses.* **(C)** *The catheters are withdrawn while lacing the entire length of thrombus using pulse-spray technique with concentrated UK (25,000 IU/mL) and heparin (500 U/mL). Mosquito clamps are laid across the catheter entry sites of the catheters to avoid pulling the proximal holes in the catheters (metal markers) out of the graft. In this case, clot was lysed entirely with the pulse-spray technique. In other cases, an infusion of UK after pulse-spray lacing of the thrombus may be necessary to lyse ≥90% of the clot.* **(D)** *After lysis, a stenosis is evident just distal to the venous anastomosis.* **(E)** *A 6 mm × 3 cm balloon catheter is used to dilate the stenosis.* **(F)** *Region of the arterial anastomosis. The graft is now free of clot and has rapid*

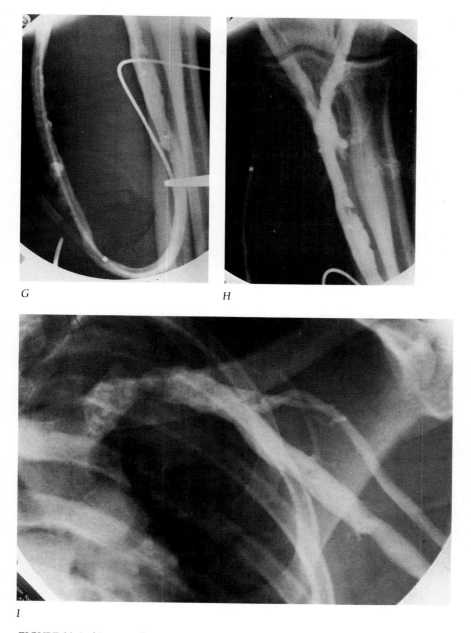

G

H

I

FIGURE 23-1. *(Continued).*

flow. **(G)** *The midgraft is patent with rapid flow of contrast material. There are residual graft defor-mities from previous punctures.* **(H)** *The venous anastomosis region, after lysis and angioplasty, shows no remaining stenosis. The mural filling defect in the graft may represent a small residual mural thrombus or a deformity from previous punctures; it does not interfere with flow and was not treated further.* **(I)** *Injection of contrast material into the now-patent graft with filming over the subclavian region confirm that there is no other significant stenosis more centrally.*

gical revision of successfully lysed cases, has been suggested as an alternative means of managing thrombosed accesses. In a report of 43 thrombosed accesses with a 58% successful lysis rate, 34% patency was attained with a mean follow-up of 33 weeks.[108] However, the protocol does not provide the potential to save future access sites, as does angioplasty.

Another proposed approach for thrombosed PTFE access sites is surgical thrombectomy followed by intraoperative balloon angioplasty.[83,109] Among 21 patients treated with this approach, success was obtained in 16 (76%), and secondary patency at 5 or more months was 58% among the successfully treated patients. These results appear similar to treatment with lysis/PTA and surgical thrombectomy/revision, suggesting that the means of ridding the access site of thrombus does not affect outcome or long-term patency once flow is reestablished and the underlying lesion is corrected with dilation.

Complications of Lysis

The most common complication of access salvage with thrombolytic therapy and angioplasty is a local hematoma due to extravasation through recent punctures for dialysis. Often the bleeding will cease with local manual tamponade and thus does not require immediate discontinuation of thrombolysis. The crossed-catheter administration of high doses of UK offers the advantage of rapid lysis and reestablishment of flow, usually in 30 to 90 minutes,[53,98] and reduces the incidence of this complication. The patient can be observed continuously during the procedure so that tamponade can be applied promptly and maintained to any expanding hematoma. Distant bleeding is much less frequent. Reported distant sites have included the gastrointestinal tract and recent surgical sites. To our knowledge, there have been no life-threatening hemorrhages. Embolic complications have been reported in several studies.[86,88,90,98,108] There may be some increased risk of clot embolization by mechanical thrombolysis or intrathrombus injection of UK, but the experience of Valji and associates[53] suggests that clinical pulmonary embolism is extremely rare, since they

saw only 2 patients in 117 procedures who had transient chest pain. We had 1 patient in 83 procedures with the same complaint. In no instance was the pain long-lived or of any clinical significance. There was no cardiopulmonary decompensation in any case. There have been a few reported cases of distal arterial embolization with clinical manifestations. All these emboli lysed with continued thrombolytic therapy,[53] without long-term sequelae. Thrombolytic therapy with manual access massage has been associated with a 7.6% incidence of asymptomatic emboli.[90] Recanalization of an infected graft can produce sepsis.[98] Graft infection is a contraindication for thrombolytic treatment.

ANGIOPLASTY FOR MAINTENANCE OF ACCESS PATENCY

Access Stenoses

While the traditional method of surgical revision of a failing or thrombosed hemodialysis access site is reasonably effective in prolonging the life of the access site, the problems of loss of usable vein by the revision, the need for interim placement of a subclavian catheter until the revision is healed, the recognition that repeated surgical revisions will be necessary to maintain patency in most patients, and the expense of surgical revision have led to the exploration of alternative means of maintaining vascular access. Percutaneous balloon angioplasty of arterial anastomotic and venous outflow stenoses can be performed in 20 to 30 minutes on an outpatient basis after dialysis, with the guidewires and subsequent balloon catheters being inserted through the indwelling needles after a dialysis run. Schwab and colleagues[34] investigated the value of prophylactic angioplasty among a group of patients who had rising venous pressures as an indication that their PTFE grafts were failing. These patients were evaluated with fistulography through indwelling dialysis needles; patients who had outflow stenoses (89% of those having fistulography) underwent balloon angioplasty of the stenotic lesions at the same time. Eighteen percent of patients had unsuccessful angioplasty and underwent surgical revision. Using this approach, the incidence of access thrombosis per patient-year decreased threefold compared with patients from the same institution before these measures were instituted. Replacement of the access decreased $3\frac{1}{2}$-fold during the same period. Patients with elevated venous pressures who underwent elective fistulography and outpatient percutaneous angioplasty of the venous stenoses had the same rate of access thrombosis as patients who had normal venous pressures (0.13 thromboses per patient-year and 0.15 thromboses per patient-year, respectively), while patients with elevated pressures who had no treatment had an incidence of 1.4 thromboses per patient-year, a 10-fold difference ($p < 0.001$). While stenoses treated with PTA had a higher recurrence rate than stenoses treated with surgery in this study, multiple PTA procedures allowed equivalent results with surgery and prolonged the life of the original fistula without extending the fistula further up the arm. Beathard[22] recently reported the long-term results of 536 percutaneous angioplasties in 285 patients. Eighty-three percent of the patients had PTFE grafts; the remainder had AVFs. Angioplasty was technically successful in 94% of 536 access PTAs. The unassisted patency rates at 180 and 360 days were 67.2% and 43.9% for anastomotic stenoses and 55.9% and 17.8% for midgraft stenoses. The unassisted patency rates following angioplasty of various types of venous stenoses of the upper extremity were slightly lower than the patency rate with anastomotic stenoses.

Three different groups of investigators compared the results of surgical revision and angioplasty and arrived at different conclusions. In a series of patients who had failing or failed hemodialysis access sites, both PTFE and AVFs, reported by Dapunt et al.,[110] retrospective comparison was made of the cumulative patencies of those sites treated with angioplasty and those treated with surgical revision. For angioplasty and surgery, respectively, the cumulative patency rates were 94.5% and 78.1% after 1 week, 72.3% and 64.1% at 1 month, 41.2% and 28.9% at 5 months, and 31.3% and 19.3% at 1 year ($p < 0.001$). The differences were due mainly to the early reocclusions after surgery. They concluded that translu-

minal angioplasty achieved at least as good results as surgical revision. Cada and coworkers[84] performed 47 angioplasties on 40 patients with a variety of failing fistula sites, principally native AVFs, with a 91.5% initial success rate and a mean patency after angioplasty of 10.5 months. In comparison, patients treated with surgical revision had a slightly shorter functional patency (9.93 months) and a higher need for repeat surgical intervention (56%) after surgical revision than after angioplasty. The percentage of fistulas with long-term functional patency after revision with angioplasty was almost twice as great as after surgical revision. They also favored balloon angioplasty as the method of choice to correct failing fistulas. In contrast, Brooks et al.,[111] in a prospective study on PTFE and bovine graft stenoses treated with inpatient angioplasty or surgical revision, found significantly longer patencies favoring the surgically revised patients.

As mentioned, in Brescia-Cimino fistulas, transluminal angioplasty has been performed in patients whose AVFs are deteriorating due both to stenoses and to total occlusions. Balloon dilation of poorly functioning arteriovenous fistulas is beneficial when the malfunctioning fistula is a mature one and when poorly functioning shunts (primary flow rates of less than 150 mL/min) are excluded. Success in the hands of Gmelin et al.,[103] defined by them as persistent patency of the shunt for at least 1 month, was 70% overall and was higher with stenoses (89%) than with occlusions (46%). Follow-up patency among the two groups was similar, although favoring the stenosis group. Secondary patency at 6 months, 1 year, and 2 years was 93%, 91%, and 57% for stenoses and 80%, 50%, and 14% for occlusions. Of their patients whose initial treatment was successful, 52% required only a single angioplasty, while 48% required two to five repeat dilatations during the follow-up. Turmel-Rodriguez et al.[69] recently reported a similar long-term assisted patency rate following angioplasty of stenotic Brescia-Cimino fistulas, with additional angioplasty as indicated. Assisted patencies were 82%, 76%, and 66% at 1, 2, and 3 years. Their repeat angioplasty rate was only 0.4 PTA procedures per stenosis per year, significantly lower than the restenosis rate they had with grafts (1.5 PTA procedures per stenosis per year). Surgical repair of stenoses in AVFs is difficult and sometimes impossible.

Central Venous Stenoses

Angioplasty is the principal method of treating central venous stenoses. Typically, the angioplasty can be performed on an outpatient basis.[16] The central stenosis can be crossed either antegrade or retrograde. Either the access or the efferent vein may be punctured for an antegrade approach. Since the stenosis may be relatively resistant to angioplasty, a high-pressure angioplasty balloon ought to be used. High initial success rates, 76% to 100%,[14,112,113] have been reported for PTA of central venous stenoses. However, restenosis is frequent. Despite repeated angioplasty, but without the benefit of stent placement, Glanz et al.[112] have reported a 1-year patency rate of 35% and a 2-year patency rate of 6% for axillary and subclavian stenoses in 19 patients, 16 of whom had hemodialysis accesses in the involved extremity.

The use of percutaneously placed intravascular stents for PTFE grafts, AVFs, and proximal upper extremity and central venous stenoses thus far has been only modestly successful, being limited by the early development of intimal hyperplasia in or immediately adjacent to the stent.[114,115] Patency may be extended with repeat PTA or additional stent placement or both.[69,113,116–118] Following placement of stents for venous anastomotic and proximal venous stenoses, unassisted and assisted access patency rates at 2 years of 25% and 42%, respectively, have been reported.[116]

Complications

There is a low incidence of complications of angioplasty of arterial and venous stenoses associated with AVFs and PTFE grafts. In almost all series, the reported complication rate is less than 8% and is usually 0% to 2%.[20,83,84,103,119–121] The most commonly reported complications are access thrombosis and vascular rupture. In the latter case, bleeding can be controlled by manual and dressing compression and seldom requires surgical intervention. Less frequent complications in-

cluded angina, pseudoaneurysm, cellulitis, and hemorrhage at the puncture site. There are insufficient published data to determine whether complication rates for angioplasties of stenoses associated with AVFs in comparison with those associated with PTFE grafts are different.

Angioplasty can be repeated many times on venous and arterial stenoses. In one of our patients, a total of 4 fibrinolyses and 27 angioplasties have been performed to maintain patency of the patient's last access site. Because stenoses have a high likelihood of recurrence with either surgical revision or balloon dilatation, we and others[34,84,110,120] have concluded that outpatient angioplasty is the preferred treatment to preserve these failing sites. As noted earlier, if a complication develops within the access or efferent vessel that is not amenable to correction with angioplasty, such as a nondilating stenosis or aneurysmal disease, surgical revision of the access should be performed. Subsequently, thrombolysis and PTA can again be used, as needed, to maintain patency of the access. Use of a combination of interventional radiologic and surgical techniques will yield the longest access patency.

SUMMARY

Angioplasty is a valuable alternative to surgical revision of failing hemodialysis access sites and may be the treatment of choice because no further vein is compromised during the revision and because patency rates with repeat dilations approach or equal those of surgical revision. Thrombolysis/angioplasty is a worthy substitute for surgical thrombectomy/revision because dialysis can be resumed immediately, without the need of placement of a temporary subclavian vein access catheter, and lysis can be performed on an outpatient basis. Long-term secondary patency also approaches that of surgical therapy. Again, future access sites are not compromised. Either with percutaneous catheter or surgical therapy, it must be recognized that repeat treatment will be necessary to maintain patency of the access site after it has thrombosed and that a combination of both approaches is likely to yield the longest patency. Close follow-up of these patients to look for signs of recurring deterioration is mandatory. Since the number of vascular access sites is limited, the preservation of each site for as long as possible is important in the long-term management of these patients.

Acknowledgment

We would like to thank Ms. Francille Randolph for her tireless efforts in all phases of the preparation of this manuscript.

References

1. Shackelton CR, Taylor DC, Buckley AR, et al. Predicting failure in polytetrafluoroethylene vascular access grafts for hemodialysis: a pilot study. Can J Surg 1987;30(6):442.
2. Rittgers SE, Garcia-Valdez C, McCormick JT, Posner MP. Noninvasive blood flow measurement in expanded polytetrafluoroethylene grafts for hemodialysis access. J Vasc Surg 1986;3:635.
3. Haimov M. Circulatory access for hemodialysis. In: Rutherford R, ed. Vascular surgery. 3d ed. Philadelphia: WB Saunders, 1989:1073.
4. Wilson SE. Complications of vascular access procedures. In: Wilson SE, Owens ML, eds. Vascular access surgery. Chicago: Year Book Medical Publishers, 1980:185.
5. Swedberg SH, Brown BG, Sigley R, et al. Intimal fibromuscular hyperplasia at the venous anastomosis of PTFE grafts in hemodialysis patients. Circulation 1989;80:1726.
6. Kherlakian GM, Roedersheimer LR, Arbaugh JJ, et al. Comparison of autogenous fistula versus expanded polytetrafluoroethylene graft fistula for angioaccess in hemodialysis. Am J Surg 1986; 152:238.
7. Hakim RM, Lazarus JM. Medical aspects of hemodialysis. In: Brenner BM, Rector FC, eds. The Kidney. Philadelphia: WB Saunders, 1986:1799.
8. Kjellstrand C. The Achilles' heel of the dialysis patient. Arch Intern Med 1978;138:1063.
9. Quinton W, Dillard D, Scribner B. Cannulation of blood vessels for prolonged hemodialysis. Trans Am Soc Artif Intern Organs 1960;6:104.
10. Cross AS, Steigbigel RT. Infective endocarditis and access site infections in patients on hemodialysis. Medicine 1976;55:453.
11. Keane WF, Shapiro FL, Raij L. Incidence and type of infections occurring in 445 chronic hemodialysis patients. Trans Am Soc Artif Intern Organs 1977;23:41.
12. Nsouli K, Lazarus J, Schoenbaum S, et al. Bacteremic infection in hemodialysis. Arch Intern Med 1979;139:1255.
13. Ingram T, Reid S, Tisnado J, et al. Percutaneous transluminal angioplasty of bachiocephalic vein stenoses in patients with dialysis shunts. Radiology 1988;166:45.
14. Schwab S. Hemodialysis-associated central vein thrombosis and stenosis: unresolved problems. Semin Dial 1989;2(3):141.
15. Piotrowski J, Rutherford R. Proximal vein thrombosis secondary to hemodialysis catheterization complicated by arteriovenous fistula. J Vasc Surg 1987;5:876.
16. Schwab SJ, Quarles LD, Middleton JP, et al. Hemodialysis-associated subclavian vein stenosis. Kidney Int 1988;33:1156.
17. Stalter KA, Stevens GF, Sterling WA Jr. Late stenosis of the subclavian vein after hemodialysis catheter injury. Surgery 1986;100(5):924.
18. Newman GE, Saeed M, Himmelstein S, et al. Total central vein obstruction: resolution with angioplasty and fibrinolysis. Kidney Int 1991;39:761.
19. Surratt RS, Picus D, Hicks ME, et al. The importance of preoperative evaluation of the subclavian vein in dialysis access planning. AJR 1991;156 (3):623.
20. Glanz S, Gordon DH, Butt KMH, et al. The role of percutaneous angioplasty in the management of chronic hemodialysis fistulas. Ann Surg 1987;206 (6):777.
21. Vanherweghem J, Yassine T, Goldman M, et al. Subclavian vein thrombosis: a frequent complication of subclavian vein cannulation for hemodialysis. Clin Nephrol 1986;26(5):2235.
22. Beathard GA. Percutaneous transvenous angioplasty in the treatment of vascular access stenosis. Kidney Int 1992;42:1390.
23. Brescia M, Cimino J, Appel K, Hurwich B. Chronic hemodialysis using venipuncture and a surgically created arteriovenous fistula. N Engl J Med 1966; 275:1089.
24. Kinnaert P, Vereerstraeten P, Toussaint C, Van Geertruyden JV. Nine years' experience with internal arteriovenous fistulas for haemodialysis: a study of some factors influencing the results. Br J Surg 1977;64:242.
25. DePalma JR, Vannix R, Bahuth J, Abukurah A. "Steal" syndrome, ischemia, congestive failure and peripheral neuropathy. Proc Clin Dial Transplant Forum 1973;3:9.
26. Bussell JA, Abbott JA, Lim RC. A radial steal syndrome with arteriovenous fistula for hemodialysis: studies in seven patients. Ann Intern Med 1971; 75:387.
27. Rassat J, Moskovtchenko J. 60 fistules artérioveineuses pour épuration extrarénale. Ann Chir Thorac Cardiovasc 1971;10:71.

28. Mehigan J, McAlexander R. Snuffbox arteriovenous fistula for hemodialysis. Am J Surg 1982; 143:252.

29. Buselmeier T, Rattazi L, Kjellstrand C, et al. A modified arteriovenous fistula applicable where there is thrombosis of standard Brescia-Cimino fistula vasculature. Surgery 1973;74:551.

30. May T. Saphenous vein arteriovenous fistula in regular dialysis treatment. N Engl J Med 1969; 280:770.

31. Rohr MS, Browder W, Frentz GD, McDonald JC. Arteriovenous fistulas for long-term dialysis. Arch Surg 1978;113:153.

32. Lyngaard F, Nordling J, Hansen R. Clinical experience with the saphena loop arteriovenous fistula on the thigh. Int Urol Nephrol 1981;13:287.

33. Palder SB, Kirkman RL, Whittemore AD, et al. Vascular access for hemodialysis. Ann Surg 1985; 202(2):235.

34. Schwab SJ, Raymond JR, Saeed M, et al. Prevention of hemodialysis fistula thrombosis: early detection of venous stenosis. Kidney Int 1989;63:707.

35. Haimov M. Alternatives for vascular access for hemodialysis: experience with autogenous saphenous vein autographs and bovine heterografts. Surgery 1974;75:447.

36. Abu-dalu J, Urca I, Zonder H. Hemodialysis treatment by means of a cadaver arterial allograft. Arch Surg 1972;105:798.

37. Adar R, Siegal A, Bogokowsky H. The use of arteriovenous autograft and allograft fistulas for chronic hemodialysis. Surg Gynecol Obstet 1973;136:941.

38. Piccone V Jr, Sika J, Ahmed N. Preserved saphenous vein allografts for vascular access. Surg Gynecol Obstet 1978;147:385.

39. Dardik H, Ibrahim I, Dardik I. Arteriovenous fistulas constructed with modified human umbilical cord vein graft. Arch Surg 1976;111:60.

40. Mindich B, Silverman M, Elguezabal A. Umbilical cord vein fistula for vascular access in hemodialysis. Trans Am Soc Artif Intern Organs 1975;21: 273.

41. Burdick J, Scott W, Cosimi A. Experience with Dacron graft arteriovenous fistulas for dialysis access. Ann Surg 1978;198:262.

42. Flores L, Dunn I, Frumkin E. Dacron arteriovenous shunts for vascular access in hemodialysis. Trans Am Soc Artif Intern Organs 1973;19:33.

43. Haimov M, Burrows L, Schanzer H, et al. Experience with arterial substitutes in the construction of vascular access for hemodialysis. J Cardiovasc Surg 1980;21:149.

44. Hurt V, Batello-Cruz M, Skipper J. Bovine carotid artery heterografts versus polytetrafluoroethylene graft: a prospective randomized study. Am J Surg 1983;146:844.

45. Hutchin P, Jacobs J, Devin J. Bovine graft arteriovenous fistulas for maintenance hemodialysis. Surg Gynecol Obstet 1975;141:255.

46. Johnson J, Kenoyer M, Johnson K. The modified bovine heterograft in vascular access for chronic hemodialysis. Ann Surg 1976;183:62.

47. Gross G, Hayes J. PTFE graft arteriovenous fistulae for hemodialysis access. Am J Surg 1979;45: 748.

48. Haimov M. Vascular access for hemodialysis. Surg Gynecol Obstet 1975;141:619.

49. Haimov M. Clinical experience with the expanded polytetrafluoroethylene vascular prosthesis. Angiology 1978;29:1.

50. Munda R, First RF, Alexander JW, et al. Polytetrafluoroethylene graft survival in hemodialysis. JAMA 1983;249(2):219.

51. Giacchino J, Geis W, Wittenstein B, Gandhi V. Recent trends in vascular access. Am Surg 1982; 48:501.

52. Mohaideen AH, Tanchajja S, Avram MM, Mainzer RA. Arteriovenous access for hemodialysis. NY State J Med 1980;80:190.

53. Valji K, Bookstein JJ, Roberts AC, Davis GB. Pharmacomechanical thrombolysis and angioplasty in the management of clotted hemodialysis grafts: early and late clinical results. Radiology 1991; 178:243.

54. Baker LD, Johnson JM, Goldfarb D. Expanded polytetrafluoroethylene (PTFE) subcutaneous arteriovenous conduit: an improved vascular access for chronic hemodialysis. Trans Am Soc Artif Intern Organs 1976;22:382.

55. Morgan P, Knight C, Tilnay L. Femoral triangle sepsis in dialysis patients. Ann Surg 1980;191:460.

56. Rizzuti R, Hale J, Burkart T. Extended patency of expanded polytetrafluoroethylene grafts for vascular access using optimal configuration and revisions. Surg Gynecol Obstet 1988;166:23.

57. Doyle D, Fry P. Polytetrafluoroethylene and bovine grafts for vascular access in patients on long-term hemodialysis. Can J Surg 1982;25:379.

58. Harder F, Landmann J. Trends in access surgery for hemodialysis. Surg Annu 1984;16:135.

59. Puckett J, Lindsay S. Midgraft curettage as a routine adjunct to salvage operation for thrombosed polytetrafluoroethylene hemodialysis access grafts. Am J Surg 1988;156:139.

60. Dobkin JF, Miller MH, Steigbigel NH. Septicemia in patients on chronic hemodialysis. Ann Intern Med 1978;88:28.

61. Higgins MR, Grace M, Bettcher KJ, et al. Blood access in hemodialysis. Clin Nephrol 1976;6:473.

62. Morgan A, Lazarus JM. Vascular access for dialysis. Am J Surg 1975;129:432.

63. Hansen OK, Kraft O, Mauritzen C. Biologic and semi-biologic vascular grafts. Surg Gynecol Obstet 1974;138:940.

64. Tordoir JHM, Herman JMMPH, Kwan TS, Diderich PM. Long-term follow-up of the polytetrafluoroethylene (PTFE) prosthesis as an arteriovenous fistula for haemodialysis. Eur J Vasc Surg 1987;2:3.

65. Sabanayagam P, Schwartz AB, Soricelli RR, et al. Experience with one hundred reinforced expanded PTFE grafts for angioaccess in hemodialysis. Trans Am Soc Artif Intern Organs 1980;26:582.

66. Tellis VA, Kohlberg WI, Bhat DJ, et al. Expanded polytetrafluoroethylene graft fistula for chronic hemodialysis. Ann Surg 1979;189:101.

67. Sterioff S. Salvage of the failing vascular access. In: Sommer BG, Henry ML, eds. Vascular Access for Hemodialysis. Flaggstaff, AZ: W.L. Gore & Associates, Inc., and Pluribus Press, Inc., 1989:153.

68. Jenkins AM, Buist TAS, Glover SD. Medium-term follow-up of forty autogenous vein and forty polytetrafluoroethylene (Gore-Tex) grafts for vascular access. Surgery 1980;88(5):667.

69. Turmel-Rodriguez L, Pengloan J, Blanchier D, et al. Insufficient dialysis shunts: improved long-term patency rates with close hemodynamic monitoring, repeated percutaneous balloon angioplasty, and stent placement. Radiology 1993;187:273.

70. Romero A, Polo JR, Morato EG, et al. Salvage of angioaccess after late thrombosis of radiocephalic fistulas for hemodialysis. Int Surg 1986;71:122.

71. Etheredge EE, Haid SD, Maeser MN, et al. Salvage operations for malfunctioning polytetrafluoroethylene hemodialysis access grafts. Surgery 1982;94(3):464.

72. Steed D, McAuley C, Rault R, Webster M. Upper arm graft fistula for hemodialysis. J Vasc Surg 1984;1:660.

73. Brown B, Cukingnan R, Peterson R, et al. Perianastomotic arteriosclerosis in grafted human coronary arteries: prevention with platelet-inhibiting therapy (abstract). Am J Cardiol 1982;47:968.

74. Imparato A, Bracco A, Kim G, Zeff R. Intimal and neointimal fibrous proliferation causing failure of arterial reconstructions. Surgery 1972;72(6):1007.

75. Castañeda-Zuniga W, Formanek A, Tadavarthy M, et al. The mechanism of balloon angioplasty. Radiology 1980;135:565.

76. Santiago-Delpin EA. Swelling of the hand after arteriovenous fistula for hemodialysis. Am J Surg 1976;132:373.

77. Windus DW, Audrain J, Vanderson R, et al. Optimization of high-efficiency hemodialysis by detection and correction of fistula dysfunction. Kidney Int 1990;38:337.

78. Middleton WD, Picus DD, Marx MV. Color Doppler sonography of hemodialysis vascular access: comparison with angiography. AJR 1989;152:633.

79. Tordoir JHM, de Bruin HG, Hoeneveld H, et al. Duplex ultrasound scanning in the assessment of arteriovenous fistulas created for hemodialysis access: comparison with digital subtraction angiography. J Vasc Surg 1989;10:122.

80. Raju S. PTFE grafts for hemodialysis access. Ann Surg 1987;206(5):666.

81. Fulks KD, Hyde GL. Jugular-axillary vein bypass for salvage of arteriovenous access. J Vasc Surg 1988;8(1):169.

82. Duncan JM, Baldwin RT, Caralis JP, Cooley DA. Subclavian vein-to-right atrial bypass for symptomatic venous hypertension. Ann Thorac Surg 1991;52(6):1342.

83. Smith TP, Cragg AH, Castañeda F, Hunter DW. Thrombosed polytetrafluoroethylene hemodialysis fistulas: salvage with combined thrombectomy and angioplasty. Radiology 1989;171:507.

84. Cada E, Karnel F, Mayer G, et al. Percutaneous transluminal angioplasty of failing arteriovenous dialysis fistulae. Nephrol Dial Transplant 1989;4:57.

85. Bone GE, Pomajzl MJ. Management of dialysis fistula thrombosis. Am J Surg 1979;138:901.

86. Klimas VA, Denny KM, Paganini EP, et al. Low dose streptokinase therapy for thrombosed arteriovenous fistulas. Trans Am Soc Artif Intern Organs 1984;30:511.

87. Collier PE, Saracco GM, Young JC, et al. Nonoperative salvage of subcutaneous hemodialysis fistulae. Am J Nephrol 1985;5:333.

88. Young AT, Hunter DW, Castañeda-Zuniga WR, et al. Thrombosed synthetic hemodialysis access fistulas: failure of fibrolytic therapy. Radiology 1985;154:639.

89. Zeit RM, Cope C. Failed hemodialysis shunts. Radiology 1985;154:353.

90. Zeit RM. Arterial and venous embolization: declotting of dialysis shunts by direct injection of streptokinase. Radiology 1986;159:639.

91. Rinast E, Weiss H-D. Regional angiotherapy by application of recombinant tissue-type plasminogen activator, followed by PTA and vascular endoprosthesis. Acta Radiol 1991;377(suppl):29.

92. Ahmed A, Shapiro WB, Porush JG. The use of tissue plasminogen activator to declot arteriovenous accesses in hemodialysis patients. Am J Kidney Dis 1993;21(1):38.

93. Vanholder R, Lameire NVJ, van Rattinghe R, et al. Complications of subclavian catheter hemodialysis: a 5-year prospective study in 257 consecutive patients. Int J Artif Organs 1982;5(5):297.

94. Brady HR, Fitzcharles B, Goldberg H, et al. Diagnosis and management of subclavian vein thrombosis occurring in association with subclavian

cannulation for hemodialysis. Blood Purif 1989; 7(4):210.

95. Cohen MAH, Kumpe DA, Durham JD, Zwerdlinger SC. Treatment of thrombosed hemodialysis access sites with thrombolysis and angioplasty: improved results with crossed-catheter technique and repeat interventional radiologic treatment. Submitted.

96. Clark DD, Albina JE, Chazan JA. Subclavian vein stenosis and thrombosis: a potential serious complication in chronic hemodialysis patients. Am J Kidney Dis 1990;15(3):265.

97. Bookstein J, Saldinger E. Accelerated thrombolysis: in vitro evaluation of agents and methods of administration. Invest Radiol 1985;20:731.

98. Davis GB, Dowd CF, Bookstein JJ, et al. Thrombosed dialysis grafts: efficacy of intrathrombotic deposition of concentrated urokinase, clot maceration, and angioplasty. AJR 1987;149:177.

99. Brunner MC Matalon TAS, Patel SK, et al. Ultrarapid urokinase in hemodialysis access occlusion. JVIR 1991;2(4):503.

100. Roberts A. Personal communication, 1991.

101. Kumpe DA, Cohen MAH, Durham JD. Treatment of failing and failed hemodialysis access sites: comparison of surgical treatment with thrombolysis/angioplasty. Semin Vasc Surg 1992;5:118.

102. Kumpe DA, Cohen MAH. Angioplasty/thrombolytic treatment of failing and failed hemodialysis access sites: comparison with surgical treatment. Progr Cardiovasc Dis 1992;34:263.

103. Gmelin E, Winterhoff R, Rinast E. Insufficient hemodialysis access fistulas: late results of treatment with percutaneous balloon angioplasty. Radiology 1989;171:657.

104. Poulain F, Raynaud A, Bourquelot P, et al. Local thrombolysis and thromboaspiration in the treatment of acutely thrombosed arteriovenous hemodialysis fistulas. Cardiovasc Intervent Radiol 1991;14:98.

105. Mangiarotti G, Canavese C, Thea A, et al. Urokinase treatment for arteriovenous fistulae declotting in dialysed patients. Nephron 1984;36:60.

106. Docci D, Turci F, Baldrati L. Successful declotting of arteriovenous grafts with local infusion of urokinase in hemodialyzed patients. Artif Organs 1986;10(6):494.

107. Hunter DW, So SKS, Castañeda-Zuniga WR, et al. Angiographic evaluation and percutaneous transluminal angioplasty in failing or thrombosed Brescia-Cimino arteriovenous dialysis fistulas. Radiology 1983;149:105.

108. Schilling JJ, Eiser AR, Slifkin RF, et al. The role of thrombolysis in hemodialysis access occlusion. Am J Kidney Dis 1987;10(2):92.

109. Smith T, Hunter D, Darcy M, et al. Thrombosed synthetic hemodialysis access fistulas: the success of combined thrombectomy and angioplasty. AJR 1986;147:161.

110. Dapunt O, Feurstein M, Rendl K, Prenner K. Transluminal angioplasty versus conventional operation in the treatment of haemodialysis fistula stenosis: results from a 5-year study. Br J Surg 1987;74:1004.

111. Brooks JL, Sigley RD, May KJ, Mack RM. Transluminal angioplasty versus surgical repair for stenosis of hemodialysis grafts. Am J Surg 1987;153:530.

112. Glanz S, Gordon DH, Lipkowitz GS, et al. Axillary and subclavian vein stenosis: percutaneous angioplasty. Radiology 1988;168:371.

113. Antonucci F, Salomonowitz E, Stuckman G, et al. Placement of venous stents: clinical experience with a self-expanding prosthesis. Radiology 1992;183(2):493.

114. Günther RW, Vorwerk D, Bohndorf K, et al. Venous stenoses in dialysis shunts: treatment with self-expanding metallic stents. Radiology 1989;170:401.

115. Zollikofer C, Largiader I, Brühlman W, et al. Endovascular stenting of veins and grafts: preliminary clinical experience. Radiology 1988;167:707.

116. Quinn SF, Schuman ES, Hall L, et al. Venous stenoses in patients who undergo hemodialysis: treatment with self-expandable endovascular stents. Radiology 1992;183(2):499.

117. Vorwerk D, Gunther RW, Bohndorf K, et al. Follow-up results after stent placement in failing arteriovenous shunts: a three-year experience. Cardiovasc Intervent Radiol 1991;14:285.

118. Zollikofer CL, Antonucci F, Stuckmann G, et al. Use of the wallstent in the venous system including hemodialysis-related stenoses. Cardiovasc Intervent Radiol 1992;15:334.

119. Hunter DW, Castañeda-Zuniga WR, Coleman CC, et al. Failing arteriovenous dialysis fistulas: evaluation and treatment. Radiology 1984;152:631.

120. Saeed M, Newman GE, McCann RL, et al. Stenoses in dialysis fistulas: treatment with percutaneous angioplasty. Radiology 1987;164:693.

121. Rodriguez-Perez JC, Maynar M, Rams A, et al. Percutaneous transluminal angioplasty as best treatment in stenosis of vascular access for hemodialysis. Nephron 1989;51:192.

24

THROMBOLYTIC THERAPY FOR ACUTE MYOCARDIAL INFARCTION

Joseph F. Pietrolungo

Eric J. Topol

The treatment of acute myocardial infarction (MI) has improved tremendously over the last decade. As our knowledge of the basic pathophysiology in this area has grown, so too has the development of new and improved interventional strategies. Overall mortality rates have decreased approximately 30% in patients eligible for myocardial reperfusion compared with conventional therapies. Central to this has been the widespread advancement in the use of thrombolytic therapy for the treatment of acute MI.

The rationale for use of these agents has grown as our basic understanding of myocardial injury has matured. Herrick[1] in 1912 first suggested that coronary thrombosis was the inciting event in acute MI. The subsequent work of Chazov et al.[2] and Rentrop et al.[3,4] contributed further to this concept, but it was not until the landmark study of DeWood and colleagues[5] in 1980 that acute thrombotic coronary occlusion became generally accepted as the central mechanism of myocardial injury. These investigators performed coronary angiography on 517 patients within the first 24 h of an acute MI. Coronary occlusion (presumably due to thrombus) was found in 87% of patients presenting within 4 h of symptom onset and 65% of patients studied within 12 to 24 h.

These and other similar observations have paved the way in our understanding that the final common pathway for MI associated with ST-segment elevation is thrombotic coronary occlusion. In addition to this very important finding, these investigators stressed the importance of the underlying coronary artery narrowing, with emphasis on the flow-limiting atherosclerotic lesions and their predisposition to the formation of thrombus. However, numerous studies[6–8] have demonstrated that "noncritical" coronary atherosclerotic narrowing is present in the setting of acute MI and is actually more apt to undergo plaque rupture than severe lesions. In these cases, acute coronary thrombosis was once again identified and implicated in the pathophysiologic process. Plaque rupture and fissuring expose the highly thrombogenic subintimal surface to the circulation, resulting in the activation of platelets and deposition of thrombin with subsequent coronary thrombosis.[8–11]

PLASMINOGEN ACTIVATORS

General Remarks

Thrombolytic agents are now several "generations" old. Each successive generation possesses a unique property distinguishing it from the others. The most notable distinction has been the development of *clot specificity*, which denotes that the primary site of plasminogenesis and fibrinolysis with a particular thrombolytic agent is at the clot surface. As illustrated in Figure 24-1, clot-specific agents preferentially degrade fibrin-bound plasminogen to plasmin through various mechanisms. The non-clot-specific agents exert their fibrinolytic effect on both bound and circulating plasminogen. Table 24-1 depicts the thrombolytics in their respective categories. The first-generation agents include streptokinase (SK) and urokinase (UK). These were developed first and lack

TABLE 24-1. Thrombolytic Agents

First generation
  Streptokinase
  Urokinase
Second generation
  Tissue-type plasminogen activator (t-PA)
  Anisoylated plasminogen activator–streptokinase
    complex (APSAC)
  Prourokinase (single-chain urokinase plasminogen
    activator) (scu-PA)
Third generation
  Fibrin-AB congugated scu-PA, t-PA
  NO–S–t-PA
  Bat-PA
  Deletion mutants, e.g., rt-PA
  Chimerics
  Synergistic combinations

clot specificity. The past 10 years or so has yielded the introduction of newer agents such as anisoylated plasminogen–streptokinase activator complex (APSAC), recombinant tissue-type plasminogen activator (rt-PA), and single-chain urokinase plasminogen activator (scu-PA) (also known as prourokinase). These agents are relatively more clot-specific when compared with the first-generation drugs. It was hoped that this would expedite vessel patency and decrease systemic fibrinolysis, resulting in earlier reperfusion and a reduction in untoward bleeding.

The third-generation agents are composed mainly of chimeric enzymes, hybrids, and synergistic combinations of first- and second-generation agents. These new substances have been developed in an attempt to increase thrombolytic potential, enhance fibrin specificity, and prolong the systemic half-life of currently available t-PAs. Several early experimental studies of their efficacy have already been reported.[12–14] However, any advantage over the currently recommended agents remains to be proved.

Streptokinase (SK)

The oldest and most well-known plasminogen activator, streptokinase (SK) is a 47-kDa, 415 amino acid protein produced by Lancefield group C strains of β-hemolytic streptococci. Although a relatively crude extract was first used therapeutically by Tillet and Sherry[15] in 1949 in a patient

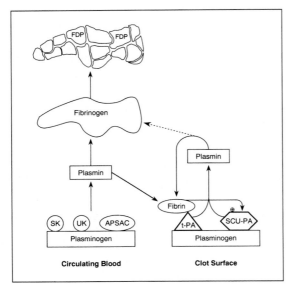

FIGURE 24-1. Schematic representation of the action of fibrinolytic enzymes. Streptokinase (SK) and urokinase (UK) and acylated plasminogen streptokinase activator complex (APSAC) interact predominately on circulating plasminogen; tissue-type plasminogen activator (t-PA) and single-chain urokinase–plasminogen activator (scu-PA) are relatively clot selective. (Reprinted with permission from Topol EJ. Clinical use of streptokinase and urokinase therapy for acute myocardial infarction. Heart Lung 16:760, 1987.)

with a fibrinous pleural effusion, difficulty with obtaining a highly purified, nonpyogenic preparation hampered rapid progression to intravascular use in humans. However, better preparations were available in the late 1950s, and Fletcher et al.[16] subsequently described the use of SK as a clot-dissolving agent in patients suffering from acute MI. Since that time, SK has been the most extensively studied thrombolytic agent to date.

SK has considerable homology with serine proteases that comprise the coagulation proteins. However, it is itself not a direct plasminogen activator, and its action depends on the formation of a 1:1 stoichiometric, noncovalent linkage with human plasminogen or plasmin. This complex results in the formation of a potent enzyme activator.[17,18]

The plasma half-life of SK is 18 minutes, with a beta elimination of 83 minutes. Once given intravenously, consumption of the natural circulating inhibitors of plasmin (α_2-antiplasmin and α_2-macroglobulin) must occur before plasmin produced by SK can lyse fibrin. Intravenous administration of SK causes a rapid reduction in fibrinogen, plasminogen, and the natural plasminogen inhibitors. In addition, coagulation factors V and VII undergo enzymatic degradation and contribute to a coagulopathy. SK does not exhibit any appreciable fibrin selectivity, and thus both circulating and bound fibrinogen is degraded, producing a systemic lytic state.[19]

Delivery of SK has come full circle since its discovery. The initial route of administration for the treatment of acute MI was intravenously,[16,20] followed later by the intracoronary route in the early 1980s when Rentrop and associates[3] showed a high recanalization rate in occluded coronary arteries. Despite the relatively good rates of reperfusion achieved by this method,[21–24] it required access to a catheterization laboratory, causing delays in administration. Furthermore, it was not associated with a significantly lower incidence of bleeding[25,26] and was found to be less effective than primary angioplasty in producing an open infarct-related artery.[27] Thus the popularity of this approach has waned considerably and is no longer a common practice.

The currently recommended mode of administration is via the intravenous route. A dose of 1.5 million units is given intravenously over 30 to 60 minutes[28,29] with optional pretreatment with antihistamines and glucocorticoids to minimize potential allergic reactions (see below). Recently, one small study has advocated that the use of 3 million units intravenously over 60 minutes may achieve increased patency rates without a concomitant increase in untoward bleeding.[30] These results, however, have yet to be validated in larger trials.

Side effects of administration are related to the bacterial origin of SK. An antigenic response has been demonstrated in all immunocompetent individuals studied to date, as evidenced by the presence of circulating neutralizing antibodies to SK.[31] The intensity of this response, however, is variable, and clinical manifestations range from fever, rash, and hives to anaphylactic reactions. These are reported to occur in approximately 2% to 6% of patients, with the more serious anaphylactic reaction being less common (0.3%).[28,32–35]

Systemic hypotension is more commonly encountered with SK administration. Although reports on the frequency of this occurrence vary widely, it probably manifests in approximately 5% to 10% of patients given the drug, and its severity is at least in part related to the rapidity of administration and the total dose of the drug given. The mechanism is likely related to kinin formation and complement activation.[36]

The antigenic properties of SK have prompted some authorities to recommend pretreatment with antihistamines and steroid preparations;[37] however, others[28] argue against the routine use of these drugs. Currently, we do not pretreat patients prior to SK administration because the majority of the adverse reactions are self-limiting or can be managed easily on a symptomatic basis.

Enthusiasm for the intravenous use of thrombolytic agents has given rise to a plethora of studies evaluating angiographic patency,[36,38–43] preservation of left ventricular function,[34,44,45] and reduction in mortality[28,33,34] associated with their use in acute MI.

Infarct artery patency rates for SK at various times are shown in Table 24-2. Early patency rates

TABLE 24-2. Patency Rates for Intravenous Streptokinase

Study	Time to Angiography*	Patency Rate % (n)
Early Patency		
ECSG-2	75–90 min	55 (34/62) (1.0 mU/1 h)
Stack (165)	90 min	44 (95/216)
TIMI-1 (97)[†]	90 min	43 (63/146)
Lopez-Sendon (40)[†]	90 min	60 (15/25)
Hogg (68)	90 min	53 (31/58)
PRIMI (84)	91 min	64 (124/194)
Charbonnier (272)	93 min	51 (27/53)
TEAM-2 (71)	126 min	73 (129/176)
Monnier (273)	150 min	64 (7/11)
Six (30)	168 min	60 (32/53)
Vought (274)	176 min	72 (21/30)
Late Patency		
PRIMI	140 min	88 (160/181)
Hogg	209 min	87 (49/56)
Lopez-Sendon[†]	90 min	75 (18/24)
Riberio (275)	180 min	80 (40/50)
Durand (276)	149 min	82 (27/30)

*Time from initiation of thrombolytic agent to angiogram. Dose equals 1.5 million units over 1 h (m U/h) unless otherwise noted.
All treatment initiated within 3–4 h unless otherwise noted.
†Presentation within 6 h.
Adapted with permission from Granger CB, Califf RM, Topol EJ. Thrombolytic therapy in acute myocardial infarction: a review. Drugs 44:293, 1992.

(90 minutes) are generally reported to be only approximately 50% when given with a mean symptom duration of 3 h.[36] While this is considerably lower than with the newer agents (see below), clear mortality reductions have been shown.[28,33] Because of the apparent paradox between low early patency rates and unequivocal mortality benefit seen with this agent, the value of assessing patency at 90 minutes with angiography has been appropriately called into question.[46] Interest in additional mechanisms by which SK (and other thrombolytic agents) may produce benefit has been growing. Substantially improved infarct-related artery patency is seen at 24 h and is due to the so-called catchup phenomenon. This fact is also illustrated in Table 24-2 and Table 24-3. Late patency is approximately 85%. Potential mecha-

nisms by which this may result in benefit are discussed further in a subsequent section. In addition to mortality benefit, improvement in ejection fraction, albeit modest, has been demonstrated with the use of SK, most notably when given in the early hours of an acute MI.[34,44,45] Again, the meager gains in left ventricular ejection fraction seem unlikely to account completely for the reduction in mortality. Rheologic and nonthrombolytic effects induced by SK administration have been postulated to contribute to its beneficial effect. These include reduction in blood viscosity,[47,48] free radical scavenger properties,[49] and antiplatelet effects.[50] However, the true significance of the rheologic factors has been disputed.[21,51]

In summation, SK is a safe and generally well-tolerated thrombolytic agent. Despite its "lackluster" performance in 90-minute angiographic

TABLE 24-3. Patency Rates for APSAC

Study	Time to Angiogram	Patency Rate % (n)
Early Patency		
Kasper (38)	60 min	64 (32/50)
TAPS (67)	60 min	60 (123/204)
Kasper	75 min	84 (42/50)
Been (69)	90 min	100 (16/16)
Lopez-Sendon (40)	90 min	86 (19/22)
Charbonnier (272)	90 min	70 (38/54)
Visser (301)	90 min	75 (107/142)
Hogg (68)	90 min	55 (32/58)
TAPS	90 min	70 (142/202)
TEAM-2 (71)	138 min	72 (132/183)
Voght (274)	156 min	77 (23/30)
Late Patency		
Hogg	24 h	81 (47/58)
Lopez-Sendon	24 h	91 (20/22)
TAPS	24 h	90 (123/137)
TEAM-3 (150)	24 h	89 (133/149)
SWIFT (277)	24 h	68 (255/373)

*Dose: 30 U intravenously over 5 minutes.
*Adapted with permission from Bates ER. Is survival from acute myocardial infarction related to thrombolytic efficacy or the open artery hypothesis? A controversy to be investigated in GUSTO. Chest 101 (suppl):140S, 1992; and Granger CB, Califf RM, Topol EJ. Thrombolytic therapy in acute myocardial infarction: a review. Drugs 44:293, 1992.

patency trials and paucity of fibrin specificity, it has been shown unequivocally to preserve left ventricular ejection fraction and reduce mortality when given in the early hours of an acute MI, particularly when accompanied by antiplatelet therapy (aspirin). Furthermore, it is easily synthesized in the laboratory and is the least expensive of the currently available thrombolytic agents.

Anisoylated Plasminogen–Streptokinase Activator Complex (APSAC)

A second-generation thrombolytic agent, anisoylated plasminogen–streptokinase activator complex (APSAC, anistreplase) is a stoichiometric combination of SK and human Lys-plasminogen which has greater fibrin specificity than the native Glu-plasminogen form.[52] It was specifically designed to improve on the efficacy of the parent compound with respect to fibrin specificity and thrombolytic potential.[41,53–60] Modification of SK–plasminogen activator complex by the reversible addition of an acyl group to the serine residue of the catalytic center on the plasminogen moiety protects it from rapid deactivation by α-antiplasmin and other plasmin inhibitors.[36,61] The plasminogen moiety undergoes slow deacylation after administration, producing a delayed onset of action and thus permitting a rapid one-time intravenous bolus of the agent.[62] Since the fibrin binding sites of plasminogen (the kringle domain) are well separated from the catalytic site and not affected by addition of the acyl group, the complex may therefore bind to forming thrombus prior to enzymatic activation.[31] This action and the enhanced fibrin affinity of Lys-plasminogen were designed to confer fibrin specificity, which is lacking in SK.[63,64]

Given at the recommended dose of 30 units intravenously over 2 to 3 minutes, deacylation occurs slowly (over approximately 90 minutes), substantially increasing the half-life as compared with SK. In addition, single-bolus dosing enhances ease of use and provides the potential for facilitated prehospital administration.[65] Unfortunately, at doses required in humans to obtain adequate reperfusion (30 units), APSAC loses any

potential for fibrin specificity and causes significant systemic fibrinogen depletion.[53,66] Furthermore, it retains considerable antigenicity, with the incidence of allergic reactions and hypotension similar to that seen with SK.[41,54–60]

Patency rates for APSAC at 60 minutes are over 60%[38,67] and at 90 minutes are over 70%[40,67–70] (see Table 24-3). These rates are more or less equivalent to those seen with tissue-type plasminogen activator (t-PA) (Table 24-4) and higher than that seen with SK (see Table 24-2). However, the rate of patency does not seem to increase between 90 and 120 minutes with APSAC, as it does with t-PA.[62] In a study published by Anderson and colleagues[71] comparing SK and APSAC given to patients presenting within 4 h of pain with electrocardiographic evidence of acute MI, patent infarct-related arteries considered to have Thrombolysis in Acute Myocardial Infarction (TIMI) Study grade 2 or 3 flow[72] were present in 72% of patients studied within 4 h of drug administration. Time from treatment to angiography also was evaluated. Overall, 72% of patients had patent infarct-related arteries when studied within 2.1 h of pain onset. The higher than average patency rate for SK in that study was attributed to early treatment with a thrombolytic agent (≤4 h) and a longer angiographic window allowing for the catchup phenomenon to occur.

Mortality after treatment with APSAC was evaluated in the British APSAC in Myocardial Infarction Study (AIMS).[73,74] In this trial, a 50% reduction in mortality was noted in patients treated with APSAC compared with placebo.

In summary, the majority of the information suggests that APSAC is a relatively safe and effective thrombolytic agent. In angiographic studies, patency rates tend to be higher at 60 and 90 minutes than with SK, and mortality is quite favorably affected. APSAC has a potential advantage over other agents in that it is given as a single bolus and has a uniform, prolonged duration of action. As with SK, its side-effect profile is related primarily to its antigenicity with common induction of hypotension, although these effects are typically self-limited. In addition, at the present time, it lacks competitive pricing with t-PA and is much more expensive than SK.

TABLE 24-4. Patency Rates for rt-PA

Study	Dose	Time to Treatment	Time to Angiogram	Patency Rate % (n)
			Early Patency	
TIMI 2A (278)	100/150 mg/6h	<4 h	84 min	82 (93/114)
RAAMI (95)	100 mg/3h	<6 h	90 min	75 (92/122)
TAMI-4 (279)	100 mg/3h	<4 h	90 min	52 (26/50)
TAMI-5 (79)	100 mg/3h	<5 h	90 min	71 (67/95)
CRAFT (80)	100 mg/3h	<6 h	90 min	63 (126/199)
KAMIT (107)	100 mg/3h	<4 h	95 min	64 (65/102)
GAUS (75)	70 mg/90 min	<6 h	97 min	69 (84/121)
Guerci (280)	80/100 mg/3h	192 min	150 min	66 (44/67)
			Late Patency	
GAUS	70 mg/90 min	<6 h	24 h	78 (82/105)
TEAM-3 (150)	100 mg/3h	<3 h	24 h	86 (128/149)
TIMI	100 mg/3h	<4 h	33 h	85 (1040/1229)
TIMI 2A (97)	100/150 mg/6h	<4 h	33 h	83 (93/114)

Adapted with permission from Granger CB, Califf RM, Topol EJ. Thrombolytic therapy for acute myocardial infartion: a review. Drugs 3:293, 1992.

Urokinase (UK)

Similar to SK, UK is one of the oldest thrombolytic agents in use today. Originally isolated from urine, it is now produced from primary cultures of fetal kidney cells and using recombinant DNA technology. A serine protease, it is produced as both high- and low-molecular-weight fractions. The latter is formed by proteolytic cleavage of the high-molecular-weight compound.[60,75,76] Both forms are highly active and can activate plasminogen directly.[77] The half-life of UK in vivo is estimated at 12 to 20 minutes. It can be given as a bolus or intravenous infusion. The degree of fibrinolysis and hemostatic abnormalities that result from its use are similar to those of both SK and APSAC, and it is lacking in fibrin specificity. Because it is an endogenous protein, it is not antigenic, and there is less hypotension with administration when it is used as either a bolus or an infusion.[78]

Dosage varies somewhat with the different studies. However, 2 million units intravenously over several minutes as a bolus has been used and was associated with a patency rate of 60% at the 60-minute (±30 minutes) arteriogram.[76] Infusion protocols generally administer 3 million units total. Three of the larger studies used a bolus dose of 1.5 million units, with the remaining dose over 90 minutes.[75,79,80] Wall et al.[81] gave 3 million units by intravenous infusion over 60 minutes. Angiographic patency rates at 1.5 h were similar with both protocols, ranging from 53% to 66%. In the large multicenter German Activator Urokinase Study (GAUS),[75] the patency rate at 120 minutes was 77% (increased from 66% at 90 minutes) and similar to that of t-PA. Of particular note in this study, UK was less effective when given later than 3 h from onset of symptoms. However, this was not the case for t-PA, although predischarge left ventricular ejection fractions were not statistically different. Ongoing studies with this agent are in progress. However, at the present time in the United States, it is not commonly used for single-drug treatment of acute MI.

Prourokinase (Single-Chain Urokinase, scu-PA)

Prourokinase is a single-chain molecule derived from urine or recombinant DNA technology. It is less active in this native state, but with cleavage of the Lys$_{158}$-Ile bond by plasmin, prourokinase becomes a two-chain molecule with markedly enhanced plasminogen activating properties. Activated prourokinase has particular affinity for clot-bound plasminogen, yielding improved fibrin specificity. In addition, prourokinase differs from UK in that it is inactivated by thrombin. The recombinant form seems to have more fibrin specificity and less systemic plasminogen activation. The half-life is short (3 to 20 minutes), and clearance is via the liver. The full thrombolytic effect, however, is attained after a long and variable latent period.[82]

Initial dose of prourokinase in early studies ranged from 50 to 70 mg given over 1 h. Coronary reperfusion rates of 50% to 70% were noted at these dosages.[83] More recently, data from the Prourokinase in Myocardial Infarction (PRIMI) Study[84] comparing prourokinase with SK showed that recombinant prourokinase given in a dose of 80 mg over 60 minutes (starting with a 20-mg bolus) achieved a patency rate of 72% at 90 minutes. Patency rates for both agents at 24 h were no different at approximately 85%. Newer dosing regimes with combinations of prourokinase and t-PA have been evaluated and are discussed in detail below.

Recombinant Tissue-Type Plasminogen Activator (rt-PA)

Tissue-type plasminogen activator (t-PA) is a second-generation thrombolytic agent. A 27 amino acid glycoprotein with a molecular weight of 70 kDa, it was initially purified from the culture fluid of a stable human melanoma cell line in sufficient quantities to study its biochemical properties. It is now synthesized by recombinant DNA technology using Chinese hamster ovary cells and designated rt-PA.[85] The native form is a single-chain molecule which upon exposure to plasmin is rapidly converted to a two-chain heterodimer. It was originally synthesized as a two-chain molecule with different pharmacokinetics but with similar pharmacodynamic and therapeutic properties to the single-chain form when used at equivalent doses. Early pharmacologic and clinical studies from 1984 to 1986 utilized this preparation. Now exclusively synthesized in the native (single-chain) form, the bulk of the clinical studies have been with this preparation.[85]

The fibrin specificity seen with this agent is due to a significantly enhanced plasminogen activation rate by rt-PA in the presence of fibrin and fibrin monomers. Fibrin-bound rt-PA has an increased affinity for plasminogen and forms a ternary complex on the clot surface.[86] The high affinity of rt-PA for plasminogen in the presence of fibrin results in efficient activation on the clot surface and relatively little activity in the plasma. Furthermore, plasmin formed on the clot surface has its lysine binding sites and active sites occupied, preventing rapid deactivation by α_2-antiplasmin.

The initial half-life ($t_{1/2,alpha}$) of this agent in plasma ranges from 3.6 to 4.6 minutes, whereas the terminal half-life ranges from 39 to 53 minutes. The activity of rt-PA is significantly affected by the circulating inhibitors present in the plasma. These include α_2-antiplasmin, α_1-antitrypsin, α-macroglobulin, C1-esterase inhibitor, and the plasminogen inhibitors (PAI-1 and PAI-2).[87,89] Unlike APSAC and scu-PA, the plasma levels of rt-PA achieved after intravenous administration are directly proportional to the rate of infusion. Thus more rapid infusions are associated with a significantly higher plasma concentration.[88,90] This observation has led to the use of accelerated dosing regimes for rt-PA (described below) designed to improve early patency. The currently recommended dosing regimen for rt-PA consists of a total dose of 100 mg given intravenously over 3 h. Administration begins with a bolus of 6 to 10 mg, followed by 50 to 54 mg during the first hour and 20 mg/h over the remaining 2 h. For patients weighing less than 65 kg, a reduced dose is given on a milligram per kilogram basis. A total of 1.25 mg/kg is recommended, with 60% given over the first hour (including bolus) and the remaining 40% over the next 2 h.[91]

Patency rates for conventionally dosed rt-PA are shown in Table 24-4. Weight-adjusted doses are depicted in Table 24-5. As illustrated, 90-minute patency is considerably higher than with the standard dose of SK and more or less equivalent to APSAC, although the interstudy variance

TABLE 24-5. Alternate Dosing Regimen for rt-PA

Study	Dose Regimen	Patency Rate 90 min % (n)
Weight Adjusted		
ECSG-1 (160)	0.75 mg/kg/90 min	70 (43/61)
ECSG-2 (281)	0.75 mg/kg/90 min	61 (38/62)
Topol (282)	1.5 mg/kg 4 h	79 (104/131)
Smalling (283)	1.2 mg/kg/1 h, then 0.8 mg/kg/2 h, 10% as bolus	84 (68/81)
TAMI-7 (284)	0.75 mg/kg 30 min, then 0.50 mg/kg/ 60 min, 10% of 1st dose as a bolus	83 (51/61)
TAMI-7	1 mg/kg/30 min, then 0.25 mg/kg/30 min, 10% of the 1st dose as a bolus	63 (24/37*)
Accelerated Doses		
TAMI-7	1.25 mg/kg/90 min, 20-mg bolus	61 (20/33)
Neuhaus (94)	50 mg/30 min, then 35 mg/1 h, 15-mg bolus	91 (67/74)
RAAMI (95)	50 mg/30 min, then 35 mg/1 h, 15-mg bolus	82 (105/128)
TAPS (67)	50 mg/30 min, then 35 mg/1 h, 15-mg bolus	84 (168/199)
Gemmill (285)	Two 35-mg boluses 30 min apart	87 (26/30)
Purvis (286)	20-mg bolus, then 50 mg	75 (15/20)
	50-mg bolus, then 20 mg	75 (15/20)
	50-mg bolus, then 50-mg	95 (18/19)

*Defined as TIMI grade 2 or 3 flow.
Adapted with permission from Bates ER. Is survival from acute myocardial infarction related to thrombolytic efficacy or the open artery hypothesis? A controversy to be investigated in GUSTO. Chest 101(suppl): 140S, 1992; and Granger CB, Califf RM, Topol EJ. Thrombolytic therapy in acute myocardial infarction: a review. Drugs 44:293, 1992.

is greater with the latter. Twenty-four-hour patency rates are similar to those of both SK and APSAC. It must be noted that anticoagulation regimes are not uniform among the studies, which may have some impact on the results. The use of adjuvant therapy with thrombolytic agents is discussed in a separate section.

At the presently recommended dose of rt-PA, patency rates at 90 minutes are greater than with SK, where a reperfusion plateau of ≤75% has been reached.[92,93] In an effort to improve on this, investigators have utilized the increased lytic potential of more rapidly administered rt-PA and have balanced this with the increased hemorrhagic complications resulting from an increased total dose. This has manifested two new dosing strategies. The first is a weight-adjusted dosing regimen with rt-PA given on a milligram per kilogram basis, and the other is an accelerated infusion ("front-loaded") of the standard dose. The latter entails a larger bolus, generally 15 mg, followed by 50 mg infused over 30 minutes, and ending with 35 mg given over the remaining 60 minutes. The major trials except for GUSTO-1 (see below) utilizing these two strategies are seen in Table 24-5. The dose-response curve seen with rt-PA is illustrated; as the dose increases from 0.75 to 1.4 mg/kg, so does the 90-minute angiographic patency rate. Although the strikingly high 90-minute arterial patency rate of 91% obtained by Neuhaus et al.[94] has not been duplicated, other studies[67,95] have reported improvement (81% to 87% patency) on the 75% plateau using the accelerated infusion protocol. Although generally encouraging, these relatively small studies lack the power to provide data on mortality.

Since this initial writing, results of the large Global Utilization of Streptokinase and Tissue Plasminogen Activator for Occluded Coronary Arteries (GUSTO) Trial[96] have become available. The findings of this important trial are discussed in a separate section at the end of this chapter.

Combination Therapy

Each of the thrombolytic agents discussed thus far have individual advantages; however, none is ideal. Recombinant t-PA achieves the highest patency rate at 90 minutes[97] but suffers from a short half-life resulting in higher reocclusion rates than non-fibrin-specific agents.[75,98–100] SK, UK, and APSAC, on the other hand, have a longer half-life than rt-PA but lack its relative fibrin specificity, causing marked systemic plasminemia. Efforts to abrogate the weakness of each of the thrombolytic agents by capitalizing on their strengths has led to the use of combination therapy. The basis of combination therapy rests on the theoretical concept of synergism between thrombolytic agents. Strictly defined, this represents a greater thrombolytic effect from a combination of agents than from either of the constituents alone. This concept has been tested both in laboratory animal and human studies. Although synergism has not been uniformly confirmed with in vitro models,[101–104] there has been considerable in vivo support for this concept in both animal and human studies. The most extensively studied combinations in acute MI include intravenous administration of either UK (including scu-PA) or SK and rt-PA. Table 24-6 compares the major combination trials in humans to date. Despite differences in methodology, patency rates with both regimes are intermediate to those found with conventional SK

and rt-PA monotherapy and "front-loaded" rt-PA therapy. Reocclusion rates for combination therapy are significantly lower (6%) than typically seen with conventional (10%) rt-PA monotherapy.[105] The lower rate of reocclusion with the combination regimen may be due to interference with fibrin polymerization,[106,107] antiplatelet effects of fibrin degradation products, or a salutary effect of prolonged fibrinogen depletion on endothelial healing.[79,108] Although enthusiasm for combination therapy is high and there is some clinical evidence of benefit, definitive data from larger mortality trials are lacking. The GUSTO Trial (see below) has now provided important data on combination therapy. Over 40,000 patients have been enrolled, of whom 10,000 received intravenous combination therapy with rt-PA (1 mg/kg) and SK (1 million units) over 60 minutes (see separate section).

TABLE 24-6. *Combination Thrombolytic Regimens*

Study	rt-PA	UK or rscu-PA	Patency 90 min	Reocclusion Rate	Comments
TAMI-2 (287)	1 mg/kg/1 h (90 mg max), 10 % total dose as bolus	0.5–2.0 m U/1 h	76% (85/112)	9% (10/110) at 7 d	IV heparin and ASA used. LVEF higher at follow-up in combination group.
TAMI-5 (79)	1 mg/kg/1 h (90 mg max), 10 % total dose as a bolus	1.5 m U/1 h	78% (75/97)	2% (2/94) at 5–10 d	IV heparin and ASA used. No difference in LVEF between groups; less clinical events in combination group.
TAMI-7 (284)	1 mg/kg/30 min (90 mg max)	1.5 m U/1 h	72% (30/42)	3% (1/42) at 5–7 d	IV heparin and ASA used. LVEF not significantly improved over other regimens.
URALMI (288)	1 mg/kg/1 h rt-PA	1.5 m U/1 h, 50-mg bolus SK	71% (55/78)	8% (5/65) at 5–7 d	
KAMIT pilot (289)	50 mg/1 h, 10-mg bolus	1.5 m U/1 h	75% (30/40)	8% (3/37) at 7 d	IV heparin and ASA used. LVEF improved from baseline to 7d.
KAMIT (107)	50 mg/1 h, 10-mg bolus	1.5 m U/1h	79% (81/102)	79% (8/102) at 7 d	IV heparin and ASA used. LVEF not significantly better than t-PA alone.
Bonnet (290)	50 mg/30 min, 20-mg bolus	1.0 m U/1 h	82% (28/34)	7% (2/28) at 24 h	Data on LVEF not reported.
GUSTO pilot (291)	1 mg/kg/30 min	1.0 m U/1 h	70% (33/47)	10% (4/51) at discharge	IV heparin and ASA used.

Adapted with permission from Granger CB, Califf RM, Topol EJ. Thrombolytic therapy for acute myocardial infarction: a review. Drugs 3:293, 1992.

Third-Generation Agents

Although the present assortment of thrombolytic agents has a broad spectrum of pharmacologic characteristics and well-established clinical efficacy, refinement and the search for new and better drugs have continued. Currently, approximately 15% to 20% of coronary thrombi are refractory to timely thrombolysis, and rethrombosis may be as high as 20% with some agents. Furthermore, the incidence of hemorrhagic complications remains at 6% to 10%. Because of these factors, efforts to improve fibrin specificity, thrombolytic activity, and overall safety have continued.[109] Experimentation with combination therapy and recombinant DNA technology have yielded a heterogeneous array of newer thrombolytic agents.[110]

Numerous mutants of t-PA, which have a higher fibrin specificity and longer in vivo half-life, constitute potentially useful thrombolytic agents. These are produced by modification, deletion, or duplication of the five t-PA functional domains.[110–112] Work with these newer forms continues, and in vitro studies and preliminary data in animals have confirmed the theorized advantages over "wild type" t-PA.[111,113–117]

Single-chain UK also has been subjected to site-specific mutagenesis.[116] Even though UK is already a relatively fibrin-specific compound, this manipulation did little to enhance the molecule's fibrin affinity, but it did prevent conversion to the enzymatically active two-chain form. The compound was unable to lyse a fibrin clot in vitro, but further amino acid substitution has led to the manufacture of a low-molecular-weight scu-PA[118] that may be preferable to intact scu-PA for large-scale production by recombinant DNA technology.[110]

In addition to site-directed mutagenesis of thrombolytic agents, hybrid molecules have been produced by numerous investigators in an effort to improve thrombolytic agents. This entails the chemical manufacture of chimeric proteins that contain sites harboring the enzymatic activity of one type of thrombolytic agent and the fibrin-specific sites of another. Linking of the catalytic site on UK (single- and double-chain forms) to fibrin binding sites of rt-PA has thus far been accomplished.[115,119,120] Although this new molecule has improved fibrin specificity, its enzymatic activity in vitro is not improved.[121] Another chimeric molecule that may possess potential for improved activity is produced by linking the K-1 and K-2 domains to the serine protease domain (Pu) of scu-PA. This agent has been shown to have preserved specificity but reduced fibrin affinity in vitro[14,111] and increased thrombolytic potency in vivo, mainly due to a reduced rate of clearance from the circulation.[14,121]

Acylation of the active center of a plasminogen molecule and its coupling to SK has produced APSAC. This has resulted in improved duration of action and ability to be given as a bolus. However, this agent still suffers from the problems of immunogenicity (allergic reaction, hypotension, etc.). Furthermore, despite hopes of improved fibrin specificity, this has not been found to be the case. Hybridization of plasminogen with rt-PA and acylation of the plasminogen-active center have resulted in a unique chimeric molecule. This agent has been shown to possess a prolonged half-life that would allow bolus administration, as well as improved thrombolytic activity and fibrin specificity in animal preparations as compared with rt-PA.[12]

Along with sophisticated genetic engineering of currently available agents, the development of totally new thrombolytic proteins continues to progress. One such agent is the plasminogen activator extracted from the salivary glands of the vampire bat, *Desmodus rotundus,* and referred to as *bat-PA.*[122] Studied primarily in vitro in animal and models, this agent, although similar to rt-PA, has a slower plasma clearance and markedly increased fibrin-dependent plasminogen activation. While these new attributes are intriguing and hold promise, questions regarding the efficacy of this agent in humans remain,[123] and it has not yet been tested thoroughly in patients.

Organic nitrates have been the cornerstone of antianginal therapy since 1867 when Brunton[124] first reported the clinical effectiveness of amyl nitrite. Since that time, nitrates have undergone numerous refinements, but the therapeutic utility of these compounds is generally thought to result from their vasculoactive properties.[125] However, there is a growing body of evidence in support of a substantial antiplatelet effect as well.[126,127] Organic nitrates as a class are metabolized to nitric oxide (or one of its *S*-nitrothiol congeners). This metabolite is a potent activator of platelet guanylate cyclase, which through the actions of increased cyclic GMP and subsequent reduction of agonist-mediated calcium flux produces an attenuation in the binding of fibrinogen to platelet glycoprotein IIb-IIIa receptors.[126,127] Inhibition of this "final common pathway" for platelet aggregation confers potent antiplatelet activity to these agents. *S*-Nitrosylation of rt-PA (via the enzymes solitary free sulfhydryl group Cys-83) to produce NO-S-rt-PA has been performed successfully in the laboratory.[128] This endows the plasminogen activator with vasodilatory as well as substantial antiplatelet properties. Importantly, this modification in no way affects the enzyme's fibrinolytic activity, fibrin specificity, or binding with its physiologic serine protease inhibitor, plasminogen activator inhibitor-1 (PAI-1). This unique and new plasminogen activator is quite provocative and should provide further insight into the role the vascular endothelium plays in the setting of thrombosis and hemostasis. Moreover, the potential for enhanced efficacy in the thrombolytic treatment of acute MI and other thrombotic disorders is present.

The development of new combinations and classes of thrombolytic agents has continued in a quest for the "ideal agent." This has led to the development of several novel and potentially useful new plasminogen activators. Enhanced fibrin selectivity and prolonged half-life may indeed be attributes of a superior agent. However, some would argue that a rapid plasma elimination is beneficial, particularly in the setting of untoward bleeding.[117] Furthermore, the systemic lytic state produced by non-fibrin-selective agents (e.g., SK) may be responsible for maintaining patency beyond the 90-minute window.[19,82] Moreover, even with the theoretical development of a totally new fibrin-specific plasminogen activator, there is as yet no way for the new molecule to distinguish between a pathologic thrombus and a protective hemostatic plug. Despite these caveats, future research and development in these areas will, at the very least, improve our knowledge and understanding of thrombolysis.[117]

MEASURED BENEFITS OF THROMBOLYTIC THERAPY

Endpoint selection for testing the benefits of thrombolytic therapy has been the subject of considerable debate.[129,130] Each of the commonly used endpoints has an inherent problem which may subsequently limit its application. Originally based on the pathophysiologic theory of early myocardial salvage associated with recanalization of an occluded coronary artery, the benefit(s) of thrombolytic therapy is(are) now known to be more complex. Thus clinically meaningful endpoints that account for both the benefits and risks associated with the administration of these agents are needed to guide their use. The most common endpoints that have been used thus far to compare the present thrombolytic agents include mortality, left ventricular ejection fraction, infarct artery patency, infarct size, and more recently, composite indices.

Mortality

Even though mortality is considered to be the most important of endpoints,[21] mortality studies are the most difficult to conduct because of the very large number of patients required to demonstrate meaningful differences between groups. Using the currently accepted statistical model (alpha: 0.05, beta: 0.20), detection of an absolute 1% reduction in mortality (e.g., from 8% to 7%, 15% relative reduction) requires approximately 15,000 to 20,000 patients. This imposes a tremendous organizational cost to the study, limiting the application of such a design. Still, mortality is generally accepted as one of the most meaningful endpoints in that it is highly objective and all other measurable variables contribute to it. Measurement of mortality typically has been divided into early (approximately 30 days) and late (1 year). This takes into account the very early (within 24 h) increase in mortality seen with thrombolytic therapy due to fatal cerebral hemorrhage, myocardial rupture, and yet unexplained factors known as the "early hazard"[28,33] as well as any survival advantage (evident during hospitalization, chiefly by 72 h, and continued for at least 1 year).[28,73,74] This finding has been confirmed recently in a large overview by Baigent and colleagues.[131] In an analysis of six large trials with over 45,500 patients, deaths were significantly higher at day 0 (day of randomization) in thrombolytic-treated patients than in controls (576 versus 456; $p < 0.00001$). However, deaths at days 2 to 35 were higher in the control group as opposed to the active treatment group (1818 versus 1328, respectively; $p < 0.00001$).

Streptokinase

Mortality reduction with the use of SK in acute MI was conclusively demonstrated in 1986 with report of the large Italian GISSI-1 study[28] and again in the ISIS-2.[33] In GISSI-1, 11,806 patients were randomized to receive either SK 1.5 million units over 60 minutes or conventional therapy. There was no specified protocol for adjuvant therapy with anticoagulants or antiplatelet agents. Entrance criteria were based on electrocardiographic evidence of ST-segment elevation or depression and onset of the symptoms within 12 h. Overall mortality for the entire population was reduced by 18%. For patients randomized within 3 and 1 h from onset of pain, mortality was reduced by 23% and a striking 49%, respectively. One year later, the results of ISIS-2 were reported. This involved a 2 × 2 factorial design in which 17,187 patients were randomized to one of four groups: (1) intravenous SK, (2) 160 mg of chewable aspirin, (3) SK and aspirin, or (4) double placebo. In contrast to GISSI-1, no electrocardiographic entry criteria were used, and the window of treatment was extended to 24 h. Mortality again was shown to be reduced in the SK group (9.2% versus 12.0%). In addition, an important finding that the combination of SK and aspirin was significantly better than either agent alone was shown, and this benefit extended throughout the 24-h treatment period. Similar to GISSI-1, there was no dedicated anticoagulant group. However, in the subgroups that received either intravenous or subcutaneous heparin, vascular deaths were less across all treatment arms when compared with double placebo.

Long-term follow-up of patients enrolled in the early Western Washington Streptokinase in Myocardial Infarction Study has been reported. Pooled results of the intracoronary and intravenous arms performed throughout the 1980s have failed to show a 3- to 8-year survival advantage between treated and placebo groups despite a trend in that direction.[132] However, the total number of patients was relatively small ($n = 618$) and may lack the power for this determination.

APSAC

Mortality benefits with APSAC were demonstrated in the APSAC Intervention Mortality Study (AIMS)[73,74] and in ISIS-3.[32] APSAC was given within 6 h of onset of symptoms as an intravenous bolus of 30 units over 5 minutes, and 30-day mortality was reduced from 12.1% in the placebo group to 6.4% in the APSAC group. This represented a 50.5% odds reduction in mortality (CI = 26% to 67%; $p = 0.0006$). Furthermore, a survival benefit was still observed. At 12 months, 69 patients (11%) treated with APSAC had died, compared with 113 patients (18%) given placebo (odds reduction 43%; $p = 0.0007$; 95% CI = 21% to 59%). This effect on mortality was not related to time between onset of symptoms and treatment or to any patient characteristic.[73] Of note, however, is that absolute benefit may be overestimated because the trial was terminated prematurely due to improved outcome identified early in the treatment arm. In retrospect, this probably represented a "high point" in terms of benefit.

Several smaller studies (less than 350 patients) also have evaluated the use of IV APSAC in acute MI. When compared with IV heparin[73,133] and intracoronary SK, these studies have either shown statistically significant benefit[134] or trends toward significance.[133,134]

Tissue-Type Plasminogen Activator

Designed to test the effects of IV rt-PA on 30-day mortality, the Anglo-Scandinavian Study of Early Thrombolysis (ASSET)[135,136] evaluated 5011 patients randomized to 100 mg of rt-PA given within 6 h of onset of symptoms in the conventional regimen (10-mg bolus followed by 50 mg over the first hour, followed by 40 mg over the next 2 h) or placebo. All patients received IV heparin for 24 h. Thirty-day all-cause mortality was reduced by rt-PA from 9.8% to 7.2%, representing a 28% odds reduction (CI = 19% to 39%; p = 0.0011). At 6 months, the mortality rates were 10.4% (alteplase) and 13.1% (placebo), representing a relative reduction of 21% (95% CI = 8% to 32%; p = 0.0026). Six-month mortality rates in patients with proven MI were 12.6% and 17.1%, respectively (relative reduction 26%; 95% CI = 14% to 37%). A smaller study, the Fourth European Cooperative Study Group (ECSG-4) Study,[137] tested the effects of rt-PA given in the conventional manner within 5 h of symptom onset against control. All patients received IV heparin for 3 days, followed by oral anticoagulation and 250 mg aspirin. Fourteen-day mortality in the placebo group was 5.7% compared with 2.8% with rt-PA (51% odds reduction; p = 0.06). An analysis of six large mortality studies comparing rt-PA with placebo revealed an overall 29% reduction in mortality (CI = 15% to 41%; p = 0.0003).[138]

Comparison of the Thrombolytic Agents

The introduction of newer thrombolytic agents other than SK and UK offered a potential for improved infarct-related artery patency and fibrin specificity while at the same time minimizing adverse bleeding and allergic complications. The development of these agents has prompted (and continues to prompt) comparative trials in an attempt to identify the best overall thrombolytic agent.

INTRAVENOUS SK, RT-PA, AND APSAC

One of the first large-scale comparative trials published, the Second Gruppo Italiano por lo Studio della Supravivienza 'nell'Infarcto Miacardio (GISSI-2)[139] was a multicenter, randomized, open-label study designed to compare the standard SK dose of 1.5 million units given IV over 30 to 60 minutes with the standard rt-PA regimen (bolus 10 mg followed by 50 mg over first hour, then 40 mg over next 2 h) given to patients within 6 h of presentation for acute MI. In addition, patients were randomized to either subcutaneous heparin (12,500 U), given every 12 h starting 12 h after the thrombolytic infusion was complete, or usual care. Aspirin and beta blockers were recommended therapy for all patients and were given in 87% and 45.3%, respectively. Hospital mortality was 8.6% in the SK group and 9.0% (p = NS) in the rt-PA group. In the original design of the GISSI-2 Study, the primary endpoint was to be a composite of mortality and left ventricular function. To detect the presence of any meaningful difference in the various subgroups, an additional 8401 patients were recruited from a second trial (the International rt-PA/SK Mortality Trial).[140] This study was carried out in several different countries using the GISSI-2 protocol. Together, a total of 20,891 patients were randomized to each of the groups. At completion, 91% of patients received aspirin and 36% received atenolol along with the respective thrombolytic agents. The results showed no difference in 5-week mortality between the SK (8.5%) and rt-PA (8.9%) groups. Concerns centered on the method of heparin administration prompted criticism of the study. The use of subcutaneous heparin given 12 h after completion of the thrombolytic regimen is deemed inadequate by many investigators, particularly for rt-PA. Critics maintain that with rt-PA, intravenous heparin is required for maximum efficacy due to its short half-life and reduced systemic fibrinolysis.[141-143] Others, however, have convincingly argued to the contrary.[46,82,144,145]

In the largest comparative trial of thrombolytic agents to date, the Third International Study of Infarct Survival (ISIS-3),[32] 46,091 patients underwent randomization to either SK, rt-PA, or APSAC. Patients presenting 6 to 24 h from onset of symptoms and without ST-segment elevation also were enrolled. As in GISSI-2, all patients were to receive aspirin (162 mg/d) started on presentation (97% did). In addition, half were randomized to subcutaneous calcium heparin (9500 U every 12 h) starting 4 h after randomization and continuing for 7 days. Oral anticoagulation was avoided unless specifically indicated.

As illustrated in Figure 24-2, the 35-day vascular mortality rate for rt-PA, SK and APSAC was 10.3%, 10.6%, and 10.5%, respectively (p = NS). Furthermore, no difference in vascular mortality was noted between the heparin and nonheparin

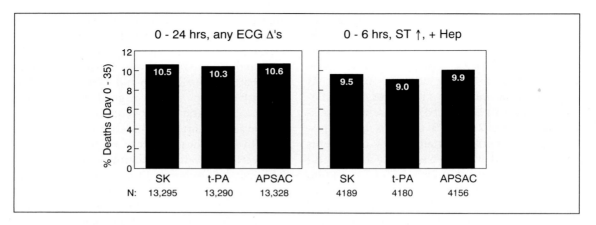

FIGURE 24-2. Thirty-five-day vascular mortality data for patients enrolled in various arms of the ISIS-3 Trial. The graph on the left depicts number of deaths in patients with any evidence of ECG abnormality enrolled within 24 h of symptom onset. The graph on the right shows number of deaths in patients with ST-segment elevation enrolled within 6 h of symptom onset and receiving heparin. The total number of patients in each group is listed at the bottom. (Reprinted with permission from Topol EJ. Which thrombolytic agent should one choose? Prog Cardiovasc Dis 3:165, 1991.)

groups (10.3% and 10.6%, respectively). However, again, advocates of rt-PA are critical of the manner in which heparin was used or not administered in half the patients. Furthermore, unlike the prototypical patient receiving thrombolysis for acute MI in the United States, the window of enrollment extended through 24 h from onset of symptoms, and in 25% of patients, the ECG was somewhat difficult to interpret. Still, when the subgroup of patients presenting within 6 h of symptom onset was analyzed separately, mortality between the groups was again not statistically different (SK = 10.0%, rt-PA = 9.6%, APSAC = 9.9%). When the data from GISSI-2 and ISIS-3 studies are analyzed together, mortality data on 48,293 patients are available for analysis. It is now clear that all three agents effectively reduce short- and long-term (at least to 1 year) mortality when given in the setting of acute MI. There are no significant differences in vascular mortality between the evaluated thrombolytic agents in the doses given and with the specified adjuvant regimens.

Optimal heparin administration within the various thrombolytic agents remains an unanswered question in the minds of many investigators. Studies to date are lacking large, prospective, direct comparisons between intravenous and sub-

cutaneous routes. Data from the recently completed Global Utilization of Streptokinase and rt-PA for Occluded Coronary Arteries (GUSTO) Study,[96] discussed at the end of this chapter, provide important insights into this issue.

Left Ventricular Function

The rationale for the use of left ventricular ejection fraction (LVEF) as an endpoint measure of thrombolytic efficacy has developed as an outgrowth of the early observations linking it directly to mortality. Indeed, the function of the left ventricle, as measured by ejection fraction, has been shown to be the most important prognostic factor in the post-MI period.[146] It is an objective variable that is easily and accurately measured by radionuclide, echocardiographic, angiographic, and now magnetic resonance imaging techniques. Furthermore, it is measured as a continuous variable, and as such, a much smaller sample population is required to show a statistical difference. It is for these reasons that some[129] argue that LVEF is the endpoint of choice in thrombolytic trials.

However, evaluation of ejection fraction after thrombolytic therapy has a number of shortcomings that limit its usefulness. First, early studies correlating LVEF and mortality after MI were not in the setting of thrombolytic administration and may not be directly applicable. Second, trials using LVEF as a primary endpoint have been weakened by large amounts of missing data points. These typically represent the more seriously ill patients who have died early in the hospital course (5% to 10% early mortality) and the technically inadequate studies (15% to 20%). Together, this may account for a significant number of patients. Thus measurements in these stud-

ies may tend to overestimate the gains in ejection fraction. Moreover, LVEF seems to be more closely associated with vessel patency[105] than with improved survival and thus may not be an ideal primary endpoint.[130] With these caveats in mind, the major studies evaluating the salutary effects of intravenously administered thrombolytic agents on preservation of left ventricular function are discussed below. Table 24-7 lists the major studies with thrombolytic agents utilizing LVEF as an endpoint.

TABLE 24-7. *Left Ventricular Function Following Intravenous Thrombolytic Therapy*

Study	Patients*	Lytic/Time to Rx	Time	Method	TX Group %	Control %	p Value
SK Trials							
ISAM (34)	1741 (848)	SK <3h 3–6 h	3–4 wks	Contrast	All 56.8 57 56.6	All 53.9 53.6 54.4	<0.005 <0.05 NS
White (44)	219 (155)	SK/<4 h	3 wks	Contrast	59	53	<0.005
Western Washington (45)	368 (170)	SK.mean 3.5 h	6–8 wks	RNA	50.8	46.6	<0.02
rt-PA Trials							
Nat'l Heart Assoc. Australia (197)	144 (103)	rt-PA/<3 h	1 wk	Contrast	57.7	51.1	0.04
Guerci (280)	85 (85)	rt-PA/<4 h	10 d	RNA	53.2	46.4	<0.02
O'Rourke (292)	145 (126)	rt-PA/<2.5 h	3 wks	Contrast	61	54	<0.006
ECSG-4 (137)	721 (577)	rt-PA/<3 h	10–22 d	Contrast	50.7	48.5	<0.05
TPAT (293)	115 (115)	rt-PA/3 h	9 d	RNA	53.6	47.8	0.017
rt-PA vs SK							
TIMI-1 (97)	290 (145)	SK/<7 h rt-PA/<7 h	Pre-discharge	Contrast	49.1 49.9	None	NS
PAIMS (148)	116 (116)	SK/<3 h rt-PA/<3 h	Hospital discharge	Echo	51 56	None	0.05
White (294)	270 (240)	SK/<3 h rt-PA/<3 h	3 wks	Contrast	58 58	None	NS
rt-PA vs UK							
GAUS (75)	157 (101)	UK/<6 h rt-PA/<6 h	10–28 d	Contrast	52 53	None	NS
rt-PA vs APSAC							
Bassand (149)	169	APSAC/<5 h rt-PA/<5 h	3–7 d	Contrast	50 52	None	NS
TEAM-3 (150)	325 (277)	APSAC/<4 h rt-PA/<4 h	7 d (pre-discharge)	RNA	51.3 54.1	None	0.04
	325 (215)	APASC rt-PA	1 mo (38 d)		50.2 54.8		0.002

*Total number of patients randomized is listed. Number in parenthesis represents the number undergoing evaluation of LVEF when available.
Adapted with permission from Cairns JA, Fuster V, Kennedy JW. Coronary thrombolysis. Chest 102(suppl):482S, 1992.

Intravenous SK versus Placebo

As shown in Table 24-7, three studies measured LVEF after intravenous SK was administered within 6 h of the onset of symptoms.[44,45,147] Left ventricular function was measured by contrast ventriculography in two studies and by radionuclide ventriculography in one. In the ISAM Trial,[34] small but significantly better left ventricular function was present only in the group treated with SK within 3 h of symptom onset. In the remaining patients treated at 3 to 6 h, no difference in LVEF was detected. Two smaller studies, White et al.[44] and the western Washington group,[45] reported somewhat greater improvement in LVEF (6% and 4.2%, respectively) between the SK-treated group as compared with placebo. Patients in these studies underwent thrombolytic therapy within 4 h of symptom onset.

Intravenous rt-PA versus Placebo

The effect of rt-PA on salvage of left ventricular function has been well studied. Five trials in all, three using contrast ventriculography and two using radionuclide angiography, have evaluated LVEF after thrombolysis and found statistically significant improvement in overall left ventricular function with treatment. Four of these studies were small, with less than 150 patients undergoing left ventricular assessment. The European Cooperative Study,[137] however, successfully evaluated over 500 patients and found a small (2.2%) but significant improvement in the rt-PA group.

Comparison Studies

The effects of intravenous SK compared with rt-PA on LVEF have been assessed in GISSI-2,[139] TIMI-1,[98] PAIMS,[148] GAUS,[75] and the study of White and colleagues.[44] Despite methodologic differences, four of these trials failed to show significant difference in LVEF between the two groups when measured by the various tests of left ventricular function. The Italian PAIMS Study, however, did show a small but significant improvement in LVEF as measured by echo at hospital discharge favoring the rt-PA group (56% versus 51%; $p = 0.05$) over the SK-treated patients. A composite endpoint of death and severe left ventricular damage was used in the large GISSI-2

Study, but no difference between the two agents was found.

Intravenous APSAC was compared with conventionally administered rt-PA within 4 h of symptom onset in a multicenter French study.[149] Ejection fraction was measured by contrast ventriculography at an average of 5.3 days and by radionuclide angiography at 18 days. No difference between the two thrombolytic agents was noted in either type of measurement with the statistical model used. However, a small 1% to 2% intergroup difference and slight improvement in regional wall motion favoring the rt-PA group was noted but did not reach statistical significance.

The recently reported Third Trial of Eminase in Acute Myocardial Infarction (TEAM-3)[150] compared the effects of standard dose intravenous APSAC and rt-PA on ejection fraction when administered to patients within 4 h of ECG-confirmed acute MI. Radionuclide ejection fractions were done at baseline soon after thrombolytic dosing (all within 4 h), at hospital discharge (or 7 to 10 days), and at 3- to 6-week follow-up. Coronary angiography was performed on average at 24 h. These investigators found that convalescent ejection fraction at the predischarge study averaged 51.3% in the APSAC group and 54.2% in the rt-PA group ($p < 0.05$). At 1 month, gains in the rt-PA group were somewhat higher, albeit still modest, at 54.8% as compared with APSAC (50.2%). This difference persisted when analysis was limited to patients presenting with first-time MI. Of note, exercise ejection fraction and exercise times were not different between the two groups at the 3- to 6-week follow-up evaluation. To account for patients who died before the follow-up study, an imputed analysis was performed. The results revealed no difference between the two thrombolytics in discharge (7- to 10-day) ejection fraction but a statistically significant improvement in the rt-PA group (rt-PA 55.5% versus APSAC 50.5%; $p = 0.007$) at 1 month follow-up. Of interest, the investigators found that the improvement in ejection fraction present in the rt-PA group at discharge was due to improved function of the myocardial segments in the infarct zone and smaller end-systolic volumes. Coronary artery patency rates were similar between the two agents at 24 h. This is the first and only trial to date to demonstrate a difference in ejection fraction between thrombolytic agents using radionuclide assessment.

In summary, modest improvement in LVEF can probably be expected after the administration of thrombolytic agents for acute MI when these drugs are given within 3 (and perhaps 4) h of symptom onset.[34,138] Until recently, no agent in the conventional dosing regimes appeared to be superior in improving posttreatment ejection fraction. The recently reported TEAM-3 Trial[150] favoring rt-PA is provocative and awaits confirmation. The use of front-loaded regimes may yield more significant gains in postthrombolytic left ventricular function, and trials are presently underway. Still, in the setting of thrombolytic administration, the clinical implications of ejection fraction measurement and its use as a marker of functional benefit, myocardial salvage, and infarct healing remain highly debated. The effects of non-infarct-zone compensatory hyperkinesis and therapeutic interventions (e.g., PTCA, etc.) confound its use as an index of benefit. Because large mortality trials to evaluate every new thrombolytic regimen are impractical to perform, the use of a composite endpoint that gives a weight-adjusted severity score for various mortal and morbid events has been proposed as an alternate way to assess clinical benefit in intermediately sized trials.[130] This was used in the TEAM-3 Study[150] and TAMI-5[79] and has been prospectively validated in the GUSTO Trial.

Postthrombolysis Infarct-Related Artery Patency

Since the early angiographic studies of patients with acute MI demonstrated the unequivocal presence of occlusive coronary thrombus, rapid lysis of clot and restoration of infarct-related artery patency have been the primary goals of thrombolytic therapy. The myocardial salvage associated with this process is generally believed to be the primary mechanism of benefit. Support for this comes from the observation that improved left ventricular function and survival are most marked when treatment is implemented within

the first hour of symptom onset,[28,137] with progressive diminution of benefit thereafter. Accordingly, numerous studies have used angiographic evidence of infarct-related artery patency to evaluate the benefit of thrombolytic compounds in the treatment of evolving acute MI. When considering this large body of data, however, it is important to realize that coronary patency is a dynamic event and that early angiographic evaluation (most notably the 90-minute endpoint) is only a transient representation of cyclic flow within the coronary artery. The clinical impact of this phenomenon has yet to be fully elucidated. Furthermore, some studies have shown that early (90-minute) coronary artery patency does not predict clinical outcome after thrombolysis.[151] Recently, the classic definition of patency (defined previously as TIMI grade 2 or 3 flow) has come under intensified scrutiny. A recent report by the TEAM investigators has found a smaller infarct size by enzymatic and ECG criteria with TIMI grade 3 flow as opposed to TIMI grade 2 flow.[71] Momentum for this observation is increasing, and similar results have been reported in a preliminary study analyzing patency data from TAMI trials 1 to 7[152] and in a review of four angiographic studies by Voght and colleagues.[153] Furthermore, the terminology used in reporting data on the efficacy of thrombolytic agents is important. The "reperfusion" rate is no longer used as an endpoint because it requires a pretreatment angiogram to assess vessel patency, thus significantly delaying time to treatment. These data are available for SK primarily from the early studies using intracoronary thrombolysis and from the initial TIMI dose-ranging trials with intravenous rt-PA.[154]

Furthermore, upon review of the studies on patency, it is important to note that spontaneous reperfusion occurs in about 10% of patients entered into angiographic trials.[155–157] Spontaneous patency is seen in 35% of patients at 12 to 24 h and 83% by 3 weeks,[158] and reocclusion is estimated to occur in 5% to 30% of vessels that are initially recanalized. The majority of these occur within the first 24 h, with fewer noted thereafter.[159] All these factors must be taken into account when interpreting the data on patency after thrombolysis.

Tables 24-2 to 24-6 list the agents and the major trials assessing infarct vessel patency. The early reperfusion studies have been omitted. In these early trials using intracoronary SK, reperfusion at 60 to 90 minutes ranged from 60% to 80% when treatment was given within 6 h of symptom onset. Intravenous SK reperfusion rates at 90 minutes range from 31% to 62%.[138] The reperfusion rate at 90 minutes with IV rt-PA given in the conventional protocol within 5 h of symptom onset was approximately 70%.[72,154]

Patency rates at 90 minutes with intravenous SK are shown in Table 24-2. They tend to range from approximately 30% to 60%[138] when given in the conventional manner within 6 h of symptom onset. As with all agents, 24-h patency rates are considerably higher.

Early patency with IV APSAC (Table 24-3) has been evaluated in a number of studies. When given as a 30-unit bolus over 5 to 15 minutes (the majority of protocols use 5 minutes) within 3 h of symptom onset, 90-minute patency rates ranging from 66% to 74% have been reported.[105]

Patency rates with IV rt-PA depend primarily on the total dose given and the interval of infusion (see Tables 24-4 and 24-5). Early reperfusion studies showed that 100 mg given over 3 h was superior to 80 mg and as efficacious as 150 mg without the increased hemorrhagic complication rates associated with the latter. Using the 100-mg dose given over 3 h, the average 90-minute patency rates for both the double-chain preparation (duteplase) and the single-chain preparation (alteplase) have been reported to be 69% and 72%, respectively.[32] The 90-minute patency rates for front-loaded regimens are improved, as shown in Table 24-5 (GUSTO-1, similar to the Neuhaus protocol) and generally range from 81% to 91%.

Patency rates for UK have been assessed in several moderately sized trials to date.[75,79,80] The most commonly used dose is 3 million units given over 90 minutes, which results in a 90-minute patency rate of 55% to 64%.

Comparative trials of the various thrombolytic agents have generally mirrored the results of noncomparative studies with regard to infarct-related artery patency. These trials[41,44,67,68,71,75,84,98,108,148,150,160] and large overviews[105] of these and smaller studies standardize treatment protocols and have confirmed that conventional dosing of rt-PA achieves a higher infarct-related artery patency rate at 90 minutes (70%) than standard-dose SK (51%), UK (60%), rscu-PA (71%), or APSAC (70%). Accelerated dosing of rt-PA (100 mg IV over 90 minutes) has been shown to achieve the highest patency rates (84%) at 90 minutes[105] and, if substantiated in the large trials now underway, holds promise as a new standard for rt-PA administration.

In addition to the stratification of thrombolytic agents with regard to early patency, these trials also have clearly shown that the advantage enjoyed by rt-PA at 90 minutes gradually declines over time. The patency rates for IV SK and APSAC exhibit a catchup phenomenon approaching 70% at 2 to 3 h and approximately 85% at 1 day.[105,138] Patency is ultimately restored in 85% to 90% of patients 3 weeks after thrombolysis regardless of the thrombolytic agent used.[105] However, ample evidence has been offered to demonstrate that a cycle of recurrent coronary thrombosis and dissolution is occurring throughout this period. This may be more prevalent with the "clot-specific" agents[161] due to the higher levels of circulating fibrinogen and reduced amount of fibrin degradation products that have potent antiplatelet and anticoagulant effects.[148] This may explain, at least partially, the apparent lack of survival despite improved early patency with the use of rt-PA. If the cycle of recurrent thrombosis (silent or not) is associated with progressive cellular damage, any benefit derived from expedient reperfusion may be lost over time until final patency is achieved.[62]

Late Thrombolysis and Infarct-Related Artery Patency

Administration of a thrombolytic agent early in the evolution of an acute MI is predicated on the belief that reperfusion within a critical time will abrogate ongoing myocardial necrosis, salvage jeopardized myocardium, and translate into improved survival.[162] This time period, derived experimentally from animal data, is generally thought to be within 4 to 6 h of symptom onset. Subsequently, numerous studies have shown that in the setting of an acute MI, patients with a patent infarct-related vessel have a very favorable prognosis compared with those who have an occluded coronary artery.[22,163–166] The observation that reperfusion therapy initiated more than 6 h from onset of symptoms may still have benefit was first alluded to in various small studies conducted throughout the mid-1980s. This concept gained considerable momentum with the report of a large meta-analysis substantiating this finding.[167] Although data from the GISSI-1 group[28] suggested that little benefit was gained after 6 h of pain, this trial only randomized approximately 2000 patients to late administration (>6 h), so the statistical power to detect a significant difference was low. Subsequent to this, data from ISIS-2 that tested about 10,000 patients assigned to late administration (>4 h) of thrombolytic therapy verified that patients treated late with SK had a significant reduction in vascular mortality.[33] However, the benefit decreased with increasing delay to treatment such that an odds reduction of $35 \pm 6\%$ at 0 to 4 h was reduced to $21 \pm 12\%$ at 12 to 24 h. The mortality reduction overall for patients treated among 6 and 24 h remained highly significant ($18 \pm 7\%; p = 0.01$) overall.

Data from the EMERAS Study[168,169] further evaluated the value of thrombolytic therapy for patients presenting between 6 and 12 h after onset of symptoms. This study showed that for patients presenting between 7 and 12 h, 5-week vascular mortality was lower in the thrombolytic as opposed to the placebo group (12.6% versus 14.6%, respectively; $p = $ NS). The benefit, however, for patients presenting between 12 and 24 h was less apparent (12.9% versus 13.5%), although this may have been attenuated by the increased risk of death within the first 24 h. When death within the first 24 h is excluded, the vascular mortality for patients treated with thrombolytic therapy is lower than that of those treated with placebo (7.5% versus 10.2%; $p < 0.01$).[170] In EMERAS, however, there was an excess of hemorrhagic complications in the SK-treated group. Combined with the lack of statistically significant benefit in the 6- to 12-h treatment group, the results were difficult to interpret insofar as adopting SK for routine therapy of late-entry patients.

The Late Assessment of Thrombolytic Effi-

cacy (LATE) Trial[171] was a multinational collaborative effort designed to further evaluate the merits of thrombolytic therapy given after the traditional 4-h time period. In this study, 5709 patients with a mean age 62.8 years (25% age > 70 years) were randomized to either rt-PA and aspirin in conventional doses (IV heparin was recommended) or placebo 4 to 24 h after the onset of symptoms. Thirty-six percent received treatment within 6 to 12 h, 34.2% within 12 to 18 h, and 29.3% at greater than 18 h. As depicted in Figure 24-3, mortality at 35 days in patients treated within 12 h was reduced from 11.9% in the placebo group to 8.7% in the rt-PA group (95% CI = 8% to 46%, RR = 27%, $p = 0.033$). In patients treated after 12 h, 35-day mortality reduction was not significant (8.7% and 9.2% in the rt-PA– and placebo-treated groups, respectively; RR = 5%, $p = 0.54$). This benefit persisted at 1 year.

Thus from these data it appears that thrombolytic therapy initiated within 6 to 12 h is definitely associated with a long-term survival benefit. Whether the accrual of this benefit is thrombolytic-specific remains unclear. Recombinant t-PA has been shown to be more effective at lysing aged thrombus.[172] Together with an improved outcome of patients enrolled in the LATE versus the EMERAS Trials, this would suggest that rt-PA may yield better results in late-entry patients, although no direct comparison studies have been done. Significant benefit when given from 12 to 24 h of symptom onset is less apparent. This benefit is presumed to be associated with a patent infarct-related artery but themechanism(s) of that benefit remain(s) largely unknown. As previously noted, the modest improvement in ejection fraction is insufficient to explain the mortality benefits associated with thrombolytic administration. Furthermore, to date, large-scale trials have failed to show that early patency rates translate into improved long- and short-term survival benefits. Nonetheless, the fact that thrombolytic therapy results in improved survival is incontrovertible. Alternate explanations for this benefit have been sought, and one such idea is the so-called open-artery hypothesis. This theory purports that the improvement in survival is related to one or more mechanism(s) favoring en-

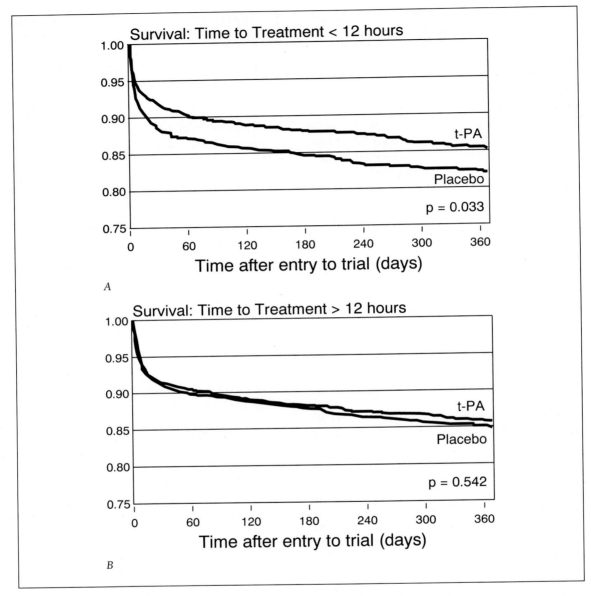

FIGURE 24-3. *Data from the Late Assessment of Thrombolytic Efficacy (LATE) Trial.* **(A)** *Survival for patients given rt-PA versus placebo within 12 h of the onset of symptoms. Percentage survival listed on the y axis shows statistically significant benefit from thrombolytic administration accruing early on and persisting through 1 year as compared with placebo.* **(B)** *Survival curve for patients treated after 12 h of symptom onset. No benefit from thrombolytic administration was realized in these patients when compared with placebo.*

hanced myocardial performance independent of ejection fraction.[173–175] Several of the postulated mechanisms are detailed below.

Acting as a source of collateral blood flow, a patent infarct-related artery may be an important reservoir of additional vascularity in patients with severe multivessel disease. Patency of this vessel may decrease ischemia in the secondary infarct zone and provide a conduit for subsequent coronary revascularization.[62]

Left ventricular remodeling is a process that occurs following Q-wave MI. Usually due to large infarcts, progressive left ventricular wall thinning and cavity dilation develop with attendant elevations in end-diastolic pressures and volume. Successive cavity enlargement and alteration in contractile function may ultimately predispose to congestive heart failure, ventricular arrhythmias, and sudden death.[175] This process of infarct expansion may be due to slippage of remaining myocytes and elongation of the myofibrils.[176] Reperfusion of the infarct segment may alter this process in one or more ways. Experimental work has shown that infarct expansion due to cell slippage may be prevented or attenuated with the preservation of a rim of viable myocardium.[177,178] Furthermore, an increase in tensile strength of the remaining infarct and peri-infarct tissue may subtend the distribution of a patent infarct-related artery. Facilitated access of inflammatory cells to the infarct area may result in less fibrosis and increased scar thickness.[179] Clinical studies have demonstrated that patients allocated to late (>4 h from symptom onset) thrombolytic therapy for acute MI have lower end-systolic and end-diastolic volumes and improved regional left ventricular function[44,172,180–182] compared with those receiving conventional treatment.

Lethal arrhythmia is a common cause of death in patients following acute MI. Several studies have shown that the propensities for spontaneous and laboratory induction of these events are reduced after successful thrombolytic administration.[183,184] A significant decrease in the number of late potentials recorded on signal-averaged ECG also has been shown following successful rt-PA administration.[185] In patients with inducible ventricular arrhythmia and sudden

cardiac death undergoing placement of an automatic implantable cardiac defibrillator, shock-free survival was significantly prolonged in those with a patent infarct-related artery as opposed to those without.[186] The mechanism(s) of this benefit is(are) largely unknown. However, improved homogeneity of myocardial substrate,[187] reduced left ventricular aneurysm formation, and improved hemodynamics all may play a role.[188]

Prehospital Thrombolysis

The benefits of thrombolytic therapy are most marked when the agent is administered within the first hour of symptom onset.[28,32,33] Thus it stands to reason that minimizing the delay to thrombolytic treatment by administration out of hospital would result in improved myocardial salvage and decreased mortality. The introduction of "in the field" or "at home" thrombolysis has been an area ongoing of investigation since the mid-1980s,[189–193] although the preliminary studies were primarily small in nature.[194] Recently, however, there have been two large trials evaluating the strategy of out-of-hospital thrombolysis, the results of which are summarized in Table 24-8.

TABLE 24-8. *Large Trials of Prehospital Thrombolysis*

EMIP (65) (5454 patients)	Prehospital Therapy	Hospital Therapy
Time from onset of pain to therapy	115 minutes	171 minutes
Prehospital hemorrhage	0	0
Prehospital ventricular fibrillation	2.5%	1.6%
Prehospital shock	6.3%	3.8%
Prehospital mortality	1.3%	0.9%
Total 30-day mortality	9.8%	11.1%

MITI (195) (360 Patients)		
Reduction in time to treatment	33 minutes	—
Prehospital arrest	<1%	<1%
LVEF after treatment	53%	54%
All-cause mortality	7%	10%

Adapted with permission from Ross AM. Prehospital thrombolysis: MITI and EMIP results. J Myocardial Ischemia 4:13, 1992.

The European Myocardial Infarction Project (EMIP)[65] is a multicenter, randomized, double-blind, placebo-controlled trial in which 5454 patients were randomized to administration of either prehospital or in-hospital IV bolus APSAC (30 U). Upon arrival to the hospital, patients allocated to placebo in the field were then given active drug, and vice versa. The time to thrombolytic administration was reduced by 58 minutes with in-the-field treatment. Total 30-day mortality was reduced from 11.1% in the hospital treatment arm to 9.8% in the prehospital group (RR = 17%, p = NS). Cardiac mortality was insignificantly reduced as well for prehospital versus hospital therapy, but this was not the prespecified primary endpoint. Furthermore, and as noted in earlier smaller studies, the incidence of cardiogenic shock, hypotension, and ventricular fibrillation was higher in the transport group. It is notable that the emergency response team in this study comprised physicians as well as paramedics.

The Seattle based Myocardial Infarction Triage and Intervention (MITI) Trial also reported on the efficacy of prehospital thrombolytic therapy.[195] In this study, 360 (5%) of 6561 patients with chest pain syndromes were randomized to receive aspirin and rt-PA (100 mg) started either in the field or in the hospital. In contrast to EMIP, all units were staffed solely with paramedic personnel who were in contact with the hospital and transmitting ECGs telephonically. In this study, time to treatment was reduced by 33 minutes in the prehospital treatment arm. This was thought to be due to the improved "door to needle" time resulting from in-field advanced briefing and preparation for hospital administered therapy. The time to treatment in hospital averaged only 19 minutes. As noted in Table 24-8, the outcomes of the two strategies were not statistically different, and the in-field complication rate was low. When the patients were stratified according to symptom duration prior to thrombolytic therapy, it was found that if treatment was given in less than 70 minutes, mortality was only 1%, ejection fraction was higher, and infarct size was smaller.[196]

Thus these studies have confirmed the findings of the previous trials using prehospital thrombolytic therapy. Although a measured clinical benefit has been demonstrated within the confines of tightly controlled trials, the number of patients benefiting from an increased outlay of resources appears to be relatively small (5% of total screened in the MITI Trial). If delay in administration of thrombolytic agent remains significantly reduced due to accurate and efficient prehospital triage with prearrival transmission of ECG, an improved outcome may follow without the need for advanced in-field training of emergency personnel and equipment. Improved patient education with emphasis on recognition of acute coronary syndromes would impact most favorably on time to therapy in acute MI. As shown in Figure 24-4, this has been the source of the greatest delay.

ADJUNCTIVE THERAPY

The benefits of thrombolytic therapy are clearly defined. Mortality reductions have been unequivocal with each of the currently available agents. However, the overall effectiveness of these thrombolytic drugs remains limited by persistent thrombotic occlusion[72,164,197] and rethrombosis[164,198] of the infarct-related artery after timely thrombolysis. Thus additional strategies consisting of antiplatelet and antithrombotic therapy have been employed concomitantly to improve on these limitations. Although there is a large body of ongoing investigation into the development of newer and more potent antithrombotic and antiplatelet agents, heparin and aspirin remain the currently accepted standards[29] and will be the focus of the ensuing discussion.

Antiplatelet Therapy

The salutary effects of antiplatelet therapy, in particular acetylsalicylic acid (aspirin, ASA), were demonstrated unequivocally in the ISIS-2 Study.[33] In this landmark trial, patients were randomized to thrombolytic therapy with conventional-dose SK and, in addition, treatment with 160 mg enteric-coated ASA per day (chewed upon admission and continued for 1 month) or placebo in a factorial design. The overall effect of ASA was a

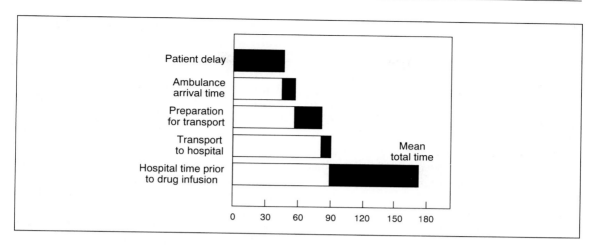

FIGURE 24-4. Cumulative causes of delay to thrombolytic administration. Time on x axis in minutes from symptom onset. As noted, delay in symptom recognition by the patient and failure of timely in-hospital administration are largely responsible for failure of very early (within 1 h) thrombolysis. (Reprinted with permission from Ross A. Prehospital thrombolysis: MITI and EMIP results. J. Myocardial Ischemia 4:13, 1992.)

marked reduction in vascular mortality from 11.8% to 9.4% ($p < 0.00001$) which persisted through 15 months of follow-up. This benefit was noted across a variety of subgroups according to age, site of infarct, and time to treatment. Importantly, this advantageous effect was achieved with only a small (0.7%) increase in minor bleeding over thrombolytic therapy alone and with a 0.5% decrease in overall stroke rate. Furthermore, the cost of this agent is minimal. These factors, coupled with its widespread availability, make administration of ASA the single most important therapeutic intervention in acute MI[199] and the current standard care. The magnitude of benefit for ASA in ISIS-2, however, remains partly unexplained. The incidence of reinfarction was reduced from 4% to 2%, but this is not enough to account for the 25% reduction in mortality.

The therapeutic benefits of ASA are related to the drug's inhibitory effect on platelet function. As noted previously, platelets are intimately related to the formation and propagation of thrombus. In addition, platelet aggregation results in release of vasoactive substances such as thromboxane A_2 that produces attendant vasoconstriction and further compromise of the vascular lumen.

Ingestion of ASA results in immediate and irreversible acetylation of the platelet cyclooxygenase enzyme system. This results in an inability of the platelet to synthesize thromboxane A_2 and other related prostaglandins, impairing their function.

Despite the use of ASA (and heparin) in patients receiving successful thrombolytic therapy, recurrent ischemia primarily due to rethrombosis occurs within 1 week in approximately 11% to 21% of patients.[200] Platelet aggregation appears to play a pivotal role in this process.[201] In this setting, recurrent platelet activity despite the presence of ASA may be mediated through stimulation of the glycoprotein IIb-IIIa receptors located in the platelet membrane. This receptor mediates the binding of platelets to sites containing various macromolecular glycoproteins along the vessel wall, including collagen, fibrinogen, fibronectin, and von Willebrand factor.[200] The passage of platelets through an area of fixed residual obstruction may result in activation of these receptors and thus platelet function.[202,203] This may occur through a number of cyclooxygenase-independent pathways resulting from the shear forces generated with this motion.[203]

Efforts to more thoroughly incapacitate

platelet activity have resulted in a search for additional agents capable of targeting areas of platelet function alternative to that effected by ASA. Among these are compounds that prevent normal function of the glycoprotein platelet receptors. Two such compounds are the murine monoclonal antibodies 7E3-F(ab')$_2$(7E3) and 10E5-F(ab')$_2$. These agents have been shown to significantly shorten time to reperfusion after thrombotic coronary occlusion[204] and prevent platelet thrombus formation after vascular injury.[205]

Compounds that share the same amino acid sequence homology as the gycloprotein IIb-IIIa receptor have been found in nature (snake venom) and synthesized in the laboratory. One of the most promising is integrelin, a highly specific heptapeptide competitive antagonist of the glycoprotein IIb-IIIa complex. This substance is a potent inhibitor of platelet aggregation in animals[206] and humans.[207] These two agents and a litany of mechanistically similar ones comprise a new and potentially very useful addition to the antiplatelet armamentarium now dominated by ASA. These new therapies may be additive to ASA or supplant its use in acute ischemic syndromes. Current studies are in progress to evaluate the therapeutic effectiveness of integrelin, 7E3 and other antiplatelet therapies in clinical practice.

Antithrombotic Therapy

The role of routine anticoagulation as adjunctive therapy to thrombolytic administration in the setting of acute MI is unclear and remains the subject of ongoing controversy. The rationale for the use of anticoagulants along with thrombolytic agents is derived from the belief that the maintenance of coronary artery patency in the infarct-related vessel is the major mechanism by which benefit is obtained and that these agents contribute to that end. In the setting of plaque disruption, intense activation of the coagulation cascade with thrombin and platelet deposition results in thrombotic occlusion of the coronary artery. The nature of reperfusion is such that dissolution and recurrent thrombosis is a cyclic phenomenon that often precedes sustained arterial patency.[208] The mechanism(s) responsible for this process

has(have) been incompletely elucidated but likely involve(s) multiple factors. The procoagulant effects of residual thrombus,[209,210] thrombin and platelet activation due to the various thrombolytic agents used,[211,212] and the underlying injured arterial surface[213,214] all may play a significant role in this process. This pathophysiology results not only in the genesis of thrombus at the time of infarction but also contributes to reocclusion that may be encountered after successful thrombolysis has been achieved. Consequently, the success of coronary thrombolysis is dependent not only on the initial clot lysis but also on prevention of reocclusive thrombus formation. Anticoagulant therapy has been proposed to enhance vessel patency by reducing procoagulation seen in the setting of thrombolysis and in the postthrombolytic period. Platelet aggregation induced by thrombin activation in the setting of thrombolytic therapy has been shown to be inhibited not by aspirin[210] but by heparin.[203,215,216]

Heparin was one of the first antithrombins used, and despite the many new and more potent drugs under investigation (see below), it currently remains the recommended antithrombotic agent.[29] Heparin is a mucopolysaccharide that binds to circulating antithrombin III. This complex greatly accelerates the inhibition of thrombin and other coagulation factors. In addition to the question regarding need for routine anticoagulation, the optimal timing, dose, and route of administration still does not have a uniform consensus. Various clinical studies have been designed to investigate some of these issues (Table 24-9).

Intravenous Heparin

In Streptokinase Trials. The earlier trials evaluating efficacy of heparin given in the setting of thrombolytic therapy generally maintained a 3 to 6-h delay in administration due to concern over potential for adverse bleeding. However, in one small randomized study,[217] patients received either intravenous heparin or placebo at the time of SK therapy. Partial thromboplastin times were maintained at 2 to 2.5 times normal, and heparin was continued for 5 days. In this trial, which utilized noninvasive endpoints as markers for reperfusion, the heparin group showed a significant in-

TABLE 24-9. Role of Heparin as Adjunctive Therapy to Thrombolytic Agents

Study	Regimen	n	Time to Angiogram after Lytic Therapy	Patency 90 Minute	Reocclusion	Recurrent Ischemia	In-Hospital Bleeding	Mortality
Topol (219)	rt-PA with heparin 10,000-U bolus, then IV	134	90 min	79	11	22	13	5
	rt-PA alone			79	5	23	18	9
HART (220)	Heparin continuous IV with rt-PA	205	18 g	82*	12	8	4	1.0
	rt-PA with ASA			85	5	2	5	4.0
Bleich (141)	rt-PA and continuous IV heparin	83	48 h	71†	Not reported	8	12	Not reported
	rt-PA alone			44		9	2	
NHF (197)	Continuous IV heparin after 24 h	202	7d	80	Not reported	10	Not reported	Not reported
	ASA and dipyridamole after 24 h			80		3.8		
SCATI (224)	Continuous subcutaneous heparin ± streptokinase	711		Not reported	Not reported			
	± streptokinase alone					17	4.4	6
						19	0.6	1

*$p < 0.05$.
†$p < 0.06$.
Adapted with permission from Popma JJ, Topol EJ. Adjuncts to myocardial reperfusion. Ann Intern Med 115:34, 1991.

crease in reperfusion as compared with placebo. In the Belgium Optimization Study of Infarct Reperfusion Investigated by ST Monitoring (OSIRIS),[218] 64 patients were randomized to intravenous bolus and continuous infusion of heparin and 1.5 million units of SK and 64 patients to placebo prior to SK therapy for acute MI. All patients received aspirin after thrombolytic therapy. Early patency rates assessed via continuous 12-lead ECG at 60 and 90 minutes were higher in the heparin-treated group than in the placebo group (60 min: heparin 65%, placebo 52%; 90 min: heparin 77%, placebo 60%; $p < 0.05$). However, patency at 24 h, incidence of reinfarction, and clinical outcome were not different.

In rt-PA Trials. The Third Thrombolysis and Angioplasty in Acute Myocardial Infarction Trial[219] investigated the utility of intermediate (within 90 minutes) IV heparin use given in the setting of rt-PA administration. In this study, the speed to reperfusion was not enhanced with heparin use. There was a 6% difference favoring heparin use, and although not statistically significant in the 170 patients studied, this could reflect a type II error. Earlier initiation of IV heparin therapy in HART[220] and the trial of Bleich et al.[141] did result in improved angiographic patency when rt-PA was the thrombolytic agent used. Data on use of IV heparin more than 24 h after thrombolytic administration were evaluated in the National Heart Foundation Trial.[197] Two-hundred and two patients were randomized to IV heparin or aspirin (300 mg/d) and dipyridamole (300 mg/d) 24 h after thrombolytic administration. Patency of the infarct-related artery, as judged by 7-day coronary angiograms, was similar in both groups. In the Sixth European Cooperative Study Group (ECSG-6) Trial,[221] 652 patients were randomized to receive either heparin (5000-U bolus followed by 1000 U/h) or placebo after treatment with rt-PA. All patients received a loading dose (250 mg) of IV aspirin followed by an oral preparation of 75 to 125 mg on alternate days. Angiographic assessment of patency between 48 and 120 h revealed a patency rate (TIMI 2 or 3 flow) in the infarct-related artery of 84% compared with 75% in the heparin-placebo group. The heparin group also tended to have a smaller infarct size and less early recurrence of chest pain, suggesting a decreased reocclusion rate.

In APSAC Trials. Routine use of heparin following APSAC therapy was evaluated in the Duke University Clinical Cardiology Studies (DUCCS-1) Trial.[222] In this randomized trial, 122 patients with acute MI received no heparin following APSAC administration, and 128 patients received IV heparin starting 4 h after treatment with APSAC. Patients under 85 years of age and within 12 h of onset of symptoms were eligible for infusion. There were no significant differences in clinical events between the two groups. The rates of reinfarction, congestive heart failure, and recurrent ischemia were similar among the heparin-treated and no-heparin patients. The overall incidence of stroke was greater in the heparin-treated group than in the no-heparin group (3% versus 0.8%), as was the incidence of hemorrhagic stroke (1.6% versus 0%). These differences were not statistically significant, however, due to the small numbers of patients. The mortality rates for the heparin and no-heparin groups were 9% and 7%, respectively. These did not achieve statistical significance. Bleeding rates, however, were significantly higher in the heparin group, with almost twice as many severe and life-threatening bleeds as compared with the no-heparin group. Thus preliminary evidence suggests that omission of IV heparin therapy with APSAC does not appear to compromise patient outcome. These results may be explained, at least in part, by several observations. First, heparin appears to be most useful for maintaining vessel patency within the first 24 h of the infarct. APSAC undergoes slow deacylation, prolonging its half-life, which may enhance protection from early rethrombosis. Second, APSAC has been shown to significantly reduce plasma viscosity during this period owing to a systemic lytic state. Third, this agent causes immediate inhibition of ex vivo platelet aggregation.[223]

Subcutaneous Heparin

The randomized trials of ISIS-3[32] and GISSI-2[139] provide a large data pool from which to examine the issue of heparin and thrombolysis. However, the majority of these patients received subcutaneous heparin because it tends to be the preferred method of administration in Europe. Several studies have compared adjunctive use of subcutaneous heparin in the setting of thrombolysis, given at various intervals after thrombolytic administration. The Italian Studio sulla Calciparina nell'Angina e nella Thrombosi ventriculre nell'Infarcto (SCATI) Trial[224] randomized patients with acute MI to no heparin or 2000 U of IV heparin followed 9 h later by 12,500 U calcium heparin subcutaneously twice daily. The anticoagulation was continued until hospital discharge and for 3 months in patients with anterior MIs. All patients presenting within 6 h were given a conventional dose of intravenous SK. Although not designed as a mortality trial with a combined primary endpoint of death and nonfatal MI, mortality was reduced in the heparin group (RR = 0.55, 95% CI = 0.32 to 0.94).

In GISSI-2 and the International Study Group,[140] patients were randomized to no heparin or subcutaneous heparin (12,500 U every 12 h) starting 12 h after SK or rt-PA administration. Combined data from these trials showed only a statistically insignificant trend toward reduced 30-day mortality in the SK- and heparin-treated group (7.9%) compared with the SK alone treatment group (9.2%). This trend was not apparent in the heparin and rt-PA (9.2%) versus the rt-PA alone (8.7%) group and may have been due simply to chance, since a difference in mortality existed between these two groups prior to the initiation of heparin.[142]

In the Third International Trial of Infarct Survival (ISIS-3),[32] a mortality benefit of 5 lives saved per 1000 treated with SK, rt-PA, and APSAC has been reported in the subcutaneous heparin groups. In this study, 12,500 U of heparin given twice daily was started 4 h after the initiation of thrombolytic therapy. All patients received oral antiplatelet therapy with aspirin.

Summary and Recommendations for Heparin Use

The data regarding heparin use with thrombolytic therapy must be interpreted cautiously in view of the diverse nature of the studies. The marked heterogeneity in the trial designs with respect to anticoagulation regimes makes direct comparison or pooling of results very difficult. The routes of administration are an obvious difference, since therapeutic heparinization is generally achieved within 24 h in patients treated with a 5000-U bolus and a 12,500-U additional infusion over the first 24 h.[143,225] However, patients receiving subcutaneous heparin in a dose of 12,500 U twice daily rarely achieve therapeutic systemic heparin levels within the first 24 h.[226] Moreover, in trials utilizing IV heparin therapy, careful attention must be paid to the percentage of patients who uniformly have partial thromboplastin times in the therapeutic range. Several analyses of larger trials have shown that in patients treated with rt-PA, coronary artery patency is significantly enhanced when PTTs are consistently therapeutic (at least 2 times baseline) compared with patients with suboptimal PTTs.[227,228] These findings may herald a new era of intensified anticoagulation monitoring that alters the results of studies utilizing present therapies. It is thus not simply adequate to administer IV heparin, but responsiveness to inadequate levels of in vivo anticoagulation appears to be critical.

Although specific consensus regarding the optimal use of anticoagulation does not as yet exist, the available data suggest that the increased procoagulant activity in patients treated with fibrinolytic agents is a principal cause of rethrombosis.[142] In patients receiving rt-PA, most, but not all,[219] of the data tend to support the use of IV heparin in maintaining early infarct-related vessel patency, and thus IV heparin has been recommended for use in this country.[29] A heparin bolus of 150 U/kg followed by an infusion rate (1000 U/h) titrated to maintain the PTT at 2 to 3 times control appears to yield acceptable results.[229] The length of anticoagulation also remains disputed. Some authors recommend a length of 3 to 5 days[230] after thrombolysis to reduce the incidence of reinfarction. Others support the same length of time followed by low-dose subcutaneous (12,500 U bid) heparin for the remainder of the hospitalization.[229] Several studies have found no additional benefit 24 h after rt-PA administration in the presence of antiplatelet therapy.[230] Given the disparate data, it seems reasonable to utilize IV heparin for approximately 72 h after thrombolysis with rt-PA unless there has been recurrent ischemia or bleeding complications.

Subcutaneous heparin does not appear to improve on rt-PA alone in patency studies when given 6 h or more after thrombolysis. Mortality, however, was improved when subcutaneous heparin was given with SK at this interval. Vascular mortality benefit has been shown with SK (rt-PA and APSAC as well) when administered 4 h after thrombolysis. A dose of 12,500 U given twice daily was standard in most trials and apparently well tolerated.[139]

In general, the tendency in the United States with regard to anticoagulation is to utilize the IV route regardless of the thrombolytic agent chosen. However, this behavior may need to be modified with regard to APSAC, as previously noted, based on the DUCCS-1 Trial.[222] This rationale is based on the premise that IV administration is more likely to produce therapeutic levels in the first 24 h than the subcutaneous route and that factors precipitating rethrombosis are independent of the thrombolytic agent. A standard protocol for dosing of IV heparin has been proposed recently to help prevent underanticoagulation and is detailed in Figure 24-5. Since this initial writing, the impact of therapeutic intravenous versus subcutaneous heparin on mortality has been investigated in the GUSTO Trial. The results are discussed in detail in a separate section. However, with respect to SK, mortality rates between the intravenous and subcutaneous heparin groups were not different. In fact, the former was associated with increased hemorrhagic sequelae, confirming earlier observations.[33]

Oral Anticoagulants

Secondary prevention of recurrent MI with the use of warfarin was evaluated in the prethrom-

Heparin Adjustment Nomogram
According to Activated Partial Thromboplastin Time (aPTT)
Goal of Therapy = therapeutic aPTT of >60 secs for first 12 hours, then 60-85 secs.

APTT (sec)	Bolus Dose	Stop Infusion (min)	* Rate Change cc / hr	Repeat aPTT
<50	5000 m	0 min	+3 cc/hr (increase by 150 u/hr)	6 hrs
50-59	0	0 min	+2 cc/hr (increase by 100 u/hr)	6 hrs
60-85	0	0 min	0 (No change)	Next am
86-95	0	0 min	-1 cc/hr (decrease by 50 u/hr)	Next am
96-120	0	30 min	-2 cc/hr (decrease by 100 u/hr)	6 hrs
>120	0	60 min	-3 cc/hr decrease by 150 u/hr)	6 hrs

* This chart is based on a concentration of 50 units of heparin in 1 cc of fluid (25,000 u/500 cc)

After initiation of thrombolytic therapy:
1. Maintain heparin infusion for at least 48 hours.
2. Draw an aPTT at 6, 12 and 24 hours

☐ For 6 & 12 hour aPTT's (post thrombolytic therapy), use only the white section of the nomogram:

1. Do **NOT** discontinue or decrease heparin unless significant bleeding occurs; high aPTT's are probably due to the effect of thrombolytic therapy itself.
2. Adjust heparin dose upward if aPTT<60 secs

☐ For ≥ 24 hour aPTT's (post thrombolytic therapy), use the entire nomogram:

Deliver the bolus, stop the infusion and/or change the rate of heparin based on the aPTT, as noted on the appropriate line of the above nomogram

Heparin should be discontinued if significant bleeding events occur, such as suspected or confirmed hemorrhagic stroke or internal bleeding.

FIGURE 24-5. Heparin adjustment nomogram.

bolytic[231-233] and the postthrombolytic[234] eras. In the Warfarin Reinfarction Study (WARIS),[235] 1214 patients were randomly assigned to receive warfarin (dose adjusted to maintain an INR of 2.8 to 4.8) or no anticoagulation starting a mean of 28 days after treatment with thrombolytic therapy. At a mean of 37 months, 94 deaths, 82 reinfarctions, and 20 strokes were present in the treatment group. In the placebo arm, there were 123 deaths, 124 reinfarctions, and 44 strokes, all highly statistically significant. Risk reduction in mortality for the anticoagulant group was calculated to be 24% ($p < 0.001$). Serious bleeding in the warfarin group was 0.6% annually.

The respective roles for ASA and anticoagulants continue to undergo exploration in the thrombolytic era and have not yet been definitely defined. Based on the preceding data, long-term (3 to 6 months) oral anticoagulation after thrombolytic therapy appears to be beneficial in patients with extensive MI, especially those with echocardiographic evidence of intracavitary thrombi.

Newer Antithrombin Agents

Efforts to improve on the antithrombin activity of heparin and enhance infarct-related artery patency have led to the investigation of newer, more powerful antithrombin agents. Hirudin, a naturally occurring component of leech saliva, now synthesized through recombinant DNA technology, prevents thrombin-induced platelet activation, conversion of fibrinogen to fibrin, and activation of factors V, VIII, and XIII by specific inhibition of thrombin.[213,236] Because of its smaller molecular profile, hirudin can penetrate into the interstices of the fibrin-bound thrombin complex and thus prevent the growth of thrombus more effectively than the larger heparin molecule.[237] In this regard, hirudin has been shown to be more effective at preventing activation of the coagulation cascade during thrombolysis.[238] This agent and its derivatives are currently undergoing clinical trials to evaluate efficacy. Several additional antithrombotic agents are in the initial stages of study. Argatroban, another synthetic thrombin inhibitor with a 5-minute half-life, has been shown to accelerate reperfusion and decrease reocclusion when used as an adjuvant to rt-PA.[239,240] Hirulog and MCI-9038 are two new thrombin inhibitors that have been found to be more effective than heparin at accelerating thrombolysis in the in vivo animal model.[241,242] These and other potent and specific inhibitors of thrombin represent a new approach to antithrombotic therapy. To determine the relative efficacy of these agents compared with conventional heparin therapy, the importance of clot-bound thrombin inhibition must be verified in clinical trials.[200]

THROMBOLYTIC THERAPY FOR UNSTABLE ANGINA

The rationale for use of thrombolytic agents in the setting of unstable anginal syndromes is related to the observation that the prevalence of coronary thrombosis in such patients ranges from 20% to 72% when angiography is undertaken within 2 weeks of the symptoms.[138] Given the fact that unstable angina is the leading cause of cardiac admissions in this country and ostensibly has a similar pathogenesis to MI, efforts to improve its treatment with the use of thrombolytic therapy seem reasonable.[243,244] However, to date, the data have been relatively unimpressive with regard to demonstrable benefit. Table 24-10 depicts the randomized, controlled trials and their outcomes. Despite a theoretical role for thrombolytic therapy in at least a subset of patients with unstable angina, support for improved outcome is lacking. Angiographic improvement is unimpressive and no better than heparin. Although some studies have shown a reduction in early ischemic episodes,[245,246] long-term outcome is not improved over heparin alone.[247] Furthermore, newer and more potent antithrombin agents such as hirudin may significantly improve on the present results of heparin without the adverse effects of thrombolytic drugs.[248]

The studies to date suffer from small sample size and marked heterogeneity in design. Moreover, the prominent salutary effects of anticoagu-

TABLE 24-10. Trials of Thrombolysis in Unstable Angina

Study	Total n	Heparin and ASA			Thrombolysis, Heparin and ASA			Thrombolytic Agent	Length of Follow-Up
		n	MI	Death	n	MI	Death		
Williams (295)	67	23	4.5%	0%	45	6.6%	0%	rt-PA	In hospital
Nicklasl (296)	40	20	10%	0%	20	10%	10%	rt-PA	In hospital
Freeman (297)	70	35	2.8%	2.8%	35	5.7%	2.8%	rt-PA	In hospital
Bar (298)	159	79	6.3%	1.2%	80	12.5%	3.7%	APSAC	In hospital
Schreiber (299)	149	53	3.8%	0%	96	8.3%	0%	UK	96 h
TIMI-3B (300)	1531	771	10.4%	2.6%	760	12.3%	2.4%	rt-PA	42 d

lants and antiplatelet agents in the setting of unstable angina may be difficult to separate from any benefit conferred by thrombolytic treatment. To address this issue, Schreiber and colleagues performed a multicenter, partially blinded three-arm study comparing UK and IV heparin, UK alone, and placebo thrombolytic and heparin. No benefit was noted in the thrombolytic groups over conventional anticoagulant treatment. The study was terminated early after randomization of only 149 patients (planned enrollment was 600 patients) due to a lack of benefit favoring active therapy. However, serious complications were comparable in all three groups, and halting the study has been considered premature by some.[249]

The reasons for the apparent lack of benefit with the use of thrombolytic agents in unstable angina are as yet undetermined but may be due to the fact that in unstable angina the thrombus is platelet-rich, transient, and nonocclusive. It is transient and not associated with myocardial damage.[249] Emphasis in treatment is directed at preventing rethrombosis, which is done effectively with conventional antithrombotic therapies.[250] The benefits of fibrinolysis are predicated on the opening of an occluded coronary artery and establishing patency. Commensurate with this is a marked procoagulant effect and platelet activation.[203,216,239,251-253] The release of free thrombin is self-perpetuating, favoring the formation of more thrombin and an increase in MIs. Perhaps without the accrued benefit derived from abrogating myocardial injury, the thrombotic tendencies may predominate in some patients.[249]

Thus thrombolytic therapy in unstable angina has not been associated with improved outcome; activation of platelets and the coagulation system may be at least partially responsible. Paradoxically, it appears that thrombolytic therapy in unstable angina poses a risk for *increased* MI for the reasons cited above (see Table 24-10). Larger trials with several thousand patients may be required to provide further insight into these issues. As seen in Table 24-10, the TIMI-IIIB Trial,[254] a large, randomized, prospective study of front-loaded rt-PA or placebo and conventional therapy has recently provided definitive evidence that thrombolytic therapy (rt-PA

in this project) is unhelpful in the setting of unstable angina.

INDICATIONS, CONTRAINDICATION, AND COMPLICATIONS

General Indications

In view of the wealth of data derived from well-done studies of thrombolytic therapy for acute MI, it is reasonable to propose that all patients with an evolving acute MI be considered for thrombolytic therapy. Patients presenting with ST-segment elevation attributable to myocardial injury represent the classic presentation. However, data from the GISSI[255] and ISIS[32,33] studies have shown benefit in patients with left bundle branch block. In those patients presenting within 6 h of symptom onset, mortality benefit is definitely present. For those presenting from 6 to 24 h from onset, mortality benefit is less but still present, particularly from 6 to 12 h. These patients should as well be considered for thrombolysis, particularly if symptoms of ongoing coronary artery occlusion and incomplete infarction (continued ischemic pain, ST-segment elevation, etc.) are present. In this group, special attention needs to be given to the individual's risk/benefit ratio.

The choice of agent at the present time remains unresolved, since equivalent benefit has been demonstrated with all the currently approved regimes. The recently proved merits of accelerated rt-PA are detailed in the separate GUSTO section. Initiation of oral aspirin (160 to 325 mg) as soon as possible is important, with chronic daily administration thereafter. Recommendations for antithrombotic therapy are less certain. Intravenous heparin appears most useful with rt-PA (particularly the accelerated regimens; see GUSTO), particularly within the first 24 h of administration. Subcutaneous regimes as previously outlined are beneficial with SK. At present, heparin is probably best avoided with the use of APSAC.

Thrombolysis in the Elderly

Although the use of thrombolytic therapy in patients over age 75 years has been the subject of ongoing debate, the majority of the evidence favors its use in this group of patients. Given the fact that this is the fastest growing part of the U.S. population[256] and that they account for 60% of the deaths attributed to MI,[257] development of an acceptably safe and efficacious strategy for their care is imperative. Although these patients as a group do tend to have more comorbid conditions with later, more atypical ECG and clinical presentations,[195,258,259] the principal reason for lack of thrombolytic administration is fear of catastrophic cerebral hemorrhage.[260] Although results of clinical trials have, for the most part, supported the notion that hemorrhagic risk with thrombolytic therapy is increased in the elderly,[261,262] it is these patient particularly that tend to derive the greatest benefit from its use. Since the early U.S. studies of thrombolysis failed to enroll elderly patients for fear of hemorrhagic complications, the large trials illustrating this point come from the European and Scandinavian studies. In ISIS-2,[33] mortality in patients less than 60 years of age was reduced from 6% to 4%, but patients 80 years of age or older had a striking reduction in mortality from 37% to 20%. In ASSET,[135] 10.8% of patients 66 to 75 years of age died in the first month following rt-PA treatment, as opposed to 16.8% of those not treated with thrombolysis. A therapeutic benefit for elderly patients treated with APSAC was demonstrated in AIMS,[73,74] where at 30 days, 30.2% of the patients aged 65 to 70 years treated with placebo had died as compared with only 12.2% of elderly patients treated with APSAC. At 1 year, 82.6% of patients in the active treatment group were alive as compared with 65.6% in the placebo arm. In a small, randomized pilot study of 69 elderly patients initiated by Feit et al.[263] and stopped prematurely due to difficult enrollment, an increase in ejection fraction and reduction in symptomatic heart failure were noted in the thrombolytic-treated group. Furthermore, a mortality reduction from 22% in the nonthrombolytic group to 16% in patients treated with thrombolytic therapy was noted. Intracranial hemorrhage was increased with a rate of 3%, a finding consistent in all evaluations of thrombolysis in the elderly. This finding has been echoed in an overview of six large thrombolytic trials.[131] Early

hazards of thrombolytic therapy outweighed benefits on day of randomization, presumably due to hemorrhagic complications, but became secondary to benefits by day 2. Early hazards corresponded to advancing age and time to presentation. However, even when these tradeoffs are taken into consideration, the risk/benefit ratio strongly favors the use of thrombolytic therapy. This was illustrated in a decision analysis composed by Krumholz and associates.[264] These investigators performed an overview of major clinical trials involving the use of thrombolytic therapy in elderly (75 years or older) patients. Making some reasonable assumptions regarding mortality in treated and untreated patients, thrombolytic therapy was found to be both beneficial and cost-effective in the elderly group.

Evidence that the principal cause of morbidity, that is, hemorrhagic stroke, may not be equal with all the currently available thrombolytic agents has been suggested,[32,139] and for the most part confirmed in a separate analysis of data from the GISSI-2 and ISG data.[140] This analysis demonstrated that in the GISSI patients over 70 years of age, the stroke rate with conventional dosing of rt-PA was 2.6% as compared with 1.6% in the SK-treated group. As has been noted,[260] the GISSI-2 trial did not provide for weight-adjusted dosing in the rt-PA arm. Body weight has been shown to be a risk factor for intracerebral hemorrhage with the use of rt-PA,[261] and in the ISIS-3 trial,[32] elderly patients given a weight-adjusted dose of duteplase had no excess clustering of hemorrhagic events.

Thus, in view of the available data to date, we recommend strongly the use of thrombolytic therapy in elderly and very elderly patients presenting with evidence of acute MI unless specific contraindications other than age are present.

Contraindications

These are based primarily on clinical experience and are subject to change as new data are accrued. Active bleeding from a noncompressible site remains the only absolute contraindication to thrombolytic therapy.

Relative Contraindications

1. History intracranial bleeding
2. Gastrointestinal or genitourinary bleeding within 6 months
3. Major surgery within past 2 to 4 weeks
4. Prolonged CPR > 10 minutes with chest trauma within past 2 to 4 weeks
5. Intracranial anatomic defect (aneurysm, neoplasm, previous surgery), proliferative diabetic retinopathy
6. Severe, uncontrolled hypertension (systolic BP > 200 mmHg, diastolic BP > 120 mmHg)
7. Pregnancy
8. Definite bleeding diathesis

In the presence of absolute or relative contraindications, revascularization of the infarct-related artery should be considered and, if possible (given the appropriate setting), attempted utilizing primary angioplasty.[265]

Complications

Complications associated with the use of thrombolytic therapy are principally those of allergic reactions and hemorrhage. The former are encountered with the use of SK and APSAC and are due to the foreign proteinaceous nature of these compounds. These have been discussed previously in the respective sections on these agents.

Hemorrhagic complications are increased in patients receiving thrombolytic therapy.[266,267] This results from the lysis of physiologic hemostatic thrombi and is enhanced by the coagulopathy induced by fibrinolysis and adjuvant therapy. In most clinical trials, bleeding is reported as a major or minor occurrence. The former has been defined by different criteria depending on the study. The requirements for transfusion, previously determined, are arbitrary fall in hemoglobin (e.g., more than 15 points)[154] and/or a clinical event (e.g., intracranial or severe gastrointestinal hemorrhage). Although any bleeding complication is generally associated with an increased morbidity, intracranial hemorrhage represents the most devastating and feared complication. Large mortality studies provide the best opportunity to assess hemorrhagic complications, but the dissimilarity in trial design makes interstudy comparison of these events difficult.

In trials without angiography, intravenous SK was generally associated with an overall bleeding rate of approximately 4%. The control patients were found to have a 3% incidence of bleeding. Major bleeds, defined by the need for transfusion, were reported in 0.5% of patients.[138] Probable cerebral hemorrhage (including strokes of uncertain type on days 0 and 1) occurred in 0.46% of SK-treated patients in the GISSI-1 study and in 0.31% in ISIS-2. Rates of intracranial hemorrhage in the control groups of these large studies were 0.13% and 0.15%, respectively.[28,33,105]

In ASSET,[135] major bleeding was reported in 1.4% of patients in the rt-PA group compared with 0.4% with placebo. Intracranial hemorrhage in the active treatment group occurred in 0.28% of patients and 0.08% in the control group. In the AIMS Trial of intravenous APSAC and heparin followed by oral warfarin for 3 months,[73] overall in-hospital bleeding complications in the thrombolytic group were reported to be 13.1%, with an intracranial hemorrhage incidence of 0.32%. Bleeding occurred in 4.1% of the control group, and cerebral hemorrhage was reported in 0.15% of these patients.

Comparison of the three agents was performed in the ISIS-3 Trial.[32] The rates of major bleeding in the groups randomized to thrombolytic plus subcutaneous heparin were not significantly different and averaged 0.8%. The rates of definite or probable cerebral hemorrhage were 0.2% for SK, 0.7% for APSAC, and 0.5% for rt-PA ($p < 0.001$). Pooled data from GISSI-2 and ISIS-3 provide a large number of similarly treated patients revealing an intracranial hemorrhage rate of 0.3% for SK and 1.4% for rt-PA.[105] Studies with all three currently approved thrombolytic agents involving invasive testing have shown a significantly higher major bleeding rate, as evidenced by an increased transfusion requirement primarily due to vascular puncture.[98,158,160]

Insight into the ischemic stroke rate after thrombolytic administration for acute MI can be derived from analysis of the large GISSI-2 and International Study Group Trials.[268] Ischemic strokes were found in 0.44% of the SK group and

0.5% of the rt-PA group (p = NS). Likewise, there was no significant increase in ischemic strokes in the heparin versus no-heparin groups.

A number of studies have evaluated and confirmed the association between increased patient age and bleeding complications.[258,269,270] Age > 70, hypertension, low body weight, and female sex are potential risk factors for intracranial hemorrhage with thrombolytic therapy. However, it is important to note that these should not preclude the use of these agents in patients with the appropriate risk/benefit ratio.

A GLOBAL RANDOMIZED TRIAL OF AGGRESSIVE VERSUS STANDARD THROMBOLYTIC STRATEGIES IN 41,021 PATIENTS WITH ACUTE MYOCARDIAL INFARCTION: THE GUSTO-1 STUDY

Designed to continue the search for improved reperfusion strategies and provide insight into many of the current controversies surrounding thrombolysis in acute MI, the Global Utilization of Streptokinase and Tissue Plasminogen Activator for Occluded Coronary Arteries Trial[96] was designed and carried out. Conceived as a mortality trial, this multinational, multicenter study effectively randomized 41,021 patients with 6 h or less of chest pain and ECG evidence of myocardial injury or bundle branch block to one of four treatment arms (see Fig. 24-6). Numerous reports from small trials[67,94,95] have suggested that infarct artery patency is more rapidly achieved with accelerated rt-PA (100 mg given over 90 minutes with a 15-mg bolus) and postreperfusion reocclusion is less with combination therapy (SK 1 million U and rt-PA 10 mg/kg over 60 minutes).[79,108,271] However, these studies lacked the statistical power to provide insight into mortality benefits (if any). These two strategies were compared with conventional SK therapy tested in GISSI-2[139] and ISIS-3[32] (1.5 million units IV over 30 to 60 minutes) followed 4 h later by subcutaneous heparin (12,500 U every 12 h). In order to provide insight into the controversy of intravenous versus subcutaneous heparin, the latter was given (5000-U bolus with infusion, 1000 to

FIGURE 24-6. Global Utilization of Streptokinase and t-PA for Occluded Coronary Arteries (GUSTO) Trial design. See text for discussion.

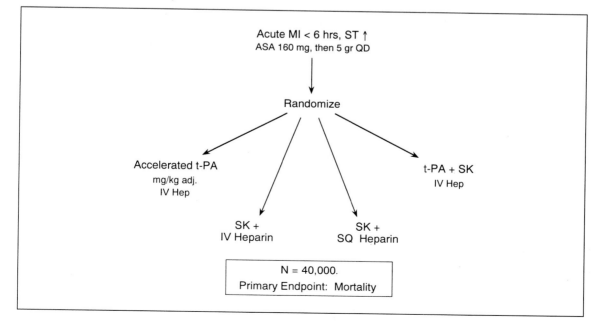

1200 U/h titrated to a PTT of 65 to 85 s) with conventional SK in a fourth arm. Intravenous heparin was similarly administered in the accelerated and combined strategies. Antiplatelet therapy consisting of aspirin 160 to 325 mg upon presentation and then daily was used. Intravenous followed by oral atenolol therapy was recommended in all patients without contraindications. All other treatment medications were left to the discretion of the physicians.

The major results are shown in Table 24-11. At 30 days, there was no significant difference in mortality between SK groups. There was a significant reduction in mortality with accelerated rt-PA when compared with other regimens with an estimated 10 lives saved per 1000 patients treated (RR = 14%; 95% CI = 5.9% to 21.3%; p = 0.001). This regimen also was significantly better in terms of mortality when compared separately with each of the SK arms. There was no significant difference between the combination regimen and the SK groups. However, the combination group fared less well than the accelerated rt-PA group (7.0% versus 6.3% mortality; RR = 10%, with 95% CI = 0.8% to 19.2%; p = 0.04). Thirty-day survival curves for each of the arms is shown in Figure 24-7.

Associated with the improved overall survival in the accelerated rt-PA arm was an excess of 2 hemorrhagic strokes per 1000 patients treated (absolute excess 0.2%) for rt-PA as compared with the SK regimens (Table 24-12). The combination of thrombolytics carried an excess of 4 hemorrhagic strokes per 1000 compared with the SK regimens. The net clinical benefit for the accelerated regimen calculated to be the prevention of death or disabling stroke in 9 patients per 1000 treated. This reduction was consistent across all prespecified subgroups (Fig. 24-8), although, as expected, most pronounced for patients with anterior infarcts and age less than 75 years.

The improved survival was felt to be due to early achievement and maintenance of infarct-related artery patency. This was evidenced by the results of an angiographic substudy of 2431 patients (approximately 600 in each treatment arm; see Fig. 24-9) integrated into the study design to test the open-artery hypothesis.[300] Patients enrolled were randomly assigned to angiography at one of four times after the initiation of thrombolytic therapy: 90 minutes, 180 minutes, 24 hours, or 5 to 7 days. All patients having angiograms at 90 minutes also received one at 5 to 7 days. As seen in Table 24-13, the analysis of these data revealed that the patency of the infarct-related artery at 90 minutes was highest in the group given accelerated rt-PA and heparin (81%) as compared with the SK and subcutaneous hep-

TABLE 24-11. Major Clinical Outcomes (Percent of Patients)

Outcome	Streptokinase and Subcutaneous Heparin (n = 9796)	Streptokinase and Intravenous Heparin (n = 10,377)	Accelerated rt-PA and Intravenous Heparin (n = 10,344)	Both Thrombolytic Agents and Intravenous Heparin (n = 10,328)	p Value, Accelerated rt-PA versus Both Streptokinase Groups
24-h mortality	2.4	2.9	2.3	2.8	0.005
30-day mortality	7.2	7.4	6.3	7.0	0.001
Or nonfatal stroke	7.9	8.2	7.2	7.9	0.006
Or nonfatal hemorrhagic stroke	7.4	7.6	6.6	7.4	0.004
Or nonfatal disabling stroke	7.7	7.9	6.9	7.6	0.006

Reproduced with permission from the GUSTO investigators. An international randomized trial comparing four thrombolytic strategies for acute myocardial infarction. N Engl J Med 392:673, 1993.

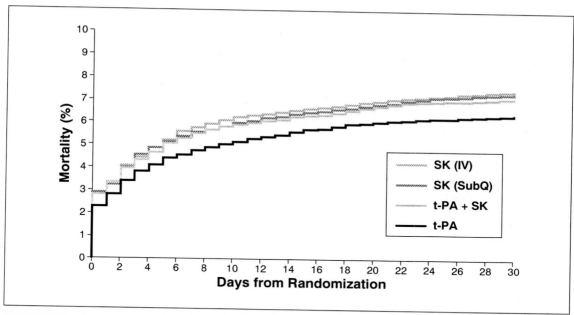

FIGURE 24-7. *Thirty-day mortality in the four treatment groups. The group receiving accelerated treatment with rt-PA had lower mortality than the two SK groups (p = 0.001) and than each individual treatment group: streptokinase and subcutaneous (SC) heparin (p = 0.009), streptokinase and intravenous (IV) heparin (p = 0.003), and rt-PA and streptokinase combined with IV heparin (p = 0.04).*

arin group (54%; $p < 0.001$) and the group given combination therapy (73%; $p = 0.032$). Flow through the infarct-related artery at 90 minutes was normal in the majority of the group given rt-PA (54%) but in less than 40% of the three other groups.

Measurements of left ventricular function paralleled the rate of patency in the four groups, with the accelerated regimen having the highest (Table 24-14). Furthermore, mortality at 30 days was lowest in those patients with normal infarct artery flow irrespective of treatment arm. As pre-

TABLE 24-12. *Incidence of Stroke and Bleeding Complications (Percent of Patients)*

Stroke	Streptokinase and Subcutaneous Heparin ($n = 9709$)	Streptokinase and Intravenous Heparin ($n = 10,314$)	Accelerated t-PA and Intravenous Heparin ($n = 10,268$)	Both Thrombolytic Agents and Intravenous Heparin ($n = 10,268$)	p Value, Accelerated t-PA versus Both Streptokinase Groups
All types	1.22	1.40	1.55	1.64	0.09
Hemorrhagic	0.49	0.54	0.71	0.94	0.03
Nonhemorrhagic	0.53	0.65	0.64	0.53	0.57
With conversion to hemorrhagic	0.04	0.05	0.06	0.080	0.62
Unknown type	0.15	0.16	0.13	0.10	0.54

Adapted with permission from the GUSTO investigators. An international randomized trial comparing four thrombolytic strategies for acute myocardial infarction. N Engl J Med 392:673, 1993.

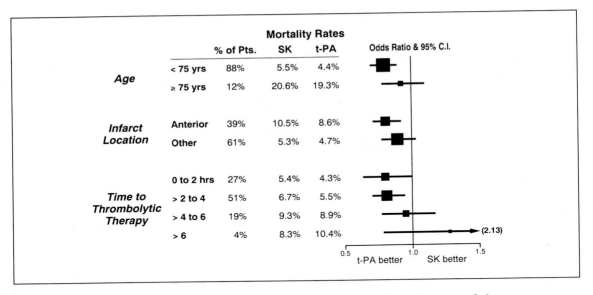

FIGURE 24-8. *Odds ratios and 95% confidence intervals (CI) for 30-day mortality in the prespecified subgroups defined by age, infarct location, and time to thrombolytic therapy.*

dicted, patients with TIMI grade 3 flow had the lowest mortality (4.4%), whereas patients with TIMI grade 2 flow (7.4%) and TIMI grade 0 to 1 flow (8.9%) had progressively higher death rates. The difference between TIMI grade 0 to 1 flow and TIMI grade 3 flow was highly significant ($p = 0.009$).

The cost differential between rt-PA and SK has been the major subject of controversy with this study. rt-PA costs $2200 to $2400 per dose.

FIGURE 24-9. *Design of GUSTO angiographic substudy: 2431 patients enrolled to study the effect of earlier and more complete reperfusion in patients with acute myocardial infarction. See text for details.*

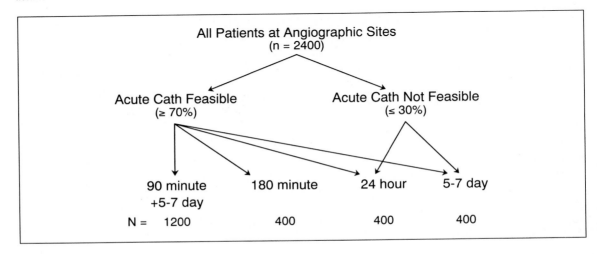

TABLE 24-13. *Patency and Reocclusion of the Infarct-Related Artery According to Treatment Group [Patients with Feature/Patients Examined (%)]*

Variable	Streptokinase + SC Heparin	Streptokinase + IV Heparin	Accelerated rt-PA	rt-PA + Streptokinase
Patency				
Open vessels, TIMI grades 2 and 3 combined				
At 90 min	159/293 (54)	170/283 (60)	236/292 (81)[*†]	218/299 (73)[†]
At 180 min	77/106 (73)	72/97 (74)	71/93 (76)	77/91 (85)
At 24 h	64/83 (77)	74/92 (80)	89/104 (86)	87/93 (94)[‡]
At 5–7 days	67/93 (72)	81/96 (84)	70/83 (84)[§]	71/89 (80)
Complete reperfusion, TIMI grade 3				
At 90 min	85/293 (29)	91/283 (32)	157/292 (54)[†¶]	114/299 (38)
At 180 min	37/106 (35)	40/97 (41)	40/93 (43)	48/91 (53)
At 24 h	42/83 (51)	38/92 (41)	47/104 (45)	56/93 (60)
At 5–7 days	47/93 (51)	56/96 (58)	48/83 (58)	49/89 (55)
Reocclusion				
From TIMI grade 2 at 90 min to grade 0 or 1 at follow-up	3/56 (5.4)	6/58 (10.3)	2/64 (3.1)	4/72 (5.6)
From TIMI grade 3 at 90 min to grade 0 or 1 at follow-up	4/54 (7.4)	1/69 (1.4)	9/121 (7.4)	4/92 (4.3)
Overall reocclusion	7/110 (6.4)	7/127 (5.5)	11/185 (5.9)	8/164 (4.9)

[*]$p = 0.032$ for the comparison of this group with the group given rt-PA with streptokinase.
[†]$p < 0.001$ for the comparison of this group with the groups given streptokinase with subcutaneous or intravenous heparin.
[‡]$p < 0.001$ for the comparison of this group with the group given streptokinase with subcuatenous heparin.
[§]$p = 0.032$ for the comparison of this group with the group given streptokinase with subcutaneous heparin.
[¶]$p < 0.001$ for the comparison of this group with the group given rt-PA with streptokinase.
Reproduced with permission from the GUSTO Angiographic Investigators. The comparative effects of tissue plasminogen activator, streptokinase, or both on coronary artery patency, ventricular function, and survival after acute myocardial infarction. N Engl J Med 329:1615, 1993.

However, an analysis performed with the GUSTO Study calculates a cost of approximately $22,000 per year of life saved owing to the average 10 years of additional quality-adjusted life years in each of the survivors. This finding compares favorably with $60,000 per year of life saved for dialysis or between $150,000 and $200,000 for some antihypertensive or hypolipidemic chronic therapies.

The results of GUSTO-1 and the angiographic substudy once again confirm the importance of early reperfusion in patients with acute MI. As this trial clearly demonstrates, improved early patency of the infarct-related artery is associated with improved left ventricular function and reduced mortality.

Thus, for patients presenting to the hospital within 6 h of chest pain and no contraindication to thrombolysis (patients with contraindications should strongly be considered for primary coronary angioplasty), management should include chewable aspirin (169 to 325 mg) and the rapid administration of a thrombolytic agent. The specifics of which agent to use are less important than the fact that one be used. Patients with large infarcts, and perhaps those less than 75 years of age, may benefit most from accelerated rt-PA and IV heparin titrated to maintain an a PTT of 60 to 85 s. If SK is used, there appears to be no benefit and perhaps increased hemorrhagic risk of associated heparin (particularly intravenous) administration.

TABLE 24-14. *Left Ventricular Function, According to Group* [a]

Variable	Streptokinase + SC Heparin	Streptokinase + IV Heparin	Accelerated rt-PA	rt-PA+ Streptokinase
At 90 min	n = 242	n = 231	n = 246	n = 248
Ejection fraction (%)	58 ± 15	57 ± 15	59 ± 15	58 ± 15
ESVI (mL/m²)	28 ± 15	30 ± 17	27 ± 16[b]	29 ± 16
Wall motion (SD/chord)	−2.5 ± 1.5	−2.7 ± 1.4[f]	−2.4 ± 1.4[c]	−2.4 ± 1.5
Abnormal chords (no.)	23 ± 17	25± 18	21 ± 19[d,e]	24 ± 19
Preserved RWM (% of group)	18	19	29[e,f]	21
At 5–7 days	n = 186	n = 171	n = 197	n = 179
Ejection fraction (%)	57 ± 14	58 ± 14	59 ± 14	58 ± 16
ESVI (mL/m²)	31 ± 14	29 ± 15	28 ± 13	30 ± 16
Wall motion (SD/chord)	−2.4 ± 1.4	−2.1 ± 1.5[g]	−2.0 ± 1.5[h]	−2.2 ± 1.6
Abnormal chords (no.)	21 ± 17	20± 19	17 ± 16[i]	21 ± 19
Preserved RWM (% of group)	21	34[j]	31	30

[a]Plus-minus values are means ± SD. ESVI denotes end-systolic volume index, and RWM indicates regional wall motion. Wall motion is expressed as the mean magnitude of depressed infarct zone chords; wall motion was considered preserved if all infarct zone chords were normal. Chords in the infarct zone were considered abnormal if they were more than 2 SD below the norm.
[b]$p = 0.037$ for the comparison of this group with the groups given streptokinase with intravenous heparin.
[c]$p = 0.018$ for the comparison of this group with the groups given streptokinase with subcutaneous or intravenous heparin.
[d]$p = 0.027$ for the comparison of this group with the groups given streptokinase with subcutaneous or intravenous heparin.
[e]$p = 0.035$ for the comparison of this group with the group given rt-PA with streptokinase.
[f]$p < 0.001$ for the comparison of this group with the groups given streptokinase with intravenous or subcutaneous heparin.
[g]$p = 0.014$ for the comparison of this group with the group given streptokinase with subcutaneous heparin.
[h]$p = 0.05$ for the comparison of this group with the group given streptokinase with subcutaneous heparin.
[i]$p = 0.05$ for the comparison of this group with the groups given streptokinase with intravenous or subcutaneous heparin.
[j]$p = 0.006$ for the comparison of this group with the groups given streptokinase with subcutaneous heparin.
Reproduced with permission from the GUSTO Angiographic Investigators. The comparative effects of tissue plasminogen activator, streptokinase, or both on coronary artery patency, ventricular function, and survival after acute myocardial infarction. N Engl J Med 329:1615, 1993.

REFERENCES

1. Herrick JB. Clinical features of sudden obstruction of the coronary arteries. JAMA 1912;59:2015.

2. Chazov EL, Matteeva LS, Mazaez AV. Intracoronary administration of fibrinolysin in acute myocardial infarction. Ter Arkh 1976;48:8.

3. Rentrop KP, Blanke H, Karsch H. Initial experience with transluminal recanalization of the recently occluded infarct-related coronary artery in acute myocardial infarction—comparison with conventionally treated patients. Clin Cardiol 1979;2:92.

4. Rentrop KP, Blanke H, Karsch KR, et al. Acute myocardial infarction: intracoronary application of nitroglycerin and streptokinase. Clin Cardiol 1979;2:354.

5. De Wood M, Spores J, Notske R, et al. Prevalence of total coronary occlusion during the early hours of transmural myocardial infarction. N Engl J Med 1980;303:897.

6. Levin DC, Fallon JT. Significance of the angiographic morphology of localized coronary stenoses: histopathologic correlations. Circulation 1982;66:310.

7. Ambrose JA, Tannenbaum MA, Alexopoulos D. An angiographic progression of coronary artery disease and the development of myocardial infarction. J Am Coll Cardiol 1988;12:56.

8. Ambrose JA. Plaque disruption and the acute coronary syndromes of unstable angina and myocardial infarction: if the substrate is similar, why is the clinical presentation different? (editorial). J Am Coll Cardiol 1992;19:1653.

9. Davies MJ, Thomas AC. Plaque fissuring: the cause of acute myocardial infarction, sudden ischaemic death, and crescendo angina. Br Heart J 1985;53:363.

10. Falk E. Plaque rupture with severe pre-existing stenosis precipitating coronary thrombosis: characterization of coronary atherosclerotic plaques underlying fatal occlusive thrombi. Br Heart J 1983;50:127.

11. Little WC, Constantinecscu M, Appelgate RJ. Can coronary angiography predict the site of subsequent myocardial infarction in patients with mild to moderate coronary artery disease? Circulation 1988;78:1157.

12. Robinson JH, Browne MJ, Carey JE, et al. A recombinant, chimeric enzyme with a novel mechanism of action leading to greater potency and selectivity than tissue-type plasminogen activator. Circulation 1992;86:548.

13. Lijnin HR, Nelles L, van Hoef B, et al. Characteri-

zation of a chimeric plasminogen activator consisting of amino acids 1–274 of tissue plasminogen activator and amino acids 138–411 of single-chain urokinase type plasminogen activator. J Biol Chem 1988;263:19083.

14. Lu HR, Wu Z, Pauwles P, et al. Comparative thrombolytic properties of tissue-type plasminogen activator (t-PA), single-chain urokinase-type plasminogen activator (u-PA) and K1K2Pu (a t-PA/u-PA chimera) in a combined arterial and venous thrombosis model in the dog. J Am Coll Cardiol 1992;19:1350.

15. Tillet WS, Sherry S. The effect in patients of streptococcal fibrinolysin (streptokinase) and streptococcal deoxyribonuclease on fibrinous, purulent, and sanguinous pleural exudations. J Clin Invest 1949;28:173.

16. Fletcher AP, Alkjaersig N, Smyrniotis FE, Sherry S. The treatment of patients suffering from early acute myocardial infarction with massive and prolonged streptokinase therapy. Trans Assoc Am Physicians 1958;71:287.

17. Davies MC, Englert ME, De Renzo EC. Interactions of streptokinase and human activator: I. Combining of streptokinase and plasminogen observed in the ultracentrifuge under a variety of experimental conditions. J Biol Chem 1964;239:2651.

18. Sherry S. The fibrinolytic activity of streptokinase human plasmin. J Clin Invest 1954;35:1054.

19. Sherry S, Marder VJ. Streptokinase and recombinant tissue plasminogen activator (rt-PA) are equally effective in treating acute myocardial infarction. Ann Intern Med 1991;114:417.

20. Fletcher AP, Alkjaersig N, Sherry S. The maintenance of a sustained thrombolytic state in man: I. Induction and effects. J Clin Invest 1959;38:1096.

21. Topol EJ. Advances in thrombolytic therapy for acute myocardial infarction. J Clin Pharmacol 1987;27:735.

22. Kennedy JW, Ritchie JL, Davis KB, et al. The western Washington randomized trial of intracoronary streptokinase in acute myocardial infarction: a 12-month follow-up report. N Engl J Med 1985;312:1073.

23. Kennedy JW, Ritchie JL, Davis KB, Fritz JK. Western Washington randomized trial of intracoronary streptokinase in acute myocardial infarction. N Engl J Med 1983;309:1477.

24. Kennedy JW, Gensini GG, Timmis GC, Maynard C. Acute myocardial infarction treated with intracoronary streptokinase: a report of the Society for Cardiac Angiography. Am J Cardiol 1985;55:871.

25. Rothbard RL, Fitzpatrick PG, Francis CW, et al. Relationship of the lytic state to successful reperfusion with standard- and low-dose intracoronary streptokinase. Circulation 1985;71:562.

26. Burkey MW, Smith MR, Walsh TE, et al. Relationship of effectiveness of intracoronary thrombolysis in acute myocardial infarction to the systemic lytic state. Am J Cardiol 1985;56:441.

27. O'Neill W, Timmis GC, Bourdillon PD, et al. A prospective, randomized clinical trial of intracoronary streptokinase versus coronary angioplasty for acute myocardial infarction. N Engl J Med 1986;314:812.

28. Gruppo Italiano por lo Studio della Streptochinasi nell'Infarcto Miacardio (GISSI). Effectiveness of intravenous thrombolytic treatment in acute myocardial infarction: Gruppo Italiano per lo Studio della Streptochinasi nell'Infarcto Miocardico (GISSI). Lancet 1986;1:397.

29. Gunnar RM, Bourdillon PD, Dixon DW, et al. Guidelines for the early management of patients with acute myocardial infarction: a report of the American College of Cardiology/American Heart Association task force on assessment of diagnostic and therapeutic cardiovascular procedures (subcommittee to develop guidelines for the management of patients with acute myocardial infarction. J Am Coll Cardiol 1990;16:249.

30. Six AJ, Louwerenburg HW, Braams R, et al. A double-blind randomized multicenter dose-ranging trial of intravenous streptokinase in acute myocardial infarction. Am J Cardiol 1990;65:119.

31. Bang NU, Wihelm OG, Clayman MD. Thrombolytic therapy in acute myocardial infarction. Annu Rev Pharmacol Toxicol 1989;29:323.

32. ISIS-3. ISIS-3: a randomized comparison of streptokinase vs tissue plasminogen activator vs anistreplase and of aspirin plus heparin vs aspirin alone among 41,299 cases of suspected acute myocardial infarction: ISIS-3 (Third International Study of Infarct Survival) Collaborative Group. Lancet 1992;339:753.

33. ISIS-2 (The Second International Study of Infarct Survival). Randomized trial of intravenous streptokinase, oral aspirin, both, or neither among 17,187 cases of suspected acute myocardial infarction: ISIS-2 (Second International Study of Infarct Survival) Collaborative Group. Lancet 1988;2:349.

34. The ISAM Study Group. A prospective trial of intravenous streptokinase in acute myocardial infarction (I.S.A.M.): mortality, morbidity, and infarct size at 21 days: the I.S.A.M. Study Group. N Engl J Med 1986;314:1465.

35. Noel J, Rosenbaum LH, Stewart J, Galen G. Serum sickness–like reaction illness and leukocytoclastic vasculitis following intracoronary arterial streptokinase. Am Heart J 1987;113:395.

36. Topol EJ. Thrombolytic interventions. In: Topol EJ, ed. Textbook of interventional cardiology. Vol 1. Philadelphia: WB Saunders, 1990:76.

37. Loscalzo J. Thrombolysis in the management of acute myocardial infarction and unstable angina. Drugs 1989;37:191.

38. Kasper W, Meinertz T, Wollschlager H, et al. Coronary thrombolysis during acute myocardial infarction by intravenous BRL 26921, a new anisoylated plasminogen-streptokinase activator complex. Am J Cardiol 1986;58:418.

39. Kasper W, Meinertz T, Wollschlager H, et al. Early clinical evaluation of the intravenous treatment of acute myocardial infarction with anisoylated plasminogen streptokinase activator complex. Drugs 1987;33(suppl 3):112.

40. Lopez-Sendon J, Seabra-Gomes R, Santos F, et al. Intravenous anisoylated plasminogen streptokinase activator complex (APSAC) versus intravenous streptokinase (SK) in myocardial infarction (AMI) a randomized multicenter study. Eur Heart J 1988;9(suppl 1):10.

41. Brochier ML, Quilit L, Kulbertus H, et al. Intravenous anisoylated plasminogen streptokinase activator complex versus intravenous streptokinase in evolving myocardial infarction. Drugs 1987;33(suppl 3):140.

42. Relik-Van Wely L, van de Pol JMJ, Visser RF, et al. A preliminary report on the angiographic assessed patency and reocclusion in patients treated with APSAC for acute myocardial infarction (AMI): a Dutch multicentre study. Eur Heart J 1988;9(suppl A):213.

43. Vogy P, Schaller MD, Monnier P, et al. Systemic thrombolysis in acute myocardial infarction: bolus injection of APSAC versus infusion of streptokinase. Eur Heart J 1988;9(suppl A):8.

44. White HD, Norris RM, Brown MA, et al. Effect of intravenous streptokinase on left ventricular function and early survival after acute myocardial infarction. N Engl J Med 1987;317:850.

45. Kennedy JW, Martin GV, Davis KB, et al. The Western Washington Intravenous Streptokinase in Acute Myocardial Infarction Randomized Trial (published erratum appears in Circulation 1988;77:1037). Circulation 1988;77:345.

46. Sherry S, Marder VJ. Mistaken guidelines for thrombolytic therapy of acute myocardial infarction in the elderly (comment). J Am Coll Cardiol 1991;17:1237.

47. Arntz R, Heitz J, Schafer H, Schroder R. Hemorrheology in acute myocardial infarction: effects of high dose intravenous streptokinase. Circulation 1985;72(III):417.

48. Reinhart JM, Chien S, et al. Altered rheologic properties of blood following administration of tissue plasminogen activator and streptokinase in patients with acute myocardial infarction. Circulation 1985;72(suppl II):417.

49. Fung AYM, Rabkin SW. Beneficial effects of streptokinase on left ventricular function after myocardial reoxygenation and reperfusion following global ischemia in the isolated rabbit heart. J Cardiovasc Pharmacol 1984;6:429.

50. Sobel BE, Gross RW, Robinson AK. Thrombolysis, clotselectivity, and kinetics. Circulation 1984;70:160.

51. Collen D, Bounameaux H, De CF, et al. Analysis of coagulation and fibrinolysis during intravenous infusion of recombinant human tissue-type plasminogen activator in patients with acute myocardial infarction. Circulation 1986;73:511.

52. Fears R, Ferres H, Standing R. Pharmacologic comparison of anisoylated Lys-plasminogen streptokinase activator complex and its Glu-plasminogen variant and streptokinase–Glu-plasminogen. Fibrinolysis 1989;93:93.

53. Marder VJ, Rothbard RL, Fitzpatrick PG, Francis CW. Rapid lysis of coronary artery thrombi with anisoylated plasminogen: streptokinase activator complex. Treatment by bolus intravenous injection. Ann Intern Med 1986;104:304.

54. Hills WS, Horning RS, Dunn FG. Coronary reperfusion following a single dose of intravenous BRL 26921. Circulation 1986;70:II-28.

55. Meinertz T, Kasper W, Schumacher M, Just H. The German multicenter trial of anisoylated plasminogen streptokinase activator complex versus heparin for acute myocardial infarction. Am J Cardiol 1988;62:347.

56. Timmis AD, Griffin B, Crick JC, Sowton E. Anisoylated plasminogen streptokinase activator complex in acute myocardial infarction: a placebo-controlled arteriographic coronary recanalization study. J Am Coll Cardiol 1987;10:205.

57. Bonnier HJ, Visser RF, Klomps HC, Hoffmann HJ. Comparison of intravenous anisoylated plasminogen streptokinase activator complex and intracoronary streptokinase in acute myocardial infarction. Am J Cardiol 1988;62:25.

58. Hills WS, Hornung RS, Hogg KJ, et al. Achievement of coronary patency by the use of anisoylated plasminogen streptokinase activator complex in acute myocardial infarction. Drugs 1987;33:117.

59. Anderson JL. Development and evaluation of of anisoylated plasminogen streptokinase activator complex (APSAC) as a second generation thrombolytic. J Am Coll Cardiol 1987;10:22B.

60. Neuhaus KL ftGAUSsg. Thrombolysis in acute myocardial infarction: results of the German-Activator-Urokinase Study. Eur Heart J 1987;8:49.

61. Muller DWM, J. TE. Reperfusion therapy for acute myocardial infarction. In: Parmely W, Chatterjee K, eds. Cardiology. Vol 1. Philadelphia: JB Lippincott, 1991:1.

62. Bates ER. Is survival in acute myocardial infarction

related to thrombolytic efficacy or the open-artery hypothesis? A controversy to be investigated with GUSTO. Chest 1992;101(suppl):140S.

63. Fears R, Ferres H, Standring R. Evidence for the progressive uptake of acylated plasminogen streptokinase activator complex by clots in human plasma in vitro. Drugs 1987;33:51.

64. Matuso O, Collen D, Verstraete M. On the fibrinolytic and thrombolytic properties of active-side p-anisoylated streptokinase plasminogen complex (BRL26921). Thromb Res 1981;24:347.

65. Boissel JP. The European Myocardial Infarct Project (EMIP): short term mortality and nonfatal outcomes. Presented at the 41st Annual Scientific Sessions of the American College of Cardiology, Dallas, Texas, April 1992.

66. Green J, Harris GS, Smith RAG, Dupe RJ. Acyenzymes: a novel class of thrombolytic agents. In: Collen D, Lijnin M, Verstraete M, eds. Thrombolysis: biologic and therapeutic properties of new thrombolytic agents. Vol 1. Edinburgh: Churchill Livingstone, 1985:124.

67. Neuhaus KL, von ER, Tebbe U, et al. Improved thrombolysis in acute myocardial infarction with front-loaded administration of alteplase: results of the rt-PA–APSAC patency study (TAPS). J Am Coll Cardiol 1992;19:885.

68. Hogg KJ, Gemmill JD, Burns JM, et al. Angiographic patency study of anistreplase versus streptokinase in acute myocardial infarction. Lancet 1990;335:254.

69. Been M, de Bono D, Muir AL, Boulton FE, et al. Coronary thrombolysis with intravenous anisoylated plasminogen-streptokinase complex BRL 26921. Br Heart J 1985;53:253.

70. Relik van Wely L, Visser RF, van der Pol JMJ, et al. Angiographically assessed coronary arterial patency and reocclusion in patients with acute myocardial infarction treated with anistreplase: results of the anistreplase reocclusion multicenter study (ARMS). Am J Cardiol 1991;68:296.

71. Anderson JL, Sorensen SG, Moreno FL, et al. Multicenter patency trial of intravenous anistreplase compared with streptokinase in acute myocardial infarction: the TEAM-2 Study investigators. Circulation 1991;83:126.

72. Chesbro JH, Knatterud G, Roberts R, et al. The Thrombolysis in Myocardial Infarction (TIMI) trial: phase I findings: TIMI study group. N Engl J Med 1985;312:932.

73. AIMS Trial Study Group. Effect of intravenous APSAC on mortality after acute myocardial infarction: preliminary report of a placebo-controlled clinical trial: AIMS Trial study group. Lancet 1988;1:545.

74. AIMS Trial Study Group. Long-term effects of intravenous anistreplase in acute myocardial infarction: final report of the AIMS study: AIMS Trial study group. Lancet 1990;335:427.

75. Neuhaus KL, Tebbe U, Gottwik M, et al. Intravenous recombinant tissue plasminogen activator (rt-PA) and urokinase in acute myocardial infarction: results of the German Activator Urokinase Study (GAUS). J Am Coll Cardiol 1988;12:581.

76. Mathey DG, Schofer J, Sheehan FH, et al. Intravenous urokinase in acute myocardial infarction. Am J Cardiol 1985;55:878.

77. Urokinase-Pulmonary Embolism Trial Study Group. The urokinase pulmonary embolism trial: phase I results. JAMA 1970;214:2163.

78. Mathey DG. Urokinase. In: Topol EJ, ed. Acute coronary intervention. Vol 1. New York: Allan R Liss, 1987:25.

79. Califf RM, Topol EJ, Stack RS, et al. Evaluation of combination thrombolytic therapy and timing of cardiac catheterization in acute myocardial infarction: results of thrombolysis and angioplasty in myocardial infarction—phase 5 randomized trial: TAMI study group. Circulation 1991;83:1543.

80. Whitlow PL, Bashore TM. Catheterization/Rescue Angioplasty Following Thrombolysis (CRAFT) study: acute myocardial infarction treated with recombinant tissue plasminogen activator versus urokinase (abstract). J Am Coll Cardiol 1991; 17:276A.

81. Wall TC, Phillips H, Stack RS, et al. Results of high dose intravenous urokinase for acute myocardial infarction. Am J Cardiol 1990;65:124.

82. Sherry S. Appraisal of various thrombolytic agents in myocardial infarction. Am J Med 1987;83(suppl 2A):31.

83. Welzel D, Wolf H. Clinical research on single-chain urokinase-type plasminogen activator (scu-PA) in Germany (abstract). Thromb Haemost 1987;58:47.

84. PRIMI Trial Study Group. Randomized double-blind trial of recombinant prourokinase against streptokinase in acute myocardial infarction: PRIMI Trial study group. Lancet 1989;1:863.

85. Collen D, Lijnin HR, Todd PA, Goa KL. Tissue-plasminogen activator: a review of its pharmacology and therapeutic use as a thrombolytic agent. Drugs 1989;38:346.

86. Hoylaerts M, Rijken DC, Lijnen HR, Collen D. Kinetics of the activation of plasminogen by human type plasminogen activator: role of fibrin. J Biol Chem 1982;257:2912.

87. Kruithof EK, Tran-Thang C, Rasijin A, Bachmann F. Demonstration of fast-acting inhibitor of plasminogen in human plasma. Blood 1984;64:907.

88. Tebbe U, Tanswell P, Seifried E, et al. Single-bolus injection of recombinant tissue-type plasminogen activator in acute myocardial infarction. Am J Cardiol 1989;64:448.

89. Lucore CL, Sobel BE. Interactions of tissue-type plasminogen activator with plasma inhibitors and their pharmacologic implications. Circulation 1988;77:660.

90. Garabedian HD, Gold HK, Leinbach RC, et al. Comparative properties of two clinical preparations of recombinant human tissue-type plasminogen activator in patients with acute myocardial infarction. J Am Coll Cardiol 1987;9:599.

91. Chaitman BR, Thompson B, Wittry MD, et al. The use of tissue-type plasminogen activator for acute myocardial infarction in the elderly: results from thrombolysis in myocardial infarction phase I, open label studies and the thrombolysis in myocardial infarction phase II pilot study: the TIMI investigators. J Am Coll Cardiol 1989;14:1159.

92. Topol EJ, George BS, Kereiakes DJ, et al. Comparison of two dose regimens of intravenous tissue plasminogen activator for acute myocardial infarction. Am J Cardiol 1988;61:723.

93. Brower RW, Arnold AE, Lubsen J, Verstraete M. Coronary patency after intravenous infusion of recombinant tissue-type plasminogen activator in acute myocardial infarction. J Am Coll Cardiol 1988;11:681.

94. Neuhaus KL, Feuerer W, Jeep TS, et al. Improved thrombolysis with a modified dose regimen of recombinant tissue-type plasminogen activator. J Am Coll Cardiol 1989;14:1566.

95. Carney RJ, Murphy GA, Brandt TR, et al. Randomized angiographic trial of recombinant tissue-type plasminogen activator (alteplase) in myocardial infarction: RAAMI Study investigators. J Am Coll Cardiol 1992;20:17.

96. The GUSTO Investigators. The international randomized trial comparing four thrombolytic strategies for acute myocardial infarction. N Engl J Med 1993;329:673.

97. Verstraete M, Bory M, Collen D, et al. Randomized trial of intravenous recombinant tissue-type plasminogen activator versus intravenous streptokinase in acute myocardial infarction. Lancet 1985;1:842.

98. Chesebro JH, Knatterud G, Roberts R, et al. Thrombolysis in Myocardial Infarction (TIMI) Trial, phase I: A comparison between intravenous tissue plasminogen activator and intravenous streptokinase. Clinical findings through hospital discharge. Circulation 1987;76:142.

99. Williams DO, Borer J, Braunwald E, et al. Intravenous recombinant tissue-type plasminogen activator in patients with acute myocardial infarction: a report from the NHLBI thrombolysis in myocardial infarction trial. Circulation 1986;73:338.

100. Johns JA, Gold HK, Leinbach RC, et al. Prevention of coronary artery reocclusion and reduction in late coronary artery stenosis after thrombolytic therapy in patients with acute myocardial infarction: a randomized study of maintenance infusion of recombinant human tissue-type plasminogen activator. Circulation 1988;78:546.

101. Lijnen HR, Zamarron C, Blaber M, et al. Activation of plasminogen by prourokinase: I. Mechanism. J Biol Chem 1986;261:1253.

102. Collen D, Stassen J, Stump DC, Verstraete M. Synergism of thrombolytic agents in vivo. Circulation 1986;74:838.

103. Collen D, De Cock F, Demarsin E, et al. Absence of synergism between tissue-type plasminogen activator (t-PA), single-chain urokinase-type plasminogen activator (scu-PA) and urokinase on clot lysis in a plasma milieu in vitro. Thromb Haemost 1986;56:35.

104. Gurewich V, Pannel R. Synergism of tissue-type plasminogen activator (t-PA) and single-chain urokinase-type plasminogen activator (scu-PA) on clot lysis in vitro and a mechanism for this effect. Thromb Haemost 1987;57:372.

105. Granger CB, Califf RM, Topol EJ. Thrombolytic therapy for acute myocardial infarction: a review. Drugs 1992;44:293.

106. Larrieu MJ. Comparative of fibrin degradation products D and E on coagulation. Br J Haematol 1973;72:719.

107. Thorsen LI, Brossad F, Gogstad G, et al. Competitions between fibrinogen with its degradation products for interaction with the platelet fibrinogen receptor. Thromb Res 1986;44:611.

108. Grines CL, Nissen SE, Booth DC, et al. A prospective, randomized trial comparing combination half-dose tissue-type plasminogen activator and streptokinase with full-dose tissue-type plasminogen activator: Kentucky Acute Myocardial Infarction Trial (KAMIT) group. Circulation 1991;84:540.

109. Haber E. Can plasminogen activators be improved? Circulation 1990;82:1874.

110. Collen D. Molecular mechanism of action of the newer thrombolytic agents. J Am Coll Cardiol 1987;10:11B.

111. Nelles L, Lijnen HR, Van Nuffelen A, et al. Characterization of domain deletion and/or duplication mutants of a recombinant chimera of tissue-type plasminogen activator and urokinase-type plasminogen activator (rt-PA/u-PA). Thromb Haemost 1990;64:53.

112. Nicolini FA, Wilmer NW, Jawahara ML, et al. Sustained reflow in dogs with coronary thrombosis with K2P, a novel mutant of tissue plasminogen activator. J Am Coll Cardiol 1992;20:228.

113. Bode C, Runge MS, Haber E. Future directions in plasminogen activator therapy. Clin Cardiol 1990;13:375.

114. Collen D. Designing thrombolytic agents: focus on safety and efficacy. Am J Cardiol 1992;69:71a.

115. Krause J. Catabolism of tissue-type plasminogen activator (t-PA), its variants, mutants, and hybrids. Fibrinolysis 1988;2:133.

116. Nelles L, Lijnen HR, Collen D, Holmes WE. Characterization of recombinant human single-chain urokinase-type plasminogen activator mutants produced by site specific mutagenesis of lysine 158. J Biol Chem 1987;262:5682.

117. Vaughan DE, Loscalzo J. New directions in thrombolytic therapy: molecular mutants and biochemical conjugates. Trends Cardiovasc Med 1991; January-February:36.

118. Stump DC, Lijnen HR, Collen D, Holmes WE. Purification and characterization of a novel low molecular weight form of single chain urokinase-type plasminogen activator. J Biol Chem 1986; 261:17120.

119. Haber E, Quertermous T, Matsueda GR, Runge MS. Innovative approaches to plasminogen activator therapy. Science 1989;243:51.

120. Lijnen HR, Collen D. Strategies for the improvement of thrombolytic agents. Thromb Haemost 1991;66:88.

121. Collen D, Stassen JM, Demarsin E, et al. Pharmacokinetics and thrombolytic properties of chimeric plasminogen activators consisting of the NH_2-terminal region of human tissue-type plasminogen activator and the COOH-terminal region of human single chain urokinase-type plasminogen activator. J Vasc Med Biol 1989;1:234.

122. Gardell SJ, Ramjit DR, Stabilito JJ, et al. Effective thrombolysis without marked plasminogenemia following bolus administration of a vampire bat salivary plasminogen activator in rabbits. Circulation 1991;84:244.

123. Bang N. Leeches, snakes, ticks, and vampire bats in today's cardiovascular drug development (editorial). Circulation 1991;84:436.

124. Brunton TL. On the use of nitrite of amyl in angina pectoris. Lancet 1867;2:97.

125. Rutherford JD, Braunwald E, Cohen PF. Chronic ischemic heart disease. In: Braunwald E, ed. Heart disease: a textbook of cardiovascular medicine. Vol 2. Philadelphia: WB Saunders, 1988:1314.

126. Stramler JS, Loscalzo J. The antiplatelet effects of organic nitrates and related nitroso compounds in vitro and in vivo and their relevance to cardiovascular disorders. J Am Coll Cardiol 1991;18:1529.

127. Loscalzo J. Antiplatelet and antithrombotic effects of organic nitrates. Am J Cardiol 1992;70 (suppl B):18B.

128. Stramler JS, Simon DI, Jaraki O, et al. S-Nitrosylation of tissue-type plasminogen activator confers vasodilatory and antiplatelet properties on the enzyme. Proc Natl Acad Sci USA 1992;89:8087.

129. Norris RM, White HD. Therapeutic trials in coronary thrombosis should measure left ventricular function as an endpoint of treatment. Lancet 1988;1:104.

130. Califf RM, Harrelson WL, Topol EJ. Left ventricular ejection fraction may not be useful as an end point of thrombolytic therapy comparative trials. Circulation 1990;82:1847.

131. Baigent C, for the Fibrinolytic Therapy Trialists' Collaboration CTS. Late benefit and early hazard associated with fibrinolytic therapy for acute myocardial infarction: results from six large randomized controlled trials. Circulation 1992;86:1643.

132. Cerqueira MD, Maynard C, Davis KB, et al. Long-term survival in 618 patients from the Western Washington Streptokinase in Myocardial Infarction Trials. J Am Coll Cardiol 1992;20:1452.

133. Ikram S, Lewis S, Bucknall C, et al. Treatment of acute myocardial infarction with anisoylated plasminogen streptokinase activator complex. Br Med J 1986;293:786.

134. Anderson JL, Rothbard RL, Hackworthy RA, et al. Multicenter reperfusion trial of intravenous anisoylated plasminogen streptokinase activator complex (APSAC) in acute myocardial infarction: controlled comparison with intracoronary streptokinase. J Am Coll Cardiol 1988;11:1153.

135. Wilcox RG, von der Lippe G, Olsson CG, et al. Trial of tissue plasminogen activator for mortality reduction in acute myocardial infarction: Anglo-Scandinavian Study of Early Thrombolysis (ASSET). Lancet 1988;2:525.

136. Wilcox RG, et al. Effects of alteplase in acute myocardial infarction: 6-month results from the ASSET study: Anglo-Scandinavian Study of Early Thrombolysis. Lancet 1990;335:1175.

137. Van de Werf F, Arnold AER. Intravenous tissue plasminogen activator and size of infarct, left ventricular function, and survival in acute myocardial infarction (ECSG-4). Br Med J 1988;287:1374.

138. Cairns JA, Fuster V, Kennedy JW. Coronary thrombolysis. Chest 1992;102:482.

139. Gruppo Italiano por lo Studio della Supravvivenza nell'Infarto Miacardio. GISSI-2: a factorial randomized trial of alteplase versus streptokinase and heparin versus no heparin among 12,490 patients with acute myocardial infarction: Gruppo Italiano per lo Studio della Sopravvivenza nell'Infarcto Miocardico. Lancet 1990;336:65.

140. The International Study Group. In-hospital mortality and clinical course of 20,891 patients with suspected acute myocardial infarction randomised between alteplase and streptokinase with or without heparin: the International Study Group. Lancet 1990;336:71.

141. Bleich SD, Nichols TC, Schumacher RR, et al. Effect of heparin on coronary arterial patency after thrombolysis with tissue plasminogen activator in

acute myocardial infarction. Am J Cardiol 1990; 66:1412.

142. Eisenberg PR. Role of heparin in coronary thrombolysis. Chest 1992;101(suppl 4):1315.

143. Prins MH, Hirsh J. Heparin as an adjunctive treatment after thrombolytic therapy for acute myocardial infarction. Am J Cardiol 1991;67:3.

144. Sherry S. Unresolved clinical pharmacologic questions in thrombolytic therapy for acute myocardial infarction. J Am Coll Cardiol 1988;12:519.

145. Sherry S. Recombinant tissue plasminogen activator (rt-PA): is it the thrombolytic agent of choice for an evolving acute myocardial infarction? Am J Cardiol 1987;59:984.

146. The Multicenter Postinfarction Research Group. Risk stratification and survival after myocardial infarction. N Engl J Med 1983;309:332.

147. Simmons ML, Serruys PW, Brand M, et al. Improved survival after early thrombolysis in acute myocardial infarction: a randomized trial by the Interuniversity Cardiology Institute in the Netherlands. Lancet 1985;2:578.

148. Magnani B. Plasminogen Activator Italian Multicenter Study (PAIMS): comparison of intravenous recombinant single-chain human tissue-type plasminogen activator (rt-PA) with intravenous streptokinase in acute myocardial infarction. J Am Coll Cardiol 1989;13:19.

149. Bassand JP, Cassagnes J, Machecourt J, et al. Comparative effects of APSAC and rt-PA on infarct size and left ventricular function in acute myocardial infarction: a multicenter randomized study. Circulation 1991;84:1107.

150. Anderson JL, Becker LC, Sherman SG, et al. Anistreplase versus alteplase in acute myocardial infarction: comparative effects on left ventricular function, morbidity, and 1-day coronary artery patency. J Am Coll Cardiol 1992;20:753.

151. Cohn P, Becker R, Goldberg R, Gore J. Early coronary artery patency does not predict clinical outcome following thrombolytic therapy: a meta-analysis (abstract). Circulation 1990;86(suppl I): I-269.

152. Lincoff AM, Ellis SG, Galeana A, et al. Is a coronary artery with TIMI grade 2 flow "patent"? Outcome in the Thrombolysis and Angioplasty in Myocardial Infarction Trial (abstract). Circulation 1992;86(suppl):I-268.

153. Voght A, Tebbe U, von Essen R, et al. 90-minute patency and optimal reperfusion of infarct-related coronary arteries (abstract). Circulation 1992;86 (suppl I):I-268.

154. Mueller HS, Rao AK, Forman SA. Thrombolysis in myocardial infarction (TIMI): comparative studies of coronary reperfusion and systemic fibrinogenolysis with two forms of recombinant tissue-type plasminogen activator. J Am Coll Cardiol 1987;10:479.

155. Leiboff RH, Katz RJ, Wasserman AG, et al. A randomized, angiographically controlled trial of intracoronary streptokinase in acute myocardial infarction. Am J Cardiol 1984;53:404.

156. Rentrop KP, Feit F, Blanke H, et al. Effects of intracoronary streptokinase and intracoronary nitroglycerin infusion on coronary angiographic patterns and mortality in patients with acute myocardial infarction. N Engl J Med 1984;311:1457.

157. Khaja F, Walton JJ, Brymer JF, et al. Intracoronary fibrinolytic therapy in acute myocardial infarction: report of a prospective randomized trial. N Engl J Med 1983;308:1305.

158. Van de Werf F. Lessons from the European cooperative recombinant tissue-type plasminogen activator (rt-PA) versus placebo trial. J Am Coll Cardiol 1988;12(suppl 16A):14a.

159. Verstraete M, Arnold AE, Brower RW, et al. Acute coronary thrombolysis with recombinant human tissue-type plasminogen activator: initial patency and influence of maintained infusion on reocclusion rate. Am J Cardiol 1987;60:231.

160. Verstraete M, Bernard R, Bory M, et al. Randomised trial of intravenous recombinant tissue-type plasminogen activator versus intravenous streptokinase in acute myocardial infarction: report from the European Cooperative Study Group for Recombinant Tissue-Type Plasminogen Activator. Lancet 1985;1:842.

161. Kwon K, Freedman SB, Wilcox I, et al. The unstable ST segment early after thrombolysis for acute infarction and its usefulness as a marker of recurrent coronary occlusion. Am J Cardiol 1991;67: 109.

162. Reimer KA, Lowe JE, Rasmeussen MM, Jennings RB. The wave front of ischemic cell death: 1. Myocardial infarct size vs duration of coronary occlusion in dogs. Circulation 1977;56:786.

163. Cigarroa RG, Lang RA, Hillis LD. Prognosis after myocardial infarction in patients with and without residual antegrade coronary blood flow. Am J Cardiol 1989;64:155.

164. Topol EJ, Califf RM, George BS, et al. A randomized trial of immediate versus delayed elective angioplasty after intravenous tissue plasminogen activator in acute myocardial infarction. N Engl J Med 1987;317:581.

165. Stack RS, O'Connor CM, Mark DB, et al. Coronary perfusion during acute myocardial infarction with a combined therapy of coronary angioplasty and high-dose intravenous streptokinase. Circulation 1988;77:151.

166. Dalen JE, Gore JM, Braunwald E, et al. Six- and twelve-month follow-up of the phase I Thrombol-

ysis in Myocardial Infarction (TIMI) trial (published erratum appears in Am J Cardiol 1988; 62:1151). Am J Cardiol 1988;62:179.

167. Yusuf S. Expanding indications for the use of thrombolytic agents in acute myocardial infarction. Clin Cardiol 1990;53:67.

168. Diaz R. EMERAS trial: study design. Presented at the 40th Annual Scientific Session of the American College of Cardiology, Atlanta, Georgia, March 1991.

169. Paolasso E. EMERAS trial: results and discussion. Presented at the 40th Annual Scientific Session of the American College of Cardiology, Atlanta, Georgia, March 1991.

170. Muller DWM. Reperfusion therapy for acute myocardial infarction. In: Topol EJ, ed. Textbook of interventional cardiology. Philadelphia: WB Saunders, 1992:59.

171. The Late Investigators. The Late Assessment of Thrombolytic Efficacy (LATE) trial. Presented at the XIV Congress of the European Society of Cardiology, Barcelona, Spain, August 1992.

172. Topol EJ, Califf RM, Vandormael M, et al. A randomized trial of late reperfusion therapy for acute myocardial infarction: Thrombolysis and Angioplasty in Myocardial Infarction-6 study group. Circulation 1992;85:2090.

173. Braunwald E. Myocardial reperfusion, limitations of infarct size, reduction of left ventricular dysfunction, and improved survival: should the paradigm be expanded? Circulation 1989;79:441.

174. Fortin DF, Califf RM. Long-term survival from acute myocardial infarction: salutary effects of an open coronary vessel. Am J Med 1990;88:1–9N.

175. Pfeffer M, Braunwald E. Ventricular remodeling after myocardial infarction. Circulation 1990;81: 1161.

176. White HD, Norris RM, Brown MA, et al. Left ventricular end-systolic volume as a major determinant of survival after recovery from acute myocardial infarction. Circulation 1987;76:44.

177. Vogel WM, Apstein CG, Briggs LL, et al. Acute alterations in left ventricular diastolic chamber stiffness: role of the "erectile" effect of coronary arterial pressure and flow in normal and damaged hearts. Circ Res 1982;51:465.

178. Kurnick PB, Courtois MR, Ludbrook PA. Diastolic stiffening induced by myocardial infarction is reduced by early reperfusion. J Am Coll Cardiol 1988;12:1029.

179. Hale SL, Kloner RA. Left ventricular topographic alterations in completely healed rat infarct caused by early and late coronary reperfusion. Am Heart J 1988;116:1508.

180. Serruys PW, Simoons ML, Suryapranata H, et al. Preservation of global and regional left ventricular function after early thrombolysis in acute myocardial infarction. J Am Coll Cardiol 1986;7:729.

181. Bonaduce D, Petretta M, Villari B, et al. Effects of late administration of tissue-type plasminogen activator on left ventricular remodeling and function after myocardial infarction. J Am Coll Cardiol 1990;16:1561.

182. Siu SC, Nidorf SM, Galambos GS, et al. The effect of late patency of the infarct-related coronary artery on left ventricular morphology and regional function after thrombolysis. Am Heart J 1992;124: 265.

183. Kersschot IE, Brugada P, Ramental M, et al. Effects of early reperfusion in acute myocardial infarction on arrhythmias induced by programed electrical stimulation: a prospective, randomized study. Am J Cardiol 1986;7:1234.

184. Sager PT, Perlmutter RA, Rosenfeld LE, et al. Electrophysiologic effects of thrombolytic therapy in patients with a transmural anterior myocardial infarction complicated by left ventricular aneurysm formation. J Am Coll Cardiol 1988;12:19.

185. Gang ES, Lew AS, Hong M, et al. Decreased incidence of ventricular late potentials after successful thrombolytic therapy for acute myocardial infarction. N Engl J Med 1989;321:712.

186. Horvitz L, Pietrolungo JF, Suri S, et al. An open infarct-related artery is associated with a lower risk of lethal ventricular arrhythmias in patients with left ventricular aneurysms. Circulation 1992; 86:I-315.

187. van der Wall E, van DP, de Roos A, et al. Diagnostic significance of gadolinium-DTPA (diethylenetriamine penta-acetic acid) enhanced magnetic resonance imaging in thrombolytic treatment for acute myocardial infarction: its potential in assessing reperfusion. Br Heart J 1990;63:12.

188. Calkins H, Maughan WL, Weisman HF, et al. Effects of acute volume load on refractoriness and arrhythmia development in isolated, chronically infarcted dog hearts. Circulation 1989;79: 687.

189. Fine DG, Weiss AT, Sapoznikov D, et al. Importance of early initiation of intravenous streptokinase therapy for acute myocardial infarction. Am J Cardiol 1986;58:411.

190. Koren G, Weiss AT, Hasin Y, et al. Prevention of myocardial damage in acute myocardial ischemia by early treatment with intravenous streptokinase. N Engl J Med 1985;313:1384.

191. Dudley CRK. Thrombolysis at home? Lancet 1987;2:1459.

192. Weiss AT, Fine DG, Applebaum D, et al. Prehospital coronary thrombolysis: a new strategy in acute myocardial infarction. Chest 1987;92:124.

193. Kennedy JW, Weaver WD. Potential use of throm-

bolytic therapy before hospitalization. Am J Cardiol 1989;64:8.

194. Ross A. Prehospital thrombolysis: MITI and EMIP results. J Myocardial Ischemia 1992;4:13.

195. Weaver WD. Myocardial Infarction Triage and Intervention (MITI) trial of prehospital initiated thrombolysis-results. Presented at the 41st Annual Scientific Session of the American College of Cardiology, Dallas, Texas, April 1992.

196. Cerqueira MD, Litwin PE, Martin JS, et al. Infarct size reduction and preservation of ejection fraction with very early thrombolytic treatment for acute myocardial infarction: radionuclide results from the Myocardial Infarction Triage Intervention Project (abstract). Circulation 1992;86(suppl I):I-643.

197. National Heart Foundation of Australia Coronary Thrombolysis Group. Coronary thrombolysis and myocardial salvage by tissue plasminogen activator given up to 4 hours after onset of myocardial infarction: National Heart Foundation of Australia Coronary Thrombolysis Group (published erratum appears in Lancet 1988;27:519). Lancet 1988;1:203.

198. Ellis SG, Topol EJ, George BS, et al. Recurrent ischemia without warning: analysis of risk factors for in-hospital ischemic events following successful thrombolysis with intravenous tissue plasminogen activator. Circulation 1989;80:1159.

199. Ohman EM, Califf RM. Thrombolytic therapy: overview of the clinical trials. In: Gersh BJ, Rahimtoola SH, eds. Acute myocardial infarction. New York: Elsevier, 1991:308.

200. Popma JJ, Topol EJ. Adjuncts to thrombolysis for myocardial reperfusion. Ann Intern Med 1991; 115:34.

201. Golino P, Ashton JH, Glas-Greenwalk P, et al. Mediation of reocclusion by thromboxane A_2 and serotonin after thrombolysis with tissue-type plasminogen activator in canine preparation of coronary thrombosis. Circulation 1988;77:678.

202. O'Brien JR. Shear-induced platelet aggregation. Lancet 1990;1:711.

203. Fitzgerald DJ, Catella F, Roy L, FitzGerald GA. Marked platelet activation in vivo after intravenous streptokinase in patients with acute myocardial infarction. Circulation 1988;77:142.

204. Gold HK, Coller BS, Yasuda T, et al. Rapid and sustained coronary artery recanalization with combined bolus injection of recombinant tissue-type plasminogen activator and monoclonal antiplatelet GPIIb/IIIa antibody in a canine preparation. Circulation 1988;77:670.

205. Coller BS, Folts JD, Smith SR, et al. Abolition of in vivo platelet thrombus formation in primates with monoclonal antibodies to GPIIb/IIIa receptor: correlation with bleeding time, platelet aggregation,

206. Song A, Scarborough RM, Phillips DR, et al. Integrelin enhances fibrinolysis and prevents arterial occlusion following thrombolysis in canine anodal current model with high grade stenosis (abstract). Circulation 1992;86(suppl I):I-410.

207. Charo IF, Scarborough RM, du Mee CP, et al. Pharmacodynamics of the GPIIb/IIIa antagonist Integrelin: phase I clinical studies in normal healthy volunteers (abstract). Circulation 1992;86 (suppl I):I-260.

208. Gold HK, Leinbach RC, Garabedian HD, et al. Acute coronary reocclusion after thrombolysis with recombinant human tissue-type plasminogen activator: prevention by a maintenance infusion. Circulation 1986;73:347.

209. Francis CW, Markham REJ, Barlow GH, et al. Thrombin activity of fibrin thrombi and soluble plasmic derivatives. J Lab Clin Med 1983;102:220.

210. Chesebro JH, Badimon L, Fuster V. New approaches to treatment of myocardial infarction. Am J Cardiol 1990;65:12.

211. Eisenberg PR, Miletich JP, Sobel BS. Induction of marked thrombin activity by pharmacologic concentrations of plasminogen activators in nonanticoagulated whole blood. Thromb Res 1989;55: 635.

212. Coller BS. Platelets and thrombolytic therapy. N Engl J Med 1990;332:33.

213. Heras M, Chesebro JH, Penny WJ, et al. Effects of thrombin inhibition on the development of acute platelet-thrombus deposition during angioplasty in pigs: heparin versus recombinant hirudin, a specific thrombin inhibitor. Circulation 1989; 79:657.

214. Eisenberg PR, Sobel BE, Jaffe AS. Activation of prothrombin accompanying thrombolysis with recombinant tissue-type plasminogen activator. J Am Coll Cardiol 1992;19:1065.

215. Seitz R, Blanke H, Pratotius G, et al. Increased thrombin activity during thrombolysis. Thromb Haemost 1988;59:541.

216. Eisenberg PR, Sherman LA, Jaffe AS. Paradoxical elevation of fibrinopeptide-A after streptokinase: evidence for continued thrombosis despite intense fibrinolysis. J Am Coll Cardiol 1987;10:527.

217. Melandri G, Branzi A, Semprini F, et al. Enhanced thrombolytic efficacy and reduction of infarct size by simultaneous infusion of streptokinase and heparin. Br Heart J 1990;64:118.

218. Col J, Decoster O, Hanique G, et al. Infusion of heparin conjunct to streptokinase accelerates reperfusion of acute myocardial infarction: results of a double blind randomized study (abstract). Circulation 1992;86:I-259.

219. Topol EJ, George BS, Kereiakes DJ, et al. A ran-

domized, controlled trial of intravenous tissue plasminogen activator and early intravenous heparin in acute myocardial infarction. Circulation 1989;79:281.

220. Hsia J, Hamilton WP, Kleiman N, et al. A comparison between heparin and low-dose aspirin as adjunctive therapy with tissue plasminogen activator for acute myocardial infarction: Heparin-Aspirin Reperfusion Trial (HART) investigators. N Engl J Med 1990;323:1433.

221. de Bono DP, Simoons ML, Tijssen J, et al. Effect of early intravenous heparin on coronary patency, infarct size, and bleeding complications after alteplase thrombolysis: results of a randomised double blind European Cooperative Study Group trial. Br Heart J 1992;67:122.

222. O'Connor CM, Meese R, Navetta F, et al. A randomized trial of heparin with anistreplase (APSAC) in myocardial infarction. Circulation 1991;84(suppl II):II-571.

223. Bonnier H, Hoffman H, Melman P, Bartholomeus I. Is there an effect of APSAC on blood viscosity, and platelet function in patients with acute myocardial infarction treated with APSAC? Circulation 1991;84(suppl II):II-524.

224. The SCATI (Studio sulla Calciparina nell'Angina e nella Trombosi Ventricolare nell'Infarto) Group. Randomised, controlled trial of subcutaneous calcium-heparin in acute myocardial infarction. Lancet 1989;2:182.

225. Hull RD, Raskob GE, Hirsh J, et al. Continuous intravenous heparin therapy compared with intermittent subcutaneous heparin in the initial treatment of proximal-vein deep venous thrombosis. N Engl J Med 1986;315:1109.

226. Turpie AG, Robinson JG, Doyle DJ, et al. Comparison of high-dose with low-dose subcutaneous heparin to prevent left ventricular mural thrombosis in patients with acute transmural anterior myocardial infarction. N Engl J Med 1989;320:352.

227. Arnout J, Simoons M, de Bono D, et al. Correlation between level of heparinization and patency of the infarct-related coronary artery after treatment of acute myocardial infarction with alteplase. J Am Coll Cardiol 1992;20:513.

228. Hsia J, Kleiman N, Aguirre F, et al. Heparin-induced prolongation of partial thromboplastin time after thrombolysis: relation to coronary artery patency. HART Investigators. J Am Coll Cardiol 1992;20:31.

229. Webster MI, Chesebro JH, Fuster V. Antithrombotic therapy in acute myocardial infarction: enhancement of thrombolysis, reduction of reocclusion, and prevention of thromboembolism. In: Gersh B, Rahimtoola S, eds. Acute myocardial infarction. New York: Elsevier, 1991:333.

230. Mahan EF, Chandler JW, Rogers WJ, et al. Heparin and infarct coronary artery patency after streptokinase in acute myocardial infarction. Am J Cardiol 1990;65:967.

231. Second Report of the Working Party on Anticoagulant Therapy in Coronary Thrombosis to the Medical Research Council. An assessment of long-term anticoagulant administration after cardiac infarction. Br Med J 1964;2:837.

232. United States Veteran Administration. Long term anticoagulation after myocardial infarction. JAMA 1965;193:157.

233. Sixty Plus Reinfarction Study Research Group. A double-blind trial to evaluate long-term anticoagulant therapy in elderly patients after myocardial infarction. Lancet 1980;2:989.

234. Schreiber TL, Miller DH, Silvasi D, et al. Superiority of warfarin over aspirin long term after thrombolytic therapy for acute myocardial infarction. Am Heart J 1990;119:1238.

235. Smith P, Arnesen H, Holme I. The effects of warfarin on mortality and reinfarction after myocardial infarction. N Engl J Med 1990;323:147.

236. Kelly AB, Hanson SR, Marzec U, Harker LA. Recombinant hirudin (r-H) interruption of platelet-dependant thrombus formation (abstract). Circulation 1988;80(suppl II):II-311.

237. Hanson SR, Harker LA. Interruption of acute platelet-dependent thrombosis by the synthetic antithrombin D-phenylalanyl-L-propyl-L-argyl chloromethyl ketone. Proc Natl Acad Sci USA 1988;85:3184.

238. Mirshahi M, Soria J, Faivre R, et al. Evaluation of the inhibition by heparin and hirudin of coagulation activation during rt-PA induced thrombolysis. Blood 1989;74:1025.

239. Kerins DM, Roy L, FitzGerald GA, Fitzgerald DJ. Platelet and vascular function during coronary thrombolysis with tissue-type plasminogen activator. Circulation 1989;80:1718.

240. Jang I-K, Gold HK, Leinbach RC. Acceleration of reperfusion by combination of rt-PA and a selective thrombin inhibitor, argatroban (abstract). Circulation 1989;80:II-217.

241. Tamao Y, Yamamoto T, Kikumoto R, et al. Effects of a selective thrombin inhibitor MCI-9038 on fibrinolysis in vitro and in vivo. Thromb Haemost 1986;56:28.

242. Klement P, Boem A, Hirsh J, et al. The effects of thrombin inhibitors on tissue plasminogen activator induced thrombolysis in the rat model. Thromb Haemost 1992;68:64.

243. Falk E. Unstable angina with fatal outcome: dynamic coronary thrombosis leading to infarction and/or sudden death. Circulation 1985;71:699.

244. Fuster V, Badimon L, Badimon J, Chesebro J. The pathogenesis of coronary artery disease and acute coronary syndromes. N Engl J Med 1992;326:310.

245. Lopez-Sendon J, Coma-Canella I, Peinado R, et al. Prolonged IV infusion of urokinase in recent onset unstable angina: a randomized study (abstract). Circulation 1992;86(suppl I):I-387.

246. Romeo F, Martuscelli E, Lacquanti B, et al. A randomized trial on combined low dose rt-PA and heparin versus heparin alone for treatment of patients with unstable angina pectoris (abstract). Circulation 1992;86(suppl I):I-387.

247. Vermeer F, Raynaud P, Materne P, et al. Thrombolytic therapy in patients with unstable angina (UNASEM): results of one-year follow-up (abstract). Circulation 192;86(suppl I):I-387.

248. Lidon R-M, Adelman B, Maraganore J, Theroux P. Hirulog, a direct thrombin inhibitor, for the management of unstable angina. Circulation 1992;86 (suppl I):I-386.

249. Waters D, Lam JYT. Is thrombolytic therapy striking out in unstable angina? Circulation 1992;86: 1662.

250. Theroux P, Watres D, Qui S, et al. Heparin prevents myocardial infarction better than aspirin during the acute phase of unstable angina. Circulation (in press).

251. Rapold HJ. Promotion of thrombin activity by thrombolytic therapy without simultaneous anticoagulation. Lancet 1990;1:481.

252. Eisenberg PR, Miletich JP. Induction of marked thrombin activity by pharmacologic concentrations of plasminogen activators in nonanticoagulated whole blood. Thromb Res 1990;55:635.

253. Aronson DL, Chang P, Kessler CM. Platelet-dependent thrombin generation after in vitro fibrinolytic treatment. Circulation 1992;85:1706.

254. The TIMI IIIB Investigators. TIMI IIIB trial of thrombolysis in unstable angina and non-Q-wave myocardial infarction. Presented at the 65th Scientific Session of the American Heart Association, New Orleans, Louisiana, November 1992.

255. Maggioni AP, Franzosi MG, Fresco C, et al. GISSI trials in acute myocardial infarction: rationale, design, and results. Chest 1990;97(suppl 4):1465.

256. Soldo BJ, Manton KG. Demography: characteristics and implications of an aging population. In: Rowe JW, Besdine RW, eds. Geriatric medicine. Vol 1, 2nd ed. Boston: Little, Brown, 1988:12.

257. Kapantais G, Powell-Griner E. Characteristics of persons dying of diseases of the heart: preliminary data from the 1986 National Mortality Followback Survey. Hyattsville, Md: Public Health Service (DHHS publication no. PHS 89–1250), 1989.

258. Muller DW, Topol EJ. Selection of patients with acute myocardial infarction for thrombolytic therapy. Ann Intern Med 1990;113:949.

259. Gurwitz JH, Goldberg RG, Gore JM. Coronary thrombolysis for the elderly? JAMA 1991;265: 1720.

260. Topol EJ, Califf RM. Thrombolytic therapy for elderly patients (editorial). N Engl J Med 1992;327: 45.

261. De Jaegere PP, Arnold AA, Balk AH, Simmons ML. Intracranial hemorrhage in association with thrombolytic therapy: Incidence and clinical predictive factors. J Am Coll Cardiol 1992;19:289.

262. Gore JM, Sloan M, Price TR, et al. Intracerebral hemorrhage, cerebral infarction, and subdural hematoma after acute myocardial infarction and thrombolytic therapy in the Thrombolysis in Myocardial Infarction Study: Thrombolysis in Myocardial Infarction, phase II, pilot and clinical trial. Circulation 1991;83:448.

263. Feit F, Breed J, Anderson JL, et al. A randomized placebo-controlled, trial of tissue plasminogen activator in elderly patients with acute myocardial infarction (abstract). Circulation 1990;82(suppl III):III-666.

264. Krumholz HM, Pasternak RC, Weinstein MC, et al. Cost effectiveness of thrombolytic therapy with streptokinase in elderly patients with suspected acute myocardial infarction. N Engl J Med 1992;327:7.

265. Grines CL, Browne KF, Vandormael M, et al. Primary Angioplasty in Myocardial Infarction (PAMI) trial. Circulation 1992;86:I-641.

266. Yusuf S, Collins R, Peto R, et al. Intravenous and intracoronary fibrinolytic therapy in acute myocardial infarction: overview of results on mortality, reinfarction, and side-effects from 33 randomized controlled trials. Eur Heart J 1985;6:556.

267. Fennerty AG, Levine MN, Hirsh J. Hemorrhagic complications of thrombolytic therapy in the treatment of myocardial infarction and venous thromboembolism. Chest 1989;95(suppl 2):885.

268. Maggioni AP, Franzosi MG, Santoro E, et al. The risk of stroke in patients with acute myocardial infarction after thrombolytic and antithrombotic treatment: Gruppo Italiano per lo Studio della Sopravvivenza nell'Infarto Miocardico II (GISSI-2) and the International Study Group. N Engl J Med 1992;327:1.

269. Kennedy JW. Expanding the use of thrombolytic therapy for acute myocardial infarction (editorial). Ann Intern Med 1990;113:907.

270. Grines CL, DeMaria AN. Optimal utilization of thrombolytic therapy for acute myocardial infarction: concepts and controversies. J Am Coll Cardiol 1990;16:223.

271. Topol EJ, Califf RM, George BS, et al. Coronary arterial thrombolysis with combined infusion of recombinant tissue-type plasminogen activator and urokinase in patients with acute myocardial infarction (TAMI-2). Circulation 1988;77:1100.

272. Charbonnier B, Cribier A, Monassier JP, et al. Etude eurpeene multicentrique et randomissee de

l'APSAC versus streptokinase dans l'infarctus du myocarde. Arch Mal Coeur 1989;82:1565.

273. Monnier P, Sigwart U, Vincent A, et al. Anisoylated plasminogen streptokinase activator complex versus streptokinase in acute myocardial infarction. Drugs 1987;33(suppl 3):175.

274. Voght P, Schaller MD, Monnier P, et al. Systemic thrombolysis in acute myocardial infarction: bolus injection of APSAC versus infusion of streptokinase. (abstract). Eur Heart J 1988;9(suppl A):213.

275. Ribeiro EE, Silva LA, Carneiro R, et al. A randomized trial of direct PTCA vs intravenous streptokinase in acute myocardial infarction (abstract). J Am Coll Cardiol 1991;17:152A.

276. Durand P, Asseman P, Pruvost P, et al. Effectiveness of intravenous streptokinase on infarct size and left ventricular function in acute myocardial infarction: prospective and randomized study. Clin Cardiol 1987;10:383.

277. SWIFT Trial Study Group. SWIFT trial of delayed elective intervention vs conservative treatment after thrombolysis with anistreplase in acute myocardial infarction. Br Med J 1991;302:555.

278. The TIMI Research Group. Immediate vs delayed catheterization and angioplasty following thrombolytic therapy for acute myocardial infarction: TIMI IIA results. JAMA 1988;260:2849.

279. Topol EJ, Ellis SG, Califf RM, et al. Combined tissue-type plasminogen activator and prostacyclin therapy for acute myocardial infarction: Thrombolysis and Angioplasty in Myocardial Infarction (TAMI) 4 study group. J Am Coll Cardiol 1989;14:877.

280. Guerci AD, Gerstenblith G, Brinker JA, et al. A randomized trial of intravenous tissue plasminogen activator for acute myocardial infarction with subsequent randomization to elective coronary angioplasty. N Engl J Med 1987;317:1613.

281. Verstraete M, Bleifeld W, Brower RW, et al. Double-blind randomised trial of intravenous tissue-type plasminogen activator versus placebo in acute myocardial infarction. Lancet 1985;2:965.

282. Topol EJ, Morris DC, Smalling RW, et al. A multicenter, randomized, placebo-controlled trial of a new form of intravenous recombinant tissue-type plasminogen activator (activase) in acute myocardial infarction. J Am Coll Cardiol 1987;9:1205.

283. Smalling RW, Schumacher R, Morris D, et al. Improved infarct-related arterial patency after high dose, weight-adjusted, rapid infusion of tissue-type plasminogen activator in myocardial infarction: results of a multicenter randomized trial of two dosage regimens. J Am Coll Cardiol 1990;15:915.

284. Wall TC, Califf RM, George BS, et al. Accelerated plasminogen activator dose regimens for coronary thrombolysis: the TAMI-7 study group. J Am Coll Cardiol 1992;19:482.

285. Gemmill JD, Hogg KJ, MacIntyre PD, et al. A pilot study of the efficacy and safety of bolus administration of alteplase in acute myocardial infarction. Br Heart J 1991;66:134.

286. Purvis JA, Trouton TG, Roberts MJ, et al. Effectiveness of double bolus alteplase in the treatment of acute myocardial infarction. Am J Cardiol 1991;68:1570.

287. Urokinase and Alteplase in Myocardial Infarction Collaborative Group (URALMI). Combination of urokinase and alteplase in the treatment of myocardial infarction. Coronary Artery Dis 1991;2:225.

288. Grines CL, Nissen SE, Booth DC, et al. A new thrombolytic regimen for acute myocardial infarction using combination half dose tissue-type plasminogen activator with full dose streptokinase: a pilot study: KAMIT study group. J Am Coll Cardiol 1989;14:573.

289. Bonnet JL, Bory M, D'Houdain F, et al. Association of tissue plasminogen activator and streptokinase in acute myocardial infarction: preliminary data (abstract). Circulation 1989;80(suppl II):II-343.

290. Granger CB, Kalbfleisch J, Califf R, et al. The global utilization of streptokinase and tissue plasminogen activator in occluded coronary arteries (GUSTO) pilot study. Circulation 1991;84(suppl II):II-573.

291. O'Rourke M, Baron D, Keogh A, et al. Limitation of myocardial infarction by early infusion of recombinant tissue-type plasminogen activator. Circulation 1988;77:1311.

292. Armstrong PW, Baigrie RS, Daly PA, et al. Tissue plasminogen activator: Toronto (TPAT) placebo-controlled randomized trial in acute myocardial infarction. J Am Coll Cardiol 1989;13:1469.

293. White HD, Rivers JT, Maslowski AH, et al. Effect of intravenous streptokinase as compared with that of tissue plasminogen activator on left ventricular function after first myocardial infarction. N Engl J Med 1989;320:817.

294. Williams DO, Topol EJ, Califf RM, et al. Intravenous recombinant tissue-type plasminogen activator in patients with unstable angina pectoris. Circulation 1990;82:376.

295. Nicklas J, Topol EJ, Kander N, et al. Randomized, double-blind, placebo-controlled trial of tissue plasminogen activator in unstable angina. J Am Coll Cardiol 1989;13:434.

296. Freeman MR, Langer A, Wilson RF, et al. Thrombolysis in unstable angina: randomized double-blind trial of t-PA and placebo. Circulation 1992;85:150.

297. Bar FW, Verheugt FW, Col J, et al. Thrombolysis in patients with unstable angina improves the an-

giographic but not the clinical outcome. Circulation 1992;86:131.

298. Schreiber TL, Rizik D, White C, et al. Randomized trial of thrombolysis versus heparin in unstable angina. Circulation 1992;86:1407.

299. TIMI-IIIB Investigators. TIMI-IIIB trial of thrombolysis in unstable angina and non-Q-wave myocardial infarction. Presented at the Annual Scientific Session of the American Heart Association, New Orleans, Louisiana, 1992.

300. The GUSTO Angiographic Investigators. The effects of tissue plasminogen activator, streptokinase, or both on coronary-artery patency, ventricular function, and survival after acute myocardial infarction. N Engl J Med 1993;329:1615.

25

THROMBOLYTIC THERAPY FOR ACUTE STROKE

Gregory J. del Zoppo

Shirley M. Otis

The hypothesis that dissolving symptom-causing thrombi in the cerebrovasculature may lead to resolution of stroke symptoms is not new. Clarke and Cliffton[1] in 1960 and Meyer and colleagues[2] in the following year described resolution of documented carotid territory occlusions with clinical improvement in selected stroke patients. In the ensuing 20 years, the observation that athero-thrombotic and thromboembolic events may contribute to focal cerebral ischemia[3–17] and are responsible for 80% to 90% of ischemic strokes within 8 to 24 h of symptom onset[18] has provided a basis for the systematic evaluation of thrombolytic agents in the treatment of acute stroke.[19] Fletcher and colleagues[20] observed no benefit in 31 patients with completed carotid territory stroke, the majority of whom received urokinase (u-PA) > 24 h from symptom onset, and reported that symptomatic hemorrhagic transformation occurred in 7 (22.8%).[21] Because of the risk of intracerebral hemorrhage associated with fibrinolytic agents and this experience,[20,21] the use of fibrinolytic agents in patients suffering a stroke has generally been contraindicated. Nonetheless, more recent efforts to evaluate the safety and efficacy of thrombolytic substances in *acute* stroke have emphasized early intervention (within 6 to 8 h of symptom onset), prospective design, vascular diagnosis, dose response and safety profile assessment, and neurologic outcome.

Little is known about the vascular responses to ischemia and reperfusion in the central nervous system, in contrast to the broad experience in myocardial ischemia. This will explain the relative paucity of clinical experience with fibrinolytic agents to date. Moreover, concerns about whether fibrin thrombi protect the ischemia-injured cerebrovasculature in the peri-ischemic zones, whether fibrinolytic agents may extend petechial hemorrhage which is common to focal ischemia, the optimal dose rates for cerebrovascular recanalization, flow restrictions in obstructed vessels (e.g., internal carotid artery or middle cerebral artery branch), and the local endothelial responses to ischemia have yet to be clearly addressed.

In this chapter we will focus on aspects of the clinical natural history of stroke which are pertinent to the use of fibrinolytic agents, diagnostic techniques that may be used for real-time assessment of vascular status, and the results of recent studies in acute stroke and the safety of the use of fibrinolytic intervention agents.

THROMBOSIS AND SPONTANEOUS THROMBOLYSIS IN ISCHEMIC STROKE

Recent prospective angiographic studies have confirmed a temporal and anatomic relationship of cerebral arterial occlusions in patients who present acutely with symptoms consistent with stroke. When angiography has been performed at later intervals after the onset of the acute neurologic deficits, the frequency of corresponding occlusions was decreased. Analogous observations have been made by De Wood and colleagues[22] regarding the incidence of acute thrombotic occlusion of coronary arteries in individuals presenting with acute myocardial infarction (MI). In separate studies, a reduction was seen in the frequency of carotid territory occlusions from 81% at 5.7 h[18] and 76% at 6 h[23] to 59% at 24 h,[24] 57% at 3 days,[25] and 44% at 7 days.[26] Whether the angiographic procedure per se contributes to recanalization is not known. However, it would seem unlikely. Because this aggregate of series represents patency information, the true incidence of recanalization is not known, but if it is assumed that 100% of patients with symptoms presenting at 6 h have occlusions as the initial event, then the patency data noted above should approximate recanalization. A better approximation would derive from serial angiographic studies in the same patient(s) with sufficient interval to allow reperfusion to occur.

Dalal and colleagues[27] reported spontaneous recanalization of carotid territory thromboembolic arterial occlusions within 10 minutes to 18 days of the control angiogram in a prospective serial angiographic study of nine acute stroke patients. Initial angiograms were performed 2 to 9 days following the stroke. Instances of spontaneous arterial recanalization with distal fragmentation emboli have been noted, most often in the middle cerebral artery (MCA) region, and fortuitously, hemorrhagic conversion of an ischemic territory associated with the arterial recanaliza-

tion does occur[28,29] (Zeumer H, personal communication). The time course of such events is not known. Of interest, among 34 patients with MCA occlusion and acute focal ischemia symptoms followed by angiography ($n = 21$) or transcranial Doppler ultrasonography ($n = 13$), MCA recanalization occurred in 21 (62%) by 48 h,[30] suggesting an occlusion frequency of 38%. This evaluation is not strictly in accord with the aggregate data derived from angiographic studies noted above.[18,23–26] Nonetheless, this database suggests that the persistence of occlusions within the carotid territory, particularly MCA-related, is beyond that currently considered threshold for intervention by a recanalization strategy. Recently, Mori and Yoneda[31] have suggested a 16.7% incidence of MCA territory recanalization among patients not treated (control cohort) between approximately 3.2 and 4.2 h after the ictus.

In the cerebral vasculature, arterial occlusions derive from in situ thrombosis on subtending atheromata, from downstream embolization of atherothrombotic material from large arteries (artery-artery emboli), from thrombi arising from a cardiac site (cardiac-source emboli), or unusually, from intrinsic hemostatic abnormalities (e.g., antithrombin III deficiency, protein C deficiency) which may be associated with arterial thrombotic events.[10,32–34] Large-artery emboli from proximal in situ thrombi originate from atheromata found in the extracranial internal carotid artery (ICA), the carotid siphon, the MCA origin, the vertebral artery (VA) origins, the vertebrobasilar junction, and the posterior cerebral artery. ICA-to-MCA embolism from a completely obstructed proximal ICA accounts for the large number of focal ischemic events in which the proximal ICA is found to be occluded and the downstream bed is unable to be visualized.

NEUROLOGIC OUTCOME

The neurologic outcome of patients with MCA occlusions may be related to some extent to the neurologic status at ictus, with milder deficits likely to fare better than severe deficits.[17,34] Fieschi and coworkers[23] observed significant improvement in patients with carotid territory acute focal ischemia whose baseline scores were ≥6.5 according to the Canadian Neurological Scale (normal = 10.0).[17,33] The 3-month mortality of patients with MCA occlusion varies with occlusion location. Whereas proximal (M1 and M2) MCA occlusions had a rather poor prognosis (33.3% 3-month mortality), more distal occlusions (M3 segment or branch) fared better (14.3% 3-month outcome) in one study.[32] However, mortality or final neurologic status is generally a poor indicator of the anatomic location of the signal occlusion.[17,32] Although the neurologic deficits reflect occlusion location, the actual deficits do not invariably correlate.[27]

Concerning the vertebrobasilar territory, the clinical outcome of brainstem infarction and angiographically proven basilar artery occlusion is poor.[3–12,19] This decrease may present two outcome profiles: either (1) early mortality or severely disabled survivors or (2) minor or transient brainstem symptoms. An 86% mortality among 22 consecutive patients with vertebrobasilar ischemia treated with antithrombotic agents (antiplatelet agents or anticoagulants) was reported by Hacke and coworkers.[35] Here, angiographically documented lesions were rather evenly distributed among the superior basilar ("top"), midbasilar artery, caudal vertebral and basilar system, and mixed patterns. Generally, it would appear that the mortality of angiographically proven vertebrobasilar territory ischemia is high.

Because of the lack of a strict correlation between specific neurologic deficits and neurologic outcome and the relative paucity of prospective vascular-based information in acute focal cerebral ischemia, studies involving angiographic or noninvasive vascular imaging techniques have been undertaken. Although the use of such techniques may be time-consuming, the presence of a vascular occlusion and its relationship to the clinical presentation would be ensured. Alternatively, symptom-based studies have relied on changes in neurologic status documented by various scoring instruments without information about the vascular status. This latter approach has the advantage of economy of time but relies heavily on the premise that clinical outcome reflects a vascular

response. In both trial types, hemorrhagic transformation has been assayed identically by computed tomography (CT) or magnetic resonance imaging (MRI). It should be noted that in comparison with prospective trials of fibrinolytic agents in acute MI, the database of organized vascular information in acute stroke is meager, and clear correlations between vascular occlusion and ultimate neurologic status are not possible. Significant residual clinical disability is the more common outcome following focal cerebral ischemia than following acute MI.

VASCULAR IMAGING TECHNIQUES

Cerebral Angiography

Cerebral angiography remains the standard method for evaluating vascular lesions in both the extra- and intracranial arteries. The transfemoral approach using selective catheterization makes it possible to demonstrate all the supraaortic arteries via one puncture site. This method allows evaluation of the origin of the great vessels, the carotid bifurcations, and the intracranial vessels. Simultaneous two-plane depictions reduce the amount of contrast material. The use of intraarterial digital subtraction angiography (IADSA) further reduces the amount of contrast infusion. Although angiography reveals valuable vascular information and has a relatively low incidence of severe complications, they do occur. Local and minor complications occur in about 1% of cases, and more severe complications, including fatalities, occur in less than 0.5%. A recent experience with angiography in acute stroke had a complication incidence (minor) of 0.4%.[18]

Once the decision to perform angiography has been made, it should be tailored to the specific clinical question and the therapeutic possibilities so that maximal information is obtained and the patient is not exposed to increased risk. Cerebral angiography has been invaluable in evaluating acute stroke patients for thrombolytic intervention. Although a number of studies have now been reported utilizing angiography in acute stroke safely, it does delay initial thrombolytic treatment in these patients significantly.[36,37]

Noninvasive Vascular Imaging

Noninvasive vascular imaging is easily performed in the acute stages of stroke.[38] Up to 20% of the patients in one recent prospective study were excluded from thrombolytic therapy on the basis of the angiographic criteria,[18] suggesting an important role for noninvasive vascular studies that give immediate, accurate anatomic and flow information so that specific intervention would not be delayed.

The so-called duplex system combines high-resolution real-time B-mode ultrasonographic information with range-gaited pulse Doppler to provide simultaneous image and flow information. This system uses the physiologic information derived from Doppler to evaluate blood flow velocities and the two-dimensional image to visualize the walls of the vessels and evaluate plaque deposits. Typical abnormalities of flow are found in areas of stenosis of the common carotid artery, ICA, and external carotid artery (ECA).[39,40] In cerebral vascular recanalization studies, the emphasis is on recognition of thrombotic occlusion and restoration of flow. Absence of detectable Doppler shift signals is an indication of arterial occlusion. However, a Doppler shift signal may not be detected in very severe stenosis (where there is only a trickle of residual flow), possibly leading to misdiagnosis. Color Doppler has helped to alleviate some of these difficulties by presenting flow information across the entire field of use superimposed on the gray-scale image. The misdiagnosis of occlusion despite the improvement of color flow remains a fairly constant problem even for the experienced technologist.[41,42] Nevertheless, color Doppler imaging has increased the accuracy of noninvasive diagnosis of carotid occlusion and stenosis and is superior to conventional duplex systems in the diagnosis of all occlusions.[41–43] When compared with angiography, color-coded Doppler flow imaging has the advantage of better measurement of carotid stenoses and evaluation of plaque morphology which may be aided by the use of slow-flow analysis.[44]

Transcranial Doppler (TCD) is an extension of these techniques to the intracranial arteries. Using 2-MHz, pulse-wave Doppler ultrasound, blood flow is detectable in all major arteries at the base of the brain.[45–47] TCD may be used to rapidly screen the acute stroke patient for intracranial high-grade stenosis or complete occlusion. Criteria for stenosis and occlusion are similar for the intracranial and extracranial arteries. Mild stenoses of the basal intracranial arteries increase peak velocity with little change in the rest of the Doppler pattern, whereas moderate or severe stenoses lead to a greater increase in peak velocity, with spectral broadening, increased diastolic velocity, and turbulent flow. A poststenotic drop in peak velocity is usually seen. Occlusion of the basal cerebral arteries can be assessed by lack of the expected arterial signal despite the presence of normal echoes from the remaining arteries of the circle of Willis. A number of errors in interpretation can occur, particularly with displacement of arteries because of space-occupying lesions, misinterpretation of hyperdynamic collateral channels as stenoses, and misdiagnosis of vasospasm for stenosis. However, with experienced personnel and the present instrumentation, these errors are becoming less significant.[46,48]

Three-dimensional localization has improved some problems of vessel identification and documentation. Here, a multiprojection sample volume unit is used for a composite diagram of the intracranial vessels produced by plotting the Doppler sample volume location and storing it in the system.[49] Duplex imaging is currently being adapted to the intracranial vessels so that, hopefully, most of the disadvantages of vessel identification with the so-called blinded TCD may be alleviated. The primary advantages of combined intracranial imaging and Doppler flow in the setting of cerebrovascular thrombolysis are the recording and continuous monitoring of quick, immediate diagnosis of vascular events, e.g., recanalization, in real time to provide a measure of treatment efficacy.[50] Two recent studies have indicated the relative accuracy of TCD compared with angiography and the ability of repetitive TCD to study the natural history of MCA occlusions.[44,51]

Computed Tomographic Scanning

Exclusion of intracranial hemorrhage, a prerequisite for the institution of fibrinolytic treatments, is possible with either CT or MRI techniques.[52] Ischemic changes may be detected differentially depending on the time after stroke onset at which the examination is performed. Within the first 8 to 12 h, well-demarcated ischemic injury may not be detected by CT, whereas large infarcts and brain swelling may be detected early. True demarcation of the infarct region begins between 8 and 24 h. A relative definition of the size of the infarct and its location in a particular vascular territory is possible after 2 to 3 days.

Two early signs of ischemia can be seen on the initial CT scans: the presence of a hyperdense MCA sign and sulcal effacement with the loss of gray–white matter differentiation. A hyperdense MCA in a non-contrast-enhanced CT scan may reflect acute MCA embolism or thrombosis and may indicate impending cerebral infarction and possibly a poor prognosis. CT is superior to MRI in this very acute phase and allows a longitudinal look at the involved MCA. For basilar artery thrombosis or embolism, MRI is more reliable. Neither technique, however, can evaluate collateral blood supply, e.g., leptomeningeal anastomoses,[53,54] a potential contributor to outcome (see below).

Effacement of the sulci, low density, and loss of gray–white matter distinction, the second sign of early ischemia, occurs in a little under a third of acute strokes compared with the MCA sign, which occurs in approximately 27% of patients.[55] Wolpert[55] recently commented on the predictive value of entry CT to outcome and recanalization following fibrinolysis[18]: Evidence of "early ischemia" on the CT had no relationship to whether recanalization occurred. This contrasts with an earlier study of 10 patients by Okada and coworkers,[37] where early signs of ischemia had a direct relationship to recanalization. However, early ischemic changes did predict a larger infarct. The hyperdense MCA sign was marginally related to infarct size, but no relationship between early ischemia and hyperdense MCA with hemorrhagic transformation was apparent.[55] Previous studies have reported the hyperdense MCA sign to be the harbinger of a large infarct in the MCA distribution.[54,56] Angiography-based studies have revealed that recanalization of occluded arteries occurred more frequently with distal than with proximal occlusions[18,57] and that recanalized arteries were

associated with small rather than large infarcts, suggesting that smaller arterial occlusions are more likely to recanalize or that smaller infarcts may result from recanalized arteries because more neuronal tissue is preserved.[18,55]

In summary, early CT evaluation of stroke patients has the advantage of being quick and decisive in ruling out evidence of hemorrhage and may have some predictive value, in that early signs of ischemia in the presence of hyperdense MCA on CT are associated with relatively large infarcts and that distal occluded arteries are more frequently recanalized than proximal. CT, however, is inferior when compared with MRI in the basilar system, but like MRI, CT is not able to demonstrate the presence of collateral arterial supply.

Magnetic Resonance Imaging

MRI is of proven value in the diagnosis of brain, spinal cord, and brainstem abnormalities. It is particularly sensitive to tumors and areas of demyelinization. The use of MRI in cerebral vascular disease is evolving. MRI may visualize ischemic changes during stroke somewhat earlier than CT.[58–61] Some of the earlier problems of distinguishing intracerebral hemorrhage from ischemia and infarct in the acute stage have been solved by gradient-echo imaging technique. MRI, however, is sensitive to tiny parenchymal hemorrhages that are invisible on CT. This limitation may pose some difficulties with current thrombolytic protocols which exclude patients with any evidence of hemorrhagic infarction.[62] The use of MRI in the acute stroke patient is still limited for the practical reason that many hospitals do not have this capability.

One modality with distinct advantages over CT scanning is MRI with MR angiography (MRA). Newer MRI scanning sequences can be accomplished in less than 30 minutes; a typical spin-echo sequence takes 15 minutes, and each MRA in the field of interest may be accomplished in less than 10 minutes. The typical bright enhancing signals of ischemic injury on T_2-weighted MRI images do not occur until approximately 8 h after stroke onset. However, other MRI phenomena are recognized earlier: absence of flow void in the vessels of interest, vessel enhancement with gadolinium, and edema.[63] With MRA, the effects of moving protons are visualized with gradient-echo sequences and three-dimensional data acquisition to demonstrate intravascular flow.[61] The technique is currently limited by a number of artifacts. With turbulent flow (which increases signal intensity), overestimation of stenosis can occur, and with slow flow, a stenosis may be missed. Also, areas of hyperintense signal associated with acute thrombosis may be misidentified as intravascular flow. With improved technology, some of these artifacts will be eliminated, and specialized sequences may be able to demonstrate collateral flow in the leptomeningeal arteries. Currently, MRA techniques add vascular flow information to the accompanying MRI anatomic information by utilizing a three-dimensional time of flight (3D TOF) process requiring less than 10 minutes for completion.[64–66]

Additionally, MR diffusion (MRD) and perfusion (MRP) techniques provide refined information about cerebral tissue. Special coil gradients in MRD are used to image very early tissue changes and may demonstrate cytotoxic edema occurring within 1 h of vascular occlusion.[63] Analysis of regional cerebral blood flow (rCBF) and flow metabolism coupling may be possible by MRP.[67]

One recent study found neither CT nor MRI superior in the early detection of ischemia.[52] Furlan[68] has suggested that despite the value and precision of angiographic data, they are impractical if intravenous thrombolytic therapy is ever to be widely applicable in the early acute stroke phase. Contrarily, nonangiographic studies are less precise and limit interpretation of clinical outcome data. A possible solution to this dilemma would be to have reliable noninvasive technology available to provide vascular anatomic information, flow data, and tissue-viability data that could be performed rapidly within the time frame of acute stroke.[68] Despite the differences of opinion regarding the need for angiography, there is general agreement that some form of imaging modality is necessary before any thrombolytic agent is given, mainly to rule out intracranial hemorrhage.

Single-Photon-Emission Computed Tomography (SPECT)

SPECT imaging provides information on tissue perfusion that allows evaluation of the disturbed metabolic processes that may occur in acute stroke.[69] [99m]Tc HMPAO is a lipophilic CBF tracer that crosses the blood-brain barrier, is then converted into a hydrophilic form, and is retained for some hours in a distribution pattern proportional to the regional CBF. This allows imaging with a rotating gamma camera. Imaging produced by CT and MRI rely on changes in the anatomy which may occur early in the acute stroke, while SPECT documents the changes in blood flow and metabolism that are present from the onset.[70] The advantage of SPECT in evaluating rCBF in acute cerebral ischemia is that there is no delay in the thrombolytic intervention, because ^{99m}Tc HMPAO is injected before the thrombolytic agent, and the time-consuming scanning can be performed later. Also, the rCBF measured by this technique provides a measure of regional tissue reperfusion that might occur with recanalization not possible by angiography. SPECT may be able to determine viable, though dysfunctional tissue, in the infarcted area.[70]

INTRACEREBRAL HEMORRHAGE AND HEMORRHAGIC TRANSFORMATION

Symptomatic intracerebral hemorrhage (ICH) is a known risk of the use of fibrinolytic agents in a number of clinical situations. For instance, among prospective studies of fibrinolytic agents (including SK, APSAC, u-PA, rt-PA, and rscu-PA) in acute MI, a rather constant 0% to 1.3% incidence of symptomatic intracerebral hemorrhage has been reported which appears independent of the specific fibrinolytic agent.[71] ICH occurred in 0.18% of patients treated with streptokinase (SK), 0.34% with anisoylated plasminogen–streptokinase activator complex (APSAC), and 0.46% with recombinant tissue-type plasminogen activator (rt-PA), compared with an ICH incidence of 0.02% among untreated or control acute MI patients.[71] The pathogenesis of ICH accompanying acute MI and other vascular disorders is often unclear because prospective CT or MRI investigations have not been routine. While an element of cerebral ischemia or cerebral embolism may underlie such hemorrhagic events, this is often uncertain; however, the rather constant incidence of symptomatic ICH in such patients implies a common pathology, which may be different from that which accompanies acute stroke.

Hemorrhagic transformation comprises hemorrhagic infarction (HI) or parenchymatous hematoma (PI) and is a common consequence of focal cerebral ischemia following atherothrombotic or thromboembolic stroke. HI refers to petechial or confluent petechial hemorrhage in the region of ischemic injury, whereas PH refers to a homogeneous discrete mass of blood that may exert a mass effect (with shift of midline structures) or extend to the ventricle. HI has been documented in less than 10% to 43% of nonanticoagulated cerebral infarction patients in prospective CT scan–based studies.[72–74] Yamaguchi and coworkers[75] have indicated that HI most commonly accompanies cardiac-source emboli. Following carotid territory embolic stroke, hemorrhagic transformation was observed in 46.4% of 140 patients, including 16 (11.4%) with PH.[76] This finding compares with 43.1% of 65 acute stroke patients, of whom 13.8% had PH, in a separate study.[77] PH, which is most often symptomatic, is uncommonly associated with cerebral embolism,[78,79] except in the setting of anticoagulant treatment.[80–82]

The long-standing concept that hemorrhagic transformation (HT) may result from arterial reperfusion is not supported by recent angiographic studies,[18,83–85] although this concept would seem intuitively correct. The finding of hemorrhagic transformation with persistent occlusion of the primary artery by Ogata and coworkers[86] has suggested that hemorrhage may occur from other vascular sources (e.g., collateral channels).[87,88] As will be seen, the time from the occlusive event to recanalization or fibrinolytic agent exposure is relevant to the incidence and perhaps severity of HT. Additionally, hypertension may contribute to the severity of HT.

From literature sources combining reports of prospective trials, the presumed incidence of symptomatic HT is approximately 10%. Well-designed prospectively, controlled trials of fibrinolytic agents in acute stroke will refine this figure.

ANIMAL MODELS OF CEREBRAL ISCHEMIA

A discussion of the nuances and vagaries of the various animal models of cerebral ischemia is beyond the scope of this chapter; however, some features of cerebral ischemia/fibrinolysis have been modeled which are relevant to clinical work. Historically, clinical studies of fibrinolytic agents have not always been preceded by discovery work in animal model systems. It is well recognized that the animal model systems employed to study problems of cerebral ischemia have specific limitations which derive as much from a poor understanding of the pathogenesis of stroke as from anatomic and practical considerations in a given species. Only a few aspects of the problems related to fibrinolysis have been modeled.[89,90] In principle, no model, by its design, has been able to examine more than two aspects of the problems raised by the use of fibrinolytic agents in this setting, e.g., infarction size and hemorrhage, neurologic size and dose rate, recanalization and hemorrhage. Insights from cerebral ischemia models in this setting have been recently summarized.[91]

Models used to explore the effect(s) of thrombolytic agents in focal cerebral ischemia have used procedures that achieve occlusion of one or more cerebral arteries by thrombosis, thromboembolism, or mechanical means to generate focal or multifocal ischemia. Small cohort sizes have limited the significance of results presented on statistically proven considerations. Few studies have simultaneously correlated intracerebral hemorrhage or hemorrhagic transformation and clinical outcome with arterial recanalization at a particular dose rate of the fibrinolytic agent studied,[91,92] and no preparation has allowed simultaneous visualization of the effects of thrombolysis (reperfusion) and neurologic outcome.

Recanalization

In a rabbit model of autologous thromboembolism, early infusion of rt-PA resulted in rapid angiographic reperfusion.[93] Other model studies have indicated that documented early cerebral arterial recanalization with rt-PA is associated with a rise in rCBF.[93–96] A reduction in the size of infarction has been suggested by local intracarotid infusion of u-PA in a nonhuman primate model,[97] and reduction in ischemia-related vascular permeability accompanied early reperfusion of in situ MCA thrombosis in a canine model.[98–100]

Clinical Outcome

Correlation between cerebral arterial reperfusion and clinical outcome has been sought in a variety of experimental preparations.[93,101,102] Recent studies with rt-PA in rodent and rabbit thromboembolic models have indicated improvement of power spectra when flow was improved[93] or a reduction in mortality (ED_{50})[101] and improvement in clinical outcome (ES_{50}).[102] In both sets of studies, the agent was given very early. Improvement in motor-weighted score was indicated following u-PA infusion in a nonhuman primate model.[97]

Hemorrhagic Transformation

This most important safety feature of thrombolysis in the central nervous system has been the subject of a number of studies of defined MCA ischemia and thromboembolism[93,102] in the rabbit[103] and of MCA ischemia in the nonhuman primate.[104] In the latter, no increase in the incidence of infarction-related petechial hemorrhage was observed following MCA occlusion and post-reperfusion rt-PA infusion (intravenous) at three dose rates.[104] Relatively early reperfusion in the presence of thrombolytic agents (in this case rt-PA) is not associated with an increase in intracerebral hemorrhage over untreated controls.

The limited experience with the several model systems described indicates that at the dose rates and with the infusion formats chosen, improvement in clinical status/mortality can be achieved following infusion with thrombus-directed fibrinolytic agents. Where the incidence of intracerebral hemorrhage was assessed in later studies of deep cortical (corpus striatal) infarction and in one early autologous thrombus model, there appeared to be no difference between control and treated animals.

THROMBOLYSIS IN ACUTE ISCHEMIC STROKE

Organized clinical experience with fibrinolytic agents in stroke patients has involved either intravenous systemic delivery or intraarterial local delivery of the agent. Among trials involving intravenous administration, the angiographically controlled format has been used for the study of streptokinase, u-PA, Thrombolysin®, and rt-PA (either alteplase or duteplase), while symptom-based trials have examined Fibrinolysin®, u-PA, and rt-PA (alteplase or duteplase). Intraarterial delivery necessitates angiographic control. In addition to anecdotes about Fibrinolysin® and plasmin, direct intraarterial infusion studies in the carotid and vertebrobasilar territories have delivered streptokinase, u-PA, or rt-PA. To date, the superiority of either approach over the other has not been shown, and the efficacy of each approach, in terms of recanalization incidence or neurologic outcome, is under scrutiny. In addition to formal phase I/II clinical studies, more recent animal model work has been undertaken to elucidate some of the factors that may be important in optimizing outcome.

CLINICAL EXPERIENCE WITH THROMBOLYTIC THERAPY IN ACUTE STROKE

Clinical experience with fibrinolytic agents (plasmin and fibrinolysin) prior to 1970 indicated successful recanalization[1] or suggested clinical improvement in certain settings.[1,105] While symptomatic HT was infrequent in several small studies,[105] it complicated others.[106] Clarke and Cliffton,[1] in a single institutional angiography-based experience, reported improvement in 5 of 7 patients (71.4%) treated with intravenous fibrinolysin in carotid territory occlusion. No central nervous system hemorrhage was described. Despite this salutary outcome, subsequent studies have, in retrospect, pointed out a number of weaknesses of those early approaches.[107] In addition to delays in treatment in the majority of patients (up to 7 days), clearly exceeding the comparatively narrow window of treatment currently considered necessary, both pretreatment and posttreatment angiography was not performed in all patients, a considerable number of patients without occlusion were included, and the interval between angiographic studies was too long to link the vascular outcome to the agent. A potentially significant limitation was that in this period before the development of CT scans and MRI, it was nearly impossible to exclude the contribution of intracerebral hemorrhage a priori. Contemporary assessment of one study concluded that although reperfusion could be achieved, there was a "significant" risk of cerebral hemorrhage associated with the therapy.[106]

In a later symptom-based clinical outcome study, Fletcher and colleagues[20] observed no benefit in 31 patients when urokinase was applied intravenously within 36 h (over 10 to 12 h) of the onset of symptoms for *completed* stroke. Intracerebral hemorrhage, which occurred in 22.6% of the treated patients, was associated with a history of definite antecedent focal neurologic deficits ($n = 2$), hypertension ($n = 2$), and atrial fibrillation and congestive heart failure ($n = 1$).[21] This experience was taken as additional evidence that the use of fibrinolytic agents (systemically) in stroke is of little benefit and may produce cerebral hemorrhage. Abe and colleagues, in two subsequent studies,[108,109] observed a lower incidence of hemorrhage and no apparent clinical benefit. Given this experience and the notion derived from prospective angiographic studies of carotid territory stroke patients that cerebral arterial occlusions underlie early territorial ischemia, a number of conditions have been imposed on recent prospective trials of fibrin(ogen)olysis in stroke. To be potentially beneficial, thrombolytic agents must be applied in the acute phase of

stroke, within 6 to 8 h of symptom onset. Infusion duration has varied but is intended to be short, from 1 to 3 h, to limit exposure of ischemic tissue to the agent. CT scan or MRI exclusion of hemorrhage within the cerebral tissue at risk is required for all patients. Other criteria derive from accepted restrictions on the use of these agents in various settings and are summarized elsewhere.[18,110,111]

Angiographically Controlled Studies

Intraarterial (Local) Infusion

Intraarterial infusions are either (1) local, employing interventional neuroradiologic techniques, or (2) regional, using diagnostic angiography catheters for territorial delivery of the agent. With regional infusion, whereby the agent may be infused in the extracranial portion of the ICA, for instance, much of the agent may be diverted to other arteries along the flowstream (e.g., ophthalmic artery or branch arteries) and away from the occlusion. Penetration of the agent into the stagnant blood column proximal to a thrombotic occlusion requires flow. Presentation of the agent at the proximal face of the occlusion via a superselective catheter constitutes local infusion and addresses this limitation of regional and systemic infusion. Zeumer and colleagues[112] have pioneered the use of flow- and guidewire-directed catheter techniques for delivery of thrombolytic agents in the cerebral (including ophthalmic) circulation. Regional and local intraarterial infusions of SK, u-PA, and rt-PA (alteplase) for angiographically demonstrable acute thrombotic carotid and vertebrobasilar artery occlusions have been reported.

In the carotid territory (Table 25-1), del Zoppo and colleagues[83] reported complete/partial recanalization in 18 of 20 patients with carotid territory thrombotic stroke with extended local intraarterial/regional infusion of u-PA or SK within 1 to 4 h of symptom onset. Eleven patients exhibited near-complete or partial clinical recovery, and no patient recovered in the absence of arterial recanalization. Hemorrhagic infarction (in the corpus striatum) was seen in 4 patients (20%), was independent of recanalization, and

TABLE 25-1. Carotid Territory: Intraarterial Delivery, Angiography-Controlled Studies

	Agent	n	Treatment		Infusion	Recanalization	
			Δ(T - 0) (h)	Duration (h)		n	%
Miyakawa (115)	P	3	—	—	R	3	100.0
del Zoppo (83)	SK/u-PA	20	1–24	1.0–4.0	I/R	18	90.0
del Zoppo/Zeumer (116)	rt-PA	3	1–24	1.0	I	2	66.7
Mori (84)	u-PA	22	0.8–7	0.2–0.5	R	10	45.5
Theron (113)	SK/u-PA	12	2–504	<1.0	I/R	12	100.0
Matsumoto (114)	u-PA	40	1–24	0.2–0.5	R	24	60.0

Legends: *Agents:* SK = streptokinase; u-PA = urokinase plasminogen activator; rt-PA = recombinant tissue plasminogen activator; C = control (placebo); *treatment:* Δ(T - 0) = interval from onset to treatment; Duration = duration of treatment; *Infusion (intraarterial):* I = interventional; R = regional; *Recanalization:* n_R = number of patients recanalized; % = percent of total number of patients who demonstrated recanalization; *Hemorrhage:* HI = hemorrhagic infarction; PH = parenchymatous hemorrhage; % = percent of total number of patients who demonstrated hemorrhagic transformation.

subsequently resolved in all patients. A parallel experience reported by Mori and coworkers[84] employing regional delivery of u-PA in 22 patients confirmed those findings, with a 45.5% incidence of recanalization and an 18.2% incidence of hemorrhagic transformation. Recently, Theron[113] and Matsumoto and Satoh[114] have extended those observations. Among the 4 uncontrolled, prospective series of u-PA or SK regional/local delivery, 84 of 94 patients (89.2%) underwent recanalization.[83,84,113,114] In his series, Mori et al.[84] noted a clear inverse relationship between the degree of recanalization and infarction size and a relative inability of proximal ICA occlusions to undergo recanalization. These observations with regional delivery have portended outcomes seen in later angiography-based systemic infusion studies.[18] Also, in 1984, Miyakawa and coworkers[115] reported successful recanalization in each of 3 patients with regional infusion of plasmin, an approach that may be of future value for patients with refractory thrombi. Finally, a limited experience with intraarterial melanoma-derived t-PA in carotid territory occlusion, which had a mixed outcome,[116] and 2 cases of intraarterial rt-PA (alteplase) infusion have appeared so far.[117,118]

In the vertebrobasilar territory (Table 25-2), Hacke and coworkers[35] compared the outcome of 22 patients with acute cerebellar and/or brainstem-related ischemia and angiographically demonstrated vertebrobasilar thrombotic occlusion who received "conventional" antithrombotic therapy with 43 individuals who received u-PA by local infusion.[119,120] Of the 43 patients, 19 achieved complete recanalization, and 14 of the 19 (73.7%) survived, while all 24 patients who did not achieve recanalization expired. These outcomes were significantly different from those of the "conventional" group. In the UK-treated cohort, 4 patients treated later than 6 h after acute symptom onset developed HI or PH, in 2 of whom large brainstem hemorrhages probably contributed to demise. HI was independent of recanalization status. Prior to this experience, Nenci and colleagues[121] demonstrated recanalization in 4 patients with acute vertebrobasilar thrombosis after local u-PA infusion.

The experience reported to date with intraarterial regional or local delivery of thrombolytic agents has been simplified by flexible guidewire-directed catheter systems, although these still represent interventional neuroradiologic approaches. For this reason, the need for interventional neuroradiologic expertise, as well as the need for early intervention and careful patient selection, has limited the widespread use of the local intraarterial approach. To theoretically reduce the risk of hemorrhage associated with u-PA and SK therapy, short-term infusions (1 to 2 h) at relatively high doses (100 to 250 × 10³ IU) have been employed in many patients, although the optimal dose rates of these agents have not been

TABLE 25-2. *Vertebrobasilar Territory: Intraarterial Delivery, Angiography-Controlled Studies*

	Agent	n	Treatment		Infusion	Recanalization	
			$\Delta(T - 0)$ (h)	Duration (h)		n	%
Nenci (121)	SK/u-PA	4	6–96	0.3–10–44	R	4	100.0
Hacke (35)	SK/u-PA	43	<24	<4/12–48	I	19	44.2
Zeumer (143)	u-PA	7	4–48	2	I	7	100.0
Mobius (144)	SK/u-PA	18	0.5–2.0	2	I	14	77.8
Matsumoto (114)	u-PA	10	3–24	0.2–0.7	R	4	40.0
Henze (117)	rt-PA	1	2.5	1.5	R	1	100.0
Buteux (118)	rt-PA	1	—	4	I	1	100.0

Note: See Table 25-1 for key to abbreviations.

worked out. It should be noted that a properly designed, prospective, controlled trial is yet to be undertaken to assess clinical outcome.

Intravenous (Systemic) Infusion

To evaluate the efficacy of intravenous infusion of thrombolytic agents on recanalization and on clinical outcome, angiographically controlled protocols have been employed. Because of the original theoretical attractiveness of the thrombus-selective agents rt-PA and scu-PA in acute cerebrovascular thrombosis, angiography-based trials of this type have been undertaken successfully and reported recently[18,111,122,123] (Table 25-3). Although the dose rates were limited and a single rt-PA (alteplase or duteplase) was used in three studies, at least partial recanalization was achieved in 34.4% to 59.1% of treated patients.[18,111,122,123] Under similar conditions, these

frequencies compare with 16.7% recanalization in 12 control patients from the prospective, placebo-controlled study of rt-PA (duteplase) in acute MCA stroke.[111] In one prospective, open, multicenter, dose-rate finding study, recanalization of ICA occlusions was infrequent at the rt-PA dose rates employed, occurring in 8% of ICA patients.[18] Here MCA division and branch occlusions displayed recanalization more frequently than ICA occlusions at the end of the rt-PA infusion period.[18]

One placebo-controlled, prospective, angiography-based study of intravenous rt-PA infusion and clinical outcome has been reported at this writing.[111] Patients receiving 30 million IU of duteplase demonstrated a better clinical improvement than those who received 20 million IU and significantly better than placebo. Patients undergoing recanalization had a better outcome than

TABLE 25-3. *Carotid Territory Occlusion: Angiography-Controlled Studies, Intravenous Infusion*

	Agent	n	Treatment		Angiography			Recanalization	
			$\Delta(T - 0)$ (h)	Duration (h)	Pre	Interval (min)	Post	n_R	%
del Zoppo (18)	rt-PA	93	<8	1.0	93	60	93	32	34.4
Mori (111)	rt-PA	19	<6	1.0	19	60	29	9	47.4
	C	12			12		12	2	16.7
Yamaguchi (137)	rt-PA	47	<6	1.0	47	60	47	10	21.3
	C	46			46		46	2	4.4
von Kummer (123)	rt-PA	22	<6	1.5	22	90	21	13	59.1

Note: See Table 25-1 for key to abbreviations.

nonrecanalized patients.[111] PH occurred equally across all treatment groups and was not related to recanalization.

von Kummer and Hacke[123] have summarized an experience with a single dose of rt-PA (alteplase). Neurologic improvement was apparently related to the presence of identifiable collateral channels. At this time, there is no extensive reported experience of systemic infusion thrombolysis with vertebrobasilar ischemia.

Symptom-Based (Clinical Outcome) Studies

Two groups of studies of thrombolytic agents with clinical outcome measures only have been undertaken: those with very low doses which were unlikely to produce thrombus lysis and those (more recent) studies with doses more likely to have a thrombus lytic effect (Table 25-4).

Among the first group are several non-angiographic systemic infusion studies using u-PA[108,109,124,125] or rt-PA (duteplase)[126,127] conducted in Japan. Two studies demonstrated equivocal clinical benefits of the treatment.[108,109,125] Clinical outcomes could not be linked to vascular reperfusion because of the very low u-PA dose rates used and the unusually long $\Delta(T - 0)$ (>3 days). Koudstaal and colleagues[128] described two

patients with fatal outcome following intravenous rt-PA (alteplase) in whom reperfusion injury was suspected but not proven.

In two parallel studies, Brott and associates have examined the clinical effect of systemic infusion rt-PA (alteplase) on neurologic outcome within 90 minutes[129] and in the interval 91 to 180 minutes[130] of focal cerebral ischemic symptoms. Thirty-four of 74 patients (45.9%) had apparent clinical improvement within 24 h of rt-PA (alteplase) treatment in relation to a neurologic outcome, but no relationship to dose was observed. The persistence of neurologic improvement was not discussed. Symptomatic intracerebral hematomas occurred in 3 of the 74 patients (4.1%).[129] Despite the intensiveness of this study, the precise nature and number of vascular events and the contributions of spontaneous recanalization remain unknown. However, the feasibility of very early intervention after focal symptom onset has clearly been shown by this study. A separate open dose-escalation study examined 20 patients who received rt-PA (alteplase) within 91 to 180 minutes of symptom onset, 3 of whom displayed improvement by 24 h.[130]

At this writing, several prospective, blinded, placebo-controlled trials are being undertaken to evaluate the effect of fibrinolysis on clinical outcome of acute stroke. These include the Aus-

TABLE 25-4. *Clinical Outcome Studies: Intravenous Delivery*

			Treatment		
	Agent	*n*	$\Delta(T - 0)$ (h)	Duration (h)	Clinical Improvement (%)
Abe (108)	u-PA	57	<720	168	70.4
	C	56			47.2
Atarashi (124)	u-PA	191	<120	168	45.0
	C	94			43.6
Otomo (125)	u-PA	176	<120	168	51.8
	C	188			41.0
Koudstaal (128)	rt-PA	2	<4	3	0.0
Otomo (126)	rt-PA	171	<120	168	59.3
	u-PA	184			54.7
Abe (127)	rt-PA	145	<72	168	66.2
	u-PA	77			44.7
Brott (129)	rt-PA	74	<1.5	1	39.0

Note: See Table 25-1 for key to abbreviations.

tralian Streptokinase Study (ASK), MAST and MAST-Italy, and the European Cooperative Acute Stroke Study (rt-PA, alteplase) or ECASS.

HEMORRHAGIC TRANSFORMATION AND THROMBOLYSIS

All thrombolytic agents carry the risk of intracranial hemorrhage.[107,131] The possibility that exposure of the focal cerebral ischemic zone to a thrombolytic agent may increase the size or severity of naturally occurring hemorrhagic transformation is the central safety issue. The actual mechanism(s) of such hemorrhages may not be different from that of hemorrhagic transformation under visual circumstances, although it has been suggested that "lysis of hemostatic plugs" may contribute.[132,133] This hypothesis, however, has not been tested.

Early studies have suggested a significant incidence of symptomatic intracranial hemorrhage and demise,[1,20,21,81,108,109,134–136] although limitations of these studies also have suggested caution in interpretation of this result.[107] The more recent angiography- and CT scan-based acute thrombol-

ysis studies have further defined the incidence of hemorrhagic transformation. In the carotid territory, the incidence of parenchymatous hematoma formation among four intraarterial u-PA or SK trials was 10.6%,[83,84,113,114] compared with 9.5% from four prospective, angiography-based trials of intravenous infusion rt-PA (duteplase or alteplase)[18,110,111,137] with similar entry criteria (Table 25-5). The respective aggregate mean frequencies of arterial recanalization were 68.1% and 35.4%. Among three intraarterial infusion trials, recanalization occurred in 5 of 9 patients with PH, and clinical deterioration was noted in 8 of the 9 patients.[83,84,113]

In a nonangiographic systemic rt-PA (alteplase) infusion study, 3 symptomatic hemorrhages (all PHs) (4.1%) were documented by CT scan among 74 patients treated.[129] Here, the symptomatic episodes seemed to be related to the higher rt-PA doses, although there was no difference in incidence from that observed in the one angiography-based rt-PA dose-escalation study[18] or two placebo-controlled trials[111,137] reported thus far. From these sources,[18,111] it has been apparent that (1) there was no relationship between intracerebral hemorrhage and recanalization,

TABLE 25-5. Hemorrhagic Transformation

| | | | | | | Hemorrhagic Transformation | | | | |
| | | | | | | | Type | | Deterioration | |
	Territory	Agent	n	$\Delta(T - 0)$ (h)	Angiography	Nil	HI	PH	n_D	%
Intraarterial u-PA, streptokinase										
del Zoppo (83)	Carotid	u-PA	20	7.6	+	16	4	0	0	0.0
Mori (84)	Carotid	u-PA	22	4.5	+	18	1	3	3*	13.3
Theron (113)	Carotid	u-PA/SK	12	<10	+	9	0	3	2*	16.6
Hacke (35)	VBA	u-PA/SK	43	<24	+	39	2	2	2*	4.7
Intravenous rt-PA										
del Zoppo (18)	Carotid	rt-PA(d)[†]	104	<8	+	72	21	11	10	9.6
Mori (111)	Carotid	rt-PA(d)[†]	19	<6	+	9	8	2	2	10.5
		C	12			7	4	1	1	8.5
von Kummer (123)	Carotid	rt-PA(a)[†]	27	<6	+	19	6	2	3	11.1
Yamaguchi (137)	Carotid	rt-PA(d)[†]	51	<6	+	23	20	4	4	7.8
		C[‡]	47			24	17	5	5	10.6
Brott (129)		rt-PA(a)[†]	74	<1.5	−	68	3	3	3	4.1

*Deterioration associated with PH.
[†] a = alteplase; d = duteplase.
[‡] C = control.

(2) PH and HI were not associated with prior antiplatelet therapy, (3) the incidence of hemorrhagic transformation increased significantly with time to treatment, particularly when rt-PA (duteplase) was initiated later than 6 h from symptom onset, (4) no difference in the incidence of symptomatic hemorrhage between rt-PA (duteplase) at two dose rates and placebo[111] or among nine dose rates[18] was observed, (5) there was no relationship between the volume of infarction and the severity of hemorrhage, and (6) the majority of ICH occurred within the ischemic territory. This does not imply that in acute focal cerebral ischemia the incidence of hemorrhagic transformation is independent of rt-PA dose above those studied. It is indeed quite possible, as observed in certain individual cases,[18] that the timing and volume of hemorrhage were different from those observed in untreated patients.

Nonetheless, acute intervention trials reported to date with similar entry criteria have suggested a rather constant incidence of hemorrhage with associated clinical deterioration that is not substantially different from literature sources.[138]

The contribution of previous hypertensive disease or acute hypertension, associated anticoagulant use, or other antithrombotics remains to be determined.

Summary

Results of the intravenous infusion studies and of the recent local infusion clinical studies and the design of prospective studies with newer agents have accentuated a number of factors that may affect the relative efficacy and safety of these approaches in acute stroke.

1. Recanalization of symptomatic carotid territory arterial occlusions within 4 to 6 h of symptom onset is feasible. Entry of patients with focal cerebral ischemia into prospective clinical trials within 1 to 5 h of symptom onset is feasible. In the vertebrobasilar territory, precise timing of symptom onset may be particularly difficult.[139]

2. Given these limits, local thrombolytic therapy may preserve tissue only within the "ischemic penumbra." In a given patient, this is related to the variability of collateral flow,[140] the location of cerebral arterial thrombotic occlusions, and the presence and extent of arteriosclerotic cerebrovascular disease.

3. A relationship between embolus location and recanalization efficacy may exist.[141,142] Occlusions of the cervical portion of the ICA by atheroma-based in situ thrombosis appear more resistant to systemic thrombolysis than cardiogenic or artery-to-artery emboli of the intracranial portion of the ICA or of the stem and major branches of the MCA.

4. Early partial or complete recanalization of symptomatic cerebral arteries correlates with a significant reduction in residual infarction volume by CT scan.

5. The incidence of cerebral arterial recanalization is apparently greater when thrombolytic agents are delivered by direct intraarterial infusion than by systemic infusion.

6. To date, the incidence of symptomatic hemorrhagic transformation following intraarterial or intravenous fibrinolysis appears to be quite similar to that suggested by literature sources for natural history at dose rates recently studied.

Certainly, long-term, prospective, placebo-controlled studies will be important to evaluate the clinical efficacy of these approaches in acute cerebral ischemia. The relationship of the best timing of intervention, the location of the occlusion, and the optimal dose rate to neurologic outcome will be important variables to the success of this as yet experimental approach.

Acknowledgment

This work was supported in part by Grant NS 26945 of the National Institutes of Health and the Roon Foundation.

References

1. Clarke RL, Cliffton EE. The treatment of cerebrovascular thrombosis and embolism with fibrinolytic agents. Am J Cardiol 1960;30:546.

2. Meyer JS, Herndon RM, Gotoh F, et al. Therapeutic thrombolysis. In: Millikan CH, Siekert RG, Whisnant JP, eds. Cerebral vascular diseases, third Princeton conference. New York: Grune & Stratton, 1961:160.

3. Denny-Brown D. Recurrent cerebrovascular episodes. Arch Neurol 1960;2:194.

4. Russell RWR. Observations on the retinal blood vessels in monocular blindness. Lancet 1961;2:1422.

5. Marshall J. The management of cerebrovascular diseases. Oxford: Blackwell Scientific Publications, 1976:57.

6. Ross RT. Transient mononuclear blindness. J Can Sci Neurol 1977;4:143.

7. Marshall J, Meadows S. The natural history of amaurosis fugax. Brain 1958;41:419.

8. Russell RWR. Atheromatous retinal embolism. Lancet 1963;2:1354.

9. Hollenhorst RW. Vascular status of patients who have cholesterol emboli in the retina. Am J Ophthalmol 1966;77:1159.

10. Barnett HJM. The pathophysiology of transient cerebral ischemic attacks: therapy with platelet antiaggregants. Med Clin North Am 1979;63:649.

11. Davis-Jones GAB, Preston FE, Temperly WR. Neurological complications in clinical hematology. Oxford: Blackwell Scientific Publications, 1980:176.

12. Croft RJ, Ellam LD, Harrison MJG. Accuracy of carotid angiography in the assessment of atheroma of the internal carotid artery. Lancet 1980;1:997.

13. Mohr JP, Caplan LR, Melski JW, et al. The Harvard Cooperative Stroke Registry: a prospective registry of patients hospitalized with stroke. Neurology 1978;28:754.

14. Aring CD, Merritt HH. Differential diagnosis between cerebral hemorrhage and cerebral thrombosis. Arch Intern Med 1935;56:435.

15. Whisnant JP, Fitzgibbons JP, Kurland LT. Natural history of stroke in Rochester, Minnesota, 1945 through 1954. Stroke 1971;2:11.

16. Matsumoto N, Whisnant JP, Kurland LT. Natural history of stroke in Rochester, Minnesota, 1955 through 1969: an extension of previous study, 1945 through 1954. Stroke 1973;4:20.

17. Kannel WB, Dawber TR, Cohen MS. Vascular disease of the brain—epidemiologic aspects: the Framingham Study. Am J Public Health 1973;63:52.

18. del Zoppo GJ, Poeck K, Pessin MS, 16 co-authors of the rt-PA Acute Stroke Study Group. Recombinant tissue plasminogen activator in acute thrombotic and embolic stroke. Ann Neurol 1992;32:78.

19. Solis OJ, Roberson GR, Taveras JM, et al. Cerebral angiography in acute cerebral infarction. Revist Interam Radiol 1977;2:19.

20. Fletcher AP, Alkjaersig N, Lewis M, et al. A pilot study of urokinase therapy in cerebral infarction. Stroke 1976;7:135.

21. Hanaway J, Torack R, Fletcher AP, Landau WM. Intracranial bleeding associated with urokinase therapy for acute ischemic hemispheral stroke. Stroke 1976;7:143.

22. DeWood MA, Spores J, Notske R, et al. Prevalence of coronary occlusion during the early hours of transmural myocardial infarction. N Engl J Med 1980;303:897.

23. Fieschi C, Argentino C, Lenzi GL, et al. Clinical and instrumental evaluation of patients with ischemic stroke within the first six hours. J Neurol Sci 1989;91:311.

24. Solis OJ, Roberson GR, Taveras JM, et al. Cerebral angiography in acute cerebral infarction. Revist Interam Radiol 1977;2:19.

25. Fieschi C, Bozzao L. Transient embolic occlusion of the middle cerebral and internal carotid arteries in cerebral apoplexy. J Neurol Neurosurg Psychiatry 1969;32:236.

26. Irino T, Taneda M, Minami T. Angiographic manifestations in post-recanalized cerebral infarction. Neurology 1977;27:471.

27. Dalal PM, Shah PM, Sheth SC, Deshpande CK. Cerebral embolism: angiographic observations on spontaneous clot lysis. Lancet 1965;1:61.

28. Pessin MS, Hinton RC, Davis KR, et al. Mechanisms of acute carotid stroke. Ann Neurol 1979;6:245.

29. Ringelstein EB, Zeumer H, Angelou D. The pathogenesis of strokes from internal carotid artery occlusion: diagnostic and therapeutical implications. Stroke 1983;14:867.

30. Ringelstein EB, Binieck R, Weiller C, et al. Type and extent of hemispheric brain infarctions and clinical outcome in early and delayed middle cerebral artery recanalization. Neurology 1992;42:289.

31. Mori E, Yoneda Y. Early spontaneous recanalization of thromboembolic stroke. In: del Zoppo GJ, Mori E, Hacke W, eds. Thrombolytic therapy in acute ischemic stroke II. Heidelberg: Springer-Verlag, 1993.

32. Caplan LR, Hier DB, D'Cruz I. Cerebral embolism in the Michael Reese Stroke Registry. Stroke 1983;14:450.

33. Prochownik EV, Antonarakis S, Bauer KA, et al. Molecular heterogeneity of inherited antithrombin III deficiency. N Engl J Med 1983;308:1549.

34. Broekmans AW, Veltkamp JJ, Bertena RM. Congenital protein C deficiency and venous thromboembolism. N Engl J Med 1983;309:340.

35. Hacke W, Zeumer H, Ferbert A, et al. Intraarterial thrombolytic therapy improves outcome in pa-

tients with acute vertebrobasilar occlusive disease. Stroke 1988;19:1216.

36. del Zoppo GJ, Poek K, Pessin MS, et al. Recombinant tissue plasminogen activator in acute thrombotic and embolic stroke. Ann Neurol 1992;32:78.

37. Okada Y, Sadoshima S, Nakane H, et al. Early computed tomographic findings for thrombolytic therapy in patients with acute brain embolism. Stroke 1992;23:20.

38. Huk WJ. Invasive and noninvasive vascular imaging techniques and their role in clinical stroke trials. In: Hacke W, del Zoppo GJ, Hirschberg M, eds. Thrombolytic therapy in acute ischemic stroke. Heidelberg: Springer-Verlag, 1991:186.

39. Breslau P. Current status of ultrasonic techniques. In: Ultrasonic duplex scanning in the classification of carotid artery disease. Amsterdam: Heerlen, 1981.

40. Katz ML, Smalley KJ, Comerota AJ. Transcranial Doppler: prospective evaluation of hand-held vs. mapping technique. J Vasc Surg 1990;14:69.

41. Jacobs NM, Grant EG, Schellinger D, et al. Duplex carotid sonography: criteria for stenosis, accuracy, and pitfalls. Radiology 1985;154:385.

42. Taylor DC, Strandness DE Jr. Carotid artery duplex scanning. J Clin Ultrasound 1987;15:635.

43. O'Leary DH. Vascular ultrasonography. Radiol Clin North Am 1985;23:39.

44. Ley-Pozo J, Ringelstein EB. Noninvasive detection of occlusive disease of the carotid siphon and middle cerebral artery. Ann Neurol 1990;28:758.

45. Aaslid R. Transcranial Doppler sonography. Wien: Springer-Verlag, 1986.

46. Otis S, Ringelstein EB. Transcranial Doppler sonography. In: Bernstein ED, ed. Non-invasive diagnostic techniques in vascular disease. St. Louis: Mosby, 1990:59.

47. Padayachee TS, Kirkham FJ, Lewis RR, et al. Transcranial measurement of blood velocities in the basal cerebral arteries using pulsed Doppler ultrasound: a method of assessing the circle of Willis. Ultrasound Med Biol 1986;12:5.

48. Spencer MP. Intracranial carotid artery diagnosis with transorbital pulsed wave (PW) and continuous wave (CW) Doppler ultrasound. J Ultrasound Med 1983;2(suppl):61.

49. Ries F. Three-dimensional transcranial Doppler scanning. In: Bernstein EF, ed. Recent advances in noninvasive diagnostic techniques in vascular disease. St Louis: Mosby, 1990.

50. Otis SM. The role of noninvasive imaging techniques in cerebrovascular recanalization. In: Hacke W, del Zoppo GJ, Hirschberg M, eds. Thrombolytic therapy in acute ischemic stroke. Heidelberg: Springer-Verlag, 1991:98.

51. Ringelstein B. Transcranial Doppler ultrasonography in acute stroke management. Presented at the 2nd International Symposium on Thrombolytic Therapy in Acute Ischemic Stroke, La Jolla, California, 1992.

52. Mohr JP, Biller J, Hilal SK, et al. MR vs CT imaging in acute stroke (abstract). Stroke 1992;23:142.

53. Schuierer G, Huk W. The unilateral hyperdense middle cerebral artery: an early CT-sign of embolism or thrombosis. Neuroradiology 1988;30: 120.

54. Leys D, Pruvo JP, Godefroy O, et al. Prevalence and significance of hyperdense middle cerebral artery in acute stroke. Stroke 1992;23:317.

55. Wolpert SM. The relevance of angiography and CT scan to acute stroke intervention. In: del Zoppo GJ, Mori E, Hacke W, eds. Thrombolytic therapy in acute ischemic stroke II. Heidelberg: Springer-Verlag, 1993.

56. Tomsick T, Brott T, Barsan W, et al: Thrombus localization with emergency cerebral CT. Am J Neuroradiol 1992;13:257.

57. Mori E. Fibrinolytic recanalization therapy in acute cerebrovascular thromboembolism. In: Hacke W, del Zoppo GJ, Hirschberg M, eds. Thrombolytic therapy in acute ischemic stroke. Berlin: Springer-Verlag, 1991:137.

58. Bose B, Jones SC, Lorig R, et al. Evolving focal cerebral ischemia in cats: spatial correlation of nuclear magnetic resonance imaging, cerebral blood flow, tetrazolium staining, and histopathology. Stroke 1988;19:28.

59. Unger EC, Gado MH, Fulling KF, Littlefield JL. Acute cerebral infarction in monkeys: an experimental study using MR imaging. Radiology 1987; 162:789.

60. Brant-Zawadzki M, Pereira B, Weinstein P, et al. MRI of acute experimental ischemia in rats. AJNR 1986;7:7.

61. Ruggieri PM, Laub E, Masaryk T, Modic M. Intracranial circulation: pulse sequence consideration in 3-dimensional MR angiography. Radiology 1989;171:785.

62. Nabatame H, Fujimoto N, Nakamura K, et al. High intensity areas of noncontrast T_1-weighted MR images in cerebral infarction. J Comput Assist Tomogr 1990;14:521.

63. Minematsu K, Li L, Fisher M, et al. Diffusion weighted magnetic resonance imaging: rapid and quantitative detection of focal brain ischemia. Neurology 1992;42:235.

64. Masaryk TJ, Tkach J, Glicklich M. Flow radiofrequency pulse sequences and gradient magnetic fields: basic interactions and adaptations to angiographic imaging. Top Magn Reson Imaging 1991; 3:1.

65. Ross JS, Masaryk TJ, Ruggieri PM. Magnetic resonance angiography of the carotid bifurcation. Top Magn Reson Imaging 1991;3:12.

66. Ruggieri PM, Masaryk TJ, Ross JS, Modic MT. Magnetic resonance angiography of the intracranial vasculature. Top Magn Reson Imaging 1991; 3:23.

67. Moseley ME, Wedland MF, Kuchorczyk J. Magnetic resonance imaging of diffusion and perfusion. Top Magn Reson Imaging 1991;3:50.

68. Furlan AJ. The potential role of magnetic resonance angiography in acute stroke imaging. Presented at the 2nd International Symposium on Thrombolytic Therapy in Acute Ischemic Stroke, La Jolla, California, 1992.

69. Okada Y, Overgaard K. The role of SPECT in acute stroke thrombolysis. Presented at the 2nd International Symposium on Thrombolytic Therapy in Acute Ischemic Stroke, La Jolla, California, 1992.

70. Mountz JM, Modell JG, Foster NL, et al. Prognostication of recovery following stroke using a comparison of CT and technetium-99m HMPAO SPECT. J Nucl Med 1990;31:61.

71. del Zoppo GJ, Mori E. Hematologic causes of intracerebral hemorrhage and their treatment. In: Batjer HH, ed. Spontaneous intracerebral hemorrhage. Neurosurg Clin North Am 1992;3:637.

72. Ott BR, Zamani A, Kleefield J, Funkenstein HH. The clinical spectrum of hemorrhagic infarction. Stroke 1986;17:630.

73. Hart RG. Cerebral embolism study group: timing of hemorrhagic transformation of cardioembolic stroke. In: Stober T, ed. Central nervous system control of the heart. Boston: Martinus Nijhoff, 1986:229.

74. Lodder J, Krijne-Kubat B, van der Lugt PJM. Timing of autopsy-confirmed hemorrhagic infarction with reference to cardioembolic stroke. Stroke 1988;19:1482.

75. Yamaguchi T, Minematsu K, Choki J-I, Ikeda M. Clinical and neuroradiological analysis of thrombotic and embolic cerebral infarction. Jpn Circ J 1984;48:50.

76. Okada Y, Yamaguchi T, Minematsu K, et al. Hemorrhagic transformation in cerebral embolism. Stroke 1989;20:598.

77. Hornig CR, Dorndorf W, Agnoli AL. Hemorrhagic cerebral infarction: a prospective study. Stroke 1986;17:179.

78. Furlan AJ, Cavalier SJ, Hobbs RE, et al. Hemorrhage and anticoagulation after nonseptic embolic brain infarction. Neurology 1982;32:280.

79. Koller RL. Recurrent embolic cerebral infarction and anticoagulation. Neurology 1982;32:283.

80. Drake ME, Shin C. Conversion of ischemic to hemorrhagic infarction by anticoagulant administration. Report of two cases with evidence from serial computed tomographic brain scans. Arch Neurol 1983;40:44.

81. Meyer JS, Gilroy J, Barnhart MI, Johnson JF. Therapeutic thrombolysis in cerebral thromboembolism. Neurology 1963;13:927.

82. Babikian VL, Kase CS, Pessin MS, et al. Intracerebral hemorrhage in stroke patients anticoagulated with heparin. Stroke 1989;29:1500.

83. del Zoppo GJ, Ferbert A, Otis S, et al. Local intraarterial fibrinolytic therapy in acute carotid territory stroke: a pilot study. Stroke 1988;19:307.

84. Mori E, Tabuchi M, Yoshida T, Yamadori A. Intracarotid urokinase with thromboembolic occlusion of the middle cerebral artery. Stroke 1988; 19:802.

85. Mori E, Yoneda Y, Ohkawa S, et al. Double-blind placebo-controlled trial of intravenous recombinant tissue plasminogen activator (rt-PA) in acute carotid stroke. Neurology 1991;41(suppl 1):347.

86. Ogata J, Yutani C, Imakita M, et al. Hemorrhagic infarct of the brain without a reopening of the occluded arteries in cardioembolic stroke. Stroke 1989;20:876.

87. Fisher CM, Adams RD. Observations on brain embolism with special reference to the mechanism of hemorrhagic infarction. J Neuropathol Exp Neurol 1951;10:92.

88. Fisher CM, Adams RD. Observations on brain embolism with special reference to hemorrhage infarction. In: Furlan AJ, ed. The Heart and stroke: exploring mutual cerebrovascular and cardiovascular issues. New York: Springer-Verlag, 1987:17.

89. Waltz AG. Clinical relevance of models of cerebral ischemia. Stroke 1979;10:211.

90. Diaz FA, Ausman JI. Experimental cerebral ischemia. Neurosurgery 1980;6:436.

91. del Zoppo GJ. Relevance of focal cerebral ischemia models: experience with fibrinolytic agents. Stroke 1990;21:IV-155.

92. Kissel P, Chehrazi B, Seibert JA, Wagner FC. Digital angiographic quantification of blood flow dynamics in embolic stroke treated with tissue-type plasminogen activator. J Neurosurg 1987;67:399.

93. Phillips DA, Fisher M, Smith TW, Davis MA. The safety and angiographic efficacy of tissue plasminogen activator in a cerebral embolization model. Ann Neurol 1988;23:391.

94. Phillips DA, Fisher M, Davis MA, et al. Delayed treatment with a t-PA analogue and streptokinase in a rabbit embolic stroke model. Stroke 1990; 21:602.

95. Papadopoulos SM, Chandler WF, Salamat MS, et al. Recombinant human tissue-type plasminogen activator therapy in acute thromboembolic stroke. J Neurosurg 1987;67:394.

96. Penar PL, Greer CA. The effect of intravenous tissue-type plasminogen activator in a rat model of embolic cerebral ischemia. Yale J Biol Med 1987;60:233.

97. del Zoppo GJ, Copeland BR, Waltz TA, et al. The

beneficial effect of intracarotid urokinase of acute stroke in a baboon model. Stroke 1986;17:638.

98. Hirschberg M, Hofferberth B. Rapid fibrinolysis of different time intervals in a canine model at acute stroke. Stroke 1987;18:292.

99. Hirschberg M, Hofferberth B. Thrombolytic therapy with urokinase and prourokinase in a canine model of acute stroke. Neurology 1987;37:133.

100. Hirschberg M, Korves M, Koc I, et al. Thrombolysis of cerebral thromboembolism by urokinase in an animal model. Schweiz Med Wochenschr 1987; 117:1811.

101. Zivin JA, Fisher M, De Girolami U. Tissue plasminogen activator reduces neurological damage after cerebral embolism. Science 1985;320:1289.

102. Zivin JA, Lyden PD, De Girolami U, et al. Tissue plasminogen activator reduction of neurologic damage after experimental embolic stroke. Arch Neurol 1988;45:387.

103. Slivka A, Pulsinelli WA. Hemorrhagic complications of thrombolytic therapy in experimental stroke. Neurology 1987;37(suppl 1):82.

104. del Zoppo GJ, Copeland BR, Anderchek K, et al. Hemorrhagic transformation following tissue plasminogen activator in experimental cerebral infarction. Stroke 1990;21:596.

105. Herndon RM, Nelson JN, Johnson JF, Meyer JS. Thrombolytic treatment in cerebrovascular thrombosis. In: MacMillan RL, Mustard JF, eds. Anticoagulants and fibrinolysins. Philadelphia: Lea & Febiger, 1961:154.

106. Meyer JS, Gilroy J, Barnhart ME, Johnson JF. Therapeutic thrombolysis in cerebral thromboembolism: Randomized evaluation of intravenous streptokinase. In: Millikan CH, Siekert RG, Whisnant JP, eds. Cerebral vascular diseases, fourth Princeton conference. New York: Grune & Stratton, 1965:200.

107. del Zoppo GJ, Zeumer H, Harker LA. Thrombolytic therapy in acute stroke: possibilities and hazards. Stroke 1986;17:595.

108. Abe T, Kazawa M, Naito I. Clinical effect of urokinase (60,000 units/day) on cerebral infarction—comparative study by means of multiple center double blind test. Blood Vessels 1981;12:342.

109. Abe T, Kazama M, Naito I, et al. Clinical evaluation for efficacy of tissue culture urokinase (TCUK) on cerebral thrombosis by means of multicenter double-blind study. Blood Vessels 1981; 12:321.

110. von Kummer R, Hacke W. Safety and efficacy of intravenous tissue plasminogen activator and heparin in acute middle cerebral artery. Stroke 1992;23:646.

111. Mori E, Yoneda Y, Tabuchi M, et al. Intravenous recombinant tissue plasminogen activator in acute

carotid artery territory stroke. Neurology 1992; 42:976.

112. Zeumer H, Freitag H-J, Knospe V. Acute central retinal artery occlusion and the role of thrombolysis. In: del Zoppo GJ, Mori E, Hacke W, eds. Thrombolytic therapy in acute ischemic stroke. Heidelberg: Springer-Verlag, 1993.

113. Theron J, Courtheoux P, Casaseo A, et al. Local intraarterial fibrinolysis in the carotid territory. Am J Neuroradiol 1989;10:753.

114. Matsumoto K, Satoh K. Topical intraarterial urokinase infusion for acute stroke. In: Hacke W, del Zoppo GJ, Hirschberg M, eds. Thrombolytic therapy in acute ischemic stroke. Heidelberg: Springer-Verlag, 1991:207.

115. Miyakawa T. The cerebral vessels and thrombosis. Rinsho Ketsueki 1984;25:1018.

116. del Zoppo GJ. Thrombolysis: new concepts in the treatment of stroke. In: Hennerici M, Sitzer G, Weger H-D, eds. Carotid artery plaques. Basel: Karger, 1988:247.

117. Henze TH, Boeer A, Tebbe U, Romatowski J. Lysis of basilar artery occlusion with tissue plasminogen activator. Lancet 1987;1:1391.

118. Buteux G, Jubault V, Suisse A. Local recombinant tissue plasminogen activator to clear cerebral artery thrombosis developing soon after surgery. Lancet 1988;1:1143.

119. Zeumer H. Survey of progress: vascular recanalizing techniques in interventional neuroradiology. J Neurol 1985;231:287.

120. Bruckmann H, Ferbert A, del Zoppo GJ, et al. Acute vertebral-basilar thrombosis: angiologic-clinical comparison and therapeutic implications. Acta Radiol 1987;369(suppl):38.

121. Nenci GG, Gresele P, Taramelli M, et al. Thrombolytic therapy for thromboembolism of vertebrobasilar artery. Angiology 1983;34:561.

122. Yamaguchi T. Intravenous rt-PA in acute embolic stroke. In: Hacke W, del Zoppo GJ, Hirschberg M, eds. Thrombolytic therapy in acute ischemic stroke. Berlin: Springer-Verlag, 1991:168.

123. von Kummer R. Intravenous tissue plasminogen activator in acute stroke. In: Hacke W, del Zoppo GJ, Hirschberg M, eds. Thrombolytic therapy in acute ischemic stroke. Berlin: Springer-Verlag, 1991:161.

124. Atarashi J, Otomo E, Araki G, et al. Clinical utility of urokinase in the treatment of acute stage of cerebral thrombosis: multicenter double-blind study in comparison with placebo. Clin Eval 1985;13:659.

125. Otomo E, Araki G, Itoh E, et al. Clinical efficacy of urokinase in the treatment of cerebral thrombosis: multicenter double-blind study in comparison with placebo. Clin Eval 1985;13:711.

126. Otomo E, Tohgi H, Hirai S, et al. Clinical efficacy of AK-124 (tissue plasminogen activator) in the treatment of cerebral thrombosis: study by means of multicenter double blind comparison with urokinase. Yakuri To Chiryo 1988;16:3775.

127. Abe T, Terashi A, Tohgi H, et al. Clinical efficacy of intravenous administration of SM-9527 (t-PA) in cerebral thrombosis. Clin Eval 1990;18:39.

128. Koudstaal PJ, Stibbe J, Vermeulen M. Fatal ischemic brain oedema after early thrombolysis with tissue plasminogen activator in acute stroke. Br Med J 1988;297:1571.

129. Brott TG, Haley EC, Levy DE, et al. Urgent therapy for stroke: I. Pilot study of tissue plasminogen activator administered within 90 minutes. Stroke 1992;23:632.

130. Haley EC, Levy DE, Brott TG, et al. Urgent therapy for stroke: II. Pilot study of plasminogen administered 91–180 minutes from onset. Stroke 1992; 23:641.

131. Aldrich MS, Sherman SA, Greenberg HS. Cerebrovascular complications of streptokinase infusion. JAMA 1985;253:1777.

132. Sherry S. Tissue plasminogen activator (t-PA): will it fulfill its promise? N Engl J Med 1985;313:1014.

133. Marder VJ. Fibrinolytic agents: are they feasible for stroke therapy? In: Plum F, Pulsinelli WA, eds. Cerebrovascular diseases, fourteenth research conference. New York: Raven Press, 1986:241.

134. Sussman BJ, Fitch TSP. Thrombolysis with fibrinolysin in cerebral arterial occlusion. JAMA 1958;167:1705.

135. Herndon RM, Meyer JS, Johnson JF, Landers J. Treatment of cerebrovascular thrombosis with fibrinolysin: preliminary report. Am J Cardiol 1960; 30:540.

136. Meyer JS, Gilroy J, Barnhart MI, Johnson JF. Anticoagulants plus streptokinase therapy in progressive stroke. JAMA 1964;189:373.

137. Yamaguchi T. Intravenous tissue plasminogen activator in acute thromboembolic stroke: a placebo-controlled, double-blind trial. In: del Zoppo GJ, Mori E, Hacke W, eds. Thrombolytic therapy in acute ischemic stroke II. Heidelberg: Springer-Verlag, 1993.

138. del Zoppo GJ, Pessin MS, Mori E, Hacke W. Thrombolytic intervention in acute thrombotic and embolic stroke. Semin Neurol 1991;11:368.

139. Caplan LR. Patterns of posterior circulation infarctions: correlation with vascular pathology. In: Berguer R, Bauer RB, eds. Vertebrobasilar arterial occlusive disease: medical and surgical treatment. New York: Raven Press, 1984:15.

140. Wood JH, Kee DB Jr. Clinical rheology of stroke and hemodilution. In: Barnett HJM, Mohr JP, Stein BM, Yatsu FM, eds. Stroke: pathophysiology, diagnosis and management. New York: Churchill Livingstone, 1986:100.

141. rt-PA Acute Stroke Study Group. An open safety/efficacy trial of rt-PA in acute thromboembolic stroke: final report. Stroke 1991;22:153.

142. Mori E. Fibrinolytic recanalization therapy in acute cerebrovascular thromboembolism. In: Hacke W, del Zoppo GJ, Hirschberg M, eds. Thrombolytic therapy in acute ischemic stroke. Heidelberg: Springer-Verlag, 1991:137.

143. Zeumer H, Freitag HJ, Grzyka U, Neunzig HP. Local intraarterial fibrinolysis in acute vertebrobasilar occlusion: technical developments and recent results. Neuroradiology 1989;31:336.

144. Möbius E, Berg-Dammer E, Kühne D, Ahser HC. Local thrombolytic therapy in acute basilar artery occlusion: experience with 18 patients. In: Hacke W, del Zoppo GJ, Hirschberg M, eds. Thrombolytic therapy in acute ischemic stroke. Berlin: Springer-Verlag, 1991:213.

26

Thrombolytic Treatment of Acute Stroke Secondary to Arterial or Venous Occlusion

Fong Y. Tsai

Kenneth M. Alfieri

Local infusion of thrombolytic agents is receiving widespread acceptance for the treatment of the acute occlusion of intracranial arterial and venous vessels. Streptokinase (SK) and urokinase (UK) are two thrombolytic agents that have been applied successfully in the clinical setting of acute thrombosis of blood vessels outside the central nervous system. This includes acute occlusions of the coronary[1-7] and pulmonary[8-10] arteries, as well as peripheral arteries and veins.[11-15] Recently, tissue-type plasminogen activator (t-PA), which is an endogenous fibrinolytic substance with a short half-life, has been introduced for clinical study.[16,17] t-PA has the potential to induce rapid thrombus dissolution with a low risk of systemic hemorrhagic complications.

These agents hold great promise for the treatment of ischemic neurologic events in the acute stage. This is particularly important in light of the fact that there is no unequivocal proof of the efficacy of standard anticoagulation therapy with heparin in the setting of progressive ischemic stroke.[18-20] The rationale for thrombolytic therapy is to salvage the ischemic penumbra of viable neural tissue and subsequently reverse clinical neurologic deficits.

PATHOPHYSIOLOGY

A stroke from an acute cerebrovascular occlusion may result from either an arterial or venous thrombosis. The majority of ischemic strokes are the result of a thromboembolic event involving the arterial supply of brain. The source of the thromboembolism is most commonly an atherosclerotic plaque in the carotid artery bifurcation or vertebrobasilar system or a cardiac abnormality such as an arrhythmia. If regional cerebral blood flow is reduced to 25% of normal, an ischemic event is initiated.[21] This may be mild with reversal of symptoms within 24 h; this is termed a *transient ischemic attack* (TIA). If remission occurs beyond 24 h, these symptoms are termed *reversible ischemic neurologic deficits* (RIND). With complete anoxia, irreversible neuron damage and death occur within a few minutes. However, clinical experience has shown that an ischemic stroke is frequently progressive. This provides a variable time interval in the acute setting in which thrombolytic intervention may reverse clinical deficits.[22,23]

Spontaneous fibrinolysis can occur but may not do so early enough to avoid a permanent deficit. It is estimated that cerebrovascular emboli are detected less than 50% of the time during angiography. This is probably due to the fact that angiography frequently is not performed earlier than 12 to 24 h after the event, allowing the intrinsic fibrinolytic system to lyse the clot during this interval. However, if arteriography is performed earlier than 12 h after the onset of an acute stroke, the causative occlusion can be identified in as many as 90% of cases.[22,23]

In addition to arterial ischemia, a stroke may result from venous occlusion. Venous stroke had not received its share of medical attention until recently and is primarily the result of venous congestion rather than arterial ischemia.[24,25] What follows is a description of the patient evaluation and thrombolytic techniques used at our institution in the setting of an acute arterial or venous stroke.

PRELIMINARY PATIENT EVALUATION

Before thrombolytic treatment is initiated, the patient must be evaluated for risk factors for hemorrhagic complications. Baseline laboratory values and a coagulation profile must be obtained, including hemoglobin, hematocrit, platelet count, fibrinogen level, prothrombin, and activated partial thromboplastin time.

Magnetic resonance imaging (MRI) and/or computed tomography (CT) are modalities that are almost invariably utilized in the preangiogram patient evaluation. MRI is more sensitive in the evaluation of cerebrovascular occlusion than CT, yet MRI may not be practical in the superacute stage of a stroke because of instability of the patient. We prefer to have CT scans done immediately after complete physical and neurologic examinations. We reserve MRI examination, including MR angiography and venography, for those patients with a suspected cerebrovenous occlusion. After the CT scan, the patient is then

transferred directly to a neuroangiographic room for cerebral angiography. The cerebral angiography must include arch aortography as well as extra- and intracranial carotid and vertebral angiography.

Contraindications to treatment include active hemorrhaging, recent cerebrovascular hemorrhage, and intracerebral tumor or vascular malformation. Relative contraindications are recent major surgery (less than 10 days ago), recent serious trauma or internal hemorrhage, and severe uncontrolled hypertension.[30]

In an early pilot study utilizing systemic (rather than intraarterial) UK in patients with completed strokes, a 25% intracerebral hemorrhage rate was observed with no demonstrable therapeutic benefit.[33,34] However, more recent studies using microcatheter techniques and local infusions directly into the thrombus or between the thrombus and the wall of the vessel have demonstrated generally lower hemorrhagic complication rates of approximately 13%. The observed risk factors for intracerebral hemorrhagic complications were brainstem infarction, occlusion of lenticulostriate arteries, and late (beyond 6 h) initiation of thrombolytic therapy.[35–39]

TECHNIQUES OF THROMBOLYSIS

With recent advances in catheter techniques, superselective local application of thrombolytic agents to the thromboembolus has become practical for extra- and intracranial vessels. The procedure begins with a routine angiographic examination, usually by way of a transfemoral approach with a no. 5 French catheter to delineate the location of the thrombus. By using a coaxial technique, a no. 2 or no. 3 French Tracker catheter (Target Therapeutics, San Jose, CA) can be advanced into intracranial branches of the carotid or vertebrobasilar artery[26,27] (Figs. 26-1, 26-9, and 26-10). The catheters utilized generally have multiple sideholes, which enhance the thrombolytic effect.

If a cerebrovenous occlusion is suspected, a no. 5 French catheter is advanced to the jugular bulb from the transfemoral vein approach. A Tracker catheter is introduced coaxially through

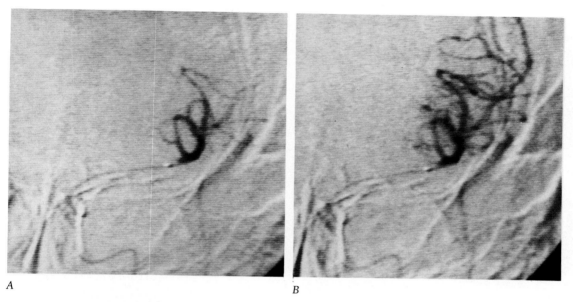

*FIGURE 26-1. Tracker catheter placement. (**A**) Digital subtraction arteriography (DSA) showed distal occlusion of branches of the left middle cerebral artery. DSA was performed with the tip of a tracker catheter in the trifurcation of the MCA. (**B**) Follow-up DSA after thrombolysis demonstrated reopening of the occluded branches of the MCA.*

the no. 5 French catheter. The Tracker catheter is then navigated to the occluded dural sinus for direct dural sinus venography and thrombolysis.[28,29]

Once the occlusion or thrombus is identified, 5000 units of IV heparin is given, and if it is needed, an additional 1000 units of heparin will be given every hour. The infusion catheter is slowly advanced to the thrombosed area with a soft-tipped guidewire positioned just beyond the end of the catheter. The catheter and guidewire are then gently pushed into the thrombus. A thrombolytic agent is administered with intermittent injections rather than with a continuous infusion. We prefer to inject 250,000 IU UK immediately and then 80,000 IU every 15 minutes in a concentration of about 8000 IU/mL until thrombolysis is completed.[26–29]

Extracranial Carotid Artery

Acute occlusion of the internal carotid artery usually is associated with a proximal stenosis, which results in progressive propagation of clot and partial or complete occlusion (Fig. 26-2). An occluded internal carotid artery may contain fresh and aged thrombus. Segments of these clots may dislodge and occlude distal intracranial branches after the major thrombus is broken up. Routine intracranial angiography is needed to search for these distal occlusions (see Fig. 26-2D). Superselective catheterization of involved intracranial vessels is then performed in a manner similar to the technique for extracranial thrombolysis (Fig. 26-3).

Middle Cerebral Artery (MCA)

The clinical symptoms of MCA occlusion may be somewhat different depending on the site of the occlusion and the possible existence of collaterals. Dense hemiplegia usually results from the occlusion of lenticulostriate branches. The lenticulostriate territory has no collateral vasculature; therefore, the timing of thrombolysis is more urgent when these vessels are involved than with distal MCA occlusion (Figs. 26-4 and 26-5).

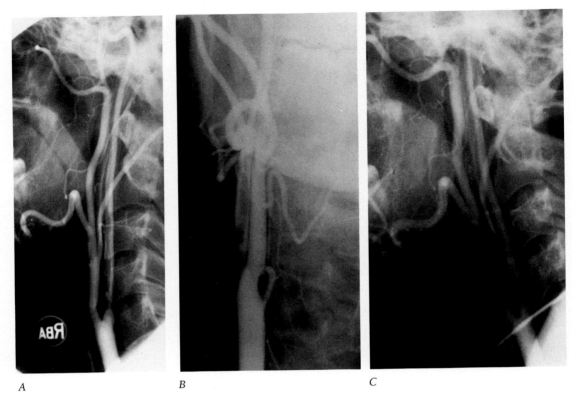

A

B

C

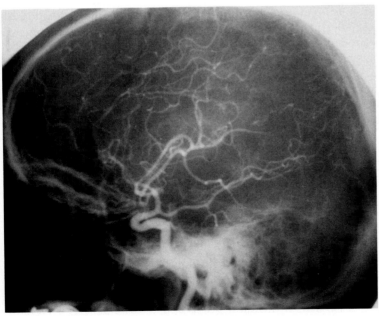

D

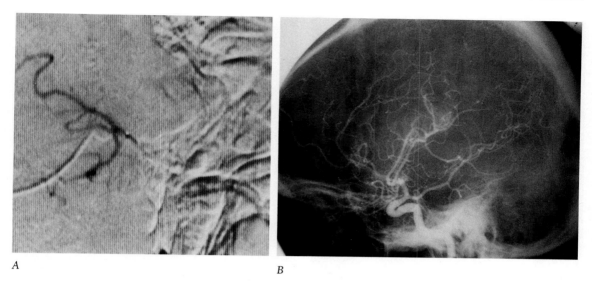

A   B

FIGURE 26-3. Intracranial migration of dislodged thrombus from the internal carotid artery. (A) Superselective angular artery DSA was performed with a tracker catheter. (B) Repeat cerebral arteriography showed that the aged thrombus could not be dissolved, but more small branches were seen after additional thrombolysis.

In our experience, the continuous infusion technique can result in inadvertent delivery of the thrombolytic agent into vessels that are not thrombosed. Two cases in our series illustrate this. One patient had occlusions of the proximal MCA and lenticulostriate arteries, and the other had involvement of the supraclinoid carotid artery and thalamoperforators (Figs. 26-6 and 26-7). As a general rule, satisfactory dissolution of a thrombus cannot be achieved if the tip of the catheter is not directly in the clot or between the clot and the vessel wall. However, in these two patients, the catheter tip could not be advanced into the thrombus. Under these circumstances, the continuous infusion technique was overinfusing unclotted vessels rather than delivering the thrombolytic agent directly into the clot. In one

instance, the infusion was shunted to the posterior cerebral artery (see Fig. 26-6), and in the other, to the anterior cerebral artery (see Fig. 26-7). Hemorrhagic complications arose in both these patients.

The intermittent infusion technique allows incremental advancement of the catheter (if this is technically possible) as the clot dissolves. Frequent digital subtraction arteriography (DSA) imaging can be used to monitor this process. We believe that this method minimizes the infusion of uninvolved vessels and minimizes the risk of hemorrhage. The risk of hemorrhage can be significant when treating thromboses of the lenticulostriate and thalamoperforator arteries. Since we have adopted the intermittent infusion technique,

(Text continued on page 427)

FIGURE 26-2. Internal carotid artery thrombosis. (A,B) Common carotid arteriography demonstrated a large thrombus extending from the proximal to the midportion of the internal carotid artery (arrow). Severe stenosis is seen proximal to the thrombus just above the bifurcation. (C) The thrombus was dissolved after UK treatment. (The patient had endarterectomy several months later for the stenosis.) (D) Dislodged thrombus migrated to the intracranial artery from the internal carotid artery. Intracranial cerebral angiography showed a dislodged small thrombus occluding the angular branch of the middle cerebral artery from the internal carotid artery.

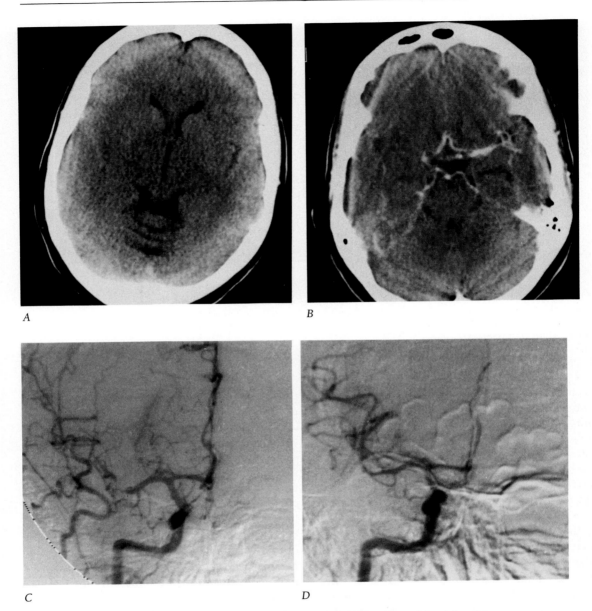

A

B

C

D

FIGURE 26-4. Middle cerebral artery occlusion. (A) CT scan showed obliteration of the right sylvian fissure. This patient had a dense hemiplegia. (B) Contrast CT showed occlusion of the right middle cerebral artery. (C) Carotid arteriography confirmed the diagnosis. (D) Repeat arteriography demonstrated reopening of the middle cerebral artery.

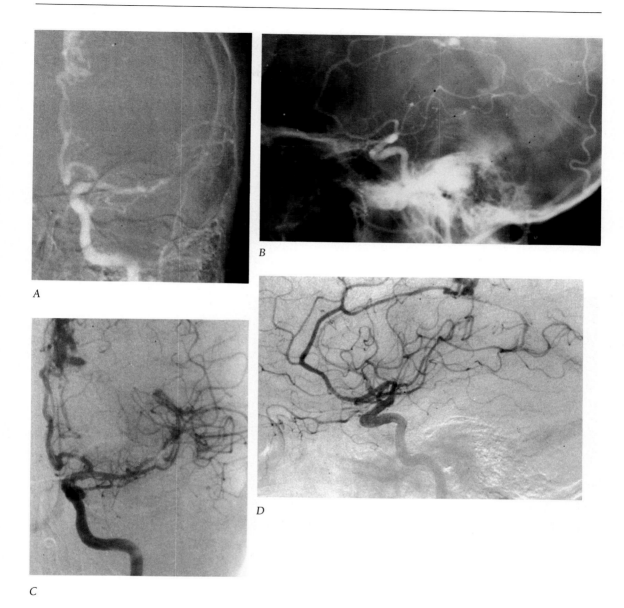

FIGURE 26-5. *Middle cerebral artery thrombosis. (A,B) Frontal and lateral views of left carotid angiogram demonstrated thrombosis of the middle cerebral artery just distal to the trifurcation. (C,D) The thrombosed middle cerebral artery was reopened after thrombolysis. (Incidentally noted is an AVM being fed by the pericallosal artery.)*

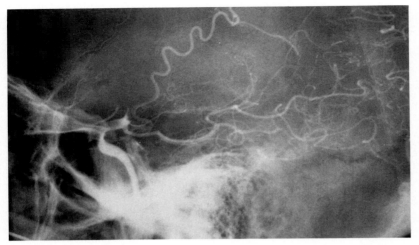

A

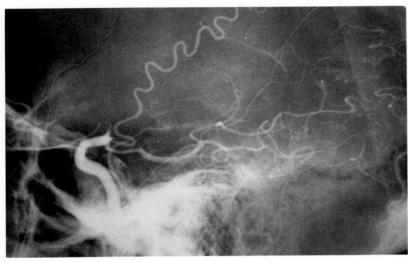

B

FIGURE 26-6. Hemorrhagic complication. (A) Lateral view of carotid arteriography showed thrombus in the cavernous portion of the internal carotid artery with a total occlusion of the supraclinoid portion of the distal internal carotid artery. (B) The thrombus of the cavernous portion of the carotid artery was dissolved after initial thrombolysis. (C,D) CT scan showed hemorrhagic complications of the basal ganglia and thalamus after continuous infusion of thrombolytic agent.

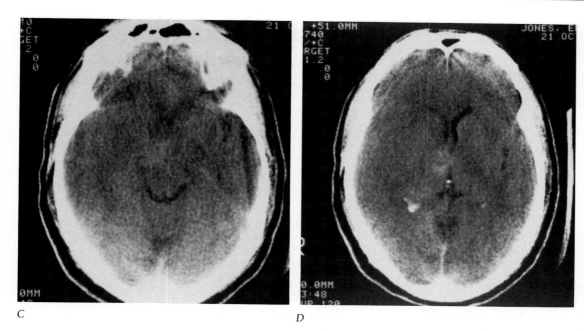

C   D

FIGURE 26-6. (Continued).

we have not experienced hemorrhagic complications in these territories.

Thrombosis of the MCA is frequently associated with an underlying stenosis. Occasionally, angioplasty of the stenosis is required to prevent rethrombosis after thrombolysis is completed.

Ophthalmic and Central Retinal Arteries

The occlusion of branches of the ophthalmic artery or central retinal artery often leads to blindness if immediate treatment is not instituted. After our initial report of superselective ophthalmic angiography,[24] we were able to apply thrombolytic techniques to those patients with acute visual loss due to occlusion of the central retinal artery. A no. 2 French microcatheter is generally used in this setting (Figs. 26-8 and 26-9).

Vertebrobasilar Artery

Vertebrobasilar artery occlusion may be due to a dislodged embolus from the heart or a proximal vertebral artery stenosis with distal proliferation of thrombus. Distal vertebral artery stenosis can lead to propagation of thrombus, resulting in occlusion of the PICA (Figs. 26-10 and 26-11).

The coma center is supplied by thalamoperforators, which are branches of the posterior cerebral artery. The comatose patient with a basilar artery occlusion may not regain consciousness if the occlusion of the thalamoperforators is not reopened.

Dural Sinus Occlusion

Less is known about the natural history of occlusive disease involving the intracranial dural sinuses and veins than about arterial thrombosis. There are a wide variety of septic and aseptic etiologies for this condition, including tumors (meningiomas, meningeal metastasis, leukemia), trauma (subdural or epidural hematoma), infection (mastoiditis, subdural or epidural empyema, meningitis, encephalitis, brain abscess, sinusitis, disseminated intravascular coagulation), low-flow states, and coagulopathies, as well as numerous

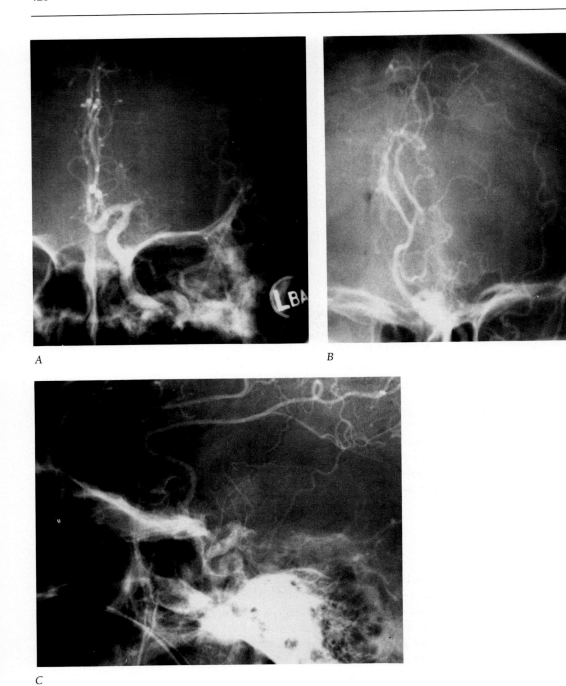

A

B

C

FIGURE 26-7. Hemorrhagic complication. **(A)** Left carotid arteriography showed a total occlusion of the proximal MCA just off the supraclinoid portion of the internal carotid artery. **(B,C)** Repeat carotid arteriography showed massive shift of anterior cerebral artery with more opacification of the lenticulostriates. The hematoma was believed to result from overinfusion of urokinase to those lenticulostriate branches.

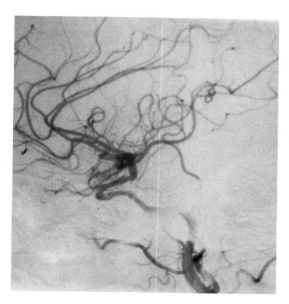

FIGURE 26-8. Ophthalmic artery occlusion. Common carotid arteriography showed occlusion of the distal ophthalmic artery. Arteriosclerotic stenosis is also seen at the distal internal carotid artery.

There are several reports of successful treatment of acute dural sinus thrombosis in adults and infants with UK. By using an approach through the femoral vein, a coaxial catheter system identical to the one used for arterial procedures can be employed to bring the tip of the microcatheter into the involved dural sinus. A typical dose of UK in this setting is 4000 IU/h until the clot is dissolved, which may take several hours. An intermittent injection technique of UK may be used as well. The microcatheter is repeatedly advanced into the remaining clot as lysis proceeds (Figs. 26-12 and 26-13). Systemic anticoagulation with heparin is administered with the UK. At the conclusion of clot lysis, the catheter system may be removed from the venous access site with little risk of local bleeding complications.[29–35] In the setting of dural venous thrombosis, the timing of thrombolytic therapy is very important. The optimal time of thrombolysis for an acute dural sinus thrombosis is at the first sign of clinical deterioration. If the patient's clinical condition deteriorates, thrombolysis must be initiated as soon as possible because these patients may suddenly lapse into a coma.[28,29] The dose of the thrombolytic agent for dural sinus thrombosis is the same as for patients with arterial thromboses.

miscellaneous conditions (diabetes, postoperative state, oral contraceptives, pregnancy and the postpartum state, etc.).[25,30] Venous sinus thrombosis can be diagnosed noninvasively with contrast-enhanced CT (by the "empty delta" sign, which is a triangular filling defect at the posterior confluence of the dural sinuses) and by a persistent loss of normal signal void in the involved dural sinus on MRI (an increased signal in the sinus lumen suggests the presence of slow, turbulent flow or thrombus in the vessel). It is estimated that parenchymal hemorrhages accompany approximately 20% of dural sinus thromboses.[26]

An acutely thrombosed dural sinus may have an isointense appearance on regular MRI and may be isodense on CT. Therefore, routine MRI might miss the finding of an intracranial acute dural sinus thrombosis. Thrombus in the superior sagittal sinus can be identified more easily than transverse sinus, sigmoid sinus, or vein of Galen thromboses.[29,30]

COMPLICATIONS AND RESULTS

Most of the patients who received local thrombolytic treatment had moderate or severe deficits at the end of the thrombolysis. However, it is common for these patients to improve progressively. Frequently, patients recover completely within a few days. Those patients with an early recovery usually have a better prognosis. Even if patients do not have a complete recovery, the thrombolytic treatment can be beneficial by halting clinical deterioration. Patients with dural sinus thrombosis have a much better prognosis than those patients with arterial stroke. Generally, the earlier thrombolysis begins, the better the result

(Text continued on page 433)

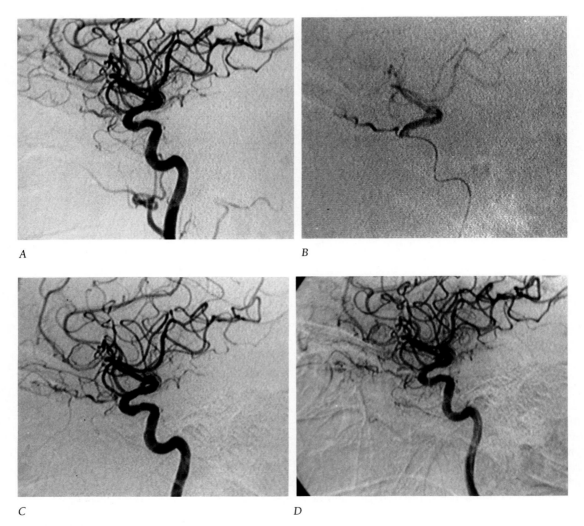

FIGURE 26-9. Ophthalmic and retinal artery occlusion. (A) Common carotid arteriography showed occlusion of ophthalmic artery just distal to the turn of optic nerve. (B) Superselective ophthalmic arteriography showed stenosis at the proximal portion just off the carotid artery. (C,D) Internal carotid arteriography showed reopening of the ophthalmic artery and a good choroidal blush after UK treatment.

FIGURE 26-10. A complete occlusion of the basilar artery. (A) Vertebral arteriography showed a total occlusion of the basilar artery. (B) Lateral view of arteriography showed the tip of the Tracker catheter in the proximal basilar artery. (C) Repeat vertebral arteriography showed complete dissolution of the thrombus. (D) Follow up MRI showed a small residual infarct at the superior vermis.

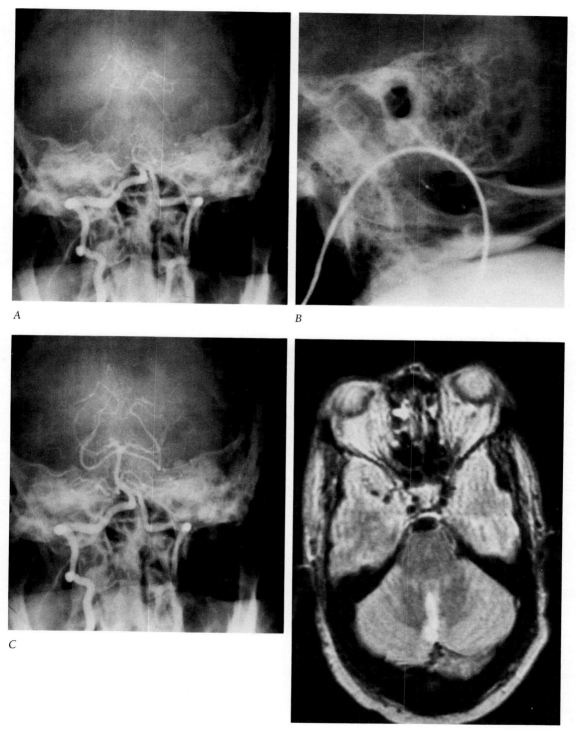

A

B

C

D

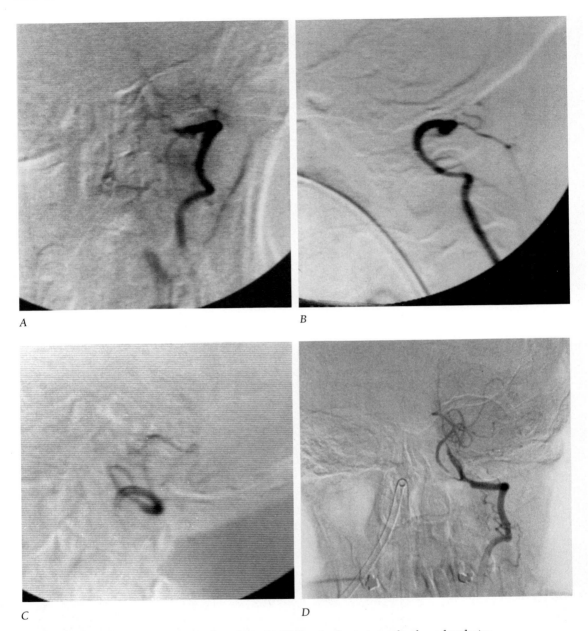

FIGURE 26-11. Distal vertebral artery thrombosis. (**A,B**) Vertebral arteriography showed occlusion at the distal vertebral artery. (**C**) Lateral view of superselective vertebral artery DSA with Tracker catheter showed reopening of the distal vertebral artery and PICA. (**D**) Vertebral arteriography shows the thrombosis being reopened, and the stenosis that caused the thrombosis.

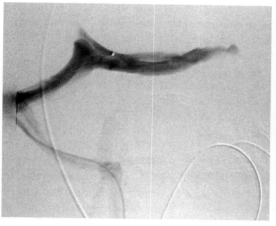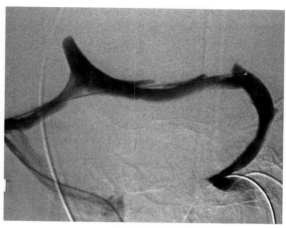

A   B

FIGURE 26-12. *Left transverse sinus thrombus.* (A) *Superselective venography showed occlusion at the distal left transverse sinus.* (B) *The left transverse sinus reopened after thrombolysis.*

will be. Earlier treatment also results in fewer complications.[27,28,36–47]

The main complication of arterial thrombolytic treatment is hemorrhage. Three patients in our series had hemorrhage during thrombol-

ysis using a continuous infusion.[36–47] This represents about 3% of all patients who received thrombolysis. Fifty percent of patients had partial or complete recoveries. Thirty-three percent had moderate deficits, and 14% had severe deficits. No

FIGURE 26-13. *Superior sagittal sinus thrombosis.* (A) *Superselective dural sinus venography showed thrombosis of the superior sagittal sinus (SSS).* (B) *Venography after thrombolysis showed reopening of the SSS.*

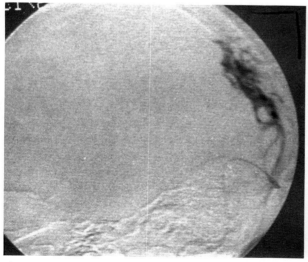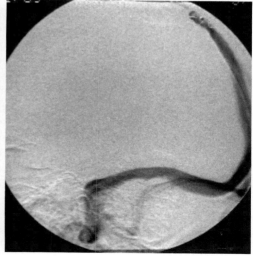

A   B

hemorrhagic complication was noted in those patients with dural sinus thrombosis. All our patients with dural sinus thrombosis recovered completely with one exception; this patient had a moderate deficit from a large cerebellar infarct. In this individual there was a 4-day interval between clinical deterioration and the institution of thrombolytic therapy.[29,30]

DISCUSSION

The traditional treatment for acute cerebrovascular occlusion has been anticoagulation. The results of anticoagulation have not been encouraging. Anticoagulation may enhance spontaneous lysis of a thrombus; however, the outcome is not predictably favorable.[1-3]

The end result of ischemic stroke is frequently catastrophic. It is one of the leading causes of death in the United States. It also can produce a severe burden to patients, their families, and society as a whole. Effective treatment of acute stroke is essential to prevent these catastrophic sequelae. This is especially important for those patients with progressive symptoms of a stroke. The use of heparin for the treatment of progressive ischemic stroke has been widespread for the past 30 years. However, 25% to 36% of patients continue to deteriorate while receiving heparin treatment.[47]

The demonstration of an acute thrombosis with angiography performed early in the process (within 12 h) provides a theoretical basis for the use of thrombolytic agents in the treatment of acute stroke. Thrombolytic agents increase the perfusion to the infarct and adjacent cerebral tissue by dissolving the thrombus, and they prevent thrombus propagation. Intravenous systemic thrombolytic therapy has been attempted to treat acute cerebrovascular thromboembolic disease for nearly 20 years, and the results have not been satisfactory. There are high rates of morbidity and mortality associated with intravenous therapy in those series using high doses; those series using low doses of thrombolytic treatment demonstrated no apparent clinical benefit.[36-49] The most recent experience with intravenous t-PA was in a 16-center clinical trial.[50] This trial had unsatisfac-

tory clinical results and unacceptable hemorrhagic complication rates.[50] With recent improvements in catheter techniques, local intraarterial or intra-dural sinus thrombolysis has become acceptable. Different thrombolytic agents have been evaluated, and experience favors UK over SK because of its shorter half-life and fewer systemic effects. In the near future, t-PA will probably be the agent of choice for this application. The timing of thrombolytic treatment of arterial occlusions is somewhat different from that for dural sinus thrombosis. The "golden grace" period for an arterial stroke is a more critical factor than in venous occlusions.[27-30] From our experience, dural sinus thrombosis has a longer grace period before thrombolysis needs to be performed. The initial treatment for acute dural sinus thrombosis is anticoagulation, and thrombolysis is given only if clinical deterioration occurs. However, arterial ischemia requires immediate attention. Thrombolysis should be started within 6 h in order to have the optimal effect.[27,28,40,41,43-47] Once there is obvious edema or hemorrhage, thrombolysis is contraindicated. This is not true with dural sinus thrombosis. Thrombolytic treatments in dural sinus thrombosis are not contraindicated if edema is seen on CT or MRI.

CONCLUSIONS

Until now, there has been little in the way of effective treatment for patients experiencing an acute ischemic stroke. Up to 25% of patients with an acute stroke treated with heparin demonstrate progression of their symptoms during therapy.[47] With the advent of effective fibrinolytic agents and the development of suitable microcatheters, there now appears to be a beneficial treatment strategy available for ischemic stroke patients. It has been shown that in the setting of an evolving acute stroke, rapid intervention with local infusion of these agents can rescue neurons in the ischemic penumbra, reverse or halt the progression of clinical neurologic deficits, and do so with an acceptable local and systemic complication rate. This approach offers a clear advantage over traditional anticoagulation with heparin.

REFERENCES

1. Duke RJ, Block RF, et al. Intravenous heparin for the prevention of stroke progression in acute partial stable stroke: a randomized controlled trial. Ann Intern Med 1986;105:825.
2. Haley EC, Kassell NF, et al. Failure of heparin to prevent progression in progressing ischemic infarction. Stroke 1988;19:10.
3. Slivka A, Levy D. Natural history of progressive ischemic stroke in a population treated with heparin. Stroke 1990;21:1657.
4. Rentrop P, Blanke H, et al. Selective intracoronary thrombolysis in acute myocardial infarction and unstable angina pectoris. Circulation 1981;63:307.
5. Ganz W, Buchbinder N, et al. Intracoronary thrombolysis in evolving myocardial infarction. Am Heart J 1981;101:4.
6. Timmis GC, Gangadharan V, et al. Intracoronary streptokinase in clinical practice. Am Heart J 1982;104:925.
7. Smalling RW, Fuentes F, et al. Beneficial effects of intracoronary thrombolysis up to eighteen hours after onset of pain in evolving myocardial infarction. Am Heart J 1982;104:912.
8. Kennedy JW, Ritchies JL, et al. Western Washington randomized trial of intracoronary streptokinase in acute myocardial infarction. N Engl J Med 1983;309:1477.
9. Leiboff RH, Katz RJ, et al. A randomized, angiographically controlled trial of intracoronary streptokinase in acute myocardial infarction. Am J Cardiol 1984;53:404.
10. TIMI Study Group. Special report: the thrombolysis in myocardial infarction (TIMI) trial. N Engl J Med 1985;312:932.
11. Walsh P, Greenspan RH, et al. Urokinase-pulmonary embolisms trial. Circulation 1978;67 (suppl II):1.
12. Urokinase-streptokinase embolism trial. JAMA 1974;16:1606.
13. Tibbutt DA, Javies JA, et al. Comparison by controlled clinical trial of streptokinase and heparin in treatment of life-threatening pulmonary embolism. Br Med J 1974;1:343.
14. Mavor GE, Dhall DP. Streptokinase therapy in deep-vein thrombosis. Br J Surg 1973;60:468.
15. Kakkar VV, Lewis M, et al. Treatment of deep-vein thrombosis with intermittent streptokinase and plasminogen infusion. Lancet 1975;1:674.
16. Seaman AJ, Common HH, et al. Deep vein thrombosis treated with streptokinase and heparin: a randomized study. Angiology 1976;27:549.
17. Serradimigni A, Bory M, et al. Treatment of venous and pulmonary embolism by streptokinase. Angiology 1978;29:825.
18. D'Angelo A, Mannuci PM. Outcome of treatment of deep-vein thrombosis with urokinase: relationship to dosage, duration of therapy, age of the thrombus and laboratory changes. Thromb Haemost 1984;51:236.
19. Agnelli G, Buchanan MR: A comparison of the thrombolytic and hemorrhagic effects of tissue-type plasminogen activator and streptokinase in rabbits. Circulation 1985;72:178.
20. Risius B, Graor RA, et al. Recombinant human tissue-type plasminogen activator for thrombolysis in peripheral arteries and bypass grafts. Radiology 1986;160:183.
21. Larsen B, Lassen NA. Regulation of cerebral blood flow in health and disease. In: Goldstein M, Bolis L, et al, eds. Advances in neurology. Vol 25. New York: Raven Press, 1979.
22. Solis OJ, Roberson GR, et al. Cerebral angiography in acute cerebral infarction. Rev Int Radiol 1977;2:19.
23. Mohr JP, Caplan LR, et al. The Harvard Cooperative Stroke Registry. Neurology 1978;28:754.
24. Tsai FY, Wadley D, Angle JF, et al. Superselective ophthalmic angiography for diagnostic and therapeutics use. AJNR 1990;11:1203.
25. Chuang S, Harwood-Nash D, Blaser S. Vascular occlusive disease: veins and dural sinuses. In: Taveras J, Ferrucci J, eds. Radiology: diagnosis, imaging, intervention. Vol 2. Philadelphia: JB Lippincott Co, 1992.
26. Rao CVK, Knipp HC, Wagner EJ. Computed tomographic findings in cerebral sinus and venous thrombosis. Radiology 1981;140:391.
27. Siepmann G, Muller-Jensen M, et al. Local intraarterial fibrinolysis in acute middle cerebral artery occlusion. Neuroradiology 1991;33(suppl):69.
28. Zeumer H, Freitag HJ, et al. Intravascular thrombolysis in central nervous system cerebrovascular disease. Neuroimaging Clin North Am 1992;2:359.
29. Tsai FY, Higashida RT, Matovich V, Alfieri KM. Acute thrombosis of the intracranial dural sinus: direct thrombolytic treatment. AJNR 1992;13:1137.
30. Tsai FY, Wang AM, Meoli C, et al. The optimal timing for thrombolytic treatment of acute cranial dural sinus thrombosis. Presented at Annual Meeting of ASNR, St Louis, June 1–5, 1992.
31. Scott JA, Pascuzzi RM, et al. Treatment of dural sinus thrombosis with local urokinase infusion. J Neurosurg 1988;68:284.
32. Higashida RT, Helmer E, et al. Direct thrombolytic therapy for superior sagittal sinus thrombosis. AJNR 1989;10:S4.
33. Eskridge JM, Wessbecher FW. Thrombolysis for superior sagittal sinus thrombosis. J Vasc Intervent Radiol 1991;2:89.

34. Barnwell SL, Higashida R, et al. Direct endovascular thrombolytic therapy for dural sinus thrombosis. Neurosurgery 1991;28:135.

35. Grotta JC. Current medical and surgical therapy for cerebrovascular disease. N Engl J Med 1987; 317:1505.

36. Verstraete M. Biochemical and clinical aspects of thrombolysis. Semin Hematol 1978;15:35.

37. Heimburger N. Basic mechanism of action of streptokinase and urokinase. Thromb Diatherm Haemorr Suppl 1971;47:21.

38. MacFarlane RG, Philling J. Fibrinolytic activity of normal urine: Nature 1974;159:779.

39. Sherry S, Lindemeyer RI, et al. Studies on enhanced fibrinolytic activity in man. J Clin Invest 1959;38:810.

40. Del Zoppo GJ, Ferbert A, et al. Local intraarterial fibrinolytic therapy in acute carotid artery stroke. Stroke 1987;19:307.

41. Hacke W, Del Zoppo GJ, et al. Thrombosis and cerebrovascular disease. In: Poeck U, Ringelstein EB, Hacke W, eds. New trends in diagnosis and management of stroke. Berlin: Springer-Verlag, 1987:59.

42. Thrombolytic therapy in thrombosis. National Institutes of Health Consensus Development Conference. Stroke 1981;12(1):17.

43. Fletcher AP, Alkjaersig N, et al. A pilot study of urokinase therapy in cerebral infarction. Stroke 1976;7:135.

44. Hanaway J, Torak R, et al. Intracranial bleeding associated with urokinase therapy for acute ischemic hemispheral stroke. Stroke 1976;7:143.

45. Mori E, Tabuchi M, et al. Intracarotid urokinase with throboembolic occlusion of the middle cerebral artery. Stroke 1988;19:802.

46. Theron J, Courthroux P, et al. Local intraarteral fibrinolysis in the carotid territory. AJNR 1989; 10:753.

47. Fieschi C, Argentino C, et al. Clinical and instrumental evaluation of patients with ischemic stroke within the first six hours. J Neurol Sci 1989; 91:311.

48. Kakkar VV, Scully MF. Thrombolytic therapy. Br Med Bull 1978;34:191.

49. Sharma GVRK, Cella G, et al. Drug therapy: thrombolytic therapy. N Engl J Med 1982;306: 1268.

50. The rt-PA Acute Stroke Study Group. An open safety/efficacy trial of rt-PA in acute thromboembolic stroke: final report. Stroke 1991;22:153.

Anthony J. Comerota (Ed.). *Thrombolytic Therapy for Peripheral Vascular Disease*. Copyright © 1995 J. B. Lippincott Company.

27

Hemorrhagic Complications of Thrombolytic Therapy

Victor J. Marder

Considered in the context of standard anticoagulant therapy, fibrinolytic agents provide an added dimension in the treatment of thrombosis, namely, a more rapid return to the physiologic state and prevention of immediate and late sequelae of disease. The major problem for the physician is to identify reliably the patient who will benefit from thrombolytic therapy but who is unlikely to suffer a serious hemorrhagic complication. In the past decade, there has been an enormous expansion of interest and application of this approach to thrombotic disease, due primarily to the impressive evidence of survival benefit in patients with acute myocardial infarction (MI). This discussion will consider the hemorrhagic complications attendant to thrombolytic therapy, specifically with regard to practical aspects of drug administration, effects on the blood (lytic state), and laboratory monitoring.

The Agents and Their Mode of Action

The rationale for inducing rapid thrombolysis by administration of plasminogen activators is shown schematically in Figure 27-1. Whatever the distinction between the currently available agents—streptokinase (SK), urokinase (UK), tissue-type plasminogen activator (t-PA), and anistreplase (APSAC)—and the newer agents at various stages of development and testing, they all share the potential for producing greater plasmin action on fibrin contained within the thrombus. Degradation of fibrin produces the beneficial effect of reducing thrombus size (thrombolysis), but at the same time the activators induce the side effect of a plasma proteolytic state (*lytic state*) (Table 27-1), with resultant lysis of hemostatic plugs. The relationship of these three biologic actions remains a controversial issue, especially with regard to the contribution of the lytic state to bleeding. Much of the energy directed toward the development of new plasminogen activators has been directed toward finding *fibrin-specific* agents, i.e., those which minimize the lytic state, as well as toward more potent agents for clot dissolution.

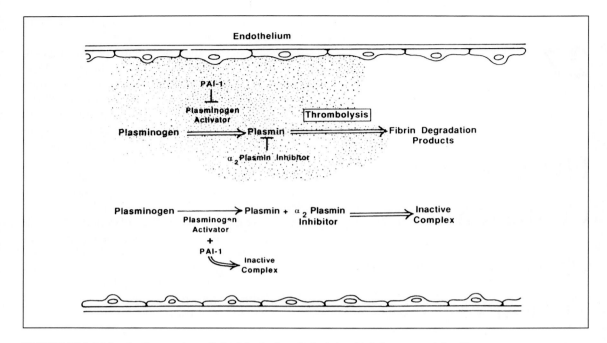

FIGURE 27-1. *Molecular interactions of physiologic thrombolysis in which the process is locally augmented yet systemically inhibited. Plasminogen and plasminogen activator (t-PA, UK, SK:plasmin complex, APSAC) bind to fibrin in the thrombus (shaded area) that is formed adjacent to an area of endothelial cell injury or in an area of vascular stasis. The inhibitors, plasminogen activator inhibitor 1 (PAI-1) and α_2-plasmin inhibitor, are not efficient inhibitors of thrombus-bound plasminogen activators and plasmin. Therefore, fibrin facilitates the conversion of plasminogen to plasmin in the thrombus, which is degraded to soluble fibrin degradation products. Under physiologic conditions in the blood, plasminogen activator (t-PA) and plasmin are efficiently inhibited by PAI-1 and α_2-plasmin inhibitor, and systemic fibrinogenolysis is prevented. However, with infusion of therapeutic quantities of plasminogen activator, virtually all the plasma plasminogen is converted to plasmin, overcoming the neutralizing capacity of antiplasmin and leading eventually to fibrinogenolysis (the lytic state). APSAC has less potential to activate plasma plasminogen than does SK or UK, but at therapeutic dosages, a striking lytic state is produced with all three agents. The "fibrin-specific" agents such as t-PA and scu-PA have the same action, but to a lesser degree, with the result being less prominent fibrinogen degradation. (From Williams et al. Hematology, 5th Ed. New York: McGraw-Hill, in press, with permission.)*

TABLE 27-1. *Principal Biologic Effects of Thrombolytic Therapy*

Effect	Event	Pathogenesis
Clinical benefit	Thrombolysis	Degradation (solubilization) of fibrin in the thrombus
Side effect	Systemic lytic state	Degradation of plasma fibrinogen by circulating plasmin
Complication	Bleeding	Degradation of fibrin in hemostatic plugs (possibly also the hypocoagulable state) adversely influenced by prolonged duration of treatment

From Marder VJ, Francis CW. An assessment of regional versus systemic thrombolytic treatment of peripheral and coronary artery thrombosis. Prog Hemost Thromb 7:325, 1984, with permission.

The plasminogen activators can be classified into three generations, according to their degree of development and clinical usage. The first generation of agents includes those which were the first to be approved by governmental agencies for routine clinical use (SK and UK). Two second-generation agents (t-PA and APSAC) are now approved for clinical use in patients. Prourokinase (single-chain urokinase-type, scu-PA) and all the third-generation agents are still in various stages of development and testing. Each of the plasminogen activators currently approved for clinical use (Table 27-2) possesses inherent advantages and limitations. Agents derived in whole or in part from bacterial sources (SK, APSAC, staphylokinase) will have an unavoidable side effect of allergic reactions, including anaphylaxis, which has required termination of treatment in about 0.1% of cases but has not resulted in a lethal outcome in megatrial reports.[1,2] Side effects such

TABLE 27-2. *Comparison of Thrombolytic Agents Approved for Clinical Use*

	Agent[a]			
	SK	UK[g]	t-PA	APSAC
Purification[b]	Cell culture (*Streptococcus*)	Cell culture (human fetal kidney)	Recombinant	Cell culture (*Streptococcus*) and plasma extraction
Cost[c]	$300	$2000	$2300	$1600
Half-life (min)[d]	23	16	5–8	90
Infusion duration (min)[d]	30–60	5–15	90–180	2–5
Fibrin enhancement[d]	1+	2+	3–4+	1+
Lytic state[d]	4+	3+	1–2+	4+
Thrombus specificity[e]	0	0	0	0
Bleeding complications[e]				
Noncerebral	4.5%	—	5.2%	5.4%
Transfused	0.9%	—	0.8%	1.0%
Cerebral	0.24%	—	0.66%	0.55%
Side effects[f]				
Hypotension, total	11.8%	—	7.1%	12.5%
Hypotension, drug treatment	6.7%	—	4.4%	7.0%
Allergy, total	3.6%	—	0.8%	5.1%
Allergy, persistent	0.3%	—	0.1%	0.5%

[a]SK: Streptase (Astra Pharmaceutical Products, Inc., Westboro, MA) and Kabikinase (Kabi Pharmacia, Piscataway, NJ); UK: Abbokinase (Abbott Laboratories, N. Chicago, IL); t-PA: Activase (Genentech, Inc., S. San Francisco, CA); APSAC: Eminase (SmithKline Beecham Pharmaceuticals, Philadelphia, PA).

[b]UK prepared by recombinant technology is under clinical trial but not yet certified for clinical use. APSAC (anistreplase) prepared by chemical processing (anisoylation) of an SK–human plasmin(ogen) complex. Recombinant t-PA exists as both single-chain (alteplase) and two-chain (duteplase) forms, the current approved agent being primarily of single-chain form. Dosages differ somewhat, with slightly greater amounts of alteplase needed for equivalent thrombolytic potential of duteplase.

[c]For a single intravenous treatment of acute MI, using recommended dosages as noted in the *Physician's Desk Reference*. UK is included for purposes of cost comparison only, since it is approved only for intracoronary administration in such patients.

[d]The agents with long circulation half-lives are administered over shorter infusion times and tend to cause a more potent plasma lytic state (more pronounced hypofibrinogenemia). *Fibrin enhancement* refers to the degree to which the presence of fibrin (or appropriate substrate) accentuates the thrombolytic potential. The agents of high fibrin enhancement react poorly with plasma plasminogen and therefore have a lesser tendency for a plasma lytic state (relative sparing of plasma fibrinogen).

[e]None of the currently approved or investigational plasminogen activators dissolve the thrombus without similarly affecting the hemostatic plug that seals traumatized vessels. Bleeding complications result primarily from lysis of these hemostatic plugs.

[f]Incidence of side effects as recorded in the ISIS-3 Trial[2] which compared SK, t-PA, and APSAC but not UK in the treatment of acute MI. Hypotension requiring drug treatment occurred in 1.5% of patients who were not treated with any plasminogen activator (because of uncertain indication). The incidence of such "profound blood pressure fall" was threefold increased with t-PA, fourfold with SK, and just under fivefold with APSAC. About 60% of instances of hypotension required drug treatment. Only a small proportion of allergic reactions (about 10%) caused persistent symptoms. Anaphylaxis occurred in about 0.1% of patients receiving SK or APSAC, but rarely, patients who received t-PA suffered bronchospasm or angioedema.

[g]Results with UK are limited, but the incidence of bleeding complications and side effects would be expected to approximate the results obtained with t-PA.

as emesis and hypotension occur more frequently with SK and APSAC than with UK and t-PA. A major impetus to the development of new agents has been to avoid the lytic state. To different degrees, this approach has been successful, with each rationale founded on different principles of the molecular mechanisms of fibrinolysis.[3] However, there is a limit to the fibrin specificity of the agents. For example, as the dose and treatment duration of t-PA were steadily increased to find an optimal regimen for dissolving coronary artery thrombi,[4] the threshold for the lytic state was exceeded. Thus the plasma fibrinogen level fell to a mean of 57% in 101 patients treated with rt-PA at a dosage of 0.75 mg/kg/90 minutes, not as severe as the decrease to 7% with SK treatment (1.5 × 10^6 U/60 min), but nevertheless, clearly affecting the blood coagulation proteins.[5,6] An additional distinguishing feature of the agents is their half-life in blood. The most fibrin-specific agents (t-PA and scu-PA) are cleared very rapidly after intravenous injection, with a half-disappearance time of about 5 minutes,[7,8] and induce a milder degree of lytic state. On the contrary, APSAC has relatively low fibrin specificity in comparison with t-PA. Its slow half-deacylation rate of 40 minutes and slow plasma half-disappearance time of 70 minutes[9] allow for long-lasting thrombolytic potential after a short 2- to 5-minute bolus injection, but the lytic state associated with APSAC use is striking. The plasma half-disappearance times of UK and free SK-plasminogen complex are of intermediate duration (16 and 25 minutes, respectively), but the lytic state induced by these agents is closer to that of APSAC than to that of t-PA or scu-PA.

Continued efforts are being made to develop new agents and/or regimens which might have superior pharmacologic properties and clinical benefit over existing ones. For example, a more accelerated dosage schedule of t-PA (100 mg over 60 minutes instead of 90 minutes) induces better coronary artery patency rates after acute MI,[10–12] and this regimen was used in the GUSTO trial.[13] Different SK dosage regimens also have been assessed, but the effects of infusions of 500,000 units to 3 billion units on coronary artery patency have not been in agreement.[14,15] "Short" injections of a thrombolytic agent may be advantageous in

the treatment of acute pulmonary embolism (PE). Thus a "bolus" UK infusion was suggested for PE in the early 1970s,[16,17] and a recent report shows that 2-h infusions of t-PA and UK provide excellent thrombolytic results,[18] equivalent to historical experience with longer infusions of 12 or 24 h of UK or SK.[19] A number of combinations of thrombolytic agents have been proposed and tested, mostly for effects on coronary artery patency. The rationale has generally been to combine t-PA for its rapid, early thrombolytic effect with less-fibrin-specific agents for their longer-lasting effects to prevent reocclusion. Thus half-dose t-PA plus full-dose SK[20] induced a higher patency rate than full-dose t-PA alone (79% versus 64%; $p < 0.05$). However, a similar regimen (90 mg t-PA over 60 minutes plus reduced-dose SK) was shown to be inferior to "front-loaded" t-PA (100 mg over 90 minutes, with the first 50 mg administered over 30 minutes) and no better than SK in the GUSTO mortality trial.[13] None of these innovations has avoided the occurrence of significant hemorrhagic events, as observed with routine dosage regimens.

Inventive approaches to improve on the plasminogen activators provided by nature have produced a plethora of potential agents, primarily by use of molecular biology and chemical fusions of monoclonal antibodies with activators.[21,22] Included in these approaches are mutants of activators, chimeras of two activators, and conjugates of part or all of an activator with a selected antibody that directs its action to a particular substrate. To date, improvements in biochemical parameters that could translate into clinical advantage have been more hopeful than realizable. The conjugation of monoclonal antibodies to activators has been attempted primarily to better direct the thrombolytic activity to a specific substrate, e.g., by binding antifibrin antibody to t-PA,[23] anti-fragment D-dimer to scu-PA,[24] or anti-glycoprotein IIb-IIIa antibody (7E3) to UK.[25] All these exquisite chemical achievements are still to be proven superior to the four approved agents (SK, UK, t-PA, and APSAC). Generally, thrombolytic therapy of venous thromboembolic disease utilizes a plasminogen activator without simultaneous heparin administration, while arterial thrombosis in association with acute MI has been managed with combinations of plasminogen activator and aspirin with or without heparin. The principal reason for a multidrug approach has been to reduce the potential for reocclusion of the coronary artery after discontinuing activator infusion, especially after the use of t-PA,[4,26] and to accelerate vascular reperfusion during the activator infusion, as for the use of SK.[27] The first definitive demonstration of antiplatelet efficacy in the treatment of an acute thrombotic event was the use of a simple aspirin regimen of 160 mg/day for 30 days to decrease mortality after acute MI (ISIS-2),[28] achieved without a significant increase in risk of bleeding complications. Whether the addition of heparin to a regimen of plasminogen activator plus aspirin will further improve the clinical outcome has yet to be definitively determined.[29] However, it seems clear that heparin does increase the incidence of overall hemorrhage as well as that of intracranial hemorrhage.[2,30] The application of adjunctive antiplatelet and antithrombin therapy also depends largely on the type of plasminogen activator utilized. For example, intravenous heparin may be critical to the use of t-PA but of negative value when APSAC is used along with heparin.[31] Newer antithrombotic agents may prove to be superior to heparin and aspirin as adjuncts to plasminogen activator therapy.[32–35] Certainly, there is room for greater efficacy (more rapid lysis and less reocclusion) and fewer complications of a hemorrhagic, thrombocytopenic, and thrombotic nature than occur with heparin. Among these potential antiplatelet agents/approaches, the best studied and perhaps most likely to have significantly increased antithrombotic potential over aspirin is the 7E3 monoclonal antibody against glycoprotein IIb-IIIa fibrinogen receptor.[36] Experience has been obtained in individual patients, for example, to dramatically reverse postangioplasty coronary artery closure[37] and in prospective trials to prevent coronary artery reocclusion after thrombolytic treatment without a significant increase in bleeding complications.

Heparin use requires laboratory monitoring, may allow thrombus extension in some patients, and induces hemorrhagic complications as well as thrombocytopenia and even acute arterial occlusion. Among the potential antithrombotic approaches that could be exploited as a replacement for heparin is the inhibition of thrombin or activated factor X (factor Xa). The agent that is closest to approval for clinical application is hirudin, the highly specific antithrombin derived from the medicinal leech (*Hirudo medicinalis*) salivary gland.[38,39] There is ample evidence in animals that hirudin, hirugen, and hirulog are superior to heparin[40–44] without an increase in bleeding events.

Since factor Xa converts prothrombin to thrombin, it is reasonable to hypothesize that factor Xa inhibitors might be better anticoagulants than inhibitors of thrombin. Nature provides factor Xa inhibitors of great specificity from the salivary gland secretions of blood-sucking animals such as the leech, the tick, and the black fly, all of which synthesize unique anti-factor Xa proteins. Tick anticoagulant peptide (TAP) and antistasin (leech *H. officinalis*) have been cloned,[45,46] and sufficient quantities have been produced to allow their assessment in experimental models. Both hirudin and TAP reperfused vessels twice as quickly as heparin, and TAP was superior to hirudin in preventing reocclusion. Clinical trials are yet to be performed, however, and antidotes are still lacking. The immediate therapy of a bleeding complication due to these agents will have to rely on rapid clearance from the blood and on supportive measures.

MECHANISMS OF ACTION OF THROMBOLYTIC AGENTS

Thrombolytic therapy induces a marked hemostatic defect by means of combined action on blood components, the vessel wall, and the hemostatic plug.[26,50] Hypofibrinogenemia and increased fibrinogen degradation products inhibit fibrin polymerization[51,52] and prolong measures of clotting activity such as the thrombin time. Newly formed fibrin undergoes rapid lysis during hemostatic responses, since activation of plasminogen proceeds efficiently in the presence of nascent fibrin fibrils,[53] essentially rendering the formation of hemostatic plugs useless. Impaired hemostatis also may be caused by dysfunction which is due partly to fibrinogenolysis, since fibrinogen is a necessary cofactor for adenosine diphosphate–induced platelet aggregation.[54] At the same time, activation of plasminogen bound to the platelet[55] leads to impaired adhesion and a decrease in the aggregation response to agonist,[56] and the effects of plasmin formed on the endothelial cell surface[57] and possibly on the subendothelial matrix[58] similarly impair the adhesion of platelets and fibrin in regions of vascular injury. Additionally, plasmin-induced cleavage of fibrin can disrupt the interplatelet matrix and cause platelet disaggregation.[59] During thrombolytic therapy, these actions mediate the dissolution of hemostatic plugs at sites of previous vascular injury. Plasminogen activation on blood and vessel wall components impairs the physiologic response to new vascular injury but also increases the severity and duration of bleeding induced by disintegration of a hemostatic plug.

Information obtained as a result of the clinical use of heparin suggests that a hypocoagulable state is itself well tolerated and an unlikely initiator of bleeding in patients with an intact vascular system—that is, in the absence of such risk factors as recent surgery, duodenal ulcer, thrombocytopenia, or administration of other antithrombotic medication.[60,61] The same is true of the use of defibrinating agents, which induce profound hypofibrinogenemia and a high concentration of fibrin degradation products.[62]

The idea that vascular injury rather than changes in blood coagulation is the main cause of bleeding is supported by three pieces of evidence. First, the principal source of hemorrhage in all studies involving arterial catheterization is the site of invasive procedures,[63,64] and extracranial bleeding was the same for SK and t-PA in the three megatrials comparing these agents.[2,13,30] Second, there is a poor correlation between the extent of hypofibrinogenemia and hemorrhagic events, with bleeding being equally frequent in patients with a marked decrease in fibrinogen concentration and in those with a minimal decrease[65] (see below). Experience with SK in patients with acute MI[66] confirms the previous studies of SK in deep vein thrombosis (DVT)[67] and of SK and UK in pulmonary embolism (PE).[63,68] Third, although the phase I TIMI Study showed a weak correlation between hypofibrinogenemia and the incidence of bleeding, hemorrhagic events were equally com-

mon in those treated with SK and those given t-PA even though fibrinogen levels drop more during treatment with SK than with t-PA (to 43% versus 74% of initial concentration).[66] That the diminished lytic state produced by t-PA fails to protect against bleeding is further confirmed by the frequency of intracranial hemorrhage (ICH) occurring without any drop in plasma fibrinogen.[69]

RISK OF HEMORRHAGE

The risk of hemorrhage caused by thrombolytic therapy is greater than that induced by anticoagulation using heparin and coumarin agents. This increase in risk occurs not only because of the potential for active disruption of previously stable hemostatic plugs but also because the plasminogen activators cause profound changes in blood coagulation that are equal to or exceed those caused by heparin and coumarin.

Determination of the rate of hemorrhagic complication using thrombolytic agents is not straightforward, since several factors may simultaneously contribute to the risk of bleeding. First, patients may manifest underlying conditions that predispose to bleeding, such as recent surgery, advanced age, coexisting pathologic lesions such as duodenal ulcer, or additional antithrombotic treatment. Second, the duration of exposure to thrombolytic treatment varies not only for a given indication (contrast the 12 h of SK used for treating acute MI in 1975[70] with the 1 h of SK used in 1986[71]) but also for thrombotic occlusions at different sites. A considerably longer treatment interval of 12 to 24 h has been used for PE[63,68] (although recent trials have used only 2 h of t-PA or UK[72]) and up to 4 to 6 days for DVT,[73] as opposed to the several minutes to 3 h now used for acute MI.[26] Third, small studies that have used invasive vascular procedures have reported high rates of bleeding in patients with acute PE and acute MI.[26] Fourth, small studies that emphasize invasive vascular procedures and hematologic measurements will necessarily differ from large-scale clinical trials of mortality. The former studies[63,64] provided detailed observations and used procedures that predispose to hemorrhagic complications, while the latter reflected general clinical practice with an emphasis on major endpoints of benefit (survival) and risk (transfusion, stroke).[1,2,28,30,74,75]

Table 27-3 records the incidence of bleeding complications in five large trials of 1000 or more patients which assessed the value and side effects of a thrombolytic agent relative to "standard" treatment (at that time, without a thrombolytic agent) in patients with acute MI. All the trials allowed a comparison of bleeding risk with a control (nonthrombolytic) group of patients that was largely, though not invariably, treated with anticoagulants and/or aspirin. The rate of bleeding complications was invariably greater in the thrombolytic groups, for overall bleeding (4–8% versus 1–2%), "severe" bleeding (0.4–2% versus 0–1.8%), and intracranial hemorrhage (ICH) (0.1–1.0% versus 0–0.3%).

A direct comparison of thrombolytic with anticoagulant hemorrhagic risk can be inferred from results of the UPET data, which compared UK followed by heparin with UK therapy alone in patients with acute PE[63] (Table 27-4). In this trial of 160 patients, the overall incidence of hemorrhage in the UK group was about twice that in the non-UK group (45% versus 27%), with most of the bleeding occurring at vascular injury sites and during the first 24 h of observation. After elimination of "nonmeaningful" bleeding (see notes to Table 27-4), the incidence was reduced significantly by 80% or more, but the hemorrhagic rate was still twice as high in the UK group (9% versus 4%). The data suggest that the thrombolytic agent causes a higher incidence and more significant bleeding in treated patients, both spontaneously from remote sites and from vascular invasion sites such as that which follows phlebotomy, arteriotomy, or intramuscular injection. These results are supported by a conglomerate analysis in patients receiving SK or heparin treatment for DVT, which suggests a three-fold increased risk of bleeding in those patients receiving SK.[76]

The incidence of major bleeding complications appears to be higher in all "invasive" studies, whatever the duration of therapy—witness the rates of 15% to 30% in patients undergoing coronary angiography after thrombolytic treatment for acute MI[77–80] and the equivalent rates in the invasive trials in patients with PE.[63,68] As to whether the length of treatment represents an independent risk factor for thrombolytic bleeding, there are no trials that have been designed to specifically test this question. The results from large-scale, noninvasive trials of MI and DVT suggest a lower incidence of severe bleeding with the shorter duration of therapy used for MI than for DVT[67] (0–10% versus 5–30%), but no clear-cut

TABLE 27-3. *Bleeding Complications in Large Studies of Thrombolytic Treatment (vs placebo) in Patients with Acute MI**

Study	Year	Agent	No. of Patients	Bleeding Complications (%)		
				Overall	Severe	ICH
ISAM[102]	1986	SK	859	5.9	—	0.5
		Control	882	1.5	—	0
GISSI[1]	1986	SK	5860	3.6	0.4	0.1[†]
		Control	5852	—	—	0
ISIS-2[28]	1988	SK	8592	4.0	0.6	0.1
		Control	8595	1.2	0.2	0
ASSET[100]	1988	rt-PA	2516	7.6	1.4	0.3
		Control	2495	0.8	0.5	0.1
AI[101]	1990	APSAC	624	13.8	4.2	0.3
		Control	634	4.1	2.4	0.16

* Large trials include those of 1000 patients or larger, in which active agent administered over 5 minutes to 3 h duration was compared prospectively with a control group treated without a thrombolytic agent. The control groups received anticoagulation according to local practice considerations, which differed for these studies. "Severe" bleeding complications included those requiring blood transfusion and intracranial hemorrhage (ICH) but excluded hematuria, hemoptysis, ecchymoses, or GI bleeding or at a vascular invasive site that did not require replacement transfusion. Dash marks (—) indicate that the information is not available in the report.
† Total CVA reported to be 0.2% in SK-treated groups, 50% of which are assumed to represent ICH.

TABLE 27-4. Bleeding Associated with Fibrinolytic or Heparin Therapy of Pulmonary Embolism*

	Heparin (78)		Urokinase (82)	
	Severe	Moderate	Severe	Moderate
Early overt bleeding	6	4	14	15
Late overt bleeding	6	6	8	0
Location				
Cutdown	5	3	8	13
Gastrointestinal	3	3	6	0
Retroperitoneal	3	2	1	0
Intramuscular	1	0	3	0
Other	0	2	4	2
Total incidence	27%		45%	
Meaningful incidence	4%		9%	

* *Meaningful* bleeding is defined as that occurring during the initial 12- or 24-h infusion of drug and serious enough to cause discontinuation of therapy, replacement transfusion, or a drop in hematocrit of greater than 5%.

conclusion can be drawn from these noncomparable studies.

Comparison of Thrombolytic Agents

A number of trials provide information on the rate of major hemorrhage (requiring transfusion and/or a life-threatening bleed) in patients with acute MI who were randomized to treatment comparing two thrombolytic agents.[2,64,71,74,75,81–89] There was a wide range of sample size, adjunctive antithrombotic treatment, and therapeutic approach (invasive versus noninvasive) in these trials. In most studies, the incidence of major bleeds was the same for the two or three thrombolytic agents compared. Thus the rate of hemorrhage was identical for SK and t-PA in five trials,[64,71,86,87,90] for SK and APSAC in two trials,[2,85] for APSAC and t-PA,[2,89] and for t-PA and UK.[81,83] In studies with demonstrated differences, t-PA had fewer major bleeding episodes than APSAC[83,88] and SK,[74,75] and pro-UK had less than SK.[82] Overall, there was little to choose between the bleeding risk of different agents (see Table 27-1), and greater differences occurred between studies than between agents.

Intracranial hemorrhage (ICH) has occurred more frequently in patients who received t-PA or APSAC rather than SK, best illustrated by the ISIS-3 data[2] (see Table 27-1) but supported by many other studies (see refs. 69 and 91–95 for summaries) in which 100 or more patients received thrombolytic agents for acute MI.[2,28,64,74,75,77–86,88,96–115] The combined ISG/GISSI-2[74,75,114] and ISIS-3[2] data indicate a statistically significant increase in total cerebrovascular accidents (CVAs) (1.35% versus 1.0%; $p < 0.001$) and ICH (0.6% versus 0.3%; $p = 0.06$) in patients receiving t-PA rather than SK, and ISIS-3[2] indicates a similarly increased rate for APSAC over SK for CVA (1.26% versus 1.04%; $p = 0.08$) and for ICH (0.55% versus 0.24%; $p = 0.0001$). The summary frequencies noted in the many other trials (including the megatrials) do not alter these trends, namely, a consistently lower frequency of ICH for SK, between 0% and 0.5% (0.2% in 40,712 patients), and higher rates (0% to 2.0%) for both t-PA (0.6% in 31,936 patients) and APSAC (0% to 1.9%) (0.6% in 21,185 patients). The increased incidence of ICH is therefore approximately 4 in 1000 patients treated with t-PA or APSAC rather than SK. Results for UK and pro-UK are limited, indicating only that ICH does occur, but the rates relative to SK cannot be stated with confidence. The lower incidence of ICH with SK was independent of adjunctive therapies, whether these were developed to maximize thrombolytic potential,[83] to limit hemorrhagic risk,[74,75] or to mimic standard antithrombotic use in Europe[2] or in the United States.[79]

Several other aspects of ICH besides that related to the specific thrombolytic agent utilized are worth separate mention. First, the duration of treatment may increase the risk of such bleeding. This tentative conclusion is based on the overall expectation of ICH in approximately 1% of patients receiving SK for DVT or PE,[116] as contrasted with a rate of 0.2% in more than 40,000 patients with acute MI who received a shorter course of SK treatment.

Second, the dose of agent may influence the rate of ICH. This is less apparent for modern therapeutic dosages of SK, all of which clearly exceed the amount required to overcome antistreptococcal antibodies[117,118] than is the case for t-PA, which has a more evident dose-response relationship for thrombolysis[4,119,120] and for which 150 mg (two-chain form) induces ICH at a higher rate than does 100 mg (1.6% versus 0.6%)[121,122] (1.3% versus 0.4%; $p < 0.01$).[96]

Third, advanced age increases the risk of CVA and ICH resulting from thrombolytic treatment.[2,74,75,95,96,114] The ISG/GISSI-2[114] data show a higher overall CVA rate with t-PA than with SK (1.3% versus 0.9%; $p = 0.008$), the difference being largely due to the very high rate in elderly patients (2.6% versus 1.6%). The difference in total CVAs between t-PA and SK holds as well for ICH (0.7% versus 0.3% for elderly patients), but similar rates (0.4% versus 0.3%) are seen in patients under age 70. The data from ISIS-3 and GUSTO also show a higher rate of ICH for t-PA than SK, especially in patients over 70 years of age (1.16% versus 0.25%; $p < 0.00001$).[2,13] Interestingly, the rate of ICH after SK was the same for both age groups (0.23% versus 0.25%).[114]

Fourth, while treated hypertension represents a potential but uncertain added risk of ICH,[114] a positive history of transient ischemic attack or CVA in a patient undergoing thrombolytic treatment with t-PA significantly increases the risk of ICH (3.4% versus 0.5%; $p = 0.01$).[96]

Fifth, the ISIS-3 trial used anticoagulant treatment with subcutaneous heparin every 12 h beginning at 4 h after the start of thrombolytic treatment, in addition to daily aspirin, and the incidence of ICH was increased slightly from 0.4% to 0.56% ($p < 0.005$).[2]

Sixth, while hypofibrinogenemia may be marked in some patients with ICH treated with either SK[116] or t-PA,[69] this laboratory manifestation of thrombolytic treatment is not useful as a predictor of ICH. For example, there is no difference in plasma fibrinogen concentration in patients manifesting either a cerebral infarction or an ICH after 100 mg of t-PA treatment,[115] and 3 of 4 patients with ICH in the ECSG trial[105] who had fibrinogen values determined showed no change at 2 or 24 h after the start of t-PA.

Seventh, while combination therapy, for example, with t-PA plus UK (TAMI-5),[83] has a low rate of ICH (none of 194 patients), the results in other similar trials have shown rates of 1.5% (2 of 132 patients)[123] and 5% (2 of 42 patients).[111] Results in the t-PA/SK combination in the GUSTO trial[13] document this increased risk of ICH, higher than with SK or t-PA alone.

Last, the clinical course of patients who suffer a CVA during or after thrombolytic treatment with any plasminogen activator is generally the following: half die of the CVA, one-quarter have permanent disability, and one-quarter recover without disability.[2]

Combined Heparin Anticoagulation with Thrombolytic Therapy

The contribution of heparin to the incidence of bleeding during the first day after initiation of thrombolytic treatment is best documented in the ISIS-3 report, which used (in addition to aspirin) a modest 12-h subcutaneous heparin regimen beginning at 4 h after the start of SK, t-PA, or APSAC treatment.[2] The effect on the rate of total CVA was nil (1.28% versus 1.18%), but the incidence of ICH was slightly but significantly increased (0.56% versus 0.4%; $p < 0.05$). The incidence of ICH was lower with SK than with t-PA or APSAC in both the aspirin and the aspirin plus subcutaneous heparin groups.[2] This difference was not apparent in ISG/GISSI-2 (0.4% versus 0.3%; $p = $ NS), perhaps because the subcutaneous heparin was delayed until 12 h after the start of thrombolytic treatment.[114] The overall incidence of bleeding showed a clear-cut effect of added heparin being associated with bleeding that required transfusion approximately 30% more often (0.7% versus 1.0%).[74,75,114] In the GUSTO Study,[13] the rates of hemorrhagic stroke were 0.49% in the SK/SC heparin group, 0.54% in the SK/IV heparin group, and 0.072% in the t-PA group, representing a significant excess of events in patients treated with t-PA compared with SK. Although there was no difference in hemorrhagic stroke in SK patients treated with either subcutaneous (SC) or intravenous (IV) heparin, a significant number of patients randomized to receive subcutaneous heparin actually received IV heparin (26% on day 1 in the United States). Thus the effect of IV heparin on the rate of intracranial hemorrhage in patients receiving SK awaits detailed analysis of these data. Since GUSTO did not include a t-PA arm without IV heparin, the issue of an increase in intracranial hemorrhage due to IV versus SC heparin in t-PA–treated patients cannot yet be answered.[13]

OTHER COMPLICATIONS AND SIDE EFFECTS

Table 27-1 indicates the incidence of allergic and hypotensive reactions to SK, t-PA, and APSAC, as reported in the ISIS-3 Study.[2] Allergic reactions were 4 to 6 times more frequent with SK or APSAC than with t-PA, and persistent symptoms of allergic reaction occurred 3 times more often with SK and 5 times more often with APSAC than with t-PA. One possible explanation for the higher incidence with APSAC is that early symptoms could not be curtailed by slowing or discontinuing the bolus injection. Of interest was the occurrence of allergic symptoms in 0.8% (0.1% persistent) of patients receiving t-PA, consistent with rare reports of bronchospasm[124] and angioneurotic edema[125] in patients receiving t-PA. The allergic manifestations following SK or APSAC treatment have not been lethal, nor have they influenced overall mortality.

The second major side effect of thrombolytic treatment is hypotension, especially in those with acute MI, occurring in approximately 12% of those exposed to SK or APSAC and 7% of those exposed to t-PA. Somewhat more than half of these patients require drug therapy for the hypotensive episode, 7% for SK and APSAC and just over 4% for t-PA. The observation relative to t-PA probably represents an effect of the drug itself rather than the underlying acute MI, since only 1.5% of patients not treated with a thrombolytic agent had this reaction.[2]

Two serious complications that have been linked to thrombolytic therapy deserve special mention. First, cardiac rupture occurs infrequently but regularly in 3% to 4% of patients admitted with acute MI but may occur more commonly in patients treated with thrombolytic agents. This conclusion was reached by a retrospective analysis of thrombolytic trials that linked late treatment (delay more than 12 h) with a higher propensity for cardiac rupture,[126] but the data are not nearly conclusive, and the assumptions, calculations, and association have been challenged.[127] The second unusual complication is that of cholesterol crystal embolization, usually occurring in the setting of severe and extensive preexisting atherosclerotic disease.[128]

SELECTION OF PATIENTS

The absolute contraindications to fibrinolytic therapy are those which may result in intracranial hemorrhage or massive, life-threatening hemorrhage (Table 27-5). Although patients with thrombotic CVAs have been treated successfully with fibrinolytic agents, the possibility exists that

TABLE 27-5. Absolute Contraindications to Fibrinolytic Therapy

Risk	Condition
Intracranial bleeding	Hemorrhagic cerebrovascular accident, intracranial neoplasm, recent cranial surgery or trauma (10 days), uncontrolled severe hypertension
Massive hemorrhage	Major surgery of thorax or abdomen (10 days), prolonged cardiopulmonary resuscitation, current severe bleeding (e.g., gastrointestinal)

hemorrhage may result from an unrecognized small hemorrhagic locus, and patients with a history of neurologic disease such as transient ischemic attack or a prior nonhemorrhagic stroke are at increased risk of ICH as a result of thrombolytic therapy.[96] Patients with recent head trauma or with an intracranial neoplasm have an increased risk of a fatal complication secondary to ICH. The risk of major bleeding such as that following recent surgery of the head, thorax, or abdomen or after prolonged and difficult cardiopulmonary resuscitation (CPR) likewise is to be avoided,[129] as is the risk with currently active major bleeding sites such as duodenal ulcers. The risk of serious bleeding due to CPR is probably less than feared, the actual incidence of such events being virtually nil in 102 patients so managed, especially when CPR lasts less than 10 minutes.[130,131] Some patients with obvious life-threatening thrombotic disease (e.g., massive pulmonary embolism with profound shock or a large anterior wall MI) may warrant potentially lifesaving thrombolytic therapy even in the face of serious contraindications.

Bleeding is sometimes unavoidable, but many instances are preventable by careful selection of patients and by avoiding trauma to the patient once treatment is instituted. Clinical situations that might be associated with an increased risk of bleeding include slight abnormalities of hemostasis discovered by screening coagulation studies, recent superficial wounds or an invasive arteriotomy or venotomy, the postpartum state, minor surgical or biopsy procedures, and patients with a history of gastrointestinal or genitourinary tract bleeding. Most instances of bleeding in these situations are neither life-threatening nor difficult to control, and these predisposing conditions are relevant to both heparin and thrombolytic therapy. Therefore, the risks of minor bleeding or even of the possible need to transfuse blood after external loss of blood or bleeding into a nonvital area are not absolute contraindications to the use of fibrinolytic agents. Decisions regarding their use must be weighed against the expected severity of the complication, with the indication and potential benefit associated with accelerated thrombolysis.

Elderly Patients

Since some of the early large trials in patients with acute MI excluded patients who were elderly (>70 years), a misconception arose that advanced age was a strong contraindication to therapy.[132] While the elderly do have a higher risk of bleeding, especially ICH, they also have a much higher risk of death from the acute MI. Therefore, the survival benefit in patients older than age 70 is much greater (80 lives saved per 1000 treated) than it is in patients under 60 years of age (25 lives saved per 1000 treated).[1,28] The importance of treating the elderly, after taking into account risk factors that may preclude therapy, has been emphasized by several groups recently.[133–136]

EMBOLIC PHENOMENA

Special consideration should be given to the question of embolic phenomena induced by thrombolytic therapy. This is not an unreasonable concern, but careful distinction should be made as to whether the underlying thrombotic disorder is of venous or arterial origin, since the risks are significantly different. The UPET Study[63] showed a presumed recurrence rate for pulmonary embolus of about 15% with either UK or heparin, but this conclusion was verified only by lung scan and not by repeat pulmonary angiography. Despite an enormous literature on the therapy of deep vein thrombosis and pulmonary embolus with SK or UK, the number of cases of fatal embolus associated with such treatment is minuscule.[137]

The opposite may be true for thrombolytic therapy of arterial thromboembolic disease. In this situation, the possibility that an initial embolic event would be followed by a subsequent embolus (e.g., from an intracardiac source) or that a reopened high-flow arterial system would dislodge part of an existing thrombus seems more realistic. One case report[138] describes a nonlethal cerebral artery embolus during therapy of two peripheral arterial emboli. The new embolus occurred 36 h into therapy, which was continued despite the event, and presumably originated from the "same detached intracardiac thrombus."

This possibility should be considered and in some cases evaluated by appropriate echocardiographic study of the heart chambers and valves, but the actual incidence is quite low, and treatment may be required even in the presence of documented thrombus. More common is distal embolization of known arterial thromboemboli,[139–144] occurring in up to 10% of cases.[141] The event is manifested by sudden new ischemia of the distal portion of the limb, but continued local thrombolytic administration is almost invariably successful in dissolving the embolus.

TREATMENT OF BLEEDING

Termination of treatment may be necessitated by allergic or pyrogenic side effects or by a hemorrhagic complication. The former are managed by immediately discontinuing drug administration, specific measures such as corticosteroids, antihistamines, or adrenergic agents for anaphylaxis, and antipyretics to counteract fever. Minor bleeding need not be an indication to stop therapy. For instance, bleeding from superficial wounds usually can be controlled by local measures such as manual pressure or pressure dressings. Hematoma formation in the region of an arteriotomy may reach significant proportions that require blood replacement, but seldom are these severe enough to require curtailment of fibrinolytic treatment. In patients who have life-threatening bleeding or who have sudden emergencies that require surgical intervention, normal hemostasis can quickly be reestablished by discontinuing administration of the activator and replenishing plasma fibrinogen by the infusion of either whole plasma or cryoprecipitate and by providing fresh platelets to supplement those which have been exposed to the plasminogen activator or to aspirin. The activator is cleared rapidly, but if clearance is not complete, it can be neutralized by ϵ = aminocaproic acid (5 g IV over 20 to 30 minutes, then 1 g/h as needed).

A limited number of reports on postthrombolytic surgical intervention exist,[145–149] but controlled studies of management are not available. Clinical studies indicate that an operation can be performed immediately after SK therapy but that it results in increased bleeding and more transfusions compared with operations on patients who had not undergone prior thrombolytic therapy. Similar results apply to invasive procedures after t-PA treatment.[78] Judging by the progress of the hypocoagulable state (Fig. 27-2) induced by plasminogen activators,[150–152] it would not be unrea-

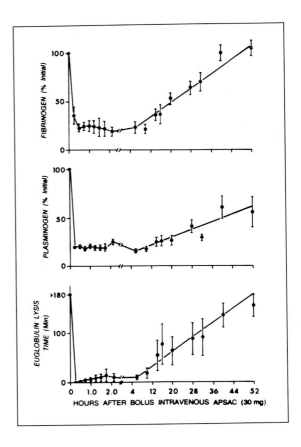

FIGURE 27-2. Plasma euglobulin lysis time and plasminogen and fibrinogen concentrations measured before (time 0) and after treatment with 30 mg of anisoylated plasminogen–streptokinase activator complex (APSAC). Values are mean ± SE obtained for all 15 patients in this group; the lines starting at the 6-h values were calculated by least-squares fit. (Reprinted with permission from Marder VJ, Rothbard RL, Fitzpatrick PG, Francis CW. Rapid lysis of coronary artery thrombi with anisoylated plasminogen:streptokinase activator complex: treatment by bolus intravenous injection. Ann Intern Med 104:304, 1986.)

TABLE 27-6. *Management of Hypocoagulable State Induced by Plasminogen Activators*

	During Treatment	Immediately After Treatment	6–36 Hours Later
Plasma fibrinogen	Low	Nadir	Progressive recovery
Need for cryoprecipitate	Yes	Yes	Yes
Platelet function	Abnormal	Abnormal	Abnormal
Need for platelets	Yes	Yes	Yes
Circulating activator	Present	Variable duration	Absent
Need for antifibrinolytic agent	Yes	Yes	Yes

sonable if cryoprecipitate replacement were needed routinely during plasminogen activator infusion as well as during the recovery phase, perhaps until more than 50% of the initial fibrinogen concentration has been recovered. In addition, antifibrinolytic therapy should be administered prophylactically if activator is still present in the blood, an expected situation for variable times after the infusion is stopped[153] (see Table 27-1). Since platelet function can be deranged by cleavage of membrane receptors or inhibition of biochemical reactions by circulating activators or by aspirin,[33] transfusion of platelets in patients with current or anticipated serious bleeding problems is reasonable. Care must be taken to normalize the coagulation status after treatment regardless of the activator used, since levels of fibrinogen regularly decrease to below 50% of initial levels even after t-PA,[154] and the molecular structure of clottable protein[155] indicates that little or no intact fibrinogen circulates during therapy with SK[151] or t-PA[152] (Table 27-6).

LYTIC STATE

Hypofibrinogenemia

Figure 27-1 summarizes the physiology of activation of plasma plasminogen and of plasminogen bound to fibrin. SK and UK have equal propensity for both forms, while APSAC and especially t-PA and scu-PA tend to favor fibrin-bound plasminogen, inducing fibrin degradation while limiting the lytic state. The lytic state is a general description of the effects of plasmin activity in the circulation,[51,156,157] but there is disagreement on a precise definition. The reason for this is the number of reactions that result from plasminogen activator administration and the variety of laboratory parameters that could reflect the presence of activator in the blood. The sequence of events starts with a shortening of the whole-blood or plasma euglobulin lysis time, which measures primarily free activator separated from plasma inhibitors (Table 27-7). A hypocoagulable state is the final stage, manifested principally by prolongation of screening coagulation tests, such as the thrombin time. Between these two landmarks are intervening events that reflect the progression of the fibri-

TABLE 27-7. *Development of the Plasma Proteolytic State*

Biochemical Step	Laboratory Parameter
Circulating plasminogen activator	Short euglobulin lysis time
Plasminogen converted to plasmin	Decreased plasminogen
Antiplasmin complexes with and inhibits plasmin	Plasmin-antiplasmin complexes, decreased antiplasmin
Free plasmin	Increased fibrin lysis or chromogenic substrate (S-2251) activity
Plasmin degradation of fibrinogen	Decreased clottable protein, circulating fibrinogen/fibrin degradation products
Degradation of other plasma clotting factors	Decreased Factors V and VIII
Hypocoagulable state	Prolonged thrombin time

From Marder VJ, Francis CW. An assessment of regional versus systemic thrombolytic treatment of peripheral and coronary artery thrombosis. Prog Hemost Thromb 7:325, 1984, by permission.

nolytic cascade, and the lytic state can be monitored with an assay that measures any aspect of the biochemical sequence. Thus various reports have utilized a combination of a short euglobulin lysis time (to 30 minutes or less) plus a 50% decrease in plasma plasminogen,[63] a striking (>50%) decrease in antiplasmin or plasma fibrinogen,[158] or simply a prolongation of the thrombin time beyond the normal range[116] to document the presence of a lytic state. It might be best to limit the definition of the lytic state to a decrease in plasma fibrinogen, specifically the quantity of thrombin-clottable protein,[159] since this is the most relevant substrate for plasmin once it has overcome the antiplasmin inhibition (Fig. 27-2). Since hemostatic plug dissolution and fibrinolytic hemorrhagic can occur with a minimal lytic state, even a 10% to 20% drop in plasma fibrinogen concentration would be an important documentation of the lytic state.[50] Whether supplemental plasmin inhibitor will have a clinical effect as well as an effect on blood coagulation assays[160] remains to be determined, although animal studies suggest a selective effect to decrease bleeding without inhibiting thrombolysis.[161]

Platelets

Free plasmin also affects platelet function, specifically to decrease aggregation induced by adenosine diphosphate (ADP), thrombin, and collagen.[59,162,163] In addition, plasmin cleaves membrane glycoprotein Ib, which includes the binding site for von Willebrand factor,[164] and reduces ristocetin-induced platelet aggregation.[165] Although this cleavage could affect hemostasis adversely, evidence for this is limited and inconclusive (see below).[166]

However, the effect of plasminogen activators on platelets is not a straightforward decrease in functional integrity. In fact, the reactions are complex and variable with time and type of activator,[167] and both platelet hyperactivity and hypoactivity may occur in the same subject.[168] It is likely that the activators (SK and t-PA) promote hyperaggregability[169] with initial exposure to platelets and that, after a variable interval, the platelets are rendered hypoaggregable.[168,170] This sequence of

events could have relevance for both reocclusion and bleeding, depending on the state of reactivity of the platelets.

The hyperreactive state of platelets could contribute to thrombotic problems attendant on therapy by promoting thrombin generation, such as has been noted for t-PA exposure in vitro and in patient samples.[171,172] Independently or as a consequence of platelet activation, thrombin action on fibrinogen can occur in patients receiving thrombolytic treatment with either fibrin-specific (t-PA) or nonspecific (SK) agents.[173,174]

PREDICTIVE VALUE OF LABORATORY CHANGES

General

The actions of plasminogen activator in the blood and the thrombus are best considered as parallel but separate events in either a fluid- or solid-phase reaction system.[156] Assuming that an adequate dose of activator has been administered, successful dissolution of the pathologic thrombus by fibrin degradation does not correlate with the extent of fibrinogenolysis. Likewise, bleeding probably results from disruption of a hemostatic plug rather than from changes in the hemostatic parameters in the blood[50] (see Table 27-1). The hypocoagulable state is a potential contributor to bleeding over and above what is induced by dissolution of hemostatic plugs. This is a controversial issue that is most relevant for the second-generation plasminogen activators, which have the potential for thrombolysis without a lytic state. If bleeding is due solely to lysis of hemostatic plugs by the plasminogen activator, then the fibrin-specific agents would still cause bleeding complications even in the absence of a lytic state. On the other hand, if the hypocoagulable state contributes to bleeding, then the fibrin-specific agents would be safer to use. It is now clear that the established clinical precautions to avoid serious and catastrophic bleeding pertain for any fibrinolytic agent used in humans[116] (see Table 27-1).

The relevance of laboratory changes for clinical events is a complex issue, since the endpoints may not be surrogates for clinical events, and value judgments regarding a hemorrhagic complication can influence the conclusion, e.g., whether a small hematoma is an indication of bleeding or an unimportant event that can be disregarded.

Tests

The lytic state can be monitored by any of a number of laboratory assays (see Table 27-7). The presence of free plasmin in the blood can be measured by chromogenic assay[175] or by lysis assays, such as the shortening of whole-blood or plasma euglobulin lysis times, fibrin plate assays, or radioactive fibrin clot lysis. The concentration of plasma inhibitors of plasmin decreases consequent to their binding with the free enzyme, and this change can be measured by immunologic or functional tests. Plasmin degrades fibrinogen, resulting in a decrease in the concentration of thrombin–clottable protein and the appearance of increased concentrations of fibrinogen and cross-linked fibrin degradation products.[176] Both these latter effects influence the screening tests of coagulation, especially the thrombin time. By far the simplest and most widely recommended assay is the thrombin time, a test that provides a rapid indication of the functional state of fibrinogen and

the presence of anticoagulant degradation products that inhibit its conversion to fibrin.[177] Heparin also prolongs the thrombin time, so the fibrinogen concentration is better determined by a clottable protein assay[159] to assess the functional state of fibrinogen and clottable plasmic derivatives[177] than by the "Clauss" technique,[178] which depends on a thrombin time measurement, or by a chemical precipitation method[179] which detects some large, nonclottable plasmic derivatives in addition to fibrinogen and clottable derivatives.

Figure 27-3 illustrates how fibrinogen could be acted on by thrombin, plasmin, and/or factor XIII to produce circulating derivatives that would reflect the biochemical action. Thus fibrinogen degradation products or a decrease in plasma fibrinogen concentration could reflect the lytic state, an increased concentration of fibrinopeptides or soluble fibrin could reflect a prothrombotic tendency, and plasmin action on fibrin could produce cross-linked degradation products (D-dimer). Theoretically, the measure of fibrinogen could predict a bleeding complication, fibrinopeptide A could reflect clot growth or vascular reocclusion, and D-dimer could reflect vascular reperfusion. Unfortunately, the data do not support these predictions, although some progress toward this end has been made, and

FIGURE 27-3. *Schematic representation of biochemical actions of thrombin, plasmin, and factor XIII or combinations of these enzymes on fibrinogen and fibrin substrates as a foundation for laboratory monitoring of clinical events. See text for details.*

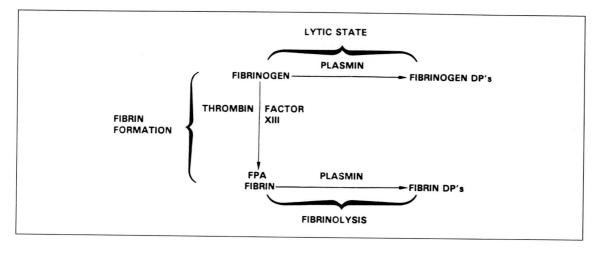

detailed analyses of laboratory results have been reported.[50,180–183]

Relation of Laboratory Findings to Bleeding

Although patients who receive thrombolytic agents are at risk of bleeding, such complications are at best only weakly correlated with laboratory parameters of the lytic state. Thus patients with a demonstrated lytic state but without susceptible hemostatic plugs usually have a therapeutic course that is unmarked by bleeding complication. Conclusions in patients with deep vein thrombosis[67] and pulmonary embolism[63] indicate that none of the laboratory results (fibrinogen concentration, plasminogen, euglobulin lysis time) has a significant correlation for a hemorrhagic occurrence in patients treated with SK or UK. Furthermore, no laboratory parameter has been shown to be useful as a predictor of bleeding. Similarly, intracoronary SK usage in patients with acute MI caused laboratory changes of plasma fibrinogen concentration that were no different in patients who did or did not have a bleeding complication,[184] and intravenous SK treatment induced the same lack of correlation.[181,182] Although a fall in fibrinogen has been reported in association with bleeding following t-PA treatment, the association has been weak[181,185] or inconsistent[183] and is of no predictive value. Of great relevance is the analysis which showed no difference in fibrinogen concentration in patients who suffered an ICH or a cerebral infarction after t-PA treatment for acute MI.[96]

In the report by Stump et al.,[182] a lower nadir fibrinogen concentration (100 versus 130 mg/dL; $p = 0.066$) and higher peak fibrin degradation product concentration (300 versus 280 μg/mL; $p = 0.081$) were noted in patients with major bleeding episodes. However, the difference between values noted in bleeders and nonbleeders was small, and neither the fibrinogen nor the fibrin degradation product concentration has a predictive value. By contrast, there was a striking difference in plasma t-PA antigen concentration (3.4 versus 2.2 μg/mL; $p = 0.002$). The higher value noted in bleeders suggests a direct effect of t-PA

on susceptible hemostatic plugs and vascular abnormalities that could lead directly to bleeding, independent of the effect on the blood. Such a scenario also would help to explain the higher rate of ICH with 150 versus 100 mg of t-PA,[121,122] independent of any difference in plasma fibrinogen concentration.[96] These findings are all in support of the concept illustrated in Table 27-1, in which bleeding is considered as an independent outcome of plasminogen activator effect occurring in a distinctly different vascular location from events in the blood.[50]

Limited information is available on the evaluation of the template bleeding time[186] as a predictor of hemorrhage. One report concludes that there is a significant correlation of a prolonged bleeding time (equal to or greater than 9 minutes) with spontaneous bleeding,[166] but no convincing information is provided that a prolonged bleeding time is a useful predictor for a clinically important bleeding event.

Relation of Laboratory Findings to Thrombolysis

Laboratory results clearly do not correlate with thrombolysis (vascular patency). For instance, the UPET Study,[63] which administered a large systemic dose of UK, showed no correlation of laboratory results with shrinkage of the embolus, as measured by change in physiologic, angiographic, or lung perfusion parameters. Two trials in DVT showed a lack of correlation of venographic change after 3 days of large-dose systemic therapy with changes in fibrinogen, thrombin time, plasminogen, or fibrin(ogen) degradation products.[67,187] A more limited dose of SK by the intracoronary route for treatment of MI showed no difference in the degree of change in plasma fibrinogen or concentration of degradation products in patients who did or did not reperfuse.[188] More recent analyses of patients with acute MI receiving t-PA support this contention that neither the nadir fibrinogen concentration nor the concentration of fibrin degradation products correlates with posttreatment coronary artery patency.[182] Although there is not universal agreement on this issue,[189] it seems that with the administration of SK, UK, or t-PA, the degree to which a laboratory test is outside the normal range does not influence the degree to which a pathologic clot is dissolved.

A possible noninvasive assay to reflect successful thrombolysis would be the measurement of the concentration of cross-linked fibrin degradation products, presumably appearing in the circulation at elevated concentration as a result of clot dissolution (see Fig. 27-4). While early "washout" enzyme activity and other cardiac-specific observations may be of value for patients with acute MI,[190] studies of fibrin-related markers potentially could be used to measure lysis of thrombus in any vessel. The data are thus far inconclusive, with some studies claiming high predictability of results for successful vascular reperfusion[191,192] and others failing to document such a correlation.[193–195] Since plasma-soluble fibrin could represent a source of D-dimer during thrombolytic treatment,[196] in vitro refinements of the system could allow better predictive assays, as has been found in preliminary evaluations of patients with DVT.[197] Other blood markers are reported to correlate with vascular patency after thrombolytic treatment of acute MI, such as von Willebrand factor, plasminogen activator inhibitor 1 (PAI-1), and C-reactive protein,[198] but none of these has been shown to be a useful predictor of vascular patency.

Relation of Laboratory Findings to Reocclusion

The value of laboratory results for predicting vascular (coronary artery) reocclusion in an individual patient is not established, but the data from trials using t-PA are instructive.[182] Among the 55 patients who suffered reocclusion, the decrease in fibrinogen was significantly less (120 versus 180 mg/dL; $p = 0.0003$) than in patients who did not reocclude. The concentrations of fibrin degradation products were likewise correlated (200 versus 310 μg/mL; $p = 0.038$), being higher in patients with patent arteries. The data suggest that a more profound lytic state protects against reocclusion and may help to explain the lower reocclusion rates with UK, SK, and APSAC than with

t-PA.[89,199,200] Additional factors that contribute to reocclusion is the short half-life of t-PA[201] (see Table 27-2) and the local prothrombotic influences at the site of the original vascular injury or plaque rupture.[26,202]

The application of coronary artery patency data as a substitute for clinical outcome (survival) has been reasonable, but until recently, the interpretation of such data has been problematic, partly because data on patency and survival were not collected from the same study. Thus patency studies comparing SK or APSAC with t-PA[64,71] have shown that t-PA is more effective in producing early patency, yet studies using mortality as the outcome reported no difference in the efficacy between SK, APSAC, and t-PA.[2,30] The GUSTO Study[13] is the first to evaluate patency in a large subgroup of patients (2000 of 41,000) who were assessed for survival. In the total group of patients treated at a median delay of less than 3 h after the onset of chest pain, there was a 2:1 higher 90-minute patency rate (TIMI-3) for t-PA over SK (54% versus 30%), albeit only a 1.18:1 difference in mortality (6.3% versus 7.2%). However, the patency data at 90 minutes do not fully explain the relatively small difference in survival, since the results at 180 minutes are the same for t-PA and SK (TIMI-3:42% versus 35%), as predicted on the basis of other data.[203] The propensity for the various activators to lyse thrombi and hemostatic plugs, to induce a lytic state, and to allow reocclusion is shown schematically in Figure 27-4.

LABORATORY MONITORING

Despite the complexity of biochemical reactions that occur during thrombolytic therapy, treatment regimens and laboratory testing have been simplified. Although debate still exists regarding the importance or lack thereof for the antistreptococcal titer, admonitions to carefully control drug dosage by laboratory testing have not proved to be essential. Although "standard" treatment has been available for decades,[117,118,204] considerable variations still occur, and ideal regimens are still under development. While SK dosage seems to be accepted uniformly for MI, the dose of t-PA and

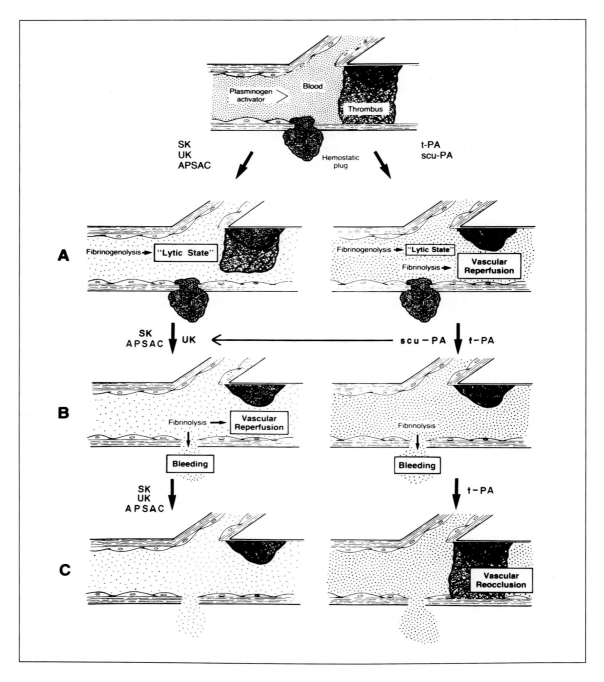

FIGURE 27-4. *Relative effects of plasminogen activators in a vessel occluded with thrombus and in which a site of prior trauma is sealed with a hemostatic plug. Two groups of plasminogen activators are compared, those with the attribute of greater "fibrinogen-sparing" (fibrin selectivity) (t-PA and scu-PA) and those with more potent effects on the blood coagulation and fibrinolytic proteins (SK, UK, and APSAC). The latter group causes a greater decrease in plasma fibrinogen, as indicated schematically by the lower density of dots, but both types of plasminogen activator induce bleeding at the same*

UK may be shortened to 2 h for pulmonary embolism, and t-PA dosages for acute MI may be more "front-loaded" than heretofore.

Once a lytic state has been attained, there is no need to regulate the dose of plasminogen activator. This is so because any degree of laboratory derangement is evidence that a lytic state has been established, and alterations of dose based on the degree of this derangement neither improve the chance of thrombolysis nor decrease the risk of hemorrhagic complications. Further, time constraints in patients with MI require commitment to a given dosage, with little chance to react to a laboratory result during the acute phase of the illness. The major role for monitoring thrombolytic therapy is to document that a given dose of SK or UK has achieved a lytic state, indicating that high-titer neutralizing antibody is not present. If after 2 h the laboratory test shows that a lytic state does not exist, then the treatment should be reevaluated with regard to possible technical problems with administration of the agent, high levels of inhibitor, or rare situations such as an abnormal plasminogen that resist conversion to plasmin. Failure to achieve a lytic state despite higher doses of activator requires cessation of the infusion and prompt administration of heparin anticoagulant therapy.

Local Administration

A recurrent concern regarding the administration of fibrinolytic agents relates to the wisdom of local therapy delivered through a catheter directly on or into a thrombus, a treatment that was tested as early as 1960 for peripheral artery occlusion[205] and for MI.[206] The rationale for such regional therapy is compelling for arterial occlusions of all types, since the offending thrombus is usually localized to a single vessel downstream from the catheter tip, and catheterization for angiographic diagnosis provides ready access to the site of occlusion. Additionally, it is the continued hope of the practitioner to confine treatment to the thrombus site alone, thereby avoiding any systemic drug effect, and to maximize local treatment to a degree that delivery from a distant venous site could not achieve.

Groundbreaking observations have been the angiographically documented instances of peripheral artery thrombolysis by Dotter and colleagues[207] and coronary artery thrombolysis by Rentrop and colleagues[208] after selective catheterization and infusion of SK. Attempts at local therapy of venous thromboembolic disease have been reported,[16,209–211] but these have a less compelling

---

rate and to the same degree by virtue of hemostatic plug dissolution. Assuming that the occluded vessel is a coronary artery in a patient with acute MI, reperfusion is more rapid with the more fibrinogen-sparing (fibrin-selective) agents, especially when thrombi are older than 3 h. Thus, at phase A (approximately 90 minutes after initiation of treatment), t-PA and scu-PA will have achieved a higher rate of vascular reperfusion than SK, UK, and APSAC, whereas with t-PA the blood fibrinogen concentration will not have decreased as much. However, this does not occur with scu-PA, because it is partially converted to UK in the circulation, resulting in a potent lytic state. By 3 to 24 h after treatment initiation (phases B and C), thrombus exposed to the non-fibrinogen-sparing agents also dissolves, producing a stable condition of a striking lytic state and persistent vascular patency. With t-PA, there is a higher tendency for vascular reocclusion (shown in phase C) related to the lesser degree of fibrinogen degradation and blood hypocoagulability. However, scu-PA therapy is associated with blood hypocoagulability and a low incidence of rethrombosis. The final patency status (70% to 80%) resulting from slower, progressive, and stable reperfusion induced by SK, UK, and APSAC is equivalent to that which follows more rapid reperfusion counterbalanced by increased rethrombosis associated with rt-PA or scu-PA. Application of more intensive anticoagulation with heparin, newer anticoagulants such as hirudin or hirulog, more potent antiplatelet strategies, and other adjunctive antithrombotic agents may alter this schematic representation, for example, by accelerating reperfusion with SK or by decreasing reocclusion with t-PA. (Reproduced from Sherry S, Marder VJ. Thrombosis, fibrinolysis and thrombolytic therapy: a perspective. Prog Cardiovasc Dis 34:89, 1991, with permission.)

rationale and less likelihood of advantage over systemic treatment.

Regional treatment of arterial thrombosis does achieve better thrombolysis than systemic therapy, but such treatment is not restricted to the pathologic thrombus. The volumes typically delivered for regional therapy of coronary artery thrombosis far exceed what could be limited to the local area of infusion, and the dose (of SK) is not very different[212] from that administered by the systemic route in the first 2 h of treatment for DVT or PE. During the period of infusion, therefore, the biochemical events occurring in the blood are comparable with those which follow systemic administration.[188,212–219] Thus a lytic state occurred in 22 of 25 patients who received 119,000 units of intracoronary SK, with a mean decrease in plasminogen to 7% of baseline and a mean decrease in fibrinogen from 342 to 87 mg/dL.[216] This high incidence of a systemic lytic state in patients receiving intracoronary UK or SK is confirmed by others[217,218] and further suggests that the lytic state is correlated with successful reperfusion and in patients with acute peripheral arterial occlusion.[219] The dose of intravenous t-PA that had been used also regularly produces a lytic state.[6] In a recent trial of regional UK for patients with acute occlusion of peripheral arterial grafts, about 11% of patients had a bleeding complication, all but one at the catheterization site,[144] despite only a modest decrease in plasma fibrinogen[220] of 25% to 30% rather than 70%, as would be expected for systemic UK therapy,[200,221] compatible with the lack of correlation of fibrinogen decrease with incidence of hemorrhage. A situation of truly fibrin-specific therapy is not yet available, but perhaps the use of bat-PA will achieve this end and determine whether such therapy can in fact avoid bleeding complications such as those which accompany regional infusions.[207]

REFERENCES

1. Gruppo Italiano per lo Studio Della Streptochinasi Nell'infarto Miocardico. Effectiveness of intravenous thrombolytic treatment in acute myocardial infarction. Lancet 1986;1:397.
2. Third International Study of Infarct Survival Collaborative Group. ISIS-3: a randomised comparison of streptokinase vs tissue plasminogen activator vs anistreplase and of aspirin plus heparin vs aspirin alone among 41,299 cases of suspected acute myocardial infarction. Lancet 1992;1:753.
3. Collen D. On the regulation and control of fibrinolysis. Thromb Haemost 1980;43:77.
4. Collen D, Topol EJ, Tiefenbrunn AJ, et al. Coronary thrombolysis with recombinant human tissue-type plasminogen activator: Prospective randomized placebo-controlled trial. Circulation 1984;70:1012.
5. Collen D, Bounameaux H, De Cock F, et al. Analysis of coagulation and fibrinolysis during intravenous infusion of recombinant human tissue-type plasminogen activator in patients with acute myocardial infarction. Circulation 1986;73:511.
6. Topol EJ, Bell WR, Weisfeldt ML. Coronary thrombolysis with recombinant tissue-type plasminogen activator: a hematologic and pharmacologic study. Ann Intern Med 1985;103:837.
7. Gurewich V, Pannell R, Louie S, et al. Effective and fibrin-specific clot lysis by a zymogen precursor form of urokinase (pro-urokinase): a study in vitro and in two animal species. J Clin Invest 1984;73:1731.
8. Collen D, DeCock F, Lijnen HR. Biological and thrombolytic properties of proenzyme and active forms of human urokinase: II. Turnover of natural and recombinant urokinase in rabbits and squirrel monkeys. Thromb Haemost 1984;52:24.
9. Staniforth DH, Smith RAG, Hibbs M. Streptokinase and anisoylated streptokinase plasminogen complex—their action on haemostasis in human volunteers. Eur J Clin Pharmacol 1983;24:751.
10. Tebbe U, Tanswell P, Seifried E, et al. Single-bolus injection of recombinant tissue-type plasminogen activator in acute myocardial infarction. Am J Cardiol 1989;64:448.
11. Neuhaus K-L, von Essen R, Tebbe U, et al. Improved thrombolysis in acute myocardial infarction with front-loaded administration of alteplase: results of the rt-PA–APSAC patency study (TAPS). J Am Coll Cardiol 1992;19:885.
12. Wall TC, Califf RM, George BS, et al. Accelerated plasminogen activator dose regimens for coronary thrombolysis. J Am Coll Cardiol 1992;19:482.
13. The GUSTO Investigators. An international randomized trial comparing four thrombolytic strategies for acute myocardial infarction. N Engl J Med 1993;329:673.
14. Col JJ, Col-De Beys CM, Renkin JP, et al. Pharmacokinetics, thrombolytic efficacy and hemorrhagic risk of different streptokinase regimens in heparin-treated acute myocardial infarction. Am J Cardiol 1989;63:1185.
15. Six AJ, Louwerenburg HW, Braams R, et al. A dou-

ble-blind, randomized multicenter dose-ranging trial of intravenous streptokinase in acute myocardial infarction. Am J Cardiol 1990;65:119.

16. Edwards IR, MacLean KS, Dow JD. Low-dose urokinase in major pulmonary embolism. Lancet 1973;2:409.

17. Dickie KJ, deGroot WJ, Cooley RN, et al. Hemodynamic effects of bolus infusion of urokinase in pulmonary thromboembolism. Am Rev Respir Dis 1974;109:48.

18. Goldhaber SZ, Kessler CM, Heit JA, et al. Recombinant tissue-type plasminogen activator versus a novel dosing regimen of urokinase in acute pulmonary embolism: a randomized controlled multicenter trial. J Am Coll Cardiol 1992;20:24.

19. Bell WR. Streptokinase and urokinase in the treatment of pulmonary thromboemboli: from a National Cooperative Study. Thromb Haemost 1976;35:57.

20. Grines CL, Nissen SE, Booth DC, et al. A prospective, randomized trial comparing combination half-dose tissue-type plasminogen activator and streptokinase with full-dose tissue-type plasminogen activator. Circulation 1991;84:540.

21. Runge MS, Quertermous T, Haber E. Plasminogen activators: the old and the new. Circulation 1989; 79:217.

22. Lijnen HR, Collen D. Towards the development of improved thrombolytic agents. Br J Haematol 1991;77:261.

23. Bode C, Matsueda GR, Hui KY, Haber E. Antibody-direction urokinase: a specific fibrinolytic agent. Science 1985;229:765.

24. Dewerchin M, Vandamme A-M, Holvoet P, et al. Thrombolytic and pharmacokinetic properties of a recombinant chimeric plasminogen activator consisting of a fibrin fragment D-dimer specific humanized monoclonal antibody and a truncated single-chain urokinase. Thromb Haemost 1992; 68:170.

25. Bode C, Meinhardt G, Runge MS, et al. Platelet-targeted fibrinolysis enhances clot lysis and inhibits platelet aggregation. Circulation 1991;84: 805.

26. Marder VJ, Sherry S. Thrombolytic therapy: current status. N Engl J Med 1988;318:1512.

27. Sherry S, Marder VJ. Thrombosis, fibrinolysis, and thrombolytic therapy: a perspective. Prog Cardiovas Dis 1991;34:89.

28. ISIS-2 (Second International Study of Infarct Survival) Collaborative Group. Randomized trial of intravenous streptokinase, oral aspirin, both, or neither among 17, 187 cases of suspected acute myocardial infarction: ISIS-2. Lancet 1988;2:349.

29. Sherry S, Marder VJ. Thrombolytic therapy: reocclusion rates with adjunctive aspirin and its relation to heparin therapy. J Am Coll Cardiol 1992; 19:678.

30. Gruppo Italiano per lo Studio Della Sopravvivenza Nell'Infarto Miocardico. GISSI-2: a factorial randomized trial of alteplase versus streptokinase and heparin versus no heparin among 12,490 patients with acute myocardial infarction. Lancet 1990; 336:65.

31. O'Connor C, for the DUCCS Study Group. Randomized trial of heparin in conjunction with anistreplase (APSAC) in acute myocardial infarction: the DUCCS-1 study. J Am Coll Cardiol 1993; 23:11.

32. Popma JJ, Topol EJ. Adjuncts to thrombolysis for myocardial reperfusion. Ann Intern Med 1991; 115:34.

33. Coller BS. Platelets and thrombolytic therapy. N Engl J Med 1990;322:33.

34. Willerson JT, Golino P, McNatt J, et al. Role of new antiplatelet agents as adjunctive therapies in thrombolysis. Am J Cardiol 1991;67:12A.

35. Becker RC. Thrombin antagonists and antiplatelet agents. Am J Cardiol 1992;69:39A.

36. Coller BS, Folts JD, Scudder LE, Smith SR. Antithrombotic effect of a monoclonal antibody to the platelet glycoprotein IIb/IIIa receptor in an experimental animal model. Blood 1986;68:783.

37. Anderson HV, Revana M, Rosales O, et al. Intravenous administration of monoclonal antibody to the platelet GPIIb/IIIa receptor to treat abrupt closure during coronary angioplasty. Am J Cardiol 1992;69:1373.

38. Markwardt F. Development of hirudin as an antithrombotic agent. Semin Thromb Hemost 1989; 15:269.

39. Markwardt F. Hirudin. Semin Thromb Hemost 1991;17:79.

40. Heras M, Chesebro JH, Penny WJ, et al. Effects of thrombin inhibition on the development of acute platelet-thrombus deposition during angioplasty in pigs: heparin versus recombinant hirudin, a specific thrombin inhibitor. Circulation 1989; 79:657.

41. Kelly AB, Marzec UM, Krupski W, et al. Hirudin interruption of heparin-resistant arterial thrombus formation in baboons. Blood 1991;77:1006.

42. Cadroy Y, Maraganore JM, Hanson SR, Harker LA. Selective inhibition by a synthetic hirudin peptide of fibrin-dependent thrombosis in baboons. Proc Natl Acad Sci USA 1991;88:1177.

43. Lidon RM, Theroux P, Bonan R, et al. Hirulog as adjunctive therapy to streptokinase in acute myocardial infarction (abstract). J Am Coll Cardiol 1993;21:419.

44. Cannon CP, McCabe CH, Henry TD, et al for the TIMI-5 Investigators. Hirudin reduces reocclusion compared to heparin following thrombolysis in acute myocardial infarction: results of the TIMI-5 trial (abstract). J Am Coll Cardiol 1993;21:136A.

45. Neeper MP, Waxman L, Smith DE, et al. Charac-

terization of recombinant tick anticoagulant peptide: a highly selective inhibitor of blood coagulation factor Xa. J Biol Chem 1990;265:17746.

46. Han JH, Law SW, Keller PM, et al. Cloning and expression of cDNA encoding antistasin, a leech-derived protein having anti-coagulant and anti-metastatic properties. Gene 1989;75:47.

47. Vlasuk GP, Ramjit D, Fujita T, et al. Comparison of the in vivo anticoagulant properties of standard heparin and the highly selective factor Xa inhibitors antistasin and tick anticoagulant peptide (TAP) in a rabbit model of venous thrombosis. Thromb Haemost 1991;65:257.

48. Schaffer LW, Davidson JT, Vlasuk GP, Siegl PKS. Antithrombotic efficacy of recombinant tick anticoagulant peptide: a potent inhibitor of coagulation factor Xa in a primate model of arterial thrombosis. Circulation 1991;84:1741.

49. Sitko GR, Ramjit DR, Stabilito II, et al. Conjunctive enhancement of enzymatic thrombolysis and prevention of thrombotic reocclusion with the selective factor Xa inhibitor, tick anticoagulant peptide: comparison of hirudin and heparin in a canine model of acute coronary artery thrombosis. Circulation 1992;85:805.

50. Marder VJ. The use of thrombolytic agents: choice of patient, drug administration, laboratory monitoring. Ann Intern Med 1979;90:802.

51. Fletcher AP, Alkjaersig N, Sherry S, et al. The development of urokinase as a thrombolytic agent: maintenance of a sustained thrombolytic state in man by its intravenous infusion. J Lab Clin Med 1965;65:713.

52. Marder VJ, Shulman NR. High molecular weight derivatives of human fibrinogen produced by plasmin: II. Mechanisms of their anticoagulant activity. J Biol Chem 1969;244:2120.

53. Hirsh J, Buchanan M, Glynn MF, Mustard JF. Effect of streptokinase on hemostasis. Blood 1968; 32:726.

54. Marguerie GA, Thomas-Maison N, Larrieu M-J, Plow EF. The interaction of fibrinogen with human platelets in plasma milieu. Blood 1982; 59:91.

55. Miles LA, Plow EF. Binding and activation of plasminogen on the platelet surface. J Biol Chem 1985;260:4303.

56. Stricker RB, Wong D, Shiu DT, et al. Activation of plasminogen by tissue plasminogen activator on normal and thrombasthenic platelets: effects on surface proteins and platelet aggregation. Blood 1986;68:275.

57. Hajjar KA, Harpel PC, Jaffe EA, Nachman RL. Binding of plasminogen to cultured human endothelial cells. J Biol Chem 1986;261:11656.

58. Knudsen BS, Silverstein RL, Leung LLK, et al. Binding of tissue plasminogen activator to cultured human endothelial cells. J Biol Chem 1986; 261:10765.

59. Loscalzo J, Vaughan DE. Tissue plasminogen activator promotes platelet disaggregation in plasma. J Clin Invest 1987;79:1749.

60. Kernohan RJ, Todd C. Heparin therapy in thromboembolic disease. Lancet 1966;1:621.

61. Pitney WR, Pettit JE, Armstrong L. Control of heparin therapy. Br Med J 1970;4:139.

62. Bell WR, Pitney WR, Goodwin JF. Therapeutic defibrination in the treatment of thrombotic disease. Lancet 1968;1:490.

63. The urokinase pulmonary embolism trial: a national cooperative study. Circulation 1973;47 (suppl II):1.

64. The TIMI Study Group. The thrombolysis in myocardial infarction (TIMI) trial: phase I findings. N Engl J Med 1985;312:932.

65. Marder VJ. Clinical guidelines and expectations for current and future thrombolytic agents in the therapy of deep vein thrombosis. In: Mannucci PM, D'Angleo A, eds. Urokinase: basic and clinical aspects. London: Academic Press, 1982:95.

66. Rao AK, Pratt C, Berke A, et al. Thrombolysis in myocardial infarction (TIMI) trial—phase I: hemorrhagic manifestations and changes in plasma fibrinogen and the fibrinolytic system in patients treated with recombinant tissue plasminogen activator and streptokinase. J Am Coll Cardiol 1988; 11:1.

67. Marder VJ, Soulen RL, Atichartakarn V, et al. Quantitative venographic assessment of deep vein thrombosis in the evaluation of streptokinase and heparin therapy. J Lab Clin Med 1977;89:1018.

68. Urokinase-streptokinase embolism trial: phase 2 results: a cooperative study. JAMA 1974;229: 1606.

69. Kase CS, Pessin MS, Zivin JA, et al. Intracranial hemorrhage after coronary thrombolysis with tissue plasminogen activator. Am J Med 1992;92:384.

70. European Cooperative Study Group for Streptokinase Treatment in Acute Myocardial Infarction. Streptokinase in acute myocardial infarction. N Engl J Med 1979;301:797.

71. Verstraete M, Bernard R, Bory M, et al. Randomised trial of intravenous recombinant tissue-type plasminogen activator versus intravenous streptokinase in acute myocardial infarction: report from the European Cooperative Study Group for recombinant tissue-type plasminogen activator. Lancet 1985;1:842.

72. Goldhaber SZ, Kessler CM, Heit JA, et al. Recombinant tissue-type plasminogen activator versus a novel dosing regimen of urokinase in acute pulmonary embolism: a randomized controlled multicenter trial. J Am Coll Cardiol 1992;20:24.

73. Trubestein G, Brecht T, Ludwig M, et al. Fibri-

nolytische therapie mit streptokinase und urokinase bei tiefer venenthrombose. In: Trubestein G, Etzel F, eds. International symposium on fibrinolytic therapy, Bonn 1982. Stuttgart: Shattauer-Verlag 1983:193.

74. White HD. Comparative safety of thrombolytic agents. Am J Cardiol 1991;67:30E.

75. The International Study Group. In-hospital mortality and clinical course of 20,891 patients with suspected acute myocardial infarction randomised between alteplase and streptokinase with or without heparin. Lancet 1990;336:71.

76. Goldhaber SZ, Buring JE, Lipnick RJ, Hennekens CH. Pooled analyses of randomized trials of streptokinase and heparin in phlebographically documented acute deep venous thrombosis. Am J Med 1984;76:393.

77. Topol EJ, Califf RM, George BS, et al. A randomized trial of immediate versus delayed elective angioplasty after intravenous tissue plasminogen activator in acute myocardial infarction N Engl J Med 1987;317:581.

78. The TIMI Research Group. Immediate vs delayed catheterization and angioplasty following thrombolytic therapy for acute myocardial infarction: TIMI-IIA results. JAMA 1988;260:2849.

79. TIMI Study Group. Comparison of invasive and conservative strategies after treatment with intravenous tissue plasminogen activator in acute myocardial infarction: results of the thrombolysis in myocardial infarction (TIMI) phase II trial. N Engl J Med 1989;320:618.

80. SWIFT (Should We Intervene Following Thrombolysis?) Trial Study Group. SWIFT trial of delayed elective intervention vs consecutive treatment after thrombolysis with anistreplase in acute myocardial infarction. Br Med J 1991;302:555.

81. Neuhaus K-L, Tebbe U, Gottwik M, et al. Intravenous recombinant tissue plasminogen activator (rt-PA) and urokinase in acute myocardial infarction: results of the German activator urokinase study (GAUS). J Am Coll Cardiol 1988;12:581.

82. PRIMI Trial Study Group. Randomised double-blind trial of recombinant pro-urokinase against streptokinase in acute myocardial infarction. Lancet 1989;1:863.

83. Califf RM, Topol EJ, Stack RS, et al. Evaluation of combination thrombolytic therapy and timing of cardiac catheterization in acute myocardial infarction. Circulation 1991;83:1543.

84. Neuhaus KL, Von Essen R, Tebbe U, et al. Improved thrombolysis in acute myocardial infarction with front-loaded administration of alteplase. Results of the rt-PA–APSAC patency study (TAPS). J Am Coll Cardiol 1992;19:885.

85. Anderson JL, Sorensen SG, Moreno FL, et al and the TEAM-2 Study Investigators. Multicentre patency trial of intravenous antistreplase compared with streptokinase in acute myocardial infarction. Circulation 1991;83:126.

86. White HD, Rivers JT, Maslowski AH, et al. Effect of intravenous streptokinase as compared with that of tissue plasminogen activator on left ventricular function after first myocardial infarction. N Engl J Med 1989;320:817.

87. Magnmani B, and the Plasminogen Activator Italian Multicentre Study (PAIMS) Group. Comparison of intravenous recombinant single-chain human tissue-type plasminogen activator (rt-PA) with intravenous streptokinase in acute myocardial infarction. J Am Coll Cardiol 1989;13:19.

88. Anderson JL, Becker LC, Sorensen SG, et al for the TEAM-3 Investigators. Anistreplase versus alteplase in acute myocardial infarction: comparative effects on left ventricular function, morbidity, and 1 day patency: the TEAM-3. J Am Coll Cardiol 1992;20:753.

89. Bassand J-P, Cassagnes J, Machecourt J, et al. Comparative effects of APSAC and rt-PA on infarct size and left ventricular function in acute myocardial infarction: a multicenter randomized study. Circulation 1991;84:1107.

90. Prowse CV, Dawes J, Lane DA, et al. Proteolysis of fibrinogen in healthy volunteers following major and minor in vivo plasminogen activation. Thromb Res 1982;27:91.

91. Kase CS, O'Neal AM, Fisher M, et al. Intracranial hemorrhage after use of tissue plasminogen activator for coronary thrombolysis. Ann Intern Med 1990;112:17.

92. O'Connor CM, Califf RM, Massey EW, et al. Stroke and acute myocardial infarction in the thrombolytic era: clinical correlates and long-term prognosis. J Am Coll Cardiol 1990;16:533.

93. Sloan MA, Plotnick GD. Stroke complicating thrombolytic therapy of acute myocardial infarction. J Am Coll Cardiol 1990;16:541.

94. Vaitkus PT, Berlin JA, Schwartz JS, Barnathan ES. Stroke complicating acute myocardial infarction: a meta-analysis of risk modification by anticoagulation and thrombolytic therapy. Arch Intern Med 1992;152:2020.

95. DeJaegere PP, Arnold AA, Balk AH, Simoons ML. Intracranial hemorrhage in association with thrombolytic therapy: incidence and clinical predictive factors. J Am Coll Cardiol 1992;19:289.

96. Gore JM, Sloan M, Price TR, et al. Intracerebral hemorrhage, cerebral infarction, and subdural hematoma after acute myocardial infarction and thrombolytic therapy in the thrombolysis in myocardial infarction study: thrombolysis in myocardial infarction, phase II, pilot and clinical trial. Circulation 1991;83:448.

97. The SCATI Group. Randomised controlled trial of

subcutaneous calcium-heparin in acute myocardial infarction. Lancet 1989;2:182.

98. Topol EJ, George BS, Kereiakes DJ, et al and the TAMI 7 Group. A randomized controlled trial of intravenous tissue plasminogen activator and early intravenous heparin in acute myocardial infarction. Circulation 1989;79:281.

99. De Bono DP, Simoons ML, Tijssen J, et al for the European Cooperative Study Group (ECSG). Effect of early intravenous heparin on coronary patency, infarct size and bleeding complications after alteplase thrombolysis: results of a randomised double blind European cooperative group trial. Br Heart J 1992;67:122.

100. Wilcox RG, von Der Lippe G, Olsson CG, et al. Trial of tissue plasminogen activator for mortality reduction in acute myocardial infarction: Anglo-Scandinavian study of early thrombolysis (ASSET). Lancet 1988;2:525.

101. AIMS Trial Study Group. Long-term effects of intravenous anistreplase in acute myocardial infarction: final report of the AIMS study. Lancet 1990; 335:427.

102. ISAM Study Group. A prospective trial of intravenous streptokinase in acute myocardial infarction (ISAM): mortality, morbidity and infarct size at 21 days. N Engl J Med 1986;314:1465.

103. White HD, Norris RM, Brown MA, et al. Effect of intravenous streptokinase on left ventricular function and early survival after acute myocardial infarction. N Engl J Med 1987;317:850.

104. Anderson JL, Rothbard RL, Hackworthy RA, et al. Multicenter reperfusion trial of intravenous anisoylated plasminogen activator complex (APSAC) in acute myocardial infarction: controlled comparison with intracoronary streptokinase. J Am Coll Cardiol 1988;11:1153.

105. Van de Werf F, Arnold AE. Intravenous tissue plasminogen activator and size of infarct, left ventricular function, and survival in acute myocardial infarction. Br Med J 1988;297:1374.

106. Bassand J-P, Machecourt J, Cassagnes J, et al. Multicenter trial of intravenous anisoylated plasminogen streptokinase activator complex (APSAC) in acute myocardial infarction: effects on infarct size and left ventricular function. J Am Coll Cardiol 1989;13:988.

107. Boissel J-P. European Myocardial Infarction Project (EMIP). Presented at the American College of Cardiology Meeting, 1993;329:383.

108. Meinertz T, Kasper W, Schumacher M, Just H, for the APSAC Multicenter Trial Group. The German multicenter trial of anisoylated plasminogen streptokinase activator complex versus heparin for acute myocardial infarction. Am J Cardiol 1988; 62:347.

109. Wall TC, Phillips HR III, Stack RS, et al. Results of

high dose intravenous urokinase for acute myocardial infarction. Am J Cardiol 1990;65:124.

110. Kennedy JW, Martin GV, Davis KB, et al. The western Washington intravenous streptokinase in acute myocardial infarction randomized trial. Circulation 1988;77:345.

111. Wall TC, Califf RM, George BS, et al. Accelerated plasminogen activator dose regimens for coronary thrombolysis. J Am Coll Cardiol 1992;19:482.

112. Simoons ML, Arnold AER, Betriu A, et al. Thrombolysis with tissue plasminogen activator in acute myocardial infarction: no additional benefit of immediate PTCA. Lancet 1988;1:197.

113. Carney RJ, Murphy GA, Brandt TR, et al, for the RAAMI Study Investigators. Randomized angiographic trial of recombinant tissue-type plasminogen activator (alteplase) in myocardial infarction. J Am Coll Cardiol 1992;20:17.

114. Maggioni AP, Franzosi MG, Santoro E, et al and the International Study Group. The risk of stroke in patients with acute myocardial infarction after thrombolytic and antithrombotic treatment. N Engl J Med 1992;327:1.

115. Califf RM, Fortin DF, Tenaglia AN, Sane DC. Clinical risks of thrombolytic therapy. Am J Cardiol 1992;69:12A.

116. National Institutes of Health Consensus Panel. Thrombolytic therapy in thrombosis: a National Institutes of Health consensus development conference. Ann Intern Med 1980;93:141.

117. Hirsh J, O'Sullivan EF, Martin M. Evaluation of a standard dosage schedule with streptokinase. Blood 1970;35:341.

118. Verstraete M, Vermylen J, Amery A, et al. Thrombolytic therapy with streptokinase using a standard dosage scheme. Br Med J 1966;1:454.

119. Mueller HS, Rao AK, Forman SA, and the TIMI Investigators. Thrombolysis in myocardial infarction (TIMI): comparative studies of coronary reperfusion and systemic fibrinogenolysis with two forms of recombinant tissue-type plasminogen activator. J Am Coll Cardiol 1987;10:479.

120. Garabedian HD, Gold HK, Leinbach RC, et al. Comparative properties of two clinical preparations of recombinant human tissue-type plasminogen activator in patients with acute myocardial infarction. J Am Coll Cardiol 1987;9:599.

121. TIMI Operations Committee, Braunwald E, Knatterud GL, Passamani ER, Robertson TL. Announcement of protocol change in thrombolysis in myocardial infarction trial. J Am Coll Cardiol 1987;9:467.

122. TIMI Operations Committee, Braunwald E, Knatterud GL, Passamani E, Robertson TL, Solomon R. Update from the thrombolysis in myocardial infarction trial. J Am Coll Cardiol 1987;10:970.

123. The Urokinase and Alteplase in Myocardial Infarc-

tion Collaborative Group. Combination of urokinase and alteplase in the treatment of myocardial infarction. Coronary Artery Dis 1991;2:225.

124. Goldhaber SZ, Heit J, Sharma GVRK, et al. Randomised controlled trial of recombinant tissue plasminogen activator versus urokinase in the treatment of acute pulmonary embolism. Lancet 1988;2:293.

125. Francis CW, Brenner B, Leddy JP, Marder VJ. Angioedema during therapy with recombinant tissue plasminogen activator. Br J Haematol 1991;77:562.

126. Honan MB, Harrell FE, Reimer KA, et al. Cardiac rupture, mortality and the timing of thrombolytic therapy: a meta-analysis. J Am Coll Cardiol 1990;16:359.

127. Massel D. Cardiac rupture and time to thrombolytic treatment. J Am Coll Cardiol 1991;17:1671.

128. Queen M, Biem HJ, Moe GW, Sugar L. Development of cholesterol embolization syndrome after intravenous streptokinase for acute myocardial infarction. Am J Cardiol 1990;65:1042.

129. Haugeberg G, Bonarjee V, Dickstein K. Fatal intrathoracic haemorrhage after cardiopulmonary resuscitation and treatment with streptokinase and heparin. Br Heart J 1989;62:157.

130. Tenaglia AN, Califf RM, Candela RJ, et al. Thrombolytic therapy in patients requiring cardiopulmonary resuscitation. Am J Cardiol 1991;68:1015.

131. Scholz KH, Tebbe U, Herrmann C, et al. Frequency of complications of cardiopulmonary resuscitation after thrombolysis during acute myocardial infarction. Am J Cardiol 1992;69:724.

132. Guidelines for the early management of patients with acute myocardial infarction: a report of the American College of Cardiology/American Heart Association Task Force on Assessment of Diagnostic and Therapeutic Cardiovascular Procedures (Subcommittee to Develop Guidelines for the Early Management of Patients with Acute Myocardial Infarction). J Am Coll Cardiol 1990;16:249.

133. Sherry S, Marder VJ. Special note: mistaken guidelines for thrombolytic therapy of acute myocardial infarction in the elderly. J Am Coll Cardiol 1991;17:1237.

134. Gurwitz JH, Goldberg RJ, Gore JM. Coronary thrombolysis for the elderly? JAMA 1991;265:1720.

135. Yusuf S, Furberg CD. Are we biased in our approach to treating elderly patients with heart disease? Am J Cardiol 1991;68:954.

136. Krumholz HM, Pasternak RC, Weinstein MC, et al. Cost effectiveness of thrombolytic therapy with streptokinase in elderly patients with suspected acute myocardial infarction. N Engl J Med 1992;327:7.

137. Goldsmith JC, Lollar P, Hoak JC. Massive fatal pulmonary emboli with fibrinolytic therapy. Circulation 1982;64:1068.

138. Earnshaw JJ, Hopkinson BR, Makin GS. Cerebral embolus as a complication of streptokinase therapy. Clin Radiol 1985;36:658.

139. Sicard GA, Schier JJ, Totty WG, et al. Thrombolytic therapy for acute arterial occlusion. J Vasc Surg 1985;2:65.

140. Kakkasseril JS, Cranley JJ, Arbaugh JJ, et al. Efficacy of low-dose streptokinase in acute arterial occlusion and graft thrombosis. Arch Surg 1985;120:427.

141. Hallett JW Jr, Greenwood LH, Yrizarry JM, et al. Statistical determinants of success and complications of thrombolytic therapy for arterial occlusion of lower extremity. Surg Gynecol Obstet 1985;161:431.

142. Pernes JM, Brenot P, Raynaud A, et al. Results of in situ arterial thrombolysis by the combination of urokinase and lysyl plasminogen in acute arterial occlusive diseases of the lower limb. J Radiol 1985;66:385.

143. McNamara TO, Fischer JR. Thrombolysis of peripheral arterial and graft occlusions: improved results using high-dose urokinase. AJR 1985;144:769.

144. Ouriel K, Shortell CK, DeWeese JA, et al. A comparison of thrombolytic therapy with operative revascularization in the treatment of acute peripheral arterial ischemia. J Vasc Surg 1994;19.

145. Skinner JR, Phillips SJ, Zeff RJ, Kongtahworn C. Immediate coronary bypass following failed streptokinase infusion evolving myocardial infarction. J Thorac Cardiovasc Surg 1984;87:567.

146. Kay P, Ahmad A, Floten S, Starr A. Emergency coronary artery bypass surgery after intracoronary thrombolysis for evolving myocardial infarction. Br Heart J 1985;53:260.

147. Anderson JL, Battistessa SA, Clayton PD, et al. Coronary bypass surgery early after thrombolytic therapy for acute myocardial infarction. Ann Thorac Surg 1986;41:176.

148. Mantia AM, Lolley DM, Stullken EJ Jr, et al. Coronary artery bypass grafting within 24 hours after intracoronary streptokinase thrombolysis. J Cardiothorac Anesth 1987;1:392.

149. Lee KF, Mandell J, Rankin JS, et al. Immediate versus delayed coronary grafting after streptokinase treatment: postoperative blood loss and clinical results. J Thorac Cardiovasc Surg 1988;95:216.

150. Marder VJ, Rothbard RL, Fitzpatrick PG, Francis CW. Rapid lysis of coronary artery thrombi with anisoylated plasminogen: streptokinase activator complex: treatment by bolus intravenous injection. Ann Intern Med 1986;104:304.

151. Mentzer RL, Budzynski AZ, Sherry S. High-dose,

brief-duration intravenous infusion of streptokinase in acute myocardial infarction: description of effects in the circulation. Am J Cardiol 1986;57:1220.

152. Owen J, Friedman KD, Grossman BA, et al. Quantitation of fragment X formation during thrombolytic therapy with streptokinase and tissue plasminogen activator. J Clin Invest 1987;79:1642.

153. Nunn B, Esmail R, Fears R, et al. Pharmacokinetic properties of anisoylated plasminogen streptokinase activator complex and other thrombolytic agents in animals and in humans. Drugs Suppl 1987;3:88.

154. Verstraete M, Miller GAH, Bounameaux H, et al. Intravenous and intrapulmonary recombinant tissue-type plasminogen activator in the treatment of acute massive pulmonary embolism. Circulation 1988;77:353.

155. Marder VJ. Comparison of thrombolytic agents: selected hematologic, vascular and clinical events. Am J Cardiol 1989;64:2A.

156. Fletcher AP, Alkjaersig N, Sherry S. Fibrinolytic mechanisms and the development of thrombolytic therapy. Am J Med 1962;33:738.

157. Sherry S, Fletcher AP, Alkjaersig N. Fibrinolysis and fibrinolytic activity in man. Physiol Rev 1959;39:343.

158. Collen D, Verstraete M. α_2-Antiplasmin consumption and fibrinogen breakdown during thrombolytic therapy. Thromb Res 1979;14:631.

159. Ratnoff OD, Menzie C. A new method for the determination of fibrinogen in small samples of plasma. J Lab Clin Med 1951;37:316.

160. Leebeek FWG, Kluft C, Knot EAR, et al. Plasmin inhibitors in the prevention of systemic effects during thrombolytic therapy: specific role of the plasminogen-binding form of α_2-antiplasmin. J Am Coll Cardiol 1990;15:1212.

161. Weitz JI, Leslie B, Hirsh J, Klement P. α_2-Antiplasmin supplementation inhibits tissue plasminogen activator-induced fibrinogenolysis and bleeding with little effect on thrombolysis. J Clin Invest 1993;91:1343.

162. Miller JL, Katz AJ, Feinstein MB. Plasmin inhibition of thrombin-induced platelet aggregation. Thromb Diatherm Haemorrh 1975;33:286.

163. Terres W, Umnus S, Mathey DG, Bleifeld W. Effects of streptokinase, urokinase, and recombinant tissue plasminogen activator on platelet aggregability and stability of platelet aggregates. Cardiovasc Res 1990;24:471.

164. Jenkins CSP, Phillips DR, Clemetson KJ, et al. Platelet membrane glycoprotein implicated in ristocetin-induced aggregation. J Clin Invest 1976;57:112.

165. Adelman B, Michelson AD, Loscalzo J, et al. Plasmin effect on platelet glycoprotein IB–von Willebrand factor interactions. Blood 1985;65:32.

166. Gimple LW, Gold HK, Leinbach RC, et al. Correlation between template bleeding times and spontaneous bleeding during treatment of acute myocardial infarction with recombinant tissue-type plasminogen activator. Circulation 1989;80:581.

167. Hirsch DR, Goldhaber SZ. The bleeding time: its potential utility among patients receiving thrombolytic therapy. Am Heart J 1990;119:158.

168. Rudd MA, George D, Amarante P, et al. Temporal effects of thrombolytic agents on platelet function in vivo and their modulation by prostaglandins. Circ Res 1990;67:1175.

169. Vaughan DE, Van Houtte E, Declerck PJ, Collen D. Streptokinase-induced platelet aggregation: prevalence and mechanism. Circulation 1991;84:84.

170. Penny WF, Ware JA. Platelet activation and subsequent inhibition by plasmin and recombinant tissue-type plasminogen activator. Blood 1992;79:91.

171. Aronson DL, Chang P, Kessler CM. Platelet-dependent thrombin generation after in vitro fibrinolytic treatment. Circulation 1992;85:1706.

172. Chang P, Aronson DL, Scott J, Kessler CM. Increase in platelet support of thrombin generation after thrombolytic therapy. Am J Cardiol 1992;70:406.

173. Owen J, Friedman KD, Grossman BA, et al. Thrombolytic therapy with tissue plasminogen activator or streptokinase induced transient thrombin activity. Blood 1988;72:616.

174. Rapold HJ, deBono D, Arnold AER, et al. Plasma fibrinopeptide A levels in patients with acute myocardial infarction treated with alteplase: correlation with concomitant heparin, coronary artery patency, and recurrent ischemia. Circulation 1992;85:928.

175. Friberger P, Knös M, Gustavsson S, et al. Methods for determination of plasma, antiplasmin and plasminogen by means of substrate S-2251. Haemostasis 1978;7:138.

176. Francis CW, Connaghan DG, Marder VJ. Assessment of fibrin degradation products during fibrinolytic therapy for acute myocardial infarction. Circulation 1986;74:1027.

177. Marder VJ, Shulman NR, Carroll WR. High molecular weight derivatives of human fibrinogen produced by plasmin: I. Physicochemical and immunological characterization. J Biol Chem 1969;244:2111.

178. Clauss VA. Gerinnungsphysiologische schnellmethode zur bestimmung des fibrinogens. Acta Haematol (Basel) 1957;17:237.

179. Rampling WF, Gaffney PJ. The sulphite precipitation method for fibrinogen measurement: its use

on small samples in the presence of fibrinogen degradation products. Clin Chim Acta 1976;67: 43.

180. Marder VJ. Relevance of changes in blood fibrinolytic and coagulation parameters during thrombolytic therapy. Am J Med 1987;83:15.

181. Rao AK, Pratt C, Berke A, et al. Thrombolysis in myocardial infarction (TIMI) trial—phase I: hemorrhagic manifestations and changes in plasma fibrinogen and the fibrinolytic system in patients treated with recombinant tissue plasminogen activator and streptokinase. J Am Coll Cardiol 1988; 11:1.

182. Stump DC, Califf RM, Topol EJ, et al. Pharmacodynamics of thrombolysis with recombinant tissue-type plasminogen activator: correlation with characteristics of and clinical outcomes in patients with acute myocardial infarction. Circulation 1989;80:1222.

183. Bovill EG, Terrin ML, Stump DC, et al. Hemorrhagic events during therapy with recombinant tissue-type plasminogen activator, heparin, and aspirin for acute myocardial infarction: results of the thrombolysis in myocardial infarction (TIMI) phase II trial. Ann Intern Med 1991;115:256.

184. Timmis GC, Gangadharan V, Ramos RG, et al. Hemorrhage and the products of fibrinogen digestion after intracoronary administration of streptokinase. Circulation 1984;69:1146.

185. Collen D, Bounameaux H, DeCock F, et al. Analysis of coagulation and fibrinolysis during intravenous infusion of recombinant human tissue-type plasminogen activator in patients with acute myocardial infarction. Circulation 1986;73:511.

186. Bain G, Forster T, Baker A. An assessment of the sensitivity of three bleeding time techniques. Scand J Haematol 1983;30:311.

187. D'Angelo A, Manucci PM. Outcome of treatment of deep-vein thrombosis with urokinase: relationship to dosage, duration of therapy, age of the thrombus and laboratory changes. Thromb Haemost 1984;51:236.

188. White CW, Schwartz JL, Ferguson DW, et al. Systemic markers of fibrinolysis after unsuccessful intracoronary streptokinase thrombolysis for acute myocardial infarction: does nonreperfusion indicate failure to achieve a systemic lytic state? Am J Cardiol 1984;54:712.

189. Duckert F, Müller G, Nyman D, et al. Treatment of deep vein thrombosis with streptokinase. Br Med J 1975;1:479.

190. Hohnloser SH, Zabel M, Kasper W, et al. Assessment of coronary artery patency after thrombolytic therapy: accurate prediction utilizing the combined analysis of three noninvasive markers. J Am Coll Cardiol 1991;18:44.

191. Eisenberg PR, Jaffe AS, Stump DC, et al. Validity of

enzyme-linked immunosorbent assays of cross-linked fibrin degradation products as a measure of clot lysis. Circulation 1990;82:1159.

192. Lawler CM, Bovill EG, Stump DC, et al. Fibrin fragment D-dimer and fibrinogen Bβ peptides in plasma as markers of clot lysis during thrombolytic therapy in acute myocardial infarction. Blood 1990;76:1341.

193. Francis CW, Connaghan DG, Marder VJ. Assessment of fibrin degradation products during fibrinolytic therapy for acute myocardial infarction. Circulation 1986;74:1027.

194. Seifried E, Tanswell P, Rijken DC, et al. Fibrin degradation products are not specific markers for thrombolysis in myocardial infarction. Lancet 1987;2:333.

195. Brenner B, Francis CW, Fitzpatrick PG, et al. Relation of plasma D-dimer concentrations to coronary artery reperfusion before and after thrombolytic treatment in patients with acute myocardial infarction. Am J Cardiol 1989;63:1179.

196. Kornberg A, Francis CW, Marder VJ. Plasma crosslinked fibrin polymers: quantitation based on tissue plasminogen activator conversion to D-dimer and measurement in normals and patients with acute thrombotic disorders. Blood 1992;80:709.

197. Brenner B, Francis CW, Totterman S, et al. Quantitation of venous clot lysis with the D-dimer immunoassay during fibrinolytic therapy requires correction for soluble fibrin degradation. Circulation 1990;81:1818.

198. Andreotti F, Hackett DR, Haider AW, et al. von Willebrand factor, plasminogen activator inhibitor-1 and C-reactive protein are markers of thrombolytic efficacy in acute myocardial infarction. Thromb Haemost 1992;68:678.

199. Chesebro JH, Knatterud G, Roberts R, et al. Thrombolysis in myocardial infarction (TIMI) trial phase I: a comparison between intravenous tissue plasminogen activator and intravenous streptokinase. Clinical findings through hospital discharge. Circulation 1987;76:142.

200. Neuhaus KL, Tebbe U, Gottwik M, et al. Intravenous recombinant tissue plasminogen activator (rt-PA) and urokinase in acute myocardial infarction: results of the German activator urokinase study (GAUS). J Am Coll Cardiol 1988;12:581.

201. Baughman RA Jr. Pharmacokinetics of tissue plasminogen activator. In: Sobel BE, Collen D, Grossbard EB, eds. Tissue plasminogen activator in thrombolytic therapy. New York: Marcel Dekker, 1987:41.

202. Sherry S. Dissimilar systemic and local adverse effects of thrombolytic therapy. Am J Cardiol 1988; 61:1344.

203. Sherry S, Marder VJ. Streptokinase and recom-

binant tissue plasminogen activator (rt-PA) are equally effective in treating acute myocardial infarction. Ann Intern Med 1991;114:417.

204. Olow B, Johanson C, Andersson I, Eklöf B. Deep venous thrombosis treated with a standard dosage of streptokinase. Acta Chir Scand 1970;136:181.

205. Boyles PW, Meyer WH, Graff J, et al. Comparative effectiveness of intravenous and intraarterial fibrinolysin therapy. Am J Cardiol 1960;6:439.

206. Boucek RJ, Murphy WP Jr. Segmental perfusion of the coronary arteries with fibrinolysin in man following a myocardial infarction. Am J Cardiol 1960;6:525.

207. Dotter CT, Rösch J, Seaman AJ. Selective clot lysis with low-dose streptokinase. Radiology 1974;111:31.

208. Rentrop KP, Blanke H, Karsch KR, et al. Acute myocardial infarction: intracoronary application of nitroglycerin and streptokinase. Clin Cardiol 1979;2:354.

209. Becker GJ, Holden RW, Rabe FE, et al. Local thrombolytic therapy for subclavian and axillary vein thrombosis: treatment of the thoracic inlet syndrome. Radiology 1983;149:419.

210. Schwarz F, Zimmerman R, Stehr H, et al. Lokale Thrombolyse mit Urokinase bei akuter massiver Lungenembolie. Dtsch Med Wochenschr 1984;109:55.

211. Schulman S, Lockner D. Local venous infusion of streptokinase in DVT. Thromb Res 1984;34:213.

212. Marder VJ. Pharmacology of thrombolytic agents: implications for therapy of coronary artery thrombosis. Circulation 1983;68(suppl 1):2.

213. deProst D, Guerot C, Laffay N, et al. Intra-coronary thrombolysis with streptokinase or lysplasminogen/urokinase in acute myocardial infarction: effects on recanalization and blood fibrinolysis. Thromb Haemost 1983;50:792.

214. Marder VJ, Francis CW. An assessment of regional versus systemic thrombolytic treatment of peripheral and coronary artery thrombosis. Prog Haemost Thromb 1984;7:325.

215. Rogers WJ, Mantel JA, Hood WA Jr, et al. Prospective randomized trial of intravenous and intracoronary streptokinase in acute myocardial infarction. Circulation 1983;68:1051.

216. Cowley MJ, Hastillo A, Vetrovec GW, et al. Fibrinolytic effects of intracoronary streptokinase administration in patients with acute myocardial infarction and coronary insufficiency. Circulation 1983;67:1031.

217. Rothbard RL, Fitzpatrick PG, Francis CW, et al. Relationship of the lytic state to successful reperfusion with standard- and low-dose intracoronary streptokinase. Circulation 1985;71:562.

218. Burket MW, Smith MR, Walsh TE, et al. Relation of effectiveness of intracoronary thrombolysis in acute myocardial infarction to systemic thrombolytic state. Am J Cardiol 1985;56:441.

219. Kolts RL, Keuhner ME, Swanson MK, et al. Local intra-arterial streptokinase therapy for acute peripheral arterial occlusions: should thrombolytic therapy replace embolectomy? Am Surg 1985;51:381.

220. Marder VJ, Ouriel K. Assessment of plasma fibrinogen concentration as a reflection of bleeding risk in patients receiving regional urokinase for peripheral arterial or graft occlusion. Personal communication.

221. Mathey DG, Schofer J, Sheehan EF, et al. Intravenous urokinase in acute myocardial infarction. Am J Cardiol 1985;55:878.

Anthony J. Comerota (Ed.). *Thrombolytic Therapy for Peripheral Vascular Disease.* Copyright © 1995 J. B. Lippincott Company.

28

APPROPRIATE USE OF ANTICOAGULANTS FOR ARTERIAL AND VENOUS THROMBOEMBOLIC DISORDERS

Russell D. Hull

Graham F. Pineo

Gary E. Raskob

Over the past decade, clinical trials have produced major advances in anticoagulant therapy. This chapter reviews the appropriate use of anticoagulants for arterial and venous thromboembolic disorders. Recent advances from randomized clinical trials will be discussed.

ARTERIAL THROMBOEMBOLISM

Pathophysiology

Arterial thrombi (*white thrombi*) are composed predominantly of platelets and fibrin, in contrast to venous thrombi (*red thrombi*), which consist primarily of red cells and fibrin.[1,2] Arterial thromboemboli usually occur when platelets come into contact with exposed subendothelium at the site of vascular injury or with a prosthetic surface. The platelets adhere, undergo the release reaction, and aggregate; if these aggregates are sufficiently large or if the atherosclerotic stenosis is severe, an occlusive thrombus may form. Frequently, however, the platelet aggregates embolize to obstruct the arterial circulation distally. Thus the clinical manifestations of arterial thromboembolism may be the result of occlusive thrombus formation (e.g., acute coronary thrombosis), which usually occurs on a background of ruptured or ulcerated atherosclerotic plaque, or the result of peripheral embolization of platelet-fibrin aggregates (e.g., transient cerebral ischemic attacks).

Systemic embolism is an important clinical sequela of arterial thrombosis. Prosthetic cardiac valves, prosthetic vascular grafts, and implanted catheters are sites for arterial thrombus formation and are important sources of systemic emboli. The introduction of a prosthetic material into the circulation exposes blood to a foreign surface that may induce platelet adhesion, aggregation, and embolization of the aggregated platelets. Furthermore, foreign surfaces may induce the activation of blood coagulation. Systemic embolism also occurs from left ventricular thrombi that form secondary to transmural myocardial infarction. Atrial fibrillation with or without valvular heart disease (e.g., rheumatic mitral stenosis) also may lead to systemic embolism. Thrombi originating in the right side of the heart or on the surface of central venous catheters may lead to pulmonary embolism.

The various risk factors for atherosclerosis and arterial thromboembolism that have been identified include age, sex, hypertension, diabetes mellitus, smoking, obesity, hypercholesterolemia, and the inherited hyperlipidemic disorders.[3]

A tendency to arterial thrombosis, which may be massive, may be seen in the anticardiolipin syndrome or in patients who develop heparin-induced thrombocytopenia and thrombosis.

Clinical Features

The clinical manifestations of arterial thromboembolism are organ-specific and depend on the particular area of the circulation that is affected. Atherosclerotic narrowing of the coronary arteries with ruptured or ulcerated plaque may lead to thrombus formation; if a sufficient area of the lumen is occluded, myocardial infarction (MI) may result. Left ventricular mural thrombosis frequently complicates the course of patients with transmural anterior MI and poses the risk of systemic embolism.

Severe atherosclerosis of the carotid artery may progress to thrombotic occlusion and subsequent stroke; the junction of the vertebral and basilar arteries and the main bifurcation of the middle cerebral artery are common sites for thrombosis.[2] Atherosclerotic narrowing of the carotid arteries may serve as a nidus for repeated formation and embolization of platelet aggregates to the cerebral circulation or to the eye. Repeated "showers" of platelet-fibrin emboli result in transient and reversible episodes of cerebral ischemia or episodes of amaurosis fugax. These emboli usually lyse and disperse spontaneously, with resolution of the neurologic deficit during a period of hours.

Atherosclerosis frequently affects the large to medium-sized arteries of the lower limbs (e.g., the distal aorta and the iliac, femoral, and popliteal arteries); these lesions may serve as foci for the development of occlusive thrombi or as a source of distal embolization. Acute thrombotic occlusion of the large or medium-sized arteries of

the leg results in limb-threatening ischemia; untreated, it may progress to ischemic necrosis. Distal embolization of platelet-fibrin thrombi from the proximal arteries of the leg may result in multiple discrete areas of localized tissue necrosis.

Laboratory Features

A number of laboratory abnormalities have been reported in patients with arterial thromboembolism, including elevated plasma levels of β-thromboglobulin and platelet factor 4 (indicating that platelets have undergone the release reaction) and elevated plasma levels of thromboxane B_2 (indicating that the platelet prostaglandin pathway has been activated). The continuous process of platelet adhesion, aggregation, and embolization may result in an increased platelet turnover (decreased survival), which can be detected by measuring the survival of isotopically labeled platelets injected intravenously. Although these laboratory tests have been useful research techniques that have provided important information about the pathophysiology of arterial thromboembolic disease, they currently have no role in patient management. Furthermore, the laboratory changes outlined above are nonspecific, because many nonthrombogenic stimuli (e.g., trauma or sepsis) may interact with platelets, inducing platelet release and prostaglandin formation and decreased platelet survival.

VENOUS THROMBOEMBOLISM

Pathophysiology

Venous thromboembolism (venous thrombosis and/or pulmonary embolism) usually complicates the course of sick, hospitalized patients but also may affect ambulatory and otherwise apparently healthy individuals.[4–6] Pulmonary embolism remains the most common preventable cause of hospital death and is responsible for approximately 150,000 to 200,000 deaths per year in the United States. Most patients who die from pulmonary embolism succumb suddenly or within 2 h of the acute event, before therapy can be initiated or can take effect.[7,8] Effective prophylaxis against venous thromboembolism is now available for most high-risk patients.[9,10] The use of prophylaxis is more effective for preventing death and morbidity from venous thromboembolism than is treatment of the established disease.

Venous thrombi are composed predominantly of fibrin and red cells with a variable platelet and leukocyte component. The formation, growth, and dissolution of venous thromboemboli represent a balance between various thrombogenic stimuli and several protective mechanisms. The factors that predispose to the development of venous thromboemboli are venous stasis, activation of blood coagulation, and vascular damage. The protective mechanisms that counteract these thrombogenic stimuli include (1) the inactivation of activated coagulation factors by circulating inhibitors (e.g., antithrombin III, α_2-macroglobulin, α_1-antitrypsin, and activated protein C), (2) clearance of activated coagulation factors and soluble fibrin polymer complexes by the reticuloendothelial system and by the liver, and (3) dissolution of fibrin by fibrinolytic enzymes derived from plasma and endothelial cells and digestion by leukocytes.

Various risk factors predispose to the development of venous thromboembolism (Table 28-1). Other conditions that have been reported to be associated with a high risk of venous thromboembolism include homocystinuria, polycythemia vera, paroxysmal nocturnal hemoglobinuria, and the presence of the lupus inhibitor.

Pulmonary embolism originates from thrombi in the deep veins of the leg in 90% or more of patients.[11–18] Other, less common sources of pulmonary embolism include the deep pelvic veins, renal veins, inferior vena cava, right side of the heart, and axillary veins. Most clinically important pulmonary emboli arise from thrombi in the popliteal or more proximal deep veins of the leg (proximal vein thrombosis). Pulmonary embolism occurs in 50% of patients with objectively documented proximal vein thrombosis; many of these emboli are asymptomatic.[12] Usually, only part of the thrombus embolizes, and patients with angiographically documented pulmonary embolism frequently have detectable deep vein thrombosis of the legs at the time of presentation. The clinical significance of pulmonary embolism depends on the size of the embolus and the cardiorespiratory reserve of the patient.[11]

Clinical Features

The clinical features of venous thrombosis include leg pain, tenderness and swelling, a palpable cord (i.e., a thrombosed vessel that is palpable as a cord), discoloration, venous distension and prominence of the superficial veins, and cyanosis. The clinical diagnosis of venous thrombosis is highly nonspecific, because none of the symptoms or signs is unique, and each may be caused by nonthrombotic disorders. The rare exception, perhaps, is the patient with phlegmasia cerulea dolens, in whom the diagnosis of massive iliofemoral thrombosis usually is clinically obvious; this syndrome occurs in less than 1% of patients with symptomatic venous thrombosis. In most patients who present with clinically suspected venous thrombosis, the symptoms and signs are nonspecific, and in more than 50% of these patients, the clinical suspicion of venous thrombosis is not confirmed by objective testing[19] (Table 28-2). Further, patients with relatively minor symptoms and signs may have extensive deep venous thrombi, whereas in patients with florid leg pain and swelling, suggesting extensive deep vein

TABLE 28-1. *Factors that Predispose to the Development of Venous Thromboembolism*

Clinical risk factors
  Surgical and nonsurgical trauma
  Previous venous thromboembolism
  Immobilization
  Malignant disease
  Heart disease
  Leg paralysis
  Age (>40 years)
  Obesity
  Estrogens
  Parturition
Inherited or acquired abnormalities
  Protein C deficiency
  Protein S deficiency
  Antithrombin III deficiency
  Dysfibrinogenemia
  Heparin-induced thrombocytopenia

TABLE 28-2. *Alternative Diagnoses for Clinically Suspected Venous Thrombosis and Negative Venograms in 87 Consecutive Patients*[*]

Diagnosis	Percent of Patients
Muscle strain	24
Direct twisting injury to leg	10
Leg swelling in paralyzed limb	9
Lymphangitis, lymphatic obstruction	7
Venous reflux	7
Muscle tear	6
Baker's cyst	5
Cellulitis	3
Internal abnormality of knee	2
Unknown	26

* The diagnosis was made once venous thrombosis had been excluded by the finding of a negative venogram.
Reproduced with permission from Hull RD, Hirsh J, Sackett DL, et al. Clinical validity of a negative venogram in patients with clinically suspected venous thrombosis. Circulation 64:622, 1981. Copyright 1981, American Heart Association.

thrombosis, objective testing may produce negative results. Thus objective testing is mandatory to confirm or exclude a diagnosis of venous thrombosis.[20]

Pulmonary embolism may present clinically in a variety of ways, depending on the size, location, and number of emboli and on the patient's underlying cardiorespiratory reserve. The clinical manifestations of acute pulmonary embolism generally can be divided into several syndromes that overlap considerably: (1) transient dyspnea and tachypnea in the absence of other associated clinical manifestations, (2) the syndrome of pulmonary infarction or congestive atelectasis (also known as *ischemic pneumonitis* or *incomplete infarction*), including pleuritic chest pain, cough, hemoptysis, pleural effusion, and pulmonary infiltrates on chest x-ray, (3) right-sided heart failure associated with severe dyspnea and tachypnea, (4) cardiovascular collapse with hypotension, syncope, and coma (usually associated with massive pulmonary embolism), and (5) a variety of less common and highly nonspecific clinical features, including confusion and coma, pyrexia, wheezing, resistant cardiac failure, and unexplained arrhythmia.

It is now widely accepted that the clinical diagnosis of pulmonary embolism is highly nonspe-

cific. Multiple studies indicate that in more than half of all patients with clinically suspected pulmonary embolism, this diagnosis is not confirmed by objective testing. Therefore, objective testing is mandatory to confirm or exclude the presence of pulmonary embolism.[21–25]

Laboratory Features

A number of laboratory abnormalities have been associated with venous thromboembolism, including a decrease in the activated partial thromboplastin time, increased levels of fibrinopeptide A and fibrin/fibrinogen degradation product E, and a group of nonspecific laboratory changes that makes up the acute phase response to injury. Tissue injury is associated with a systemic response, including elevated levels of fibrinogen, factor VIII and α_1-antitrypsin, and increases in both the leukocyte and the platelet counts. Tissue injury is also associated with systemic activation of blood coagulation and fibrin formation, a decrease in the activated partial thromboplastin time, and increases in the levels of fibrinopeptide A and fibrin/fibrinogen degradation product E. All these changes are highly nonspecific and may occur as a result of surgical or nonsurgical trauma, infection, inflammation, or infarction. Patients with venous thromboembolism frequently have other comorbid conditions, and it is not surprising that the laboratory changes reported to be associated with venous thromboembolism are highly nonspecific.[27,28] There is currently no evidence to indicate that any of the reported laboratory changes associated with venous thromboembolism can be used to predict the development of venous thromboembolism.

Two blood tests, the fibrinopeptide A assay and the assay for fibrin/fibrinogen fragment E, are highly sensitive to venous thromboembolism in symptomatic patients but are nonspecific. Both the fibrinopeptide A assay and the assay for fragment E are performed by radioimmunoassay and require technical simplification for routine clinical use. If simplified, however, either of these assays possibly could be used to exclude a diagnosis of venous thromboembolism in symptomatic patients, but this will require formal evaluation in adequately designed and executed clinical trials.

The assay for fragment D-dimer of fibrin may overcome the technical limitations of the previous assays of fibrinopeptide A and fragment E.[29]

Differential Diagnosis

The differential diagnosis in patients with clinically suspected venous thrombosis includes muscle strain (usually associated with unaccustomed exercise), muscle tear, direct twisting injury to the leg, vasomotor changes in a paralyzed leg, venous reflux, lymphangitis, lymphatic obstruction, Baker's cyst, cellulitis, internal derangement of the knee, hematoma, and venous insufficiency. An alternate diagnosis is frequently not evident at presentation, and without objective testing, it is impossible to exclude venous thrombosis.[24,26] The cause of symptoms often can be determined by careful follow-up once a diagnosis of venous thrombosis has been excluded by objective testing. In some patients, however, the cause of pain, tenderness, and swelling remains uncertain even after careful follow-up.

ANTICOAGULANT THERAPY FOR ARTERIAL AND VENOUS THROMBOEMBOLISM

Anticoagulant drugs (heparin and/or warfarin) are the mainstay in the management of both arterial and venous thromboembolism. The treatment of these disorders depends somewhat on the their pathophysiology. Therefore, both anticoagulant and antiplatelet drugs have an important role in the management of arterial thromboembolism, but antiplatelet therapy has little, if any, role in the treatment of venous thromboembolism.

This section will concentrate on the role of heparin and warfarin in the treatment of thromboembolism and will not further discuss the role of antiplatelet drugs or thrombolysis.

The Role of Anticoagulants in the Treatment of Venous Thromboembolism

The objectives of treatment in patients with venous thromboembolism are (1) to prevent death from pulmonary embolism, (2) to prevent recurrent venous thromboembolism, and (3) to prevent the postphlebitic syndrome. Initial therapy with intravenous heparin using a heparin protocol monitored by the activated partial thromboplastin time (APTT) is the treatment of choice for most patients with pulmonary embolism or proximal venous thrombosis. In the past, continuous IV heparin was given for 7 to 10 days before warfarin therapy was commenced. Results of two randomized clinical trials comparing the effectiveness and safety of warfarin started with heparin at the time of diagnosis versus day 5 of heparin showed that the two groups were equal.[30,31] It can therefore be recommended that, in most patients, warfarin can be started at the time of diagnosis. Exceptions include patients who are unstable and who may require other interventions such as thrombolytic therapy or thrombectomy. Less intense warfarin (INR 2 to 3) should be continued for 3 months in most patients with proximal vein thrombosis.[32] Exceptions would include patients who have had massive iliofemoral thrombosis, with or without pulmonary embolism, or patients who have had recurrent episodes of venous thromboembolism. In such cases, warfarin therapy should be continued for 6 to 12 months and, in some cases, indefinitely.[33] Also, patients with known inhibitor deficiency, e.g., antithrombin III or protein C or S deficiency, who have had thromboembolic events, especially if they have commenced early in life, should be placed on lifelong oral anticoagulants.[33] On the other hand, the presence of an inhibitor deficiency state without thromboembolic events may not require lifelong anticoagulants. Concentrates of antithrombin III, protein C, and protein S are now available for treatment or prophylaxis in patients with known deficiency states, e.g., in pregnancy, major surgery, or other situations causing a high risk for venous thrombosis.

HEPARIN

Heparin is a mixture of anionic glycosaminoglycans with an average molecular weight of 10,000 to 17,000 (range 3000 to 25,000). Heparin inhibits the coagulation pathway by a number of mechanisms. The most important activity is the inhibition of activated factors XII, XI, IX, and X and prothrombin, i.e., thrombin, with the greatest inhibition being on factor Xa and thrombin.[34–36] The anticoagulant effect of heparin is also mediated by heparin cofactor II, which is independent of antithrombin III.[36] Heparin also has been known to interfere with the generation and function of factor Xa and to interfere with platelet function. Although heparin has an anticoagulant effect when taken orally or intrabronchially in very large doses, in clinical practice it must be given parenterally. Heparin is well absorbed after subcutaneous injection, with peak levels appearing after injection and lasting up to 12 h. The subcutaneous route for administration has been used in both prophylaxis and treatment, but continuous IV infusion is the preferred approach for treatment. Intermittent IV injection is associated with a greater risk of bleeding. The test most commonly used to monitor heparin therapy is the activated partial thromboplastin time (APTT). The anticoagulant response to heparin in an individual patient is unpredictable, and therefore, monitoring by the APTT is necessary to guarantee that a therapeutic effect has been achieved.

Anticoagulant Treatment of Venous Thromboembolism

The development of accurate objective tests to detect venous thromboembolism together with advances in clinical trial methodology have made it possible to perform clinical trials evaluating heparin therapy for venous thromboembolism. The results of these trials have resolved many of the uncertainties that a clinician confronts in selecting the appropriate course of heparin. The clinical trials have established the need for initial heparin treatment and have defined the optimal duration for this treatment. They have also shown that an adequate intensity of heparin is required to prevent recurrent venous thromboembolism. Although there has been concern that bleeding risk is increased with higher doses of heparin, the association of bleeding with supratherapeutic APTT levels has not been well documented. The evidence supporting the requirement of a therapeutic APTT range will be reviewed, and a heparin protocol that guarantees that patients achieve the targeted therapeutic range will be presented.

Monitoring of Heparin Therapy: The Therapeutic Range

Clinical trials have established the need for initial heparin treatment in patients with proximal vein thrombosis.[37] An adequate intensity of heparin treatment was shown to be required to prevent recurrent venous thromboembolism. As mentioned earlier, this latter finding also establishes both the need to monitor the anticoagulant response to heparin and the need for dose titration in the individual patient, because the anticoagulant response to a standard dose of heparin varies widely among patients.

It has become common clinical practice to adjust the heparin dose to maintain the result of the APTT within a defined therapeutic range. Over the years, this therapeutic range evolved based on clinical custom to the use of an upper and lower limit, i.e., an APTT of 1.5 to 2.5 × control. The use of an APTT ratio of 1.5 as the lower limit of the therapeutic range is supported by data from clinical trials. In contrast, until very recently, there has been no firm evidence from clinical trials to provide clear guidelines on the upper limit of the therapeutic range. The use of an upper limit and the clinical practice of reducing the heparin dose when the APTT result exceeded this limit have been based on clinical custom and the intuitive belief that this practice will minimize the risk of bleeding. Indeed, the dose of heparin given has been cited as one of the risk factors for bleeding on heparin, but this was based on retrospective studies.[38–40] Recently, data from rigorously designed clinical trials have become available which enable firm recommendations about the appropriate therapeutic range for the APTT. The findings indicate that failure to exceed the lower limit, i.e., APTT ratio of 1.5, is associated with an unacceptably high risk of recurrent venous thromboembolism, but in contrast, no association exists between supratherapeutic APTT responses and the risk of bleeding.

Lower Limit of Therapeutic Range
Data from two randomized trials establish an APTT ratio of 1.5 as the lower limit of the therapeutic range.[41,42] The first trial evaluated the clinical outcomes in patients with proximal vein thrombosis who were treated either with continu-

ous IV heparin or intermittent subcutaneous heparin.[41] Both treatment groups had the heparin dose adjusted to maintain the APTT ratio above the predefined lower limit of 1.5. The intravenous and subcutaneous regimens produced markedly different intensities of anticoagulant response early in the course of therapy. The subcutaneous regimen resulted in an initial anticoagulant response below the lower limit in the majority (63%) of patients and a high frequency of recurrent venous thromboembolism (11 of 57 patients, 19%) which was virtually confined to patients with a subtherapeutic APTT response. In contrast, continuous IV heparin resulted in an adequate anticoagulant response in the majority (71%) of patients and a low frequency of recurrent thromboembolic events (3 of 58 patients, 5%); the recurrences in this group also were limited to patients with an initial subtherapeutic anticoagulant response. Thus 13 of 53 patients (24.5%) with an APTT response below the lower limit for 24 h or more had recurrent venous thromboembolism, compared with only 1 of 62 patients (1.6%) in whom an APTT ratio of 1.5 or more was achieved ($p < 0.001$). This represents a relative risk for recurrent venous thromboembolism of 15:1 for patients given inadequate initial heparin treatment (APTT ratio less than 1.5).

The preceding findings are strongly supported by a recent randomized trial which compared IV heparin with oral anticoagulants alone for the initial treatment of patients with proximal vein thrombosis.[42] The latter treatment group, by the nature of their treatment, has an inadequate APTT response for at least the first 48 h, since the onset of the anticoagulant effect of oral anticoagulants is delayed. Recurrent venous thromboembolism occurred in 12 of 60 patients (20%) treated with oral anticoagulants alone, compared with 4 of 60 patients (6.7%) who received initial IV heparin adjusted to maintain the APTT above 1.5 times control ($p = 0.058$). Asymptomatic extension of venous thrombosis was observed in 39.6% of the oral anticoagulant group, compared with 8.2% of patients in the heparin plus oral anticoagulant group ($p < 0.001$). Major bleeding was infrequent and no different between the two groups.

The clinical trial findings just outlined indicate that an adequate intensity of initial heparin treatment is required to prevent recurrent venous thromboembolism. Sufficient heparin should be given to prolong the APTT ratio to 1.5 or more.

Upper Limit of Therapeutic Range

New information about the upper limit of the therapeutic range for the APTT has become available very recently.[43] This study evaluated the clinical outcomes in patients with proximal vein thrombosis who were randomized to receive initial treatment with either IV heparin alone or IV heparin with simultaneous warfarin sodium. Both regimens achieved adequate therapy in almost all patients, but the combined heparin and warfarin group received more intensive anticoagulation, with the majority of patients exceeding the predefined upper limit (APTT ratio 2.5) for sustained periods of time. Thus 69 of 99 patients (69%) in the combined group had a supratherapeutic value (ratio 2.5 or more) persisting for 24 h or more, compared with 24 of 100 patients (24%) receiving heparin alone ($p < 0.001$). Despite this more intense therapy in the combined group, bleeding complications occurred with similar frequency in the two groups: 9 of 99 patients in the combined group (9.1%) compared with 12 of 100 patients (12.0%) in the group given heparin alone. Importantly, bleeding complications occurred in 8 of 93 patients (8.6%) with supratherapeutic findings. Major bleeding occurred in 3 of 93 patients (3.2%) with supratherapeutic APTT findings (RR = 0.3; $p = 0.09$). Major bleeding occurred in 11% of patients considered to be at high risk but in only 1% of those considered to be at low risk ($p = 0.007$). These findings demonstrate a lack of association between a supratherapeutic APTT result (ratio 2.5 or more) and the risk of clinically important bleeding complications.

The Need for Quality Assurance of Heparin Therapy

Audits of heparin therapy suggest that administration of IV heparin is fraught with difficulty.[43,44] These audits indicate that the current clinical practice of using an intuitive approach to heparin dose titration frequently results in inadequate therapy. For example, an audit of physician practice at three university-affiliated hospitals documented that 60% of patients failed to achieve an adequate APTT response (ratio 1.5) during the initial 24 h of therapy, and 30% to 40% of patients remained subtherapeutic over the next 3 to 4 days.[44] A startling finding was that in one-third of patients in whom a subtherapeutic APTT was found, no change in heparin dose occurred. These findings show that physician practices in the administration of IV heparin have been dominated by a desire to avoid supratherapeutic APTT responses, due to the fear of bleeding complications, with much less concern about the risk of recurrent venous thromboembolism. Consequently, it is been common practice for many clinicians to start treatment with a low heparin dose and to cautiously increase this dose over several days to achieve the therapeutic range. This approach has been shown to result in the administration of inadequate therapy in the majority of patients; the clinical trial data indicate that it is inappropriate, and indeed dangerous, because it places the patients at unacceptably high risk for recurrent venous thromboembolism.

The audits of heparin therapy indicate a need for quality assurance. We have recently completed a randomized clinical trial evaluating a prescriptive approach to IV heparin administration.[43] Patients were randomized to initial heparin therapy alone or to heparin therapy with simultaneous warfarin sodium therapy. The objective of the prescriptive approach was to minimize the proportion of patients receiving subtherapeutic doses of heparin and to do so within 24 h in the presence or absence of oral anticoagulants. Only 2% and 1% of the patients were subtherapeutic for more than 24 h in the heparin and warfarin group and the heparin alone group, respectively. Recurrent venous thromboembolism (objectively documented) occurred infrequently in both groups (7%). The findings demonstrate that subtherapy was avoided in most patients and that the prescriptive heparin protocol resulted in effective delivery of heparin therapy in both groups.

Heparin Protocol[43]

1. Initial IV heparin bolus: 5000 units
2. Continuous IV heparin infusion: Commence at 42 mL/h of 20,000 units (1680 units/h) in 500 mL of two-thirds dextrose and one-third saline (a 24-h heparin dose of 40,320 units), except in the following patients, in whom heparin infusion will be commenced at a rate of 31 mL/h (1240 units/h) (i.e., a 24-h dose of 29,760 units):
   a. Patients who have undergone surgery within the previous 2 weeks
   b. Patients with a previous history of peptic ulcer disease or gastrointestinal or genitourinary bleeding
   c. Patients with recent stroke (i.e., thrombotic stroke within 2 weeks previously)
   d. Patients with a platelet count of less than 150×10^9 per liter
   e. Patients with miscellaneous reasons for a high risk of bleeding (e.g., hepatic failure, renal failure, or vitamin K deficiency)
3. Heparin dose is adjusted using the APTT. The APTT is performed in all patients as outlined below:
   a. 4 to 6 h after commencing heparin; the heparin dose is then adjusted according to the nomogram shown in Table 28-3.
   b. 4 to 6 h after implementing the first dosage adjustment.
   c. The APTT is then performed as indicated by the nomogram for the first 24 h of therapy.
   d. Thereafter, the APTT will be performed once daily, unless the patient is subtherapeutic, in which case the APTT will be repeated 4 to 6 h after increasing the heparin dose.
4. If heparin is interrupted for reasons other than as required by the nomogram, the following procedure should be used when recommencing heparin:
   a. If heparin therapy is interrupted for 1 h or less, then
      i. Recommence the heparin infusion at the rate that was being administered prior to the interruption.
      ii. Perform an APTT 4 to 6 h after restarting heparin, and adjust the heparin dose as indicated by the nomogram (Table 28-3).

TABLE 28-3. *Intravenous Heparin Dose-Titration Nomogram for APTT**

| APTT | IV Infusion | | Additional Action |
	Rate Change, mL/h	Dose Change, U/24 h[†]	
≤45	+6	+5760	Repeated APTT[‡] in 4–6 h
46–54	+3	+2880	Repeated APTT in 4–6 h
55–85	0	0	None[§]
86–110	−3	−2880	Stop heparin sodium treatment for 1 h; repeated APTT 4–6 h after restarting heparin treatment
>110	−6	−5760	Stop heparin treatment for 1 h; repeated APTT 4–6 h after restarting heparin treatment

* APTT = activated partial thromboplastin time.
[†] Heparin sodium concentration, 20,000 U in 500 mL = 40 U/mL.
[‡] With the use of Actin-FS thromboplastin reagent (Dade, Mississauga, Ontario).
[§] During the first 24 h, repeated APTT in 4 to 6 h. Thereafter, the APTT will be determined once daily, unless subtherapeutic.
Reproduced with permission from Hull RD, Raskob GE, Rosenbloom D, et al. Optimal therapeutic level of heparin therapy in patients with venous thrombosis. Arch Intern Med 152:1589, 1992. Copyright 1992, American Medical Association.

b. If heparin therapy is interrupted for longer than 1 h, then

   i. Administer a 5000-unit IV heparin bolus.

   ii. Recommence the heparin infusion at the rate that was being administered prior to the interruption.

   iii. Perform an APTT 4 to 6 h after restarting heparin, and adjust the heparin dose as indicated by the nomogram (Table 28-3).

Endogenous Periodicity of the APTT Responses

A striking periodicity of the APTT responses was observed[43] (Fig. 28-1). A clinically and statistically significant diurnal variation was noted ($p < 0.0001$) when the APTT findings were analyzed. The mean peak-to-trough variation in APTT was 9.5 s; 95% confidence limits were 5.9 to 13.2 s. Peak values were seen at 3:23 A.M.; 95% confidence limits were 2:01 to 4:44 A.M., and the trough was seen 12 h later. There was no diurnal variation in the heparin doses infused. A similar circadian rhythm has been noted in normal volunteers and in patients on heparin therapy, and a similar variation was seen in the thrombin time and the factor Xa levels as were seen with APTT, again unrelated to the heparin dose being infused.

Other Potential Uses of Heparin Protocol

The heparin protocol was developed and evaluated in patients with venous thrombosis. The principles applied by this prescriptive approach have the potential for broad application to the varied clinical settings in which heparin is used. Our findings provide support for expanded evaluation of the protocol by clinical trials in these settings (e.g., adjunctive heparin treatment to coronary thrombolysis or in patients undergoing coronary or peripheral angioplasty).

Subcutaneous Heparin Compared with Continuous IV Heparin

In the past, a number of randomized trials have compared the effectiveness and safety of heparin given by the subcutaneous and continuous IV routes.[46] In was concluded that subcutaneous heparin was as effective and safe as IV heparin.[47] However, this meta-analysis has been criticized because of the selection of studies for review and for the lack of data on APTT values in patients receiving subcutaneous heparin.[48] In view of the well-established need to achieve a lower limit of the APTT therapeutic range, heparin given by the subcutaneous route cannot be recommended in the initial treatment of proximal venous thrombosis.

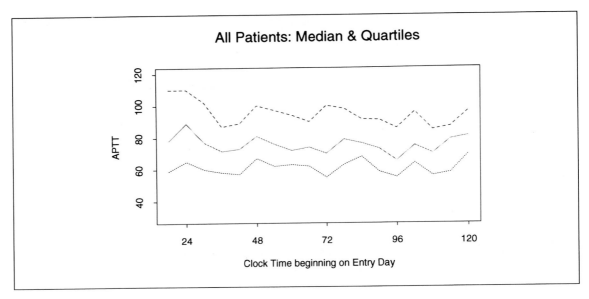

FIGURE 28-1. *Periodicity of activated partial thromboplastin time (APTT) results for all patients. The median and quartiles for the APTT values grouped within 6-h intervals show a significant diurnal variation (p < 0.0001). There was a 9.5-s variation in the mean peak to trough levels (95% CI = 5.9 to 13.2 s), with the peak level occurring at 3:23 A.M. and the trough level occurring 12 h later. (Reproduced with permission from Hull RD, Raskob GE, Rosenbloom D, et al. Optimal therapeutic level of heparin therapy in patients with venous thrombosis. Arch Intern Med 152:1589, 1992. Copyright 1992, American Medical Association.)*

Subcutaneous Adjusted-Dose Heparin for Long-Term Treatment

Adjusted-dose subcutaneous heparin is the long-term anticoagulant regimen of choice in pregnant patients, certain patients at high risk of bleeding, and patients who return to geographically remote areas in which long-term anticoagulant monitoring is unavailable or impractical (in whom the heparin dose is adjusted during the first few days of long-term therapy and then fixed).[49] The starting dose of long-term subcutaneous (SC) heparin is determined from the patient's initial IV heparin dose requirement. A starting SC dose equivalent to one-third of the patient's 24-h IV heparin dose is administered every 12 h. For example, if the patient required 30,000 units per 24 h of continuous IV heparin to maintain the APTT above 1.5 times the control value, the starting dose of long-term SC heparin would be 10,000 units every 12 h. The SC dose is adjusted during the first few days of long-term therapy to maintain the midinterval

APTT (determined 6 h after injection) at 1.5 times the control value. This level of anticoagulant response is usually achieved with a dose of 8000 to 12,000 units every 12 h (mean dose 10,000 units every 12 h). In pregnant patients, larger doses may be required, and continued monitoring is desirable because of changes in heparin requirements throughout the course of pregnancy.

Adverse Effects of Heparin Therapy

The side effects of heparin therapy include bleeding, thrombocytopenia, arterial thromboembolism, hypersensitivity, and osteoporosis. Bleeding, the most common side effect of heparin, occurs in 5% to 10% of patients during initial continuous IV heparin therapy.[38–40] At particular risk are those patients who have been exposed to recent surgery or trauma and those with an underlying hemostatic defect or predisposing clinical risk factor (such as unsuspected peptic ulcer or occult carcinoma). The risk of bleeding complications is greater in patients who receive IV heparin by intermittent injection than in those who receive a continuous infusion.

The onset of thrombocytopenia, now a well-recognized complication of heparin therapy, usually occurs 7 to 10 days after heparin treatment is commenced but may be earlier in patients previously exposed to heparin.[50] This complication has been seen with the low-molecular-weight heparins as well. Although the exact incidence of this complication with these agents is as yet undetermined, it appears to be around 1% to 2%. Heparin-induced thrombocytopenia is more common in patients receiving beef-lung heparin than in those receiving porcine-intestinal heparin. The thrombocytopenia may be moderate or severe. The precise mechanism of heparin-induced thrombocytopenia is currently unknown but probably involves immune mechanisms, particularly in the severe forms. The severe form is less common than the moderate form. It is currently unknown how frequently patients with moderate thrombocytopenia may progress to the severe form with the added complication of arterial thrombosis. This may precede or coincide with the fall in platelet count. Heparin-induced thrombocytopenia with arterial thrombosis results in a high incidence of limb amputation and mortality. It is therefore mandatory that heparin in all forms be discontinued when heparin-induced thrombocytopenia is diagnosed. Alternate approaches to treatment include insertion of an inferior vena caval filter or the use of arvin (Ancrod),[51] a defibrinogenating extract of snake venom which produces effective anticoagulation while oral anticoagulants are being instituted. A heparinoid consisting mainly of dermatan sulfate along with heparin and condroitin sulfate (ORG10172, Organon, Inc., The Netherlands) does not cross-react with heparin using in vitro immunoassays and has been used effectively in a few patients with heparin-induced thrombocytopenia.[52,53]

Osteoporosis occurs rarely in patients receiving long-term SC heparin therapy (more than 15,000 units of heparin per day for longer than 6 months).[54] The earliest clinical manifestation of heparin-associated osteoporosis is usually the onset of nonspecific low-back pain primarily involving the vertebrae or ribs; patients also may present with spontaneous fracture in these areas.

Hypersensitivity to heparin is uncommon and may take the form of a skin rash or, less commonly, anaphylaxis. Alopecia has been reported as a rare complication of heparin. Serum transaminase levels may be moderately raised. Heparin-induced hypoaldosteronism is recognized but rare.[55,56] Rarely, a bluish discoloration of the toes, associated with a burning sensation, has been reported.

Neutralization of Heparin Anticoagulant Effect

The anticoagulant effect of heparin can be immediately neutralized by the IV injection of protamine sulfate. The appropriate neutralizing dose depends on the dose of heparin, its route of administration, and the time it is given. If protamine sulfate is used within minutes of an IV heparin injection, a full neutralizing dose (1 mg protamine sulfate/100 units heparin) should be given. Because the plasma half-life of intravenously administered heparin is approximately 60 minutes, an injection of protamine sulfate in a bolus of more than 50 mg is seldom required. An occasional hypotensive response to protamine sulfate has been reported; therefore, it should be injected slowly over a 10- to 30-minute period. Treatment with protamine sulfate may need to be repeated, because protamine is cleared from the blood more quickly than is heparin. After an SC injection of heparin, repeated small doses of protamine may be required because of prolonged heparin absorption from the SC depot.

Low-Molecular-Weight Heparin and Heparinoids

In recent years, low-molecular-weight (LMW) derivatives of commercial heparin have been prepared that have a mean molecular weight of 4000 to 5000, in contrast to unfractionated heparin, which has a mean molecular weight of 10,000 to 17,000. Pharmacokinetic studies and recent small clinical trials in selected patients with venous thrombosis indicate that the bioavailability of these LMW heparin fractions following subcutaneous injection is very high.[57,58] For example, it was reported that the bioavailability of LMW heparin after an SC injection of 120 factor Xa international units per kilogram to healthy volunteers was approximately 90% of an equivalent IV dose.[59] The excellent bioavailability of LMW heparin, together with a longer half-life (anti-factor Xa activity) than unfractionated heparin, suggests that it may be possible to develop an effective regimen for initial treatment with LMW heparin using once-daily subcutaneous injection.[60,61] The anticoagulant response (factor Xa units/mL) observed with a given dose of LMW heparin is highly correlated with body weight, so LMW heparin is effective when given in standard doses (factor Xa international units/kg) without laboratory monitoring.[60,61]

Low-Molecular-Weight Heparin in the Treatment of Proximal Venous Thrombosis

The number of small trials comparing SC or IV low-molecular-weight (LMW) heparin with continuous IV heparin suggested that LMW heparin may have a role in treatment as well as in prophylaxis.[62] Within the past year there have been four randomized clinical trials comparing LMW heparin given once or twice daily subcutaneously with continuous IV heparin with or without the use of oral warfarin.[63–66] In two of the European trials, Fraxiparine was given in a fixed dose SC twice a day and compared with continuous IV heparin monitored by APTT.[63,64] Both studies used the Arnesen and Marder scales on repeat venography to assess efficacy, and in the collaborative European multicenter study, perfusion lung scans were done on days 0 and 10. Both studies suggest that Fraxiparine was at least as effective as unfractionated heparin in preventing venographic extension of thrombosis.

A randomized trial was reported in consecutive symptomatic patients with proximal vein thrombosis comparing the relative effectiveness and risk of bleeding of fixed-dose LMW heparin (Fraxiparine) with adjusted-dose IV unfraction-

ated heparin for 10 days followed by oral warfarin sodium for 3 months.[65] Patients in the LMW heparin group received SC injections every 12 h according to body weight [12,500 aXa Institute Choay (IC) units for patients weighing < 55 kg, 15,000 aXa IC units for patients weighing between 55 and 80 kg, and 17,500 aXa IC units for patients weighing > 80 kg). Patients in the adjusted-dose IV heparin group received a continuous infusion to maintain the APTT within 1.5 to 2.0 times the mean normal control value.[66] All patients had baseline perfusion lung scans and chest x-rays. In these studies as well, contrast venography was repeated on day 10 or earlier if new symptoms developed. The principal endpoint for the assessment of efficacy was symptomatic recurrent venous thrombosis or symptomatic pulmonary embolism. Secondary endpoints for efficacy assessment were changes between days 0 and 10 in the venograms and perfusion lung scans. The frequency of objectively diagnosed recurrent venous thromboembolism was comparable between the unfractioned heparin and the LMW heparin groups [12 (14%) versus 6 (7%), difference 7%; 95% CI = −3% to 15%; $p = 0.13$]. Clinically evident bleeding occurred in 3.5% of patients receiving unfractionated heparin versus 1.1% of those receiving LMW heparin ($p > 0.2$). In the 6-month follow-up period there were 12 deaths in the unfractionated heparin group versus 6 in the LMW heparin group, and this difference was largely due to cancer deaths (8 of 18 in the unfractionated heparin group versus 1 of 15 in the LMW heparin group).

In a multicenter, double-blind clinical trial, fixed-dose subcutaneous LMW heparin (Logiparin) (175 factor Xa IU/kg) was compared with intravenous heparin by continued infusion adjusted to maintain an APTT of 1.5 to 2.5 times the mean normal control value.[66] All patients had venographically proven proximal venous thrombosis and at the time of entry had ventilation-perfusion lung scans, chest radiographs, and impedance plethysmography. Outcome events included objectively documented venous thromboembolism (recurrence or extension of deep vein thrombosis or pulmonary embolism), major or minor bleeding, thrombocytopenia, and death.

New episodes of venous thromboembolism were seen in 6 of 213 patients receiving LMW heparin (2.8%) and 15 of 219 patients receiving IV unfractionated heparin (6.9%) ($p = 0.07$; 95% CI = 0.02% to 8.1%). Major bleeding associated with initial therapy occurred in 1 patient receiving LMW heparin (0.5%) and in 11 patients receiving IV unfractionated heparin (5.0%), a reduction in risk of 95% ($p = 0.006$). During long-term warfarin therapy, major hemorrhage was seen in 5 patients who had received LMW heparin (2.3%) and in none of those receiving IV heparin ($p = 0.028$). Ten patients who received LMW heparin (4.7%) died, as compared with 21 patients who received IV unfractionated heparin (9.6%), a risk reduction of 51% ($p = 0.049$). The most striking difference was in abrupt deaths in patients with metastatic carcinoma, and the majority of these deaths occurred within the first 3 weeks. It is possible that the long-term use of LMW heparin in place of warfarin sodium may have a greater impact on recurrent thromboembolic events, bleeding, and death, particularly in patients with metastatic carcinoma.

Taken together, the results of these studies provide strong evidence that LMW heparin given subcutaneously is as effective and as safe as unfractionated heparin in the treatment of proximal venous thrombosis. The decreased mortality rate, particularly in patients with metastatic carcinoma, was unexpected and requires confirmation in further prospective, randomized trials.[67]

Management of Calf Vein Thrombosis

The management of patients with calf vein thrombosis remains more complex. It is known that 20% to 30% of thrombi confined to the calves may propagate proximally and thus present a significant risk of pulmonary embolism. To avoid such propagation, treatment with heparin and warfarin, as for proximal vein thrombosis, is commonly prescribed.[68] Where feasible, an acceptable option is to monitor the patient with serial objective tests for proximal venous thrombosis for a period of 10 days from the time of diagnosis.[69,70] If the tests remain negative, no further treatment is required. This option may be particularly useful

in patients at high risk for bleeding. The tests most commonly used are impedance plethysmography and duplex ultrasound.

Inferior Vena Cava Interruption

The transvenous placement of a filter in the vena cava, if possible below the level of the renal veins, may be used in the following circumstances: (1) in the patient with acute venous thromboembolism and an absolute contraindication to anticoagulant therapy, (2) in the patient with massive pulmonary embolism who survives but in whom recurrent embolism may be fatal, and (3) in the very rare patient who suffers from objectively documented recurrent venous thromboembolism during adequate anticoagulant therapy. With the modern filters available, the risk of complications, such as perforation of the vena cava, embolism, and infection, is low.[71] Therefore, all major centers should have the capability of implanting inferior vena cava filters in the appropriate circumstances.

Management of Massive Venous Thrombosis or Pulmonary Embolism

The role of thrombolytic therapy in such circumstances will be discussed elsewhere. Pulmonary embolectomy by catheter devices is continuing to receive attention in the management of massive pulmonary embolism and may have a role in patients for whom fibrinolytic therapy may be contraindicated or surgery may be impossible.

Management of Superficial Thrombophlebitis

Superficial thrombophlebitis may occur with or without associated deep venous thrombosis. In the absence of associated deep vein thrombosis, the treatment of superficial thrombophlebitis is usually confined to symptomatic relief with analgesia and rest of the affected limb. The exception is the patient with superficial thrombophlebitis involving a large segment of the long saphenous vein, particularly when it occurs above the knee. These patients may benefit from treatment with anticoagulant therapy. Patients in whom superficial thrombophlebitis occurs in association with deep venous thrombosis should be treated with heparin and long-term oral anticoagulants as described above.

ORAL ANTICOAGULANT THERAPY

There are two distinct chemical groups of oral anticoagulants: the 4-hydroxy coumarin derivatives (e.g., warfarin sodium), and the indane-1,3-dione derivatives (e.g., phenindione). The coumarin derivatives are the oral anticoagulants of choice because they are associated with fewer nonhemorrhagic side effects than are the indanedione derivatives (see "Adverse Effects of Oral Anticoagulants").

Oral anticoagulants produce an anticoagulant effect by inhibiting the vitamin K–dependent γ-carboxylation of coagulation factors II, VII, IX, and X.[72,73] This results in the synthesis of immunologically detectable but biologically inactive forms of these coagulation proteins. Oral anticoagulants also inhibit the vitamin K–dependent γ-carboxylation of proteins C and S. Protein C circulates as a proenzyme that is activated on endothelial cells by the thrombin-thrombomodulin complex to form activated protein C. Activated protein C inhibits activated factor VIII activity directly, and in the presence of protein S, it also inhibits activated factor V. Therefore, vitamin K antagonists such as warfarin sodium create a biochemical paradox by producing an anticoagulant effect due to the inhibition of procoagulants (factors II, VII, IX, and X) and a potentially thrombogenic effect by impairing the synthesis of naturally occurring inhibitors of coagulation (proteins C and S).

The anticoagulant effect of the vitamin K antagonists is delayed until the normal clotting factors are cleared from the circulation, and the peak effect does not occur until 36 to 72 h after drug administration.[72,73] With a 40-mg loading dose, factor VII levels usually fall rapidly to less than 20% of normal and sometimes to less than 10% of normal for as long as 3 to 4 days. In some patients, suppression of factor VII to this level is seen within 24 h. Sick patients with impaired liver function or reduced vitamin K stores are particularly susceptible to large loading doses. Equilibrium levels of factors II, IX, and X are not reached until about 1 week after the initiation of therapy. The equilibrium levels of these factors are not achieved quicker by using a large loading dose (e.g., 40 mg). Therefore, the use of small initial daily doses (e.g., 10 mg) is the preferred approach for initiating warfarin treatment.

A 4 to 5-day overlap with IV heparin during the initiation of warfarin sodium therapy is important. In a recent trial comparing IV heparin plus oral warfarin with oral warfarin alone, the incidence of recurrent thromboembolic events was shown to be excessively high in the warfarin-only group. Experimental evidence indicates that the maximal antithrombotic effect of warfarin is delayed for as long as 5 days, even though the anticoagulant effect, reflected by an increase in the prothrombin time (due mainly to a reduction in factor VII), may be evident within 2 to 3 days. Factor VII and protein C have similar short half-lives (approximately 4 to 5 h). During the first 24 to 48 h of warfarin sodium therapy, the levels of functional factor VII and protein C fall, while the levels of functionally active factors II, IX, and X remain relatively normal. Thus, during the first 24 to 48 h of therapy, oral anticoagulants have the potential to be thrombogenic, because the anticoagulant effect of low functional factor VII is counteracted by the potentially thrombogenic effect of low levels of functional protein C with near-normal levels of functional factors II, IX, and X. After 72 to 96 h, the levels of functional factors II, IX, and X fall, and the optimal anticoagulant activity of warfarin therapy is expressed. For these reasons, it is important to overlap oral anticoagulant therapy with heparin therapy for 4 to 5 days even though the prothrombin time may be prolonged into the therapeutic range after 2 to 3 days.

Monitoring of Oral Anticoagulants

The laboratory test most commonly used to measure the effects of warfarin is the one-stage prothrombin time, which is sensitive to reduced activity of factors II, VII, and X but is insensitive to reduced activity of factor IX. The optimal therapeutic range for oral anticoagulant therapy monitored using the prothrombin time has been controversial because, until recently, it had not been adequately evaluated in clinical trials. Further confusion about the appropriate therapeutic range occurred because the different tissue thromboplastins used for measuring the prothrombin time vary considerably in sensitivity to the vitamin K–dependent clotting factors and in response to warfarin. Rabbit brain thromboplastin, which is widely used in North America, is less sensitive than is standardized human brain thromboplastin, which has been used widely in the United Kingdom and other parts of Europe. A prothrombin time ratio of 1.5 to 2.0 using rabbit brain thromboplastin (i.e., the traditional therapeutic range in North America) is equivalent to a ratio of 4.0 to 6.0 using human brain thromboplastin. Conversely, a 2- to 3-fold increase in the prothrombin time using standardized human brain thromboplastin is equivalent to a 1.25- to 1.5-fold increase in the prothrombin time using a rabbit brain thromboplastin such as Simplastin or Dade-C.

The optimal therapeutic range for oral anticoagulant therapy in patients with venous thrombosis has recently been established. The findings of randomized trials indicate that venous thrombosis can be treated effectively and more safely with a therapeutic range of 1.25 to 1.5 times control using a rabbit brain thromboplastin such as Simplastin or Dade-C rather than the range of 1.5 to 2.0 times control conventionally recommended in North America.

To promote standardization of the prothrombin time for monitoring oral anticoagulant therapy, the World Health Organization (WHO) has developed an international reference thromboplastin from human brain tissue and has recommended that the prothrombin time ratio be expressed as the *international normalized ratio* (INR).[74] The INR is the prothrombin time ratio obtained by testing a given sample using the WHO reference thromboplastin. For practical clinical purposes, the INR for a given plasma sample is equivalent to the prothrombin time ratio obtained using a standardized human brain thromboplastin known as the *Manchester comparative reagent,* which has been widely used in the United Kingdom. The currently recommended therapeutic range of 1.25 to 1.5 times control using a rabbit brain thromboplastin such as Simplastin or Dade-C corresponds to an INR of 2.0 to 3.0.

In a survey of 53 hospital laboratories, only 21% reported prothrombin times as INR results, and 30% of hospitals could not provide data on the *international sensitivity index* (ISI) of the thromboplastin being used. This study indicated that the current recommendations regarding ISI and INR are being disregarded by the majority of laboratories involved in the study and that anticoagulant monitoring would therefore be substandard.[75]

Oral Anticoagulant (Warfarin Sodium) Protocol

Warfarin sodium is administered in an initial dose of 10 mg/day for the first 2 days, and the daily dose is then adjusted according to the INR. Heparin therapy is discontinued on the fourth or fifth day following initiation of warfarin therapy, provided the INR is prolonged into the therapeutic range (prothrombin time 1.25 to 1.5 times control value, INR 2.0 to 3.0).

Once the anticoagulant effect and the patient's warfarin dose requirements are stable, the INR is monitored weekly throughout the course of oral anticoagulant therapy. However, if there are factors that may produce an unpredictable response to warfarin (e.g., concomitant drug therapy), the INR should be monitored more frequently to minimize the risk of complications due to poor anticoagulant control.

Attempts have been made to improve the control of oral anticoagulants while at the same time decreasing the risk of bleeding complications. These have included the use of warfarin protocols to predict dosing requirements,[76,77] the development of anticoagulant clinics, or the use of a prothrombin home monitor device.[78] An alternative to measurement of the INR is the use of an immunoassay to detect native prothrombin antigen. Early clinical trials indicate that ultralow-dose warfarin therapy (1 mg/day) may be effective prophylaxis in certain settings, e.g., in the prevention of catheter thrombosis in patients with long-term central venous catheters.[79] Such treatment does not significantly prolong the INR, and if dose titration is done, other methods must be used, such as the measurement of prothrombin fragments 1.2 or an assay of activated factor VII.

Adverse Effects of Oral Anticoagulants

The major side effect of oral anticoagulant therapy is bleeding.[80] Bleeding during well-controlled oral anticoagulant therapy is usually due to surgery or other forms of trauma or to local lesions such as peptic ulcer or carcinoma.[80] Spontaneous bleeding may occur if warfarin sodium is given in an excessive dose, resulting in marked prolongation of the INR; this bleeding may be severe and even life-threatening. The risk of bleeding can be substantially reduced by adjusting the warfarin dose to achieve a less intense anticoagulant effect than has traditionally been used in North America (PT 1.25 to 1.5 times control using a rabbit brain thromboplastin such as Simplastin or Dade-C, INR 2.0 to 3.0).[32,81–83]

Nonhemorrhagic side effects of oral anticoagulant differ according to whether the coumarin derivatives (e.g., warfarin sodium) or indanediones are administered. Nonhemorrhagic side effects of coumarin anticoagulants are uncommon, and the coumarins are the oral anticoagulants of choice. Nonhemorrhagic side effects occur more frequently with the indanedione derivatives and include skin necrosis, dermatitis, and a syndrome of painful blue toes. Hypersensitivity reactions have been reported to occur in 1% to 3% of patients receiving indanedione derivatives and include rash, fever, hepatitis, leukopenia, renal failure, and diarrhea; these side effects are sometimes fatal. The indanedione derivatives also produce in many patients red discoloration of the urine that may be confused with hematuria.

Coumarin-induced skin necrosis is a rare but serious complication that requires immediate cessation of oral anticoagulant therapy.[84,85] It usually occurs between 3 and 10 days after therapy has commenced, is more common in women, and most often involves areas of abundant subcutaneous tissues such as the abdomen, buttocks, thighs, and breast. The mechanism of coumarin-induced skin necrosis, which is associated with microvascular thrombosis, is uncertain but appears to be related, at least in some patients, to the depression of protein C. Patients with congenital deficiencies of protein C may be particularly prone to the development of coumarin skin necrosis.

It has been shown recently that oral anticoagulants may have an impact on bone mineral metabolism.[86–88] Two major components of bone matrix require vitamin K for γ-carboxylation [osteocalcin and matrix Gla protein (MGP)], and levels of these proteins as well as mean bone mass are decreased in patients on long-term oral anticoagulants when compared with age-matched controls. Many patients with osteoporosis with fracture of the femur or vertebral bodies have decreased levels of circulating vitamin K, and the administration of vitamin K will correct low osteocalcin levels.[86] Studies are currently under way to further assess the impact of oral anticoagulants on bone mineral metabolism, particularly in elderly females or patients being placed on lifelong oral anticoagulants.

Oral anticoagulants cross the placenta and may cause fetal malformations when used during pregnancy.[89–91] Two specific fetopathic syndromes are associated with oral anticoagulant administration during pregnancy. Treatment with oral anticoagulants during the sixth to twelfth weeks of gestation may induce the syndrome of *warfarin embryopathy* in the fetus. This syndrome consists of skeletal abnormalities ranging from stippled epiphyses to frank skeletal hypoplasia. Although most of the reported cases have occurred in infants of mothers receiving warfarin, it also has been reported as a result of phenindanedione or acenocoumarin administration. Oral anticoagulant administration during the second or third trimester of pregnancy may result in central nervous system abnormalities in the fetus, including abnormalities of the ventricular system (the Dandy-Walker malformation), dorsal midline dysplasia, and optic atrophy. Therefore, the use of oral anticoagulants is contraindicated at any time during pregnancy, and they should not be used in women planning a pregnancy. Adjusted-dose heparin can be given safely throughout pregnancy in patients with venous thromboembolism, and this observation has been extrapolated to patients requiring anticoagulation to prevent systemic embolism from prosthetic heart valves.[90]

Oral anticoagulants may be secreted in the milk of nursing mothers, and the use of these agents in lactating women remains controversial. Recent studies in small numbers of patients have indicated that the prothrombin time and levels of factors II, VII, and X in breast-fed infants were normal, even though the nursing mother received therapeutic doses of warfarin sodium. Further studies are required to make firm clinical recommendations about the use of warfarin in lactating women.

A recent report assessed quality-of-life parameters in patients on low-intensity warfarin compared with those not on warfarin.[92] Oral anticoagulants did not affect quality-of-life parameters except in those patients who experienced bleeding complications. The patients in this study were older (mean age 68 years), and the outcomes may not be applicable to younger patients on long-term anticoagulants, who may experience more inconvenience and lifestyle changes. It has been shown recently that warfarin sensitivity increases with advancing age, emphasizing the need for closer monitoring in older patients.[93]

Factors that Interact with the Effect of Oral Anticoagulant Therapy

A large number of drugs interact with oral anticoagulants and may produce either a prolongation or a reduction in the anticoagulant effect (Table 28-4). Special care should be taken to adjust the dose of oral anticoagulant therapy during the time that other drugs are being taken to minimize the risk of inadequate anticoagulant control.

Increased sensitivity to oral anticoagulants occurs in vitamin K deficiency and impaired liver function and in thyrotoxicosis due to the more rapid metabolism of the vitamin K–dependent clotting factors.

TABLE 28-4. *Drug Interactions with Oral Anticoagulants*

Increase Anticoagulant Effect	Decrease Anticoagulant Effect
Allopurinol	Barbiturates
Anabolic steroids	Cholestyramine
Clofibrate	Diuretics
Cotrimoxazole (trimethoprim and sulphamethoxazole)	Estrogens
Dextrothyroxine	Glutethimide
Neomycin	Griseofulvin
Nortriptyline	Phenytoin
Phenyramidol	Rifampicin
Quinidine	
Salicylate	
Sulphinpyrazone	

Antidote to Oral Anticoagulants

The antidote to the vitamin K antagonists is vitamin K_1. If there is an excessive increase of the INR, the treatment depends on the degree of increase and whether or not the patient is bleeding. If the increase is mild and the patient is not bleeding, no specific treatment is necessary other than reduction in the warfarin dose. The INR can be expected to decrease during the next 24 h with this approach. With a more marked increase in the INR in patients who are not bleeding, treatment with small doses of vitamin K_1, given either orally or by SC injection (2.5 to 5.0 mg), could be considered. With a very marked increase in the INR, particularly in a patient who is either actively bleeding or at risk of bleeding, the coagulation defect should be corrected.

Reported side effects of vitamin K include flushing, dizziness, tachycardia, hypotension, dyspnea, and sweating. Intravenous administration of vitamin K_1 should be done with caution, to avoid inducing an anaphylactoid reaction. The risk of anaphylactoid reaction can be reduced by giving vitamin K_1 slowly, at a rate no faster than 1 mg/min IV. In most patients, IV administration of vitamin K_1 produces a demonstrable effect on the INR within 6 to 8 h and corrects the increased INR within 12 to 24 h. Because the half-life of vitamin K_1 is less than that of warfarin sodium, a repeat course of vitamin K_1 may be necessary. If bleeding is very severe and life-threatening, vitamin K therapy can be supplemented by using concentrates of factors II, VII, IX, and X.

Second-generation rodenticides known as *superwarfarins* have an extremely long half-life. Accidental or intentional consumption of these agents requires repeated injection of vitamin K and fresh frozen plasma for up to 1 to 2 years to completely overcome their effects.

The Role of Anticoagulant Therapy in Patients with Arterial Thromboembolism

The objective of treating patients with arterial thromboembolism with anticoagulants is to prevent the clinical sequelae that occur as a consequence of thrombosis and systemic embolism. Evidence from prospective, randomized clinical trials has demonstrated the effectiveness of anticoagulants in the prevention of recurrent MI and death following an initial MI and in the prevention of systemic embolism following transmural MI, in patients with prosthetic heart valves, and in patients with nonvalvular atrial fibrillation. The role of anticoagulant therapy in the management of individual clinical disorders of arterial thromboembolism is discussed below.

Traditionally, patients with arterial thromboembolism have been treated using a more intense oral anticoagulant regimen (prothrombin time 2.0 to 2.5 using rabbit brain thromboplastin, INR 4.0 to 10.0) than that used in patients with venous thromboembolism. Randomized clinical trials support the use of a less intense therapeutic range (INR 2.0 to 3.0) for the prevention of systemic embolism in patients with MI, atrial fibrillation, and prosthetic cardiac valves.

Myocardial Infarction

Anticoagulant therapy was recommended as part of the routine management of patients with MI in the 1950s but later fell into disrepute because of the fear of bleeding complications and because of doubt about its effectiveness. The objectives of anticoagulant treatment in patients with MI are (1) to improve survival, (2) to prevent recurrent infarction, mural thrombosis, and systemic embolism, and (3) to prevent the complication of venous thromboembolism. Although there is a consensus that anticoagulant therapy should be used for preventing systemic embolism, the use of long-term anticoagulant therapy for improving survival and preventing recurrent MI has been controversial. This long-standing debate has been resolved by the findings of recent randomized clinical trials. These findings have renewed interest in the role of long-term anticoagulant therapy following MI.[94–96] The Sixty-Plus Reinfarction Study Research Group reported a 55% reduction in fatal and nonfatal reinfarction in elderly patients (over 60 years) treated with long-term oral anticoagulant therapy following MI.[95]

In a more recent trial, warfarin treatment was associated with a 24% reduction in total mortality over a 3-year period (from 20% to 15.5%).[96] The beneficial effect of warfarin persisted in patients who also were taking beta blockers on a long-term basis. Both trials evaluating long-term warfarin after MI used relatively intense warfarin therapy (INR 2.7 to 4.8), and trials are currently under way using less intense warfarin or very low intensity warfarin plus low-dose aspirin in this setting.

Anticoagulant therapy is effective for preventing systemic embolism in patients with MI. Cerebral embolism occurs in 2% to 4% of nonanticoagulated patients following MI. Patients with transmural anterior MI are at particularly high risk of mural thrombosis (30%) and systemic embolism (2% to 6%) and should be treated with anticoagulant therapy for the period of risk. Full-dose continuous IV heparin followed by warfarin sodium for up to 1 year is a current practical regimen. Further studies are required to definitively establish the most appropriate duration of anticoagulant therapy. Heparin is administered in full therapeutic doses to maintain the APTT at 1.5 to 2.0 times the control value; the protocol for heparin administration and the adverse effect of heparin were outlined previously in the section discussing the treatment of venous thromboembolism. Therapeutic doses of heparin are used because the effectiveness of low-dose subcutaneous heparin for preventing systemic embolism is currently uncertain. Warfarin sodium is overlapped with IV heparin for 4 or 5 days and then continued long term. Warfarin is administered according to the protocol outlined previously for venous thromboembolism to maintain the INR between 2.0 and 3.0.

Antiplatelet agents, primarily aspirin, have been used in patients with cardiovascular diseases as an adjunct to thrombolytic therapy in the prevention of MI in patients with unstable angina, for secondary prophylaxis after an initial myocardial infarction, and as primary prophylaxis.[97] When compared with placebo or no treatment, ASA has been shown to be superior in all these situations. A meta-analysis performed by the Antiplatelet Trialists Collaboration Group reviewed 25 randomized trials of antiplatelet treatment in patients with a history of transient ischemic attacks, occlusive stroke, unstable angina, or MI.[98] There was a 15% risk reduction in vascular mortality and nonfatal vascular events (stroke or MI). The addition of dipyridamole to aspirin had no benefit. A larger meta-analysis of antiplatelet drug therapy is currently under review by the same group.

Cerebrovascular Disease

For practical purposes, patients with thromboembolic cerebrovascular disease can be divided into three categories: (1) those with attacks of transient cerebral ischemia, (2) those with stroke in evolution (progressing thrombotic stroke), and (3) those who have suffered a completed stroke (thrombotic infarction).

The aim of treating patients who have had transient ischemic attacks with anticoagulants is to prevent further episodes of transient cerebral ischemia, to prevent stroke, and to improve survival.[99] The use of anticoagulant therapy in patients with transient ischemic attacks is highly controversial, owing to doubt about its effectiveness and the fear of bleeding complications. Further clinical trials are required to definitively establish the place of anticoagulant treatment in patients with transient ischemic attacks.[100] Antiplatelet therapy with aspirin or ticlopidine is partially effective for preventing stroke and death in patients with transient ischemic attacks.

In patients with stroke in evolution, the objective of treatment with anticoagulants is to arrest the thrombotic process and prevent its progression to completed infarction, to improve survival, and to prevent venous thromboembolism.[101,102] The effectiveness of anticoagulant therapy for these purposes is currently uncertain, with the exception of prophylaxis of deep vein thrombosis. In patients with completed stroke, anticoagulant therapy is without benefit and is potentially dangerous.

Review of the published literature indicates that the risk of major bleeding complications associated with long-term anticoagulant therapy for patients with completed strokes was high using the high-intensity warfarin regimens.[80] As in the treatment of other conditions, the use of less intense warfarin therapy should reduce the bleeding risk in these patients.

Prosthetic Cardiac Valves

The goal of anticoagulant therapy in patients with artificial cardiac valves is to prevent thrombus formation on the valve surface and subsequent systemic embolism. In the absence of anticoagulant treatment, patients with prosthetic cardiac valves have a yearly risk of systemic embolism of approximately 5% to 30% or more, depending on the type of valve and its position. Mechanical valves are associated with a higher frequency of systemic embolism than are tissue (bioprosthetic) valves. Mitral prosthetic valves are associated with a greater risk of systemic embolism than are aortic valves. The risk of systemic embolism appears to be increased by the presence of coexistent atrial fibrillation. In anticoagulated patients, the frequency of systemic embolism with mechanical valves is approximately 4% per year for valves in the mitral position and 2% per year for aortic placement.

The clinical practice of treating patients with prosthetic heart valves with long-term oral anticoagulant therapy is now well established. The use of warfarin sodium to maintain an INR of 2 to 3 has been the standard approach for patients with bioprosthetic (tissue) valves, and in the past, an INR of 3.0 to 4.5 has been recommended for patients with mechanical valves, particularly if they have been complicated by systemic embolism. However, lower-intensity regimens of warfarin alone (INR 1.9 to 3.6) or warfarin (INR 2.0 to 3.0) plus aspirin and dipyridamole have been shown to be as effective as higher-dose warfarin with fewer bleeding complications.[81–83] The addition of aspirin, 100 mg/day, to warfarin (INR 3.0 to 4.5), when compared with warfarin alone, resulted in a marked improvement in efficacy without an increase in major bleeding or cerebral hemorrhage.[103] Dipyridamole in addition to warfarin may be of benefit in patients who suffer systemic embolism during adequate warfarin treatment.[104,105]

In pregnant patients with prosthetic heart valves, subcutaneous heparin in therapeutic doses (e.g., 15,000 units every 12 h) that maintain the APTT to 1.5 to 2.0 times the control value is a practical anticoagulant regimen that avoids the risk of fetopathic effects associated with warfarin therapy during pregnancy. To date, however, the effectiveness of this regimen for preventing systemic embolism in patients with prosthetic valves has not been formally evaluated by randomized clinical trials. A recent study indicates that lower doses of subcutaneous heparin (5000 units every 12 h) are ineffective in preventing valve thrombosis and systemic embolism in pregnant women with prosthetic cardiac valves.[91] The use of long-term subcutaneous heparin exposes the patient to the potential risk of osteoporosis.

Nonvalvular Atrial Fibrillation

Nonvalvular atrial fibrillation is a well-known cause of systemic embolism. Recent studies have shown that warfarin can significantly reduce this complication in such patients. Four randomized clinical trials have recently compared the use of less intense or moderately intense warfarin therapy with aspirin or placebo[108] (Table 28-5).

In the Copenhagen AFASAC Study, patients were randomly assigned to warfarin with a targeted INR of 2.8 to 4.2, aspirin 75 mg/day, or placebo.[107] Thromboembolic complications occurred in 21 of 336 patients (6.25%) given placebo, compared with 5 of 335 patients (1.49%)

TABLE 28-5. Warfarin for Prevention of Stroke in Nonvalvular Atrial Fibrillation

	AFASAC	BAATAF	SPAF
Total patients randomized	1007	420	1330
Warfarin protocol, INR	2.8–4.2	1.5–2.7	2–4.5
Strokes, n	5/335	2/212	6/210[†]
Risk reduction, %	76	86	67
Intracranial hemorrhage, n (%)	1 (0.4)	1 (0.2)	2 (0.9)
Major bleeding, n (%)	1 (0.4)	8 (3.8)	3 (1.2)
Control	ASA 75 mg/d	Placebo	ASA 325 mg/d
Strokes, n	21/366*	13/208	26/552[‡]
Intracranial hemorrhage, n (%)	0 (0)	0 (0)	2 (0.4)
Major bleeding, n (%)	0 (0)	8 (3.8)	5 (0.9)

* Includes 3 patients with TIA and 2 patients with visceral embolism.
[†] Stroke or systemic embolism compared with 18/211 patients given placebo (p = 0.01)
[‡] Stroke or systemic embolism compared with 46/568 patients given placebo (p = 0.02)
Adapted with permission from Albers GW, Atwood JE, Hirsh J, et al. Stroke prevention in nonvalvular atrial fibrillation. Ann Intern Med 115:727, 1991.

who received warfarin (RR = 76%; p < 0.05). There was no observed risk reduction with aspirin, 75 mg/day [20 of 336 patients (5.95%) had thromboembolism]. Serious bleeding was seen in 2 patients on warfarin with none on aspirin or placebo.

The Boston Area Anticoagulation Trial for Atrial Fibrillation (BAATAF) was a randomized trial comparing warfarin with a targeted INR of 1.5 to 2.7 with an identical placebo.[108] The incidence of strokes was reduced from 2.98% per year with placebo to 0.41% per year with warfarin, a risk reduction of 86% (p = 0.002). Major bleeding was seen in eight patients on warfarin, with one of these being intracranial hemorrhage.

In the Stroke Prevention in Atrial Fibrillation (SPAF) Study, warfarin with a targeted INR of 2 to 4.5 was compared with enteric-coated aspirin 325 mg/day and placebo.[109] Warfarin reduced the incidence of stroke and systemic embolism from 7.4% per year on placebo to 2.3% per year, a risk reduction of 67% ($p = 0.01$). Aspirin therapy reduced the incidence of stroke and systemic embolism to 3.6% per year as compared with 6.3% per year in the placebo group, a risk reduction of 42% ($p = 0.02$). The incidence of major bleeding was low and comparable in the three groups (about 1.5% per year).

The Canadian Atrial Fibrillation Anticoagulation (CAFA) Study was stopped on ethical grounds because other trials had demonstrated the efficacy of warfarin treatment in nonvalvular atrial fibrillation as compared with placebo.[110]

On review of the data from SPAF, certain predictors of thromboembolism in atrial fibrillation were identified.[111,112] Clinical features of patients at risk included recent congestive heart failure, a history of hypertension, and previous arterial thromboembolism.[111] Echocardiographic features of patients at risk included left ventricular dysfunction and the size of the left atrium from M-mode echocardiograms.[112]

Based on the information from these well-designed clinical trials in nonvalvular atrial fibrillation, it is clear that less intense warfarin therapy is effective in the prevention of stroke and systemic embolism with a low incidence of major bleeding. Aspirin at 325 mg/day resulted in a significant risk reduction when compared with placebo, whereas aspirin at 75 mg/day had no benefit. In patients in whom oral anticoagulants are contraindicated, aspirin 325 mg daily provides a useful alternative for the prevention of stroke and systemic embolism in atrial fibrillation.

ANTITHROMBOTIC AGENTS IN PERIPHERAL VASCULAR DISEASE

The role of anticoagulant therapy in the management of patients with arterial occlusive disease of the legs is limited. Anticoagulant therapy is effective in preventing recurrent distal embolism in patients with acute arterial occlusion. Continuous IV heparin should be commenced immediately in patients with acute arterial occlusion of the limb and continued after embolectomy until full therapeutic oral anticoagulation with warfarin is accomplished. The role of long-term anticoagulant therapy in the management of patients with intermittent claudication or ischemic rest pain is uncertain. Anticoagulant therapy may be effective in improving the long-term patency of peripheral arterial bypass procedures (e.g., femoropopliteal bypass), particularly procedures involving prosthetic graft materials, but further studies are required to adequately assess its role in this context. A recent randomized trial suggests that long-term oral anticoagulant therapy improves survival following femoropopliteal bypass surgery by reducing mortality from associated cardiovascular disease (e.g., coronary artery disease).[113] The role of less intense warfarin therapy has not been tested in patients with peripheral vascular disease.

REFERENCES

1. Freiman DG. The structure of thrombi. In: Colman RW, Hirsh J, Marder V, Salzman EW, eds. Thrombosis and hemostasis: basic principles and clinical practice. 2nd ed. Philadelphia: JB Lippincott, 1987:1123.
2. Badimon L, Badimon JJ, Fuster V. Pathogenesis of thrombosis. In: Fuster V, Verstraete M, eds. Thrombosis in cardiovascular disorders. Philadelphia: WB Saunders, 1992:17.
3. Meade TW, Miller GJ, Rosenberg RD. Characteristics associated with the risk of arterial thrombosis and the prethrombotic state. In: Fuster V, Verstraete M, eds. Thrombosis in cardiovascular disorders. Philadelphia: WB Saunders, 1992:79.
4. Dismuke SE, Wagner EH. Pulmonary embolism as a cause of death: the changing mortality in hospitalized patients. JAMA 1986;255:2039.
5. Dalen JE, Alpert JS. Natural history of pulmonary embolism. Prog Cardiovasc Dis 1975;17:259.
6. Anderson FA, Wheeler HB, Goldberg RJ, et al. A population-based perspective of the hospital incidence and case-fatality rates of deep vein thrombosis and pulmonary embolism. Arch Intern Med 1991;151:933.
7. Donaldson GA, Williams C, Scanell J, Shaw RS. A reappraisal of the application of the Trendelenburg operation to massive fatal embolism. N Engl J Med 1963;268:171.
8. Collins R, Scrimgeour A, Yusef S, Peto R. Reduction in fatal pulmonary embolism and venous thrombosis by perioperative administration of subcutaneous heparin. N Engl J Med 1988;318:1162.

9. Consensus Conference. Prevention of venous thrombosis and pulmonary embolism. JAMA 1986;256:744.

10. International Multicenter Trial. Prevention of fatal postoperative pulmonary embolism by low doses of heparin. Lancet 1975;2:45.

11. Moser KM, LeMoine JR. Is embolic risk conditioned by location of deep venous thrombosis? Ann Intern Med 1981;94:439.

12. Hull RD, Hirsh J, Carter CJ, et al. Pulmonary angiography, ventilation lung scanning, and venography for clinically suspected pulmonary embolism with abnormal perfusion lung scan. Ann Intern Med 1983;98:891.

13. Hull RD, Raskob GE, Hirsh J. The diagnosis of clinically suspected pulmonary embolism: practical approaches. Chest 1986;89(suppl):417S.

14. Sevitt S, Gallagher N. Venous thrombosis and pulmonary embolism: a clinicopathological study in injured and burned patients. Br J Surg 1961; 48:475.

15. Hull RD, Raskob GE, Coates G, et al. A new non-invasive management strategy for patients with suspected pulmonary embolism. Arch Intern Med 1989;149:2549.

16. Huisman MV, Buller HR, ten Cate JW, Vreeken J. Serial impedance plethysmography for suspected deep-vein thrombosis in outpatients: the Amsterdam General Practitioner Study. N Engl J Med 1986;314:823.

17. Kakkar VV, Howe CT, Flanc C, Clarke MB. Natural history of postoperative deep vein thrombosis. Lancet 1969;2:230.

18. Nicolaides AN, Kakkar VV, Field ES, Renney JTG. The origin of deep vein thrombosis: a venographic study. Br J Radiol 1971;44:653.

19. Hull RD, Hirsh J, Sackett DL, et al. Clinical validity of a negative venogram in patients with clinically suspected venous thrombosis. Circulation 1981; 64:622.

20. Rabinov K, Paulin S. Roentgen diagnosis of venous thrombosis in the leg. Arch Surg 1972;104:134.

21. Bone RC. Ventilation/perfusion scan in pulmonary embolism: "the emperor is incompletely attired." JAMA 1990;263:2794.

22. Secker-Walker RH. On purple emperors, pulmonary embolism, and venous thrombosis. Ann Intern Med 1983;98:1006.

23. Kelley MA, Carson JL, Palevsky HI, Schwartz JS. Diagnosing pulmonary embolism: new facts and strategies. Ann Intern Med 1991;114:300.

24. Hirsh J, Hull RD. Natural history and clinical features of venous thrombosis. In: Colman RW, Hirsh J, Marder VJ, Salzman EW, eds. Thrombosis and hemostasis: basic principles and clinical practice. 2nd ed. Philadelphia: JB Lippincott, 1987: 1208.

25. Hull RD, Secker-Walker RH, Hirsh J. Diagnosis of deep vein thrombosis. In: Colman RW, Hirsh J, Marder VJ, Salzman EW, eds. Thrombosis and hemostasis: basic principles and clinical practice. 2nd ed. Philadelphia: JB Lippincott, 1987:1220.

26. Hull RD, Hirsh J, Sackett DL, et al. Replacement of venography in suspected venous thrombosis by impedance plethysmography and ^{125}I-fibrinogen leg scanning. Ann Intern Med 1981;94:12.

27. Yudelman IM, Nossel HL, Kaplan KL, Hirsh J: Plasma fibrinopeptide A levels in symptomatic venous thromboembolism. Blood 1978;51:1189.

28. Zielinsky A, Hirsh J, Hull RD, et al. Evaluation of radioimmunoassay for fragment E in the diagnosis of venous thrombosis. Thromb Haemost 1979; 42:28.

29. Bounameaux H, Cirafici P, Moerloose P, et al. Measurement of D-dimer in plasma as diagnostic aid in suspected pulmonary embolism. Lancet 1991;337:196.

30. Gallus A, Jackaman J, Tillett J, et al. Safety and efficacy of warfarin started early after submassive venous thrombosis or pulmonary embolism. Lancet 1986;2:1293.

31. Hull RD, Raskob GE, Rosenbloom D, et al. Heparin for 5 days as compared with 10 days in the initial treatment of proximal venous thrombosis. N Engl J Med 1990;322:1260.

32. Hull R, Hirsh J, Jay R, et al. Different intensities of oral anticoagulant therapy in the treatment of proximal-vein thrombosis. N Engl J Med 1982; 307:1676.

33. Hull RD, Carter CJ, Jay RM, et al. The diagnosis of acute, recurrent, deep-vein thrombosis: a diagnostic challenge. Circulation 1983;67:901.

34. Bjork I, Lindahl U. Mechanism of the anticoagulant action of heparin. Mol Cell Biochem 1982;48:161.

35. Rosenberg, RD. The heparin-antithrombin system: a natural anticoagulant mechanism. In: Colman RW, Hirsh J, Marder V, Salzman EW, eds. Thrombosis and hemostasis: basic principles and clinical practice. 2nd ed. Philadelphia: JB Lippincott, 1987:1373.

36. Hirsh J. Heparin. N Engl J Med 1991;324:1565.

37. Salzman EW, Deykin D, Shapiro RM, Rosenberg R. Management of heparin therapy: controlled prospective trial. N Engl J Med 1975;292:1046.

38. Mant MJ, O'Brien BD, Thong KL, et al. Haemorrhagic complications of heparin therapy. Lancet 1977;1:1133.

39. Levine MN, Hirsh J, Kelton JG. Heparin-induced bleeding. In: Lane DA, Lindahl U, eds. Heparin: chemical and biological properties, clinical applications. Boca Raton, Fl: E Arnold, 1989:517.

40. Nieuwenhuis HK, Albada J, Banga JD, Sixma JJ. Identification of risk factors for bleeding during

treatment of acute venous thromboembolism with heparin or low-molecular-weight heparin. Blood 1991;78:2337.

41. Hull RD, Raskob GE, Hirsh J, et al. Continuous intravenous heparin compared with intermittent subcutaneous heparin in the initial treatment of proximal-vein thrombosis. N Engl J Med 1986; 315:1109.

42. Brandjes DPM, Buller HR, Heijboer H, et al. Comparative trial of heparin and oral anticoagulants in the initial treatment of proximal deep vein thrombosis. N Engl J Med 1992;327:1485.

43. Hull RD, Raskob GE, Rosenbloom D, et al. Optimal therapeutic level of heparin therapy in patients with venous thrombosis. Arch Intern Med 1992;152:1589.

44. Wheeler AP, Jaquiss RD, Newman JH. Physician practices in the treatment of pulmonary embolism and deep-venous thrombosis. Arch Intern Med 1988;148:1321.

45. Cruickshank MK, Levine MN, Hirsh J, et al. A standard heparin nomogram for the management of heparin therapy. Arch Intern Med 1991;151: 333.

46. Pini M, Pattachini C, Quintavalla R, et al. Subcutaneous vs intravenous heparin in the treatment of deep venous thrombosis—a randomized clinical trial. Thromb Haemost 1990;64:222.

47. Hommes DW, Bura A, Mazzolai L, et al. Subcutaneous heparin compared with continuous intravenous heparin administration in the initial treatment of deep vein thrombosis. Ann Intern Med 1992;116:279.

48. Moser KM, Fedullo PF. Subcutaneous compared with intravenous heparin for deep vein thrombosis. Ann Intern Med 1992;117:265.

49. Hull R, Delmore T, Carter C, et al. Adjusted subcutaneous heparin versus warfarin sodium in the long-term treatment of venous thrombosis. N Engl J Med 1982;306:189.

50. Warkentin TE, Kelton JG. Heparin and platelets. Hematol Oncol Clin North Am 1990;4:243.

51. Demers C, Ginsberg JS, Brill-Edwards P, et al. Rapid anticoagulation using ancrod for heparin-induced thrombocytopenia. Blood 1991;78: 2194.

52. Chong BH, Ismail F, Cade J, et al. Heparin-induced thrombocytopenia: studies with a new low molecular weight heparinoid, Org 10172. Blood 1989;73:1592.

53. Ortel TL, Gockerman JP, Califf RM, et al. Parenteral anticoagulation with the heparinoid lomoparan (Org 10172) in patients with heparin induced thrombocytopenia and thrombosis. Thromb Haemost 1992;67(3):292.

54. Howell R, Fidler J, Letsky E, DeSwiet M. The risks of antenatal subcutaneous heparin prophylaxis: a controlled trial. Br J Obstet Gynecol 1983;90: 1124.

55. Lechey D, Gantt C, Lim V. Heparin-induced hypoaldosteronism. JAMA 1981;246:2189.

56. Wilson ID, Goetz FC. Selective hypoaldosteronism after prolonged heparin administration. Am J Med 1964;36:635.

57. Hirsh J, Levine MN. Low molecular weight heparin. Blood 1992;79:1.

58. Verstraete M. Pharmacotherapeutic aspects of unfractionated and low molecular weight heparin. Drugs 1990;40:498.

59. Bratt G, Tornebohm E, Widlund L, Lockner D. Low molecular weight heparin (Kabi 2165; Fragmin): pharmacokinetics after intravenous and subcutaneous administration in human volunteers. Thromb Res 1986;42:613.

60. Bergqvist D, Hedner U, Sjorin E, Holmer E. Anticoagulant effects of two types of low molecular weight heparin administered subcutaneously. Thromb Res 1983;32:381.

61. Siegbahn A, Y-Hassan S, Boberg J, et al. Subcutaneous treatment of deep venous thrombosis with low-molecular-weight heparin: a dose-finding study with LMWH-Novo. Thromb Res 1989;55: 767.

62. Albada J, Nieuwenhuis HK, Sixma JJ. Treatment of acute venous thromboembolism with low molecular weight heparin (Fragmin): results of a double-blind, randomized study. Circulation 1989;80: 935.

63. A Collaborative European Multicenter Study. A randomized trial of subcutaneous low molecular weight heparin (CY 216) compared with intravenous unfractionated heparin in the treatment of deep vein thrombosis. Thromb Haemost 1991;65: 251.

64. Lopaciuk S, Meissner AJ, Filipecki S, et al. Subcutaneous low-molecular-weight heparin versus subcutaneous unfractionated heparin in the treatment of deep vein thrombosis: a Polish multicenter trial. Thromb Haemost 1992;68:14.

65. Prandoni P, Lensing AW, Buller HR, et al. Comparison of subcutaneous low-molecular-weight heparin with intravenous standard heparin in proximal deep-vein thrombosis. Lancet 1992;339: 441.

66. Hull RD, Raskob GE, Pineo GF, et al. Subcutaneous low-molecular-weight heparin compared with continuous intravenous heparin in the treatment of proximal-vein thrombosis. N Engl J Med 1992;326:975.

67. Green D, Hull RD, Brant R, Pineo GF. Lower mortality in cancer patients treated with low-molecular-weight versus standard heparin. Lancet 1992;339:1476.

68. Lagerstedt CI, Fagher BO, Albrechtsson U, et al.

Need for long-term anticoagulant treatment in symptomatic calf-vein thrombosis. Lancet 1985;2:518.

69. Wheeler HB, Anderson FA Jr. Can noninvasive tests be used as the basis for treatment of deep vein thrombosis? In: Bernstein EF, ed. Noninvasive diagnostic techniques in vascular disease. 2nd ed. St. Louis: CV Mosby, 1982:545.

70. Hull RD, Hirsh J, Carter CJ, et al. A randomized trial of noninvasive diagnostic testing for clinically suspected deep-vein thrombosis: the diagnostic efficacy of impedance plethysmography. Ann Intern Med 1985;102:21.

71. Jones TK, Barnes RW, Greenfield LJ. Greenfield vena cava filter: rationale and current indications. Ann Thorac Surg 1986;42:S28.

72. Vermeer C. Gamma-carboxyglutamate-containing proteins and the vitamin K-dependent carboxylase. Biochem J 1990;266:625.

73. Furie B, Furie BC. Molecular basis of vitamin K-dependent gamma-carboxylation. Blood 1990;75:1753.

74. Poller L, Tabener DA. Dosage and control of oral anticoagulants: an international study. Br J Haematol 1982;51:479.

75. Bussey HI, Force RW, Bianco TM, Leonard AD. Reliance on prothrombin time ratios causes significant errors in anticoagulation therapy. Arch Intern Med 1992;152:278.

76. Fennerty A, Dolben J, Thomas P, et al. Flexible induction dose regimen for warfarin and prediction of maintenance dose. Br Med J 1984;288:1268.

77. Ovesen L, Lyduch S, Ott P. A simple technique for predicting maintenance dosage of warfarin—is it better than empirical dosing? Eur J Clin Pharmacol 1989;37:573.

78. White RH, McCurdy SA, von Marensdorff H, et al. Home prothrombin time monitoring after the initiation of warfarin therapy. Ann Intern Med 1989;111:730.

79. Bern MM, Lokich JJ, Walloch SR, et al. Very low doses of warfarin can prevent thrombosis in central venous catheters. Ann Intern Med 1990;112:423.

80. Levine MN, Raskob GE, Hirsh J. Hemorrhagic complications of long-term anticoagulant therapy. Chest 1989;95(suppl 2):26S.

81. Turpie AGG, Gunstensen J, Hirsh J, et al. Randomized comparison of two intensities of oral anticoagulant therapy after tissue heart valve replacement. Lancet 1988;1:1245.

82. Saour JN, Sieck JO, Mamo LAR, Gallus AS. Trial of different intensities of anticoagulation in patients with prosthetic heart valves. N Engl J Med 1990;322:428.

83. Altman R, Rouvier J, Gurfinkel E, et al. Compari-son of two levels of anticoagulant therapy in patients with substitute heart valves. J Thorac Cardiovasc Surg 1991;101:427.

84. Grimaudo V, Gueissaz F, Hauert J, et al. Necrosis of skin induced by coumarin in a patient deficient in protein S. Br Med J 1989;298:233.

85. Becker CG. Oral anticoagulant therapy and skin necrosis: speculation on pathogenesis. Adv Exp Med Biol 1987;214:217.

86. Hart JP, Catterall A, Dodds RA, et al. Circulating vitamin K_1 levels in fractured neck of femur. Lancet 1984;2:283.

87. Knapen MHJ, Hamulyak K, Vermeer C. The effect of vitamin K supplementation on circulating osteocalcin (bone Gla-protein) and urinary calcium excretion. Ann Intern Med 1989;111:1001.

88. Fiore CE, Tamburino C, Roti R, Grimaldi D. Reduced bone mineral content in patients taking an oral anticoagulant. South Med J 1990;83:538.

89. Hall JG, Pauli RM, Wilson KM. Maternal and fetal sequelae of anticoagulation during pregnancy. Am J Med 1980;68:122.

90. Ginsberg JS, Hirsh J. Use of anticoagulants during pregnancy. Chest 1989;95(suppl 2):156S.

91. Iturbe-Alessio I, del Carmen Fonseca M, Mutchinik O, et al. Risks of anticoagulant therapy in pregnant women with artificial heart valves. N Engl J Med 1986;315:1390.

92. Lancaster TR, Singer DE, Sheehan MA, et al. The impact of long-term warfarin therapy on quality of life: evidence from a randomized trial. Arch Intern Med 1991;151:1944.

93. Gurwitz JH, Avron J, Ross-Degnan D, et al. Aging and the anticoagulant response to warfarin therapy. Ann Intern Med 1992;116:901.

94. Neri Seneri GG, Gensini GF, Poggesi L. Effectiveness of low-dose heparin in prevention of myocardial reinfarction. Lancet 1987;2:937.

95. Sixty-Plus Reinfarction Study Research Group. A double-blind trial to assess long-term anticoagulant therapy in elderly patients after myocardial infarction. Lancet 1980;2:989.

96. Smith P, Arneson H, Holme I. The effect of warfarin on mortality and reinfarction after myocardial infarction. N Engl J Med 1990;323:147.

97. Meade TW. Low-dose warfarin and low-dose aspirin in the primary prevention of ischemic heart disease. Am J Cardiol 1990;65:7C.

98. Antiplatelet Trialists' Collaboration. Secondary prevention of vascular disease by prolonged antiplatelet treatment. Br Med J 1988;296:320.

99. Duke RJ, Bloch RF, Turpie AGG, et al. Intravenous heparin for the prevention of stroke progression in acute partial stable stroke: a randomized controlled trial. Ann Intern Med 1986;105:825.

100. Hass WK, Easton JD, Adams HP, et al. A random-

ized trial comparing ticlopidine hydrochloride with aspirin for the prevention of stroke in high-risk patients. N Engl J Med 1989;321:501.

101. Sherman DG, Dyken ML, Fisher M, et al. Antithrombotic therapy for cerebrovascular disorders. Chest 1989;95:140S.

102. Cerebral Embolism Study Group. Immediate anticoagulation of embolic stroke: brain hemorrhage and management options. Stroke 1984;15:779.

103. Turpie AGG, Gent M, Laupacis A, et al. Reduction in mortality by adding aspirin (100 mg) to oral anticoagulants in patients with heart valve replacement (abstract). Can J Cardiol 1991;7(suppl A): 95A.

104. Cheseboro JH, Fuster V, McGoon DC, et al. Trial of combined warfarin plus dipyridamole or aspirin therapy in prosthetic heart valve replacement: danger of aspirin compared to dipyridamole. Am J Cardiol 1983;51:1537.

105. Mok CK, Boey J, Wang R, et al. Warfarin versus dipyridamole-aspirin and pentoxifylline-aspirin for the prevention of prosthetic heart valve thromboembolism: a prospective, randomized clinical trial. Circulation 1985;72:1059.

106. Albers GW, Atwood JE, Hirsh J, et al. Stroke prevention in nonvalvular atrial fibrillation. Ann Intern Med 1991;115:727.

107. Peterson P, Kastrup J, Helseg-Larsen S, et al. Risk factors for thromboembolic complications in chronic atrial fibrillation: the Copenhagen AFASAK Study. Arch Intern Med 1990;150:819.

108. The Stroke Prevention in Atrial Fibrillation Investigators. Stroke prevention in atrial fibrillation study: final results. Circulation 1991;80:527.

109. The Boston Area Anticoagulation Trial for Atrial Fibrillation Investigators. The effect of low-dose warfarin on the risk of stroke in patients with nonrheumatic atrial fibrillation. N Engl J Med 1990; 323:1505.

110. Connelly SJ, Laupacis A, Gent M, et al. Canadian atrial fibrillation anticoagulation (CAFA) study. J Am Coll Cardiol 1991;18:349.

111. The Stroke Prevention in Atrial Fibrillation Investigators. Predictors of thromboembolism in atrial fibrillation: I. Clinical features of patients at risk. Ann Intern Med 1992;116:1.

112. The Stroke Prevention in Atrial Fibrillation Investigators. Predictors of thromboembolism in atrial fibrillation: II. Echocardiographic features of patients at risk. Ann Intern Med 1992;116:6.

113. Kretschmer G, Wenzl E, Schemper M, et al. Influence of postoperative anticoagulant treatment on patient survival after femoropopliteal vein bypass surgery. Lancet 1988;1:797.

29

ANTITHROMBOTIC AGENTS: THE OLD AND THE NEW

Jack Hirsh

Antithrombotic agents prevent thrombosis and recurrent thrombosis by inhibiting blood coagulation or by preventing platelet aggregation. Unlike thrombolytic agents, antithrombotic agents are not fibrinolytic in their own right but have the potential to enhance thrombolysis by preventing rethrombosis. Currently, three antithrombotic agents are in common clinical use in North America: (1) heparin, (2) coumarins, and (3) aspirin. Ticlopidine, a new antiplatelet agent, has been introduced recently, and low-molecular-weight heparins (LMWHs), which have been approved for clinical use in Europe, are presently under review by drug regulatory agencies in North America.

Interest in the development of new antithrombotic agents has been stimulated by a number of considerations. These are (1) the recognized importance of thrombosis as a leading cause of death and disability, (2) the observation that the three established antithrombotic agents are effective but that they all have limitations which are not shared by the newer compounds, and (3) advances in our understanding of thrombogenesis which provide the scientific basis for the development of more targeted and specific agents.

The pathways of blood coagulation and platelet activation which are important in thrombogenesis are shown in Figures 29-1 and 29-2. Also included in Figures 29-1 and 29-2 and Tables 29-1 and 29-2 are the sites of action of the old and new antithrombotic agents. In this chapter the mechanisms of action and limitations of the established antithrombotic agents will be reviewed first, and then the potential of the newer antithrombotic agents will be discussed in detail.

HEPARIN

Mechanism of Action

Heparin acts as an anticoagulant by catalyzing the inactivation of thrombin, activated factor X (factor Xa), and activated factor IX (factor IXa) by antithrombin III (AT III).[1] Upon binding to lysine sites on AT III, heparin produces a conformational change at the active site which markedly accelerates the rate at which AT III inhibits the co-

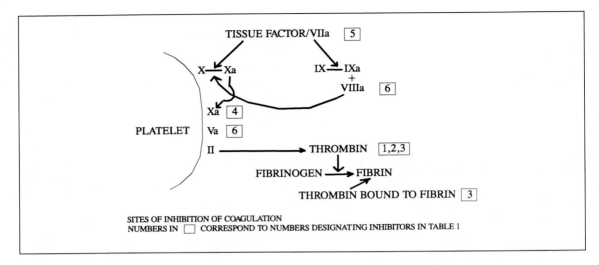

FIGURE 29-1. Sites of inhibition of coagulation. Numbers in boxes correspond to numbers designating inhibitors in Table 29-1.

agulation enzymes.[1] Heparin then dissociates from the enzyme-inhibitor complex and can catalyze other AT III molecules.[1]

Although the heparin–AT III complex can inactivate a number of coagulation enzymes,[1] recent studies in plasma suggest that the major mechanism by which heparin blocks coagulation is by catalyzing the inhibition of thrombin.[2,3] Thrombin plays a central role in hemostasis and thrombogenesis. It activates platelets and induces their aggregation, it converts fibrinogen to fibrin, and it activates factor XIII which then stabilizes the fibrin. Thrombin also amplifies coagulation by activating factors V and VIII, thereby accelerating both the generation of prothrombinase and the subsequent activation of prothrombin. By preventing thrombin-mediated activation of factors V and VIII, heparin blocks the feedback amplification of coagulation that is initiated by thrombin[4] (see Fig. 29-1 and Table 29-1). This amplification step is important in thrombogenesis because one thrombin molecule is able to catalyze the generation of many thousand thrombin molecules. Thrombin is also mitogenic for vascular smooth-muscle cells. Thus the inhibition of thrombin generation and thrombin activity is the key to prevention and treatment of both fibrin-dependent and platelet-dependent thromboembolic disorders.

Limitations

The limitations of heparin are based on its pharmacokinetic, biophysical, and antihemostatic properties. The pharmacokinetic limitations are based on its binding to plasma proteins and endothelial cells, which results in a complicated mechanism of clearance. Biophysical limitations occur because the heparin–AT III complex is unable to access and inactivate (1) factor Xa in the prothrombinase complex, (2) thrombin bound to

TABLE 29-1. Inhibitors of Coagulation

Inhibitor	Inactivates
1. Heparin	Nonbound thrombin Nonbound factor Xa (factors IXa and XIa)
2. Low Molecular Weight Heparins	Nonbound factor Xa Nonbound thrombin (factors IXa and XIa)
3. Hirudin Hirudin fragments Chlormethylketones and related small molecules	Fibrin-bound thrombin Free thrombin
4. Tick anticoagulant protein Antistasin	Factor Xa bound in prothrombinase complex Free factor Xa
5. Tissue pathway inhibitor (TIP)	Tissue factor–factor VIIa complex
6. Activated protein C (APC)	Factors Va and VIIIa

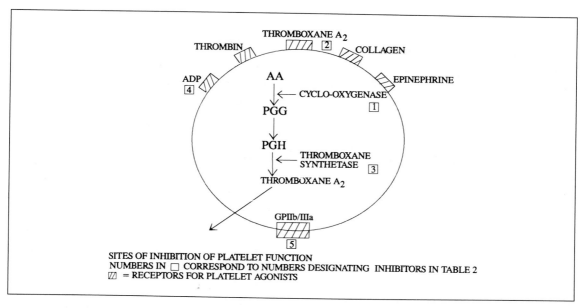

FIGURE 29-2. Sites of inhibition of platelet function. Numbers in boxes correspond to numbers designating inhibitors in Table 29-2. Hatching designates receptors for platelet agonists.

fibrin, and (3) thrombin bound to subendothelial surfaces. The limitations due to its other (non-anticoagulant) antihemostatic properties are caused by a poorly defined inhibitory. effect of heparin on platelet function.

The limitations related to the pharmacokinetic and antihemostatic properties of heparin are not shared by the LMWHs and heparinoids, while the limitations caused by the lack of accessibility of the heparin–AT III complex to fibrin-bound thrombin and factor Xa are overcome by several new classes of AT III–independent thrombin and factor Xa inhibitors.

Pharmacokinetics

The mechanisms of heparin clearance are complex. Heparin binds to a number of plasma proteins other than AT III[5] which compete with AT III for heparin binding. As a result, approximately 10-fold higher concentrations of heparin are required to inhibit identical concentrations of thrombin in normal plasma than in a buffer system containing physiologic concentrations of AT III.[6] There is evidence that binding of heparin to

plasma proteins also contributes to the variability of anticoagulant response between patients and to the heparin resistance seen in some patients with thromboembolic disorders.[7]

Heparin is cleared by a rapid phase of elimi-

TABLE 29-2. Inhibitors of Platelet Function

Inhibitor	Effect
1. Aspirin	Thromboxane A_2 synthesis Prostaglandin $G_2 + H_2$ synthesis Prostaglandin I_2 synthesis
2. Thromboxane A_2 receptor antagonists	Thromboxane A_2–mediated platelet activation
3. Thromboxane A_2 synthetase inhibitors	Thromboxane A_2 synthesis
4. Ticlopidine Clopidogrel	Inhibition of platelet aggregation by ADP and other agonists (mechanism unknown)
5. Glycoprotein IIb-IIIa inhibitors	Inhibit platelet aggregation induced by ADP, thrombin, thromboxane A_2, and collagen by inhibiting binding of fibrinogen to GPIIb-IIIa

nation followed by a more gradual disappearance, which can best be explained by a combination of a saturable and a nonsaturable, first-order mechanism of clearance.[8] The saturable phase of heparin clearance is thought to be the result of heparin binding to receptors on endothelial cells and macrophages. Once bound, the heparin is internalized, depolymerized, and metabolized into smaller, less sulfated derivatives.[9,10] When heparin binds to endothelial cells, it displaces platelet factor 4, which can then inactivate circulating heparin.[11] The slower, nonsaturable mechanism of heparin clearance probably reflects renal excretion. At therapeutic concentrations, a major proportion of the heparin is cleared by the more rapid saturable mechanism.

This complex mechanism of heparin clearance explains why the apparent biologic half-lives of heparin increases from 30 to 60 to 150 minutes with intravenous boluses of 25, 100, and 400 units/kg of heparin, respectively.[12] Heparin has decreased bioavailability when administered subcutaneously in low doses but has approximately 90% bioavailability when administered in high therapeutic doses (e.g., 35,000 units/24 h). The reduced bioavailability of heparin when it is administered subcutaneously occurs because as heparin gradually enters the circulation from the subcutaneous depot site, it binds to plasma proteins and is rapidly cleared by the saturable mechanism, resulting in reduced plasma levels and a delay in achieving a steady state. In practical terms, these pharmacokinetic properties are responsible for the 24-h delay before steady-state levels are reached with subcutaneous administration of heparin doses of 12,500 units 12 hourly and for the higher heparin requirements when administered by the subcutaneous route. These unfavorable pharmacokinetic properties of heparin provide opportunities for the LMWHs and heparinoids, which show less protein and endothelial cell binding, and, as a consequence, have a more predictable dose response, better bioavailability, and a longer plasma half-life.

Other Potential Limitations

The other potential limitations of heparin relate to the observations that the anticoagulant effect of heparin is modified by platelets, fibrin, vascular surfaces, and plasma proteins. Platelets limit the anticoagulant effect of heparin in two ways. First, factor Xa that is generated on the platelet surface is protected from inhibition by heparin–AT III.[13,14] Second, platelets release the heparin-neutralizing protein platelet factor 4.[15] Fibrin binds thrombin and protects it from inactivation by heparin–AT III.[16,17] Thus much higher concentrations of heparin are needed to inhibit thrombin bound to fibrin than are required to inactivate the free enzyme.[17] Thrombin also binds to subendothelial matrix proteins, where it is again protected from inhibition by heparin.[18] These observations not only explain why heparin is less effective than the AT III–independent thrombin and factor Xa inhibitors at preventing thrombosis in experimental animals[19,20] but also suggest that AT III–independent inhibitors may be more effective than heparin in certain clinical settings.

Heparin also inhibits platelet function, increases vascular permeability, and increases experimental microvascular bleeding. These nonanticoagulant antihemostatic properties are not shared by the LMWHs and heparinoids, which, therefore, allow them to be administered to patients in higher anticoagulant and antithrombotic doses than heparin.

The clinical limitations of heparin are listed in Table 29-3 and can be summarized as follows:

1. The dose response to heparin shows wide variations in sick patients. Since there is a close relationship between clinical efficacy of heparin and the intensity of its anticoagulant effect measured as the activated partial thromboplastin time (APTT), the dose of heparin must be monitored carefully. Heparin monitoring can be problematic because the commercial partial thromboplastin reagents vary in their sensitivity to heparin.
2. Heparin has a narrow risk/benefit ratio which is manifested as a substantial risk of bleeding when used in therapeutic concentrations. Both the need for careful laboratory monitoring and the narrow risk/benefit ratio are reduced by using LMWHs or heparinoids.
3. The failure of heparin to inactivate thrombin and factor Xa bound in complexes with fibrin

TABLE 29-3. Limitations of Heparin

Limitation	Reason for Limitation	Limitation Overcome By
Marked interpatient variability in dose response	Heparin binding to plasma proteins Variability in clearance between patients	Low-molecular-weight heparins bind less avidly and show less variability in dose response
Resistance to anticoagulant effect in some patients	High concentrations of heparin binding proteins Increased heparin clearance in some patients	Low-molecular-weight heparins bind to plasma proteins less avidly
Difficulty in monitoring anti-coagulant effect	Activated partial thromboplastin time reagents show considerable variability in their sensitivity to heparin	Low-molecular-weight heparins may not require monitoring because of their more predictable dose response
Relatively ineffective against fibrin-bound thrombin	Thrombin bound to fibrin is inaccessible to inactivation by heparin–AT III	The direct thrombin inhibitors including hirudin and hirulog and chlormethyketones
Relatively ineffective against platelet-bound factor Xa	Fractor Xa in the prothrombinase complex is inaccessible to heparin–AT III	The direct factor Xa inhibitors including tick anticoagulant protein and antistasin

and platelets, respectively, could be responsible for the failure of heparin to prevent propagation of experimental and clinical venous thrombi after heparin has been discontinued. Thus unless anticoagulant therapy is maintained for weeks to months in patients with deep vein thrombosis, clot extension occurs in 29% to 47% of patients treated with a 5- to 14-day course of heparin.[21,22] In addition, heparin is limited in its ability to prevent experimental and clinical rethrombosis after successful coronary thrombolysis with tissue-type plasminogen activator (t-PA). The new AT III–independent thrombin and factor Xa inhibitors have the potential to overcome these limitations.

ASPIRIN

Aspirin is an effective antithrombotic agent which acts by irreversibly inhibiting the enzyme cyclo-oxygenase[23–25] and so inhibiting the conversion of arachidonic acid in platelets to prostaglandin-endoperoxide precursors of thromboxane A_2 (TXA_2). In contrast, in vascular wall cells, aspirin inhibits the conversion of arachidonic acid to prostaglandin I_2 (PGI_2).[24,26–32] TXA_2 induces platelet aggregation and vasoconstriction while PGI_2 inhibits platelet aggregation and induces vasodilation.[26,33] Thus, by blocking formation of TXA_2, aspirin has the potential to be both antithrombotic and thrombogenic by blocking formation of PGI_2. Evidence from clinical trials indicates that interruption of formation of PGI_2 is unlikely to be a sufficient stimulus to initiate the thrombotic process or to interfere with the antithrombotic effect of aspirin.

Aspirin is rapidly absorbed in the stomach and upper intestine. Peak plasma levels occur 15 to 20 minutes after aspirin ingestion, and inhibition of platelet function is evident by 1 h. The plasma concentration of aspirin decays with a half-life of 15 to 20 minutes. Despite the rapid clearance of aspirin from the circulation, the platelet-inhibitory effect lasts for the lifespan of the platelet because aspirin irreversibly inactivates platelet cyclooxygenase.[23,24] Aspirin also acetylates cyclooxygenase in megakaryocytes before new platelets are released into circulation.[23,34–36] The mean lifespan of the human platelet is approximately 10 days. Therefore, approximately 10% of circulating platelets are replaced every 24 h,[37,38] and after 5 to 6 days, approximately 50% of the platelets function normally.

Aspirin is generally well tolerated, but some patients suffer side effects. The side effects of aspirin are mainly gastrointestinal, dose-related, and reduced by using low doses (325 mg/day or less).[39,40] Aspirin-induced injury to the gastrointestinal tract can be acute or chronic. Acute aspirin use produces gastric erosions and gastric hemorrhage, while chronic use can produce gastric ulcers, anemia, and gastrointestinal hemorrhage. Aspirin produces a dose-related increase in acute gastric bleeding.[41–44]

Aspirin solutions containing antacids with sufficient buffering capacity cause no measurable blood loss in normal subjects.[45] Enteric-coated aspirin results in less gastric and duodenal mucosal injury than regular aspirin,[46] and preparations are available with reliable absorption.[46]

A number of trials using aspirin in a dose of 900 mg/day or more have reported an increase in the incidence of stomach pain, heartburn, nausea, constipation, and occult gastrointestinal blood loss[39,47–52] by comparison with placebo. In one study, aspirin at a dose of 324 mg was not reported to be associated with a significant increase in gastrointestinal side effects when compared with a control group,[53] but in another, larger study,[39] there was a slight but significant increase (compared with placebo) in minor gastrointestinal side effects in patients treated with 300 mg/day of aspirin.

The exact cause of aspirin-induced gastric injury has not been elucidated. Inhibition by aspirin of prostaglandin synthesis in the gastric mucosa[54] has been proposed as an important mechanism. There is evidence that the gastric side effects of aspirin can be reduced by treatment with cimetidine,[55] by antacids,[56] and by the use of enteric-coated or highly buffered aspirin.[46,57,58]

Aspirin is effective in reducing the incidence of thrombotic complications of atherosclerosis. It has been shown to reduce the incidence of myocardial infarction and/or death in the following groups: males over age 50,[59] asymptomatic females over age 50,[60] subjects with stable angina,[61] patients with unstable angina and non-Q-wave infarction, in whom it appeared to be more effective than a short course of intravenous heparin,[62] patients with acute myocardial infarction (30-day incidence[47] and long-term incidence),[63] and patients with cerebrovascular disease.[39,63,64]

ORAL ANTICOAGULANTS

Oral anticoagulants are vitamin K antagonists which produce their anticoagulant effect by interfering with the cyclic interconversion of vitamin K and its 2,3-epoxide (vitamin K epoxide). Vitamin K is a cofactor for the posttranslational carboxylation of glutamate residues to γ-carboxyglutamates (Gla) on the N-terminal regions of vitamin K–dependent proteins.[65–70] The process of γ-carboxylation permits the coagulation proteins to undergo a conformational change[71–73] which is necessary for calcium-dependent complexing of vitamin K–dependent proteins to their cofactors on phospholipid surfaces and for their biologic activity. Carboxylation of vitamin K–dependent coagulation factors is catalyzed by a carboxylase, which requires the reduced form of vitamin K (vitamin KH_2), molecular oxygen, and carbon dioxide. During this reaction, the vitamin KH_2 is oxidized to vitamin K epoxide, which is recycled to vitamin K by vitamin K epoxide reductase, which in turn is reduced to vitamin KH_2 by vitamin K reductase. The vitamin K antagonists exert their anticoagulant effect by inhibiting vitamin K epoxide reductase[65–67] and possibly vitamin K reductase.[66] This process leads to the depletion of vitamin KH_2 and limits the γ-carboxylation of the vitamin K–dependent coagulant proteins (prothrombin, factor VII, factor IX, and factor X). In addition, the vitamin K antagonists limit the carboxylation of the regulatory proteins (protein C and protein S) and as a result impair the function of these anticoagulant proteins. By inhibiting the cyclic conversion of vitamin K, oral anticoagulants result in the hepatic production and secretion of partially carboxylated and descarboxylated proteins.[74,75]

Pharmacokinetics and Pharmacodynamics

Warfarin (a 4-hydroxycoumarin compound) is the most widely used oral anticoagulant in North America because its onset and duration of action are predictable and because it has excellent bioavailability.[76,77] Warfarin is almost always administered by the oral route, although an injectable preparation is available. It is rapidly absorbed from the gastrointestinal tract, reaches maximal blood concentrations in healthy volunteers in 90 minutes,[76,78] and has a half-life of 36 to 42 h.[79] It circulates bound to plasma proteins and rapidly accumulates in the liver.[80]

The dose-response relationship of warfarin differs between healthy subjects[81] and can vary to a much greater extent among sick patients. Because of the variations in dose response in individual patients during the course of anticoagulant therapy, their anticoagulant dosage must be monitored closely to prevent overdosing or underdosing.

The dose response to warfarin is influenced by both pharmacokinetic factors (due to differences in absorption or metabolic clearance of warfarin) and pharmacodynamic factors (due to differences in the hemostatic response to given concentrations of warfarin). Technical factors also contribute to the variability in dose response, including inaccuracies in laboratory testing and reporting, poor patient compliance, and poor communication between patient and physician.

Drugs can influence the pharmacokinetics of warfarin by reducing its absorption from the intestine or by altering its metabolic clearance (Table 29-4). Chronic alcohol use has the potential to increase the clearance of warfarin by hepatic enzyme induction, although studies have shown that even relatively high wine consumption does not influence the prothrombin time in subjects treated with warfarin.[82]

The pharmacodynamics of warfarin are affected by many factors which can influence its anticoagulant effect. Hereditary resistance to warfarin has been described in humans.[83,84] They require doses which are 5- to 20-fold higher than average to achieve an anticoagulant effect. This disorder is thought to be caused by an altered affinity of the receptor for warfarin, since the plasma warfarin levels required to achieve an anticoagulant effect are much higher than average.

Subjects receiving long-term warfarin therapy are sensitive to fluctuating levels of dietary vitamin K,[85] which is obtained predominantly from phylloquinone in plant material.[86] Important fluctuations in vitamin K intake occur in both apparently healthy and sick subjects. Increased intake

TABLE 29-4. *Factors Which Potentiate or Inhibit the Effect of Warfarin*

Drugs	Other
Potentiate Anticoagulant Effect	
Phenylbutazone	Low vitamin K intake
Metronidazole	Reduced vitamin K absorption
Sulfinpyrazone	Liver disease
Trimethoprim-sulfamethoxazole	Hypermetabolic states (fever thyrotoxicosis)
Disulfiram	
Amiodarone	
Erythromycin	
Anabolic Steroids	
Clofibrate	
Cimetidine	
Omeprazole	
Thyroxine	
Ketoconazole	
Isoniazid	
Fluconazole	
Piroxicam	
Tamoxifen	
Quinidine	
Vitamin E (megadose)	
Phenytoin	
Inhibit Anticoagulant Effects	
Reduced absorption of warfarin by *cholestyramine*	Increased vitamin K intake
Barbiturates	Alcohol
Rifampin	
Griseofulvin	
Carbamazepine	
Penicillin	

of dietary vitamin K sufficient to reduce the anticoagulant response to warfarin[85,87] occurs in patients on weight-reduction diets (rich in green vegetables) and those treated with intravenous nutritional fluid supplements rich in vitamin K. The effects of warfarin can be potentiated in sick patients with poor vitamin K intake (particularly if they are treated with antibiotics and intravenous fluids without vitamin K supplementation) and in states of fat malabsorption. Hepatic dysfunction also potentiates the response to warfarin through impaired synthesis of coagulation factors.[88] Hypermetabolic states produced by fever or hyperthyroidism increase responsiveness to warfarin probably by increasing the catabolism of vitamin K–dependent coagulation factors.[89–91] Drugs can influence the pharmacodynamics of warfarin by inhibiting the synthesis of vitamin K–dependent coagulation factors, by increasing the metabolic clearance of vitamin K–dependent coagulation factors, and by interfering with other pathways of hemostasis (Table 29-4).

Drugs such as aspirin,[25] other nonsteroidal anti-inflammatory drugs,[92] and high doses of penicillins[93,94] and moxolactam[95] can increase the risk of warfarin-associated bleeding by inhibiting platelet function (Table 29-5). Aspirin is the most important because of its widespread use and prolonged effect on hemostasis.[25] Aspirin also can produce gastric erosions, which increase the risk of serious upper gastrointestinal bleeding.[46]

Sulfonamides and many broad-spectrum antibiotics have the potential to augment the anticoagulant effect of warfarin by eliminating bacterial flora and thereby producing vitamin K deficiency, but these agents only potentiate the anticoagulant effect of warfarin in patients on a vitamin K–deficient diet.[96]

Many other drugs either interact with oral anticoagulants or have been reported to alter the prothrombin time response to warfarin,[97] but in most of these reports, convincing evidence of a causal association is lacking. Nevertheless, special care should be taken when use of any new drug is necessary in patients who are being treated with oral anticoagulants and to monitor the prothrombin time more frequently during the initial stages of combined drug therapy, with dose adjustments made when appropriate.

Oral anticoagulants have been shown to be effective in the primary and secondary prevention of venous thromboembolism, in the prevention of systemic embolism in patients with tissue and mechanical prosthetic heart valves or with atrial fibrillation, in the prevention of acute myocardial infarction in patients with peripheral arterial disease, and in the prevention of stroke, recurrent infarction, and death in patients with acute myocardial infarction.[98] Oral anticoagulants are indicated in patients with valvular heart disease to prevent systemic embolism, although their effectiveness has never been demonstrated by a randomized clinical trial.[98] For most indications, a moderate anticoagulant effect with a targeted international normalized ratio (INR) of 2.0 to 3.0 (less intense regimen) is appropriate.

The main limitations of oral anticoagulants are that they have a narrow risk/benefit ratio, the dosage requirement varies widely among patients and can fluctuate within patients because of changes in diet and concomitant use of drugs, and laboratory monitoring can be difficult and time consuming. Currently, there is no replacement for oral anticoagulants, but orally active AT III–independent thrombin inhibitors and factor Xa inhibitors are in an experimental stage of development.

LOW-MOLECULAR-WEIGHT HEPARINS AND HEPARINOIDS

The development of LMWHs for clinical use was stimulated by the observation that for equivalent antithrombotic effects in experimental models, LMWHs produce less bleeding than the heparin from which they were derived.[94–104] These observations were followed by clinical studies which demonstrated that LMWHs are effective and safe antithrombotic agents for the prevention and treatment of venous thrombosis. LMWHs have been approved for clinical use for the prevention and treatment of venous thrombosis in Europe and are currently under review in North America.

LMWHs are fragments of standard commercial-grade heparin (SH) produced by either chemical or enzymatic depolymerization.[105] SH is a heterogeneous mixture of polysaccharide chains with a wide molecular weight distribution which ranges from 3000 to 30,000, with a mean molecular weight of 15,000.[15,106,107] LMWHs are approxi-

TABLE 29-5. Factors Which Potentiate
the Antihemostatic Effect of Warfarin
by Impairing Platelet Function

Drugs	Other
Aspirin	Thrombocytopenia
Other NSAIDs	
Ticlopidine	Renal failure
Moxalactam	
Carbenicillin	

mately one-third the size of heparin. Like SH, they are heterogeneous in size with a molecular weight range of 1000 to 10,000 and a mean molecular weight of 4000 to 5000 (Table 29-6).

Depolymerization of SH results in a change in its anticoagulant profile, in its bioavailability and pharmacokinetics, and in its effects on platelet function and experimental bleeding. Two other glycosaminoglycans also have been developed for clinical use. These are dermatan sulfate and the organon heparinoid (Lomoparin), which is a mixture of heparan sulfate (the major component making up 80% of the mixture) and smaller amounts of dermatan sulfate and chondroitin sulfates.

Anticoagulant Effects

Like SH, LMWHs produce their major anticoagulant effect by binding to AT III through a unique pentasaccharide sequence.[108–120] This pentasaccharide sequence is present on approximately a third of the heparin chains and is present on less than a third of LMWH molecules. The binding of the pentasaccharide to AT III produces a conformational change in the AT III molecule[121–123] which enhances its ability to inactivate the coagulation enzymes thrombin (factor IIa) and factor Xa.[119] SH and LMWHs catalyze the inactivation of thrombin by AT III, acting as a template that binds both the plasma cofactor through the unique pentasaccharide sequence and thrombin to form a ternary complex.[108,110,119,124,125] A minimum chain length of 18 saccharides (including the pentasaccharide sequence) is required for ternary complex formation. In contrast, inactivation of factor Xa by AT III does not require binding of the heparin molecules to the clotting enzyme[108,110,119,124,125] and is therefore achieved by small-molecular-weight heparin fragments provided that they contain the high-affinity pentasaccharide. Virtually all SH molecules contain at least 18 saccharide units, while only 25% to 50% of the different LMWHs contain fragments with 18 or more saccharide units.[117,126–129] Therefore, compared with SH, which has a ratio of anti-factor Xa to anti-factor IIa activity of approximately 1:1, the various commercial LMWHs have anti-factor Xa to anti-IIa ratios which vary between 4:1 and 2:1 depending on their molecular size distribution.

Pharmacokinetics

The plasma recoveries and pharmacokinetics of LMWHs differ from those of SH because of differences in the binding properties of the two sulfated polysaccharides to plasma proteins and endothelial cells (Table 29-6).

LMWHs bind much less avidly to heparin-binding proteins than SH,[106,130–136] a property which contributes to the superior bioavailability of LMWHs at low doses and their more pre-

---

TABLE 29-6. *Comparisons Between Standard Heparin and LMWHs: Molecular Size, Anticoagulant Activity, Binding Properties, and Pharmacokinetics*

	Standard Unfractionated Heparin*	Low-Molecular-Weight Heparins*
Mean molecular weight	12,000–15,000	4000–6500
Saccharide units (mean)	40–50	13–22
Anti-Xa, anti-IIa activity	1:1	2:1 to 4:1
Protein binding	++++	+
Binds to endothelium	+++	
Dose-dependent clearance	Yes	No
Bioavailability	Poor	Good
Inhibits platelet function	++++	++
Increases vascular permeability	Yes	No
Augments microvascular bleeding	++++	++

* +, slight increase; ++, moderate increase; +++, increase; ++++, marked increase.

dictable anticoagulant response.[137] LMWHs do not bind to endothelial cells in culture,[138–140] a property that could account for their longer plasma half-life.[141–150] LMWHs are cleared principally by the renal route, and their biologic half life is increased in patients with renal failure.[143,151,152]

LMWH preparations have a lower affinity than SH for von Willebrand factor (vWF),[136] a finding which could contribute to the observation that they produce less experimental bleeding than SH for equivalent anticoagulant effects[99–104,153] (see Table 29-6).

Antithrombotic and Hemorrhagic Effects in Experimental Animal Models

The antithrombotic and hemorrhagic effects of SH have been compared with those of LMWHs, the organon heparinoid, and dermatan sulfate in a number of experimental animal models.[99–104,153–158] In these models of thrombosis, temporary venous stasis is produced by ligating an appropriate vein, and blood coagulation is stimulated by injecting either serum, factor Xa, thrombin, or tissue factor.[153,157,158] When compared on a gravimetric basis, LMWHs are slightly less effective than heparin as antithrombotic agents but produce much less bleeding than heparin in models measuring blood loss from a standardized injury.[100–103,153,155,156] The differences in the relative antithrombotic to hemorrhagic ratios among these sulfated polysaccharides could be due in part to their different effects on platelet function[99,136,159,160] and vascular permeability[161] (see Table 29-6).

Clinical Studies

LMWHs have a number of advantages over SH. The observations that LMWHs have a longer plasma half-life (see Table 29-6) and a more predictable anticoagulant response than SH allow LMWHs to be administered once daily and without laboratory monitoring. The observation in experimental animals that LMWHs produce less bleeding than SH for an equivalent antithrombotic effect has allowed patients to be treated with higher anticoagulant doses of LMWHs without compromising patient safety. This latter potential advantage of LMWHs has been demonstrated in one prophylactic study in which SH produced a significant increase in bleeding when its dose was increased to match the anticoagulant effect ex vivo of an LMWH[162] and in two studies comparing high doses of an LMWH with full doses of SH for the treatment of venous thrombosis[163,164] (Table 29-7). LMWHs have been evaluated for the prevention and treatment of venous thromboembolism and have been shown to be highly effective.

Prevention of Venous Thrombosis

General Surgery

LMWHs have been shown to be effective and safe in two well-designed randomized trials when compared with an untreated control.[165,166] In one study, there was an increase in minor bleeding (compared with placebo),[166] but in neither was there an increased incidence of major bleeding.[165,166] One study of 4498 patients[166] showed a statistically significant reduction in thromboem-

TABLE 29-7. LMWH for Established Venous Thrombosis

Study	Treatment	Dose (Anti-Xa, U)	No. of Patients	Recurrent VTE (%)	Bleeding
Prandoni (194)	Fraxiparin	12,500–17,5000 IC U bid SC	85	7.1	4 (4.7)
	SH	Continuous IV	85	12.9	9 (10.6)
Hull (193)*	Logiparin		213	3.3	7 (3.3)
	SH	175/kg OD SC Continuous IV	213	6.1	16 (7.5)

*Double-blind trial.

bolic mortality in favor of LMWH, 0.36% to 0.09% (RR = 75%). The other study demonstrated a marked risk reduction in fibrinogen scan–detected thrombi.[166]

Two studies reported that LMWHs were more effective than low-dose SH,[167,168] and the other six studies showed no significant difference in efficacy between the LMWHs and low-dose SH.[169–174] In one study, bleeding was significantly less in the LMWH group,[172] while in the other study, bleeding was significantly greater in the LMWH group.[169]

Orthopedic Surgery

Compared with placebo, LMWHs produced a risk reduction for all thrombi and for proximal vein thrombi of between 70% and 79%. This impressive reduction occurred without an increase in clinically important bleeding in two studies[175,176] and a small increase in minor bleeding in the third[177,178] (Table 29-8).

LMWHs have been compared with a variety of other methods of prophylaxis, including low-dose SH[162,179,180] (three studies), low-dose SH and dihydroergotamine (DHE)[181] (one study), adjusted-dose heparin[182,183] (two studies), dextran[184,185] (two studies), and warfarin[186] (one study).

The results of studies comparing LMWH with fixed-low-dose SH are summarized in Table 29-9. LMWHs were between 29% and 50% more effective than low-dose SH 5000 units three times daily without any apparent difference in bleeding. When, however, the dose of SH was increased to 7500 units, the difference in efficacy was only 16% (NS) in favor of LMWH, but the incidence of

bleeding was increased significantly in the SH group.

In the limited number of comparative trials, LMWHs appeared to be as effective and safe as adjusted-dose heparin[182,183] and warfarin[186] in patients having elective hip surgery and were much more effective than dextran.[185] LMWHs also were more effective than warfarin in patients having major knee surgery.[186]

There has only been one randomized trial evaluating an LMWH or heparinoid in patients with hip fracture.[184] In this study, Lomoparin was compared with dextran, both regimens commencing preoperatively. The incidence of thrombosis was 10% in the Lomoparin group and 30% in the dextran group ($p < 0.001$). The number of units of blood transfused was significantly higher in the dextran group.

Medical Patients

LMWHs are very effective and safe prophylactic agents in medical patients. LMWHs have been compared with placebo in two studies of patients with ischemic stroke[187,188] and in one study in high-risk medical patients over age 65 years.[189] LMWHs also have been compared with low-dose SH in two studies[190,191] (Table 29-10). In all the reported studies, fibrinogen leg scanning was used to detect venous thrombosis. Compared with placebo, LMWHs produced a relative risk reduction in venous thrombosis of between 40% and 86% in patients with stroke and in high-risk medical patients; this effect was seen without an increase in clinically important bleeding. In both

TABLE 29-8. Double-Blind Trials Comparing LMWH with Placebo in Orthopedic Surgery

Study	Type	Treatment	No. of Patients	DVT (%)	Bleeding[†] (%)
Turpie (177)*	Elective hip	Enoxaparin	37	10.8	4.0
		Placebo	39	51.3[‡]	4.0
Leclerc (176)*	Elective knee	Enoxaparin	41	19.5	6.1
		Placebo	54	64.8[‡]	7.6
Hoek (178)	Elective hip	Lomoparin	97	15.5	6.1
		Placebo	99	56.6[‡]	0[†]

* Prophylaxis commenced postoperatively.
[†] More patients were included in safety analysis than efficacy analysis.
[‡] $p < 0.05$.

TABLE 29-9. *Double-Blind Trials Comparing LMWH with Low-Dose SH in Orthopedic Surgery*

Study	Type	Treatment	No. of Patients	DVT Event (%)	DVT Risk Reduction %	Bleeding* (%)
Planes (179)	Elective hip	Enoxaparin	120	12.5	50	2.4
		SH	108	25.0[†]		1.8
Levine (162)[†]	Elective hip	Enoxaparin	258	19.4	16	5.6
		SH	263	23.2		9.3
Estoppey (181)	Elective hip	Lomoparin	146	17.1	47	
		SH/DHE	149	32.2[†]		
Eriksson (180)	Elective hip	Fragmin	63	30.2	29	1.5
		SH	59	42.4		7.4

* More patients were included in safety analysis than efficacy analysis.
[†] Prophylaxis commenced postoperatively.
[‡] $p < 0.05$.

studies comparing these LMWHs with SH, patients randomized to receive LMWHs showed a greater than 70% relative risk reduction in thrombosis, a statistically significant difference.[190,191]

Heparinoids. Two heparinoids are currently being investigated. These are dermatan sulfate and Lomoparin, which is a mixture of dermatan sulfate, chondroitin sulfate, and heparan sulfate. Dermatan sulfate catalyzes heparin cofactor II,[192] which is a secondary inhibitor of thrombin. Since, unlike AT III, heparin cofactor II only inhibits thrombin, dermatan sulfate has minimal anti-factor Xa activity. In contrast, because Lomoparin

contains large amounts of heparan sulfate, this preparation has both antithrombin and anti-factor Xa activity.

Treatment of Established Thrombosis

LMWHs have been compared with SH in five relatively large studies.[193–198] Most of the randomized trials used a change in thrombus size between the pretreatment and 5- to 10-day posttreatment venogram as the outcome measure. In all studies, LMWHs were at least as effective as SH in preventing extension of venous thrombosis, and in

TABLE 29-10. *Randomized Trials of Prophylactic LMWH in Medical Patients*

Study	Condition	Treatment	No. of Patients	DVT Event (%)	DVT Risk Reduction %	Bleeding (%)
Turpie (188)*	Stroke	Lomoparin	50	4.0	86	2.0
		Placebo	25	28.0[†]		8.0
Prins (187)*	Stroke	Fragmin	30	30.0	40	13.3
		Placebo	30	50.0[†]		6.7
Dahan (189)*	Elderly	Enoxaparin	132	3.0	67	1.0
		Placebo	131	9.1[†]		2.3
Turpie (191)*	Stroke	Lomoparin	45	8.9	71	0
		SH	42	31.0[†]		0
Green (190)	Spinal cord injury	Logiparin	20	0	>90	0
		SH	21	23.8[†]		9.5

* Double-blind trial.
[†] $p < 0.05$.

most studies, LMWHs were associated with a greater reduction in thrombus size than SH. In most of these studies, SH was administered by continuous intravenous infusion and was monitored to maintain the APTT in a defined therapeutic range. In most of the studies, the LMWH was administered by subcutaneous injection and without laboratory monitoring.

Two recent large studies used the more clinically relevant endpoint of confirmed symptomatic recurrent thromboembolism as an outcome measure (see Table 29-7). In the study reported by Prandoni and associates,[194] 170 patients with venographically confirmed proximal deep vein thrombosis were randomized to receive an LMWH (using a weight-adjusted regimen) or SH administered by continuous intravenous infusion adjusted to maintain the APTT at 1.5 to 2 times control. At 10 days, 4 of 85 (4.7%) patients receiving SH developed recurrence compared with 1 of 85 (1.2%) receiving LMWH ($p = 0.1$). At 6 months, 11 of 85 (12.9%) patients receiving SH developed recurrent thromboembolism compared with 6 of 85 LMWH patients (7.1%) ($p = 0.2$). Bleeding occurred in 10.6% of the SH patients compared with 3.5% of the LMWH patients ($p = 0.1$). The mortality at 6 months was 12 of 85 (14.1%) in the SH group and 6 of 85 (7.1%) in the LMWH group (NS). Most deaths were cancer-related.

The second study reported by Hull and associates[193] was a double-blind trial performed in patients with proximal vein thrombosis. A fixed dose of LMWH (175 anti-factor Xa units of Lomoparin per kilogram of body weight) given subcutaneously once daily was compared with adjusted-dose intravenous heparin given by continuous infusion. The patients in the intravenous heparin group received an initial intravenous bolus dose of 5000 units of heparin, followed by a continuous intravenous infusion of heparin. Objective tests were used to document clinical outcomes.

The initial dose of heparin was 40,320 units every 24 h for patients without the designated risk factors for bleeding and 29,760 units every 24 h for patients who had one or more designated risk factors. Fifty-three patients randomly assigned to receive intravenous heparin had one or more designated risk factors for bleeding, as compared with 56 patients randomly assigned to receive LMWH.

Six of 213 patients who received LMWH (2.8%) and 15 of 219 patients who received intravenous heparin (6.9%) had new episodes of venous thromboembolism ($p = 0.07$; 95% CI for the difference = 0.02% to 8.1%). Analysis by the log-rank test demonstrated a significant difference ($p = 0.049$) in the frequency of thromboembolic events.

Major bleeding associated with initial therapy occurred in 1 patient receiving LMWH (0.5%) and in 11 patients receiving intravenous heparin (5.0%), a reduction in risk of 91% ($p = 0.006$). Minor hemorrhagic complications occurred during or immediately after the initial therapy in 5 patients receiving LMWH (2.4%) and in 4 patients receiving intravenous heparin (1.8%).

Ten patients assigned to receive LMWH (4.7%) and 21 patients assigned to receive intravenous heparin (9.6%) died during the 3 months of follow-up ($p = 0.062$ by Fisher's exact test; $p = 0.049$ by the uncorrected chi-squared test; RR = 51%).

Three patients receiving LMWH died abruptly (1.4%), as compared with 13 patients receiving intravenous heparin (5.9%) ($p = 0.019$).

The results of these studies suggest that in patients with proximal vein thrombosis, LMWHs administered by subcutaneous injection in a fixed dose or weight-adjusted dose is at least as safe and effective as conventional SH administered by continuous infusion and monitored with the APTT.

NOVEL ANTITHROMBOTIC COMPOUNDS

A large array of new compounds designed to inhibit specific molecular interactions which are believed to be important in thrombogenesis have been developed. These include (1) inhibitors of vWF-dependent platelet adhesion to platelet glycoprotein receptor Ib (GPIb), (2) inhibitors of platelet glycoprotein receptor IIb-IIIa (GPIIb-IIIa)–dependent platelet aggregation, (3) platelet thrombin receptor antagonists, (4) inhibitors of thrombin generation—tissue pathway inhibitor (TPI), activated protein C (APC), and activated factor Xa inhibitor, and (5) direct thrombin inhibitors. The development of these inhibitors has been made possible by advances in molecular biology and in knowledge of the structural chemistry of binding sites on receptors and ligands involved in thrombogenesis. The inhibitors fall into three classes of molecules. These are monoclonal antibodies directed at specific platelet glycoprotein receptors, recombinant naturally occurring peptides derived from snakes, leeches, ticks, and toads, and synthetic competitive peptide analogues which compete with ligand-receptor or enzyme-substrate binding.

PLATELET-FUNCTION INHIBITORS

Aspirin is a very selective inhibitor of platelet function, since it only inhibits platelet aggregation mediated through activation of the arachidonic acid–TXA_2 pathway. This selective activity may explain the limited effectiveness of aspirin in inhibiting coronary reocclusion clinically[199–201] and in experimental models of thrombolysis.[202,203] Nevertheless, despite its limited selectivity, aspirin is effective in preventing death and reinfarction after coronary thrombolysis.[204] Both the effectiveness of aspirin clinically and its limitations have generated considerable interest in developing new and more potent inhibitors of platelet aggregation. These fall into four main classes (Tables 29-11 and 29-12): (1) the nonspe-

TABLE 29-11. *New Antithrombotic Strategies*

Antiplatelet Agents
1. Ticlopidine
2. Thromboxane A_2 receptor antagonists and synthetase inhibitors
3. Competitors of binding of vWF to GPIb
   a. Monoclonal antibodies
   b. vWF-like proteins
   c. Inhibition of vWF multimerization with arvin tricarboxylic acid
4. Competitors of binding fibrinogen, vWF, and other ligands to GPIIb-IIIa
   a. Monoclonal antibodies
   b. Snake venoms (RDG-containing)
   c. Synthetic cyclic peptides (RGD, KGD)
5. Thrombin receptor antagonists (TRAPs)

TABLE 29-12. *New Antithrombotic Strategies*

Anticoagulants
1. Low-molecular-weight heparins and heparinoids
2. Direct thrombin inhibitors (AT III–independent)
   a. Hirudin and derivatives
   b. Chloromethyl ketones (D-FPRCH)
   c. Benzamidine compounds
   d. Argipidine
3. Director factor Xa inhibitors (AT III–independent)
   a. Tick anticoagulant protein
   b. Antistasin
4. Activated protein C
   a. Recombinant
   b. Thrombin with selected activity
5. Tissue factor pathway inhibitor

cific inhibitor ticlopidine, (2) the TXA_2 receptor antagonists and synthetase inhibitors, (3) compounds which compete with vWF for binding to platelet GPIb, and (4) compounds which compete for binding of fibrinogen and other adhesive proteins to platelet GPIIb-IIIa. Of these, the most promising group of compounds are those which compete with fibrinogen and the other adhesive proteins for binding to the platelet glycoprotein receptor GPIIb-IIIa. Ticlopidine is currently the only one of the four classes of new compounds approved for clinical use.

Ticlopidine

Ticlopidine is a new antiplatelet drug with an entirely different mechanism of action than aspirin.[205] Ticlopidine is a thienopyridine derivative which inhibits platelet aggregation induced by a variety of agonists, including ADP, possibly by altering the platelet membrane and blocking the interaction between fibrinogen and its membrane glycoprotein receptor GPIIb-IIIa.[206] The inhibitory effect of ticlopidine is delayed for 24 to 48 h after its administration, suggesting that the anti-aggregating effects are caused by metabolites.[205] Ticlopidine has been evaluated in patients with stroke,[207] transient cerebral ischemia,[208] unstable angina,[209] intermittent claudication,[210–212] and aortocoronary bypass surgery.[213] Ticlopidine was significantly more effective than aspirin in reducing stroke in patients with transient cerebral ischemia or minor stroke,[208] was more effective than placebo in reducing the risk of the combined outcome of stroke, myocardial infarction, or vascular death in patients with thromboembolic stroke,[207] was more effective than an untreated control group in reducing vascular death and myocardial infarction in patients with unstable angina,[209] was more effective than placebo in reducing acute occlusion of coronary bypass grafts,[213] and was more effective than controls in improving walking distance[211] and reducing vascular complications in patients with peripheral vascular disease.[209,210,212]

Ticlopidine has a number of troublesome side effects, the most common of which are diarrhea and skin rash, and the most serious, neutropenia. Nevertheless, ticlopidine should be used in patients with aspirin allergy or gastrointestinal intolerance.

Inhibitors of Platelet Adhesion

Platelet adhesion occurs when glycoprotein receptors on inactivated platelets bind to the ligands in the subendothelial extracellular matrix exposed during vascular injury[214–217] (Fig. 29-3). The most important ligands are collagen and vWF, but platelets also may adhere to other subendothelial proteins, including fibronectin, laminin, vitronectin, and thrombospondin.[214–224] The platelet membrane glycoprotein receptors for the various adhesive matrix molecules are GPIb-IX, GPIa-IIa, GPIc-IIa, vitronectin receptor, and GPIV (GPIIIb).

Platelets exposed to elevated levels of fluid shear stress bind to vWF and then aggregate in the absence of exogenous agonists.[225] vWF binds to two receptors on the platelet membrane, GPIb and GPIIb-IIIa, both of which are involved in shear-stress–induced platelet aggregation.[223,226,227] Shear stress stimulates binding of vWF multimers to GPIb on the surface of inactivated platelets. This binding interaction then activates platelets and exposes functional GPIIa-IIIb integrin receptors which bind vWF multimers and undergo aggregation. Shear-stress–induced aggregation is inhibited in part by a monoclonal antibody (10E5), which inhibits vWF binding to GPIIb-IIIa.

The molecular mechanism responsible for shear-stress–induced vWF-GPIb binding is uncertain. Shear stress could either alter the structure of vWF or alter some characteristic of platelet surface GPIb and permit ligand binding to occur.[223,226,227] Whatever the mechanism, high shear stress initiates vWF-dependent transmembranous influx of Ca^{2+} and induces platelet aggregation. This platelet response is not inhibited by aspirin and requires a functional platelet GPIIb-IIIa complex.

Binding of collagen to its glycoprotein receptors also stimulates platelet activation with the exposure of the integrin GPIIb-IIIa in its functional form. Inhibition of vWF-dependent platelet adhesion can be achieved by interfering with binding of vWF to GPIb and inhibition of vWF multimerization.[218–224,228–231]

Monoclonal antibodies against GPIb or GPIb-IX have been studied in experimental animal

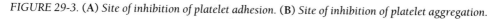

FIGURE 29-3. (**A**) *Site of inhibition of platelet adhesion.* (**B**) *Site of inhibition of platelet aggregation.*

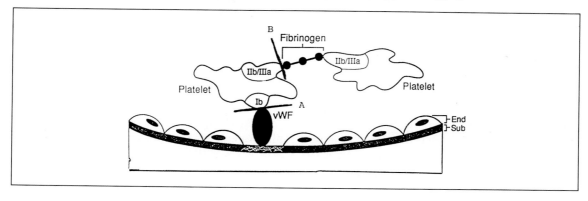

models of thrombosis.[228,231,232] Monoclonal antibodies raised against GPIb have antithrombotic effects in guinea pigs subjected to laser-induced injury to mesenteric small arteries.[228] These antibodies to GPIb produce irreversible thrombocytopenia in nonhuman primates.[232] Peptides mimicking the GPIb binding domain of vWF inhibit ristocetin-induced GPIb-dependent platelet agglutination,[219,222,229] inhibit platelet deposition in high-shear flow models in vitro,[222,229] and reduce thrombus formation under arterial flow conditions in experimental animal models.[233] The template bleeding time is prolonged at concentrations of these peptides which exhibit antithrombotic effects.[228,232,233]

Moderate antithrombotic effects are also observed in animal models of arterial thrombosis when anti-vWF neutralizing antibodies[228,230,231] are administered intravenously at doses that produce a marked prolongation of the bleeding time. Similarly, moderate antithrombotic effects are produced in animal models of arterial thrombus by inhibiting vWF multimerization using aurintricarboxylic acid at doses that produce marked prolongation of the bleeding time.[234]

Inhibitors of Platelet GPIIb-IIIa–Dependent Recruitment

Platelet aggregation can be triggered by platelet adhesion to either collagen or vWF (under conditions of high shear) or by exposure to ADP, TXA$_2$, or thrombin (Figs. 29-3 and 29-4). Platelet activation by these agonists results in the expression on the platelet surface of functional GPIIb-IIIa receptors for fibrinogen and other adhesive glycoproteins, leading to calcium-dependent interplatelet linkages.[215–217] The functional GPIIb-IIIa receptor binds with a number of adhesive glycoprotein ligands, including fibrinogen, vWF, fibronectin, vitronectin, and thrombospondin. Of these, fibrinogen is the most important because it is present in much greater concentrations in plasma than the other adhesive glycoproteins. Arg-Gly-Asp (RGD) serves as the integrin recognition sequence in the adhesive proteins interacting with this receptor.[215–217,235–237] Fibrinogen contains RGD sequences in each alpha chain.[215,217] An additional site on the carboxy-terminal dodecapep-

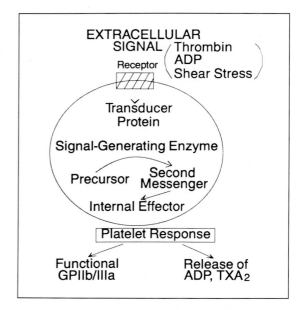

FIGURE 29-4. *The extracellular stimulus binds to its receptor and sets into motion intracellular platelet responses which culminate in the exposure of functional GPIIb-IIIa receptors for fibrinogen and the release of ADP and TXA$_2$.*

tide of each gamma chain of fibrinogen also binds to GPIIb-IIIa. This latter dodecapeptide is not found in other adhesive proteins and contains a Lys-Ala-Gly-Asp sequence.

Platelet aggregation is inhibited by anti–GPIIb-IIIa monoclonal antibodies by naturally occurring peptides containing RGD or dodecapeptide sequences and by synthetic competitive analogues.

Monoclonal Antibodies Directed Against GPIIb-IIIa. Inhibition of the platelet GPIIb-IIIa receptor by murine monoclonal antibodies prevents thrombosis in experimental models of vascular injury[232,237–244] and significantly shortens the time to reperfusion using t-PA after thrombotic coronary occlusion.[241,245] In dogs with experimental coronary thrombosis, 7E3 F(ab')$_2$ accelerates thrombolysis and prevents rethrombosis.[241,243,245]

The dosages that are required to achieve antithrombotic effects with murine monoclonal antibodies essentially eliminate GPIIb-IIIa receptor function on all circulating platelets and produce substantial experimental bleeding at sites of tissue injury in nonhuman primates.[232,240,244] Thrombocytopenia also develops in nonhuman primates following the administration of some murine monoclonal antibodies.[232,240] In patients, antithrombotic doses of these monoclonal antibodies also produce template bleeding times of greater than 30 minutes and occasionally serious thrombocytopenia, although severe spontaneous abnormal bleeding has not been reported in clinical trials to date. Preliminary studies using "humanized" anti–GPIIb-IIIa monoclonal antibodies in patients[245,246] at risk for arterial thrombotic events are reportedly free of both bleeding events and significant thrombocytopenia at doses that exhibit antiplatelet effects in patients with unstable angina[247] and myocardial infarction who are also treated with thrombolytic agents.[248]

Natural Antiplatelet Peptides. A number of naturally occurring cysteine-rich single-chain polypeptides have been isolated from snake venoms that potentially inhibit the binding of fibrinogen to GPIIb-IIIa receptors and abolish platelet aggregation. This group of RGD-containing peptides includes trigramin,[249–251] bitistatin,[252,253] echistatin,[254] kistrin,[255] and applaggin.[256,257] In experimental animals, all these polypeptides, referred to as *disintegrins,* produce dose-dependent inhibition of platelet aggregation ex vivo and thrombus formation in vivo. Accelerated t-PA–induced thrombolysis with prevention of subsequent reocclusion also has been demonstrated experimentally with some of these polypeptides.[252,253,255] For example, bitistatin[253] augments the effect of heparin in accelerating thrombolysis and prevents reocclusion following t-PA–induced thrombolysis in canine models of coronary thrombolysis.

These biologic peptides inhibit binding of all RGD-containing adhesive proteins with platelet GPIIb-IIIa receptors with affinities similar to monoclonal antibodies, although their effects are short-lived in vivo. Barbourin, a peptide isolated from the southwestern pygmy rattlesnake *Sistrurus m. barbouri,* differs from the other snake venom peptides in that it specifically inhibits the binding of adhesive proteins with human platelet GPIIb-IIIa without affecting the binding to GPIIa-IIIb on other cells.[258] This specificity is a consequence of the substitution of Arg for Lys, forming the unique recognition sequence KGD.

RGD-containing snake venom polypeptides[251,259–262] enhance and maintain coronary arterial thrombolysis with recombinant tissue-type plasminogen activator (rt-PA) in dogs.[263]

Synthetic Antiplatelet Peptides. GPIIb-IIIa antagonist peptides have been synthesized and characterized in vitro and in vivo as competitive inhibitors of platelet GPIIb-IIIa binding with the adhesive proteins.[264–268] These peptides, which are potent when synthesized in a cyclic configuration, inhibit platelet aggregation in a dose-dependent manner when tested in vitro and ex vivo and produce antithrombotic effects in experimental models of thrombosis.[264–269] In experimental animal models, the tetrapeptide analogue Arg-Gly-Asp-0-methyltyrosine amide prevents reocclusion caused by platelet-rich thrombi after successful t-PA–induced thrombolysis in the femoral arteries of dogs,[270,271] and the cyclic heptapeptide MK-852 is an effective antithrombotic compound in experimental models of arterial thrombosis.[271]

G4120, a cyclic RGD, accelerates lysis of platelet-rich arterial thrombosis with rt-PA and prevents reocclusion during and within 3 h of the infusion.[272] Synthetic cyclic peptides containing the KGD sequence also inhibit the binding of human platelets with adhesive proteins but with greater specificity for platelet GPIIb-IIIa than the integrins on other cells.[264,266]

Thrombin Receptor Antagonists

The platelet thrombin receptor is a 425 amino acid seven-transmembrane G protein–coupled molecule with an amino-terminal extracellular domain that undergoes activation by thrombin-mediated cleavage at Arg_{41} in the LDPR/S amino acid sequence.[273–276] Severance of this terminal peptide creates a neo-amino terminus that activates the receptor as a tethered ligand.[274] Thrombin interacts with an acidic region on the receptor through an anion-binding exosite in a manner analogous to its interaction with hirudin.[277] Each platelet has, on average, about a thousand copies of the thrombin receptor. The thrombin receptor is also present on endothelium and vascular smooth-muscle cells. Because the proteolytic activation of the thrombin receptor is not reversible, down-regulation of receptor function involves attenuation and inactivation after signal initiation.[274,278]

In vitro platelet thrombin receptor activity is inhibited by monoclonal antibodies and synthetic peptides targeting specific receptor sites.[275] In preliminary studies, novel synthetic thrombin receptor antagonist peptides (TRAPs) comprising portions of the neo-amino-terminal, hirudin-like binding sequence or other extramembranous domains also inhibit thrombin receptor function in vivo.[279,280] TRAPs do not inhibit the cleavage of fibrinogen by thrombin, but they may block other thrombin receptor–dependent responses at sites of vascular injury, including the mitogenic stimulation of vascular smooth-muscle cell proliferation[279,280] and leukocyte chemotaxis and cell adhesion receptor expression.[281,282]

Thromboxane A$_2$ Synthetase Inhibitors

Thrombin and TXA$_2$ are both important mediators of platelet activation.[283–287] TXA$_2$ causes platelet activation and coronary vasoconstriction. Studies in experimental animal models of thrombolysis and in humans using activation markers suggest that reocclusion after thrombolytic therapy is contributed to by TXA$_2$ production and release at the site of the lysing coronary thrombus.[245,288] There is experimental evidence that inhibition of both TXA$_2$ and thrombin activity may be more effective than inhibition of either one alone in shortening the time to reperfusion and in the prevention of reocclusion.[202,203,271,289–291] Recent studies showed that ridogrel, a combined TXA$_2$ synthetase inhibitor and receptor antagonist,[292,293] when added to hirulog, reduces the frequency of reocclusion after t-PA–induced lysis of coronary arteries of experimental thrombi in dogs more effectively than hirulog and t-PA. In this model, inhibition of thrombin alone or TXA$_2$ alone did not prevent reocclusion. Thus both TXA$_2$ and thrombin might contribute to the process of reocclusion. Ridogrel[294,295] was more effective than either a thromboxane receptor antagonist[296] or thromboxane synthetase inhibitor[297] when either of these classes of thromboxane inhibitors is used alone.

AT III–INDEPENDENT THROMBIN INHIBITORS

Several AT III–independent inhibitors are now available. These include hirudin, hirudin fragments, argatroban, and the peptide chloromethyl ketone inhibitor D-Phe-Pro-ArgCH$_2$Cl (PPACK) and its derivatives. Although all these inhibitors bind directly to thrombin, they have different mechanisms of action, as described below. The potential advantage of the AT III–independent inhibitors is that unlike heparin, these agents can access and inactive thrombin that is bound to fibrin.[17] This potential advantage appears to be real, since these inhibitors have proven to be more effective than heparin in experimental animal models of venous and arterial thrombosis[19,20,298] and as adjuncts to t-PA–induced thrombolysis using a variety of model systems.[299,300] These observations illustrate the importance of inhibiting fibrin-bound thrombin to achieve optimal antithrombotic effects.

Hirudin and Its Derivatives

Hirudin is a 65 amino acid residue protein isolated from the salivary glands of the medicinal leech. It is a potent and specific thrombin inhibitor which is now available through recombinant DNA technology. It forms an essentially irreversible stoichiometric complex with thrombin. Analysis of the crystal structure of the thrombin-hirudin complex illustrates the extensive contact that hirudin makes with thrombin as it binds to both the active center and the substrate-recognition site of the enzyme.[277] It inhibits thrombin by forming a stoichiometric complex with a dissociation constant that has been reported to be as low as 20 fmol.[301] The action of hirudin on thrombin is bivalent; it binds to both the anionic exosite (which is the substrate recognition site) and the catalytic center.

A novel class of synthetic C-terminal peptide fragments of hirudin has been developed[302–304] as thrombin inhibitors.[305,306] The first of these fragments, hirugen, is a synthetic dodecapeptide comprising residues 53 to 64 of the carboxy-terminal region of hirudin.[306] Hirugen binds only to the substrate-recognition site of thrombin but does not bind to the catalytic center of the enzyme. As a result, hirugen blocks the interaction of thrombin with fibrinogen, platelets, and other substrates. By adding D-Phe-Pro-Arg-Pro-(Gly)$_4$ to the amino-terminal region, hirugen has been converted from a weak competitive inhibitor to a potent bivalent inhibitor known as hirulog.[305] Like hirudin, hirulog blocks both the active center and the substrate-recognition site. However, active-site inhibition is transient because once complexed, thrombin can slowly cleave the Pro-Arg bond on the amino-terminal extension, thereby converting hirulog to a hirugen-like species.

In experimental animals, hirudin inhibits the formation of venous thrombi and blocks intra-vascular coagulation when administered intra-venously or subcutaneously.[307] Hirudin is much more effective than high-dose heparin[19,308] and as-pirin[309] in reducing platelet deposition and thrombosis after angioplasty in pigs. Hirudin also inter-rupts platelet-dependent thrombus formation at sites of mechanical deep arterial injury in pigs[19] and nonhuman primates,[308] although the doses required to inhibit platelet deposition also produce corresponding impairment in hemostatic function. Clinical trials are currently being conducted to evaluate the relative efficacy and safety for both venous and arterial thrombotic outcomes in patients, and preliminary findings are promising.

Argatroban

This synthetic arginine derivative of argipidine (also known as MD-805), argatroban is a competitive inhibitor of thrombin[310] which interacts with the active site of thrombin. It has a half-life of only a few minutes. Although argatroban is a relatively potent antithrombin in vitro,[310] it fails to inhibit platelet-dependent thrombus formation in vivo.

PPACK and Its Derivatives

The tripeptide chloromethyl ketone D-Phe-Pro-Arg-chloromethyl ketone (D-FPRCH or PPACK) irreversibly inhibits thrombin by alkylating the active center histidine.[311] This synthetic anti-thrombin is unique among the AT III–independent direct antithrombins because it potently and irreversibly inactivates both soluble and thrombus-bound thrombin.[312–317] Recent crystallographic studies confirm the tight interactions of this molecule with thrombin's catalytic pocket in addition to its covalent derivatization of His_{57} in the catalytic triad.[318] Since thrombin binds to fi-brin through a site distinct from its catalytic center, PPACK readily inhibits clot-bound throm-

bin.[17] Systemic infusions of $D-FPRCH_2Cl$ into nonhuman primates interrupt platelet-rich, aspirin- and heparin-resistant thrombi on Dacron vascular grafts,[312,313] vascular stents,[316] and hemo-dialyzers.[314] Transient intravenous infusions of $D-FPRCH_2Cl$ produce lasting interruption of platelet deposition at sites of surgical carotid endarterectomy by irreversibly inactivating thrombin generated by and bound to forming thrombus.[312] The lasting antithrombotic benefits following brief systemic treatment with $D-FPRCH_2Cl$ appear to result from the permanent inactivation of thrombin bound to and saturating any already formed thrombus. $D-FPRCH_2Cl$, but not competitive antithrombins such as hirudin, interrupts subsequent thrombus formation after topical application at a site of established thrombus.[315,317] The long-term toxicities associated with systemically or locally administered $D-FPRCH_2Cl$ have yet to be adequately investigated with respect to its potential as a systemic therapeutic agent in humans.

Recently, a PPACK derivative, D-Phe-Pro-Arg-borate, has been developed which is a more specific inhibitor of thrombin than the parent molecule.[319] This competitive antithrombin peptide blocks thrombin's catalytic site through a transition-state mechanism[319,320] and exhibits potent antithrombotic effects in several different animal models of arterial thrombosis.[320,321] Two additional synthetic antithrombinpeptides, D-Phe-Pro-Arg-H and D-MePhe-Pro-Arg-H, have anticoagulant and antiplatelet effects when administered both intravenously and orally in a number of animal species.[322] Benzamidine-based compounds also exhibit significant antithrombotic effects in vivo.[307]

Catalytic site–directed antithrombins are less specific than natural or bivalent antithrombin peptides. Specificity may be critical for achieving therapeutic efficacy without inducing toxic side effects.

The relative efficacy of the direct thrombin inhibitors has been compared in a number of different animal models with heparin or aspirin or platelet GPIIb-IIIa receptor antagonists in accelerating t-PA–induced thrombolysis or preventing reocclusion. In all these studies, the direct thrombin inhibitors proved to be more effective than the other antithrombotic agents. In a coronary thrombosis model in dogs, hirudin was more effective than heparin, aspirin, or a peptide RGD-containing analogue in accelerating t-PA–induced thrombolysis in which a 6-fold prolongation of the APTT by heparin failed to prevent reocclusion.[323] However, argipidine (argatroban) in doses that prolonged the APTT 2- to 4-fold was not effective in preventing coronary reocclusion in dogs. In a rat aortic thrombosis model of t-PA–induced thrombolysis, the effects of heparin, hirudin, and the synthetic hirulog were compared.[299] Compared with saline control, heparin had no significant effect on time to reperfusion or reocclusion, while the direct antithrombins decreased the number of reocclusions and accelerated thrombolysis. The superiority of hirudin over heparin in preventing thrombosis during and after thrombolysis and in permanently inactivating clot-bound thrombin also has been demonstrated in a study using a rabbit jugular vein model.[20]

Both recombinant hirudin and hirulog are undergoing clinical testing for prevention of both venous[324] and arterial[325] thrombosis during coronary angioplasty and in unstable angina. In addition, the effectiveness of these agents is being examined during coronary reperfusion therapy with thrombolytic drugs. Hirulog is also being compared with heparin in patients having routine cardiac catheterization.[325]

The relative antithrombotic and antihemostatic effects of a number of the direct antithrombins have been compared.[308,312,314,319,321,326] All direct antithrombins tested interrupt platelet and fibrin deposition and prevent thrombotic occlusion in a dose-dependent manner. The relative efficacy of the direct thrombin inhibitors has been compared with that of heparin or aspirin or platelet GPIIb-IIIa receptor antagonists in accelerating or preventing reocclusion in animal models of t-PA–induced thrombolysis. In all these studies, the direct thrombin inhibitors proved to be more effective than the other antithrombotic agents.

DIRECT FACTOR Xa INHIBITORS

Two AT III–independent factor Xa inhibitors, a tick anticoagulant peptide (TAP) and a leech anticoagulant peptide (Antistasin), have been developed. TAP is a 60 amino acid polypeptide which was originally isolated from the soft tick *Ornithodoros moubata*[327] and subsequently made recombinantly in yeast (r-TAP).[328] It is a potent and selective inhibitor of factor Xa, which, unlike heparin, can access and inhibit factor Xa in the prothrombinase complex. r-TAP has been shown to effectively prevent venous thrombus formation in rabbits,[329] to suppress systemic elevations in FPA induced by intravenous administration of thromboplastin in conscious rhesus monkeys,[328] and to inhibit thrombosis in a Silastic femoral arteriovenous shunt in baboons, a model that has been used extensively[240,312] to simulate arterial thrombosis produced under conditions of high shear.

The relative effects of recombinant TAP, recombinant hirudin, and heparin have been compared in a canine model of r-tPA–mediated coronary thrombolysis.[253,271] Both r-TAP and r-HIR but not heparin significantly accelerated r-tPA–mediated thrombolysis and prevented acute reocclusion. Heparin had a modest effect on enhancing thrombolytic reperfusion but failed to prevent or significantly delay reocclusion even in doses which elevated the APTT to approximately 8-fold over baseline values.

Like TAP, recombinant antistasin (r-ATS) is a potent and selective inhibitor of factor Xa. Antistasin was originally isolated from the Mexican leech *Haementeria officinalis*.[330-333] r-ATS has a molecular weight of 13,341 and produces potent anticoagulant properties for a period of greater than 30 h following a single subcutaneous administration. This long duration of action reflects a prolonged period of absorption coupled with a rather long plasma half-life.[334] r-ATS exhibits no detectable inhibition of thrombin at molar ratios as high at 500:1.[330] The in vivo antithrombotic effects of r-ATS following continuous intravenous infusion have been demonstrated in a rabbit model of venous thrombosis[329] and a rhesus monkey model of mild DIC.[332]

The effectiveness of both r-TAP and hirudin in preventing experimental arterial thrombosis and reocclusion in models of arterial thrombosis and thrombolysis which are resistant to the effects of heparin is likely to reflect the ability of r-TAP to directly access factor Xa assembled in the prothrombinase complexes[3,13,335,336] and of hirudin to access thrombin bound to fibrin within the residual thrombus.[17] In addition, release of platelet factor 4 by platelets in the thrombi could result in high levels of this heparin-neutralizing protein locally and so interfere with the anticoagulant effect of heparin.[129,130]

ACTIVATED PROTEIN C (APC)

Thrombin activates the natural antithrombotic zymogen protein C by cleaving the amino-terminal dodecapeptide when bound to thrombomodulin on the vascular endothelial membrane surface.[337] APC inhibits coagulation and prolongs the APTT by inactivating activated factors V and VIII (factor Va and factor VIIIa) on endothelial and platelet surfaces. By so doing, APC inhibits thrombin generation induced by thrombin and factor Xa.

Natural and recombinant forms of APC have been developed and studied in vitro and in experimental models of thrombosis and hemostasis.[338–341] APC inhibits platelet deposition in baboon models of acute arterial thrombosis,[338,341,342] prevents experimental venous thrombosis, and interrupts rethrombosis after experimental thrombolysis.[339,340] When combined with urokinase in an experimental model using a Dacron vascular graft in baboons,[342] APC had additive effects in preventing the accumulation of fibrin and platelets onto the graft.

In contrast to the findings with antiplatelet agents and the direct antithrombins, the administration of APC in effective antithrombotic doses is not associated with any detectable prolongation of bleeding times.[338,341] A soluble thrombomodulin also has been developed as a potential means for generating APC endogenously.[343] In addition, the possibility of engineering thrombin to promote selective endogenous activation of protein C is being evaluated.[344]

TISSUE FACTOR PATHWAY INHIBITOR

Exposure of blood to tissue factor contained in the depths of the lipid-rich atherosclerotic plaque is thought to be an important mechanism for reocclusion following successful thrombolysis.[269,345–347] Tissue pathway inhibitor (TPI, formerly known as lipoprotein-associated coagulation inhibitor, or LACI)[348,349] forms a complex with activated factor X which binds to and inhibits tissue factor–activated factor VII complex and so inhibits thrombin generation. TPI has been cloned, and limited studies with recombinant TPI have been performed in a canine femoral artery model. Thrombosis was induced by two methods, and recanalization was produced by t-PA infusion. TPI infusion prevented reocclusion following t-PA in the arteries subjected to intimal injury.[269] These findings support a role in reocclusion for tissue factor exposure after successful thrombolysis and suggest a new approach for adjuvant antithrombotic therapy.

REFERENCES

1. Rosenberg RD, Bauer, KA. The heparin-antithrombin system: a natural anticoagulant mechanism. In: Colman RW, Hirsh J, Marder VJ, Salzman EW, eds. Hemostasis and thrombosis: basic principles and clinical practice. 3rd ed. Philadelphia: JB Lippincott, 1994.
2. Ofosu FA, Hirsh J, Esmon CT, et al. Unfractionated heparin inhibits thrombin-catalyzed amplification reactions of coagulation more efficiently than those catalyzed by factor Xa. Biochem J 1989;257:143.
3. Beguin S, Lindbout T, Hemker HC. The mode of action of heparin in plasma. Thromb Haemost 1988;60:457.
4. Ofosu FA, Sie P, Modi GJ, et al. The inhibition of thrombin-dependent positive-feedback reactions is critical to the expression of the anticoagulant effect of heparin. Biochem J 1987;243:579.
5. Lindahl U, Hook M. Glycosaminoglycans and their binding to biological macromolecules. Annu Rev Biochem 1978;47:385.
6. Young E, Cosmi B, Weitz JI, Hirsh J. Comparison of nonspecific binding of unfractionated heparin and low molecular weight heparin to plasma proteins. Blood Thromb Haemost 1993;70:625.
7. Hirsh J, van Aken WG, Gallus AS, et al. Heparin kinetics in venous thrombosis and pulmonary embolism. Circulation 1976;53:691.
8. deSwart CAM, Nijmeyer B, Roelofs JMM, Sixma JJ. Kinetics of intravenously administered heparin in normal humans. Blood 1982;60:1251.
9. Glimelius B, Busch C, Hook M. Binding of heparin on the surface of cultured human endothelial cells. Thromb Res 1978;12:773.

10. Mahadoo J, Hiebert L, Jaques LB. Vascular seques-
    tration of heparin. Thromb Res 1977;12:79.
11. Dawes J, Smith RC, Pepper DS. The release, distri-
    bution and clearance of human β-thromboglobu-
    lin and platelet factor 4. Thromb Res 1978;12:851.
12. Olsson P, Lagergren H, Ek S. The elimination from
    plasma of intravenous heparin: an experimental
    study on dogs and humans. Acta Med Scand
    1963;173:619.
13. Marciniak E. Factor X_a inactivation by antithrom-
    bin III: evidence for biological stabilization of fac-
    tor X_a by factor V–phospholipid complex. Br J
    Haematol 1973;24:391.
14. Walker FJ, Esmon CT. The effects of phospholipid
    and factor V_a on the inhibition of factor X_a by
    antithrombin III. Biochem Biophys Res Commun
    1979;90:641.
15. Johnson EA, Mulloy B. The molecular-weight
    range of commercial heparin preparations. Carb
    Res 1979;51:119.
16. Hogg PJ, Jackson CM. Fibrin monomer protects
    thrombin from inactivation by heparin–anti-
    thrombin III: implications for heparin efficacy.
    Proc Natl Acad Sci USA 1989;86:3619.
17. Weitz JI, Hudoba M, Massel D, et al. Clot-bound
    thrombin is protected from inhibition by hep-
    arin–antithrombin III but is susceptible to inacti-
    vation by antithrombin III–independent inhib-
    itors. J Clin Invest 1990;86:385.
18. Bar-Shavit R, Eldor A, Vlodavsky I. Binding of
    thrombin to subendothelial extracellular matrix:
    protection and expression of functional proper-
    ties. J Clin Invest 1989;84:1096.
19. Heras M, Chesebro JH, Penny WJ, et al. Effects of
    thrombin inhibition on the development of acute
    platelet-thrombus deposition during angioplasty
    in pigs: heparin versus recombinant hirudin, a
    specific thrombin inhibitor. Circulation 1989;79:
    657.
20. Agnelli G, Pascucci C, Cosmi B, Nenci GG. The
    comparative effects of recombinant hirudin (CGP
    39393) and standard heparin on thrombus growth
    in rabbits. Thromb Haemost 1990;63:204.
21. Hull RD, Delmore T, Genton E, et al. Warfarin
    sodium versus low-dose heparin in the long-term
    treatment of venous thrombosis. N Engl J Med
    1979;301:855.
22. Lagerstedt CJ, Olsson CG, Fagher BO, et al. Need
    for long-term anticoagulant treatment in sympto-
    matic calf-vein thrombosis. Lancet 1985;2:515.
23. Burch JW, Stanford PW. Inhibition of platelet
    prostaglandin synthetase by oral aspirin. J Clin In-
    vest 1979;61:314.
24. Majerus PW. Arachidonate metabolism in vascu-
    lar disorders. J Clin Invest 1983;72:1521.
25. Roth GJ, Majerus PW. The mechanism of the
    effect of aspirin on human platelets: I. Acetylation

of a particulate fraction protein. J Clin Invest
    1975;56:624.
26. Moncada S, Vane JR. Pharmacology and endoge-
    nous roles of prostaglandin endoperoxides,
    thromboxane-A_2 and prostacyclin. Pharmacol Rev
    1978;30:293.
27. Moncada S, Vane JR. The role of prostacyclin in
    vascular tissue. Fed Proc 1979;38:66.
28. Weksler BB, Pett SB, Alonso D, et al. Differential
    inhibition by aspirin of vascular and platelet
    prostaglandin synthesis in atherosclerotic pa-
    tients. N Engl J Med 1983;308:800.
29. Patignani P, Filabozzi P, Patrono C. Selective cu-
    mulative inhibition of platelet thromboxane pro-
    duction by low-dose aspirin in healthy subjects.
    J Clin Invest 1982;69:1366.
30. FitzGerald GA, Oates JA, Hawiger J, et al. Endoge-
    nous biosynthesis of prostacyclin and thrombox-
    ane and platelet function during chronic adminis-
    tration of aspirin in man. J Clin Invest 1983;
    71:678.
31. Preston FE, Whipps S, Jackson CA, et al. Inhibi-
    tion of prostacyclin and platelet thromboxane A_2
    after low-dose aspirin. N Engl J Med 1981;304:76.
32. Kyrle PA, Eichler HG, Jager U, Lechner K. Inhibi-
    tion of prostaglandin and thromboxane A_2 genera-
    tion by low-dose aspirin at the site of plug forma-
    tion in man in vivo. Circulation 1987;75:1025.
33. Moncada S, Vane JR. Mode of action of aspirin-like
    drugs. In: Stollerman GH, ed. Cardiovascular
    drugs. Vol. 24. New York: Adis Press, 1982:1.
34. Demers LM, Budin R, Shaikh B. The effects of as-
    pirin on megakaryocyte prostaglandin produc-
    tion. Blood 1977;50(suppl 1):239.
35. Burch JW, Baenziger NL, Stanford N, et al. Sensi-
    tivity of fatty acid cyclooxygenase from human
    aorta to acetylation by aspirin. Proc Natl Acad Sci
    USA 1978;75:5181.
36. Burch JW, Majerus PW. The role of prostaglandins
    in platelet function. Semin Hematol 1979;16:196.
37. Cerskus AL, Ali M, Davies BJ, et al. Possible signif-
    icance of small numbers of functional platelets in a
    population of aspirin-treated platelets in vitro and
    in vivo. Thromb Res 1980;18:389.
38. O'Brien JR. Effects of salicylates on human
    platelets. Lancet 1968;1:779.
39. UK-TIA Study Group. The UK-TIA Aspirin Trial:
    interim results. Br Med J 1988;296:316.
40. Levy M. Aspirin use in patients with major upper
    gastrointestinal bleeding and peptic ulcer disease.
    N Engl J Med 1974;290:1158.
41. Prichard PJ, Kitchingman GK, Walt RP, et al.
    Human gastric mucosal bleeding induced by low
    dose aspirin, but not warfarin. Br Med J 1989;
    298:493.
42. Hawkey CJ, Somerville KW, Marshall S. Prophy-
    laxis of aspirin induced gastric mucosal bleeding

with ranitidine. Alimentary Pharmacol Ther 1988;2:245.

43. Prichard PJ, Kitchingman GK, Hawkey CJ. Gastric mucosal bleeding: what dose of aspirin is safe? Gut 1987;28:A1401.

44. Pierson RN, Holt PR, Watson RM, Keating RP. Aspirin and gastrointestinal bleeding: chromate-51 blood loss studies. Am J Med 1961;31:259.

45. Leonards JR, Levy G. Effect of pharmaceutical formulation on gastrointestinal bleeding from aspirin tablets. Arch Intern Med 1972;129:457.

46. Graham DY, Smith JL. Aspirin and the stomach. Ann Intern Med 1986;104:390.

47. ISIS-2 Collaborative Group. Randomised trial of intravenous streptokinase, oral aspirin, both or neither among 17,187 cases of suspected acute myocardial infarction: ISIS-2. Lancet 1988;318:349.

48. Cairns JA, Gent M, Singer J, et al. Aspirin, sulfinpyrazone, or both in unstable angina. N Engl J Med 1985;313:1369.

49. Persantine-Aspirin Reinfarction Study Research Group. Persantine and aspirin in coronary heart disease. Circulation 1980;62:449.

50. Coronary Drug Project Group. Aspirin in coronary heart disease. J Chron Dis 1976;29:625.

51. Breddin K, Loew D, Lechner K, et al. Secondary prevention of myocardial infarction: comparison of acetylsalicylic acid, phenprocoumon and placebo: a multicenter two-year prospective study. Thromb Haemost 1979;40:225.

52. Aspirin Myocardial Infarction Study Research Group. A randomized, controlled trial of aspirin in persons recovered from myocardial infarction. JAMA 1980;243:661.

53. Lewis HD, Davis JW, Archibald DG, et al. Protective effects of aspirin against acute myocardial infarction and death in men with unstable angina: results of a Veterans Administration cooperative study. N Engl J Med 1983;309:396.

54. Ali M, Zamecnik J, Cerskus AL, et al. Synthesis of thromboxane-B_2 and prostaglandins by bovine gastric mucosal microsomes. Prostaglandins 1977;14:819.

55. MacKercher PA, Ivey KJ, Baskin WN, et al. Protective effect of cimetidine on aspirin-induced gastric mucosal damage. Ann Intern Med 1977;87:676.

56. Bowen BK, Kraus WJ, Ivey KJ. Effect of sodium bicarbonate on aspirin-induced damage and potential difference changes in human gastric mucosa. Br Med J 1977;2:1052.

57. Mielants H, Veys EM, Verbruggen G, et al. Salicylate-induced gastrointestinal bleeding: comparison between soluble buffered, enteric-coated, and intravenous administration. J Rheumatol 1979;6:210.

58. Croft DN, Wood PHN. Gastric mucosa and susceptibility to occult gastrointestinal bleeding. Br Med J 1967;1:137.

59. Hennekens CH, Peto R, Hutchison GB, Doll R. An overview of the British and American aspirin studies. N Engl J Med 1988;318:923.

60. Manson JE, Stampfer MJ, Colditz GA, et al. A prospective study of aspirin use and primary prevention of cardiovascular disease in women. JAMA 1991;266:521.

61. Ridker PM, Manson JE, Gaziano M, et al. Low-dose aspirin therapy for chronic stable angina: a randomized, placebo-controlled clinical trial. Ann Intern Med 1991;114:835.

62. The RISC Group. Risk of myocardial infarction and death during treatment with low dose aspirin and intravenous heparin in men with unstable coronary artery disease. Lancet 1990;336:827.

63. Antiplatelet Trialists' Collaboration. Secondary prevention of vascular disease by prolonged antiplatelet treatment. Br Med J 1988;296:320.

64. The Dutch TIA Trial Study Group. The effects of 30 mg versus 300 mg acetylsalicylic acid, and of 50 mg atenolol versus placebo on mortality, stroke and myocardial infarction after TIA or minor ischemic stroke. N Engl J Med 1991;325:1261.

65. Whitlon DS, Sadowski JA, Suttie JW. Mechanisms of coumarin action: significance of vitamin K epoxide reductase inhibition. Biochemistry 1978;17:1371.

66. Fasco MJ, Hildebrandt EF, Suttie JW. Evidence that warfarin anticoagulant action involves two distinct reductase activities. J Biol Chem 1982;257:11210.

67. Choonara IA, Malia RG, Haynes BP, et al. The relationship between inhibition of vitamin K 1,2,3-epoxide reductase and reduction of clotting factor activity with warfarin. Br J Clin Pharmacol 1988;25:1.

68. Trivedi LS, Rhee M, Galivan JH, Fasco MJ. Normal and warfarin-resistant rat hepatocyte metabolism of vitamin K 2,3-epoxide: evidence for multiple pathways of hydroxyvitamin K formation. Arch Biochem Biophys 1988;264:67.

69. Stenflo J, Fernlund P, Egan W, Roepstorff P. Vitamin K–dependent modifications of glutamic acid residues in prothrombin. Proc Natl Acad Sci USA 1974;71:2730.

70. Nelsestuen GL, Zytkovicz TH, Howard JB. The mode of action of vitamin K: identification of γ-carboxyglutamic acid as a component of prothrombin. J Biol Chem 1974;249:6347.

71. Nelsestuen GL. Role of gamma-carboxyglutamic acid: an unusual transition required for calcium-dependent binding of prothrombin to phospholipid. J Biol Chem 1976;251:5648.

72. Prendergast FG, Mann KG. Differentiation of metal ion–induced transitions of prothrombin fragment 1. J Biol Chem 1977;252:840.

73. Borowski M, Furie BC, Bauminger S, Furie B. Prothrombin requires two sequential metal-dependent conformational transitions to bind phospholipid. J Biol Chem 1986;261:14969.

74. Friedman PA, Rosenberg RD, Hauschka PV, Fitz-James A. A spectrum of partially carboxylated prothrombins in the plasmas of coumarin treated patients. Biochim Biophys Acta 1977; 494:271.

75. Malhotra OP, Nesheim ME, Mann KG. The kinetics of activation of normal and gamma carboxy glutamic acid deficient prothrombins. J Biol Chem 1985;260:279.

76. Breckenridge AM. Oral anticoagulant drugs: pharmacokinetic aspects. Semin Hematol 1978;15:19.

77. O'Reilly RA. Vitamin K and other oral anticoagulant drugs. Annu Rev Med 1976;27:245.

78. Kelly JG, O'Malley K. Clinical pharmacokinetics of oral anticoagulants. Clin Pharmacokinet 1979; 4:1.

79. O'Reilly RA. Warfarin metabolism and drug-drug interactions. In: Wessler S, Becker CG, Nemerson Y, eds. The new dimensions of warfarin prophylaxis: advances in experimental medicine and biology. Vol. 214. New York: Plenum Press, 1986: 205.

80. Sutcliff FA, MacNicholl AD, Gibson GG. Aspects of anticoagulant action: a review of the pharmacology, metabolism and toxicology of warfarin and congeners. Q Rev Drugs Met Drug Interact 1987;5:225.

81. O'Reilly RA, Aggeler PM. Determinants of the response to oral anticoagulant drug in man. Pharmacol Rev 1970;22:35.

82. O'Reilly RA. Lack of effect of fortified wine ingested during fasting and anticoagulant therapy. Arch Intern Med 1981;141:458.

83. O'Reilly RA, Aggeler PM, Hoag MS, et al. Hereditary transmission of exceptional resistance to coumarin anticoagulant drugs. N Engl J Med 1983;308:1229.

84. Alving BM, Strickler MP, Knight RD, et al. Hereditary warfarin resistance. Arch Intern Med 1985;145:499.

85. O'Reilly R, Rytand D. Resistance to warfarin due to unrecognized vitamin K supplementation. N Engl J Med 1980;303:160.

86. Suttie JW, Muhah-Schendel LL, Shah DV, et al. Vitamin K deficiency from dietary vitamin K restriction in humans. Am J Clin Nutr 1988;47:475.

87. Lader E, Young L, Clarke A. Warfarin dosage and vitamin K in osmolite. Ann Intern Med 1980; 93:373.

88. Bell RG. Metabolism of vitamin K and prothrombin synthesis: anticoagulants and the vitamin K–epoxide cycle. Fed Proc 1978;37:2599.

89. Richards RK. Influence of fever upon the action of 3,3-methylene bis-(4-hydroxoycoumarin). Science 1943;97:313.

90. Owens JC, Neely WB, Owen WR. Effect of sodium dextrothyroxine in patients receiving anticoagulants. N Engl J Med 1962;266:76.

91. Loeliger EA, van der Esch B, Mattern MJ, et al. Biological disappearance rate of prothrombin, factors VII, IX and X. Thromb Diath Haemorrh 1964;10:266.

92. Schulman S, Henriksson K. Interaction of ibuprofen and warfarin on primary haemostasis. Br J Rheumatol 1989;38:46.

93. Casenave J-P, Packham MA, Guccione MA, et al. Effects of penicillin G on platelet aggregation, release and adherence to collagen. Proc Soc Exp Med 1973;142:159.

94. Brown CH, Natelson EA, Bradshaw MW, et al. The hemostatic defect produced by carbenicillin. N Engl J Med 1974;291:265.

95. Weitkamp M, Aber R. Prolonged bleeding times and bleeding diathesis associated with moxalactam administration. JAMA 1983;249:69.

96. Udall JA. Human sources and absorption of vitamin K in relation to anticoagulation. JAMA 1965;194:127.

97. Koch-Weser J, Sellers DM. Drug interactions with oral anticoagulants. N Engl J Med 1971;285:487.

98. Hirsh J, Dalen JE, Deykin D, Poller L. Oral anticoagulants; mechanisms of action, clinical effectiveness, and optimal therapeutic range. Chest 1992; 102(4):312S.

99. Andriuoli G, Mastacchi R, Barnti M, et al. Comparison of the antithrombotic and hemorrhagic effects of heparin and a new low molecular weight heparin in the rat. Haemostasis 1985;15:324.

100. Bergqvist D, Nilsson B, Hedner U, et al. The effects of heparin fragments of different molecular weight in experimental thrombosis and haemostasis. Thromb Res 1985;38:589.

101. Cade JF, Buchanan MR, Boneu B, et al. A comparison of the antithrombotic and haemorrhagic effects of low molecular weight heparin fractions: the influence of the method of preparation. Thromb Res 1984;35:613.

102. Carter CJ, Kelton JG, Hirsh J, et al. The relationship between the hemorrhagic and antithrombotic properties of low molecular weight heparins and heparin. Blood 1982;59:1239.

103. Esquivel CO, Bergqvist D, Bjork C-G, et al. Comparison between commercial heparin, low-molecular-weight heparin and pentosan polysulphate on haemostasis and platelets in vivo. Thromb Res 1982;28:389.

104. Holmer E, Matsson C, Nilsson S. Anticoagulant and antithrombotic effects of low-molecular-weight heparin fragments in rabbits. Thromb Res 1982;25:475.

105. Ofosu FA, Barrowcliffe TW. Mechanisms of action of low molecular weight heparins and heparinoids. In: Hirsh J, ed. Antithrombotic therapy, Bailliere's clinical haematology. Vol 3. London: Bailliere Tindall, 1990:505.

106. Andersson L-O, Barrowcliffe TW, Holmer E, et al. Molecular weight dependency of the heparin potentiated inhibition of thrombin and activated factor X: effect of heparin neutralization in plasma. Thromb Res 1979;115:531.

107. Harenberg J. Pharmacology of low molecular weight heparins. Semin Thromb Hemost 1990; 16:12.

108. Bjork I, Lindahl U. Mechanism of the anticoagulant action of heparin. Mol Cell Biochem 1982;48:161.

109. Rosenberg RD, Damus PS. The purification and mechanism of action of human antithrombin-heparin cofactor. J Biol Chem 1973;248:6490.

110. Rosenberg RD, Jordan RE, Favreau LV, et al. Highly active heparin species with multiple binding sites for antithrombin. Biochem Biophys Res Commun 1979;86:1319.

111. Thunberg L, Backstrom G, Lindahl U. Further characterization of antithrombin-binding sequence in heparin. Carbohydrate Res 1982;100: 393.

112. Casu B, Oreste P, Torri G, et al. The structure of heparin oligosaccharide fragments with high anti-(factor Xa) activity containing the minimal antithrombin III–binding sequence. Biochem J 1981;197:599.

113. Choay J, Lormeau JC, Petitou M, et al. Structural studies on a biologically active hexasaccharide obtained from heparin. Ann NY Acad Sci 1981;370: 644.

114. Choay J, Petitou M, Lormeau JC, et al. Structure-activity relationship in heparin: a synthetic pentasaccharide with high affinity for antithrombin III and eliciting high anti-factor Xa activity. Biochem Biophys Res Commun 1983;116:492.

115. Hook M, Bjork I, Hopwood J, et al. Anticoagulant activity of heparin: separation of high-activity and low-activity heparin species by affinity chromatography on immobilized antithrombin. FEBS Lett 1976;66:90.

116. Lindahl U, Backstrom G, Hook M, et al. Structure of the antithrombin-binding site of heparin. Proc Natl Acad Sci USA 1979;76:3198.

117. Lindahl U, Thunberg L, Backstrom G, et al. Extension and structural variability of the antithrombin-binding sequence in heparin. J Biol Chem 1984; 259:12368.

118. Petitou M. Synthetic heparin fragments: new and efficient tools for the study of heparin and its interactions. Nouv Rev Fr Hematol 1984;26:221.

119. Rosenberg RD. Actions and interactions of antithrombin and heparin. N Engl J Med 1975; 292(3):146.

120. Rosenberg RD, Lam L. Correlation between structure and function of heparin. Proc Natl Acad Sci USA 1979;76:1218.

121. Nordenman B, Bjork I. Binding of low-affinity and high-affinity heparin to antithrombin: ultraviolet difference spectroscopy and circular dichroism studies. Biochemistry 1978;17:3339.

122. Olson ST, Srinivasan KR, Bjork I, et al. Binding of high affinity heparin to antithrombin III: stopped flow kinetic studies of the binding interaction. J Biol Chem 1981;256:11073.

123. Villanueva GB, Danishefsky I. Evidence for a heparin-induced conformational change on antithrombin III. Biochem Biophys Res Commun 1977;74:803.

124. Danielsson A, Raub E, Lindahl U, et al. Role of ternary complexes in which heparin binds both antithrombin and proteinase, in the acceleration of the reactions between antithrombin and thrombin or factor Xa. J Biol Chem 1986;261:15467.

125. Olson ST, Shore JD. Demonstration of a two-step reaction mechanism for inhibition of α-thrombin by antithrombin III and identification of the step affected by heparin. J Biol Chem 1982;257: 14891.

126. Holmer E, Kurachi K, Soderstrom G. The molecular-weight dependence of the rate-enhancing effect of heparin on the inhibition of thrombin, factor Xa, factor IXa, factor XIa, factor XIIa and kallikrein by antithrombin. Biochem J 1981;193: 395.

127. Holmer E, Soderberg K, Bergqvist D, et al. Heparin and its low molecular weight derivatives: anticoagulant and antithrombotic properties. Haemostasis 1986;16(suppl 2):1.

128. Jordan RE, Oosta GM, Gardner WT, et al. The kinetics of hemostatic enzyme-antithrombin interactions in the presence of low molecular weight heparin. J Biol Chem 1980;255:10081.

129. Rosenberg RD, Rosenberg JS. Natural anticoagulant mechanisms. J Clin Invest 1984;74:1.

130. Lane DA. Heparin binding and neutralizing protein. In: Lane DA, Lindahl U, eds. Heparin, chemical and biological properties, clinical applications. London: Edward Arnold, 1989:363.

131. Lane DA, Pejler G, Flynn AM, et al. Neutralization of heparin-related saccharides by histidine-rich glycoprotein and platelet factor 4. J Biol Chem 1986;261:3980.

132. Lijnen HR, Hoylaerts M, Collen D. Heparin binding properties of human histidine-rich glycopro-

tein: mechanism and role in the neutralization of heparin in plasma. J Biol Chem 1983;258:3803.

133. Peterson CB, Morgan WT, Blackburn MN. Histidine-rich glycoprotein modulation of the anticoagulant activity of heparin. J Biol Chem 1987; 262:7567.

134. Preissner KT, Muller-Berghaus G. Neutralization and binding of heparin by S-protein/vitronectin in the inhibition of factor Xa by antithrombin III. J Biol Chem 1987;262:12247.

135. Dawes J, Pavuk N. Sequestration of therapeutic glycosaminoglycans by plasma fibrinonectin (abstract). Thromb Haemost 1991;65:829.

136. Sobel M, McNeill PM, Carlson PL, et al. Heparin inhibition of von Willebrand factor–dependent platelet function in vitro and in vivo. J Clin Invest 1991;87:1787.

137. Handeland GF, Abidgaard GF, Holm U, et al. Dose-adjusted heparin treatment of deep venous thrombosis: a comparison of unfractionated and low molecular weight heparin. Eur J Clin Pharmacol 1990;39:107.

138. Barzu T, Molho P, Tobelem G, et al. Binding and endocytosis of heparin by human endothelial cells in culture. Biochem Biophys Acta 1985;845: 196.

139. Barzu T, Molho P, Tobelem G, et al. Binding of heparin and low molecular weight heparin fragments to human vascular endothelial cell sin culture. Nouv Rev Fr Haematol 1984;26:243.

140. Barzu T, Van Rijn JLMC, Petitou M, et al. Heparin degradation in the endothelial cells. Thromb Res 1987;47:601.

141. Bara L, Billaud E, Gramond G, et al. Comparative pharmacokinetics of low molecular weight heparin (PK 10169) and unfractionated heparin after intravenous and subcutaneous administration. Thromb Res 1985;39:631.

142. Bara L, Samama MM. Pharmacokinetics of low molecular weight heparins. Acta Chir Scand 1988;543:65.

143. Boneu B, Caranobe C, Cadroy Y, et al. Pharmacokinetic studies of standard unfractionated heparin, and low molecular weight heparins in the rabbit. Semin Thromb Hemost 1988;14:18.

144. Bradbrook ID, Magnani HN, Moelker HC, et al. ORG 10172: a low molecular weight heparinoid anticoagulant with a long half life in man. Br J Clin Pharmacol 1987;23:667.

145. Bratt G, Tornebohm E, Widlund L, et al. Low molecular weight heparin (KABI 2165, FRAGMIN): pharmacokinetics after intravenous and subcutaneous administration in human volunteers. Thromb Res 1986;42:613.

146. Briant L, Caranobe C, Saivin S, et al. Unfractionated heparin and CY216: pharmacokinetics and bioavailabilities of the anti-factor Xa and IIa. Effects of intravenous and subcutaneous injection in rabbits. Thromb Haemost 1989;61:348.

147. Choay J, Petitou M. The chemistry of heparin: a way to understand its mode of action. Med J Aus 1986;144(HS):7.

148. Frydman A, Bara L, Leroux Y, et al. The antithrombotic activity and pharmacokinetics of Enoxaparin, a low molecular weight heparin, in man given single subcutaneous doses of 20 up to 80 mg. J Clin Pharmacol 1988;28:608.

149. Matzsch T, Bergqvist D, Hedner U, et al. Effect of an enzymatically depolymerized heparin as compared with conventional heparin in healthy volunteers. Thromb Haemost 1987;57:97.

150. Stiekema JC, Wijnand HP, Van Dinther TG, et al. Safety and pharmacokinetics of the low molecular weight heparinoid ORG 10172 administered to healthy elderly volunteers. Br J Clin Pharmacol 1989;27:39.

151. Caranobe C, Barret A, Gabaig AM, et al. Disappearance of circulating anti-Xa activity after intravenous injection of standard heparin and of low molecular weight heparin (CY216) in normal and nephrectomized rabbits. Thromb Res 1985;40: 129.

152. Palm M, Mattsson CH. Pharmacokinetics of heparin and low molecular weight heparin fragment (Fragmin) in rabbits with impaired renal or metabolic clearance. Thromb Haemost 1987;58:932.

153. Ockelford PA, Carter CJ, Mitchell L, et al. Discordance between the anti-Xa activity and antithrombotic activity of an ultra-low molecular weight heparin fraction. Thromb Res 1982;28:401.

154. Boneu B, Buchanan MR, Cade JF, et al. Effects of heparin, its low molecular weight fractions and other glycosaminoglycans on thrombus growth in vivo. Thromb Res 1985;40:81.

155. Henny CP, ten Cate H, ten Cate JW, et al. A randomized, blind study comparing standard heparin and a new low molecular weight heparinoid in cardiopulmonary bypass surgery in dogs. J Lab Clin Med 1985;106:187.

156. Hobbelen PM, Vogel GM, Meuleman DG. Time courses of the antithrombotic effects, bleeding enhancing effects and interactions with factors Xa and thrombin after administration of low molecular weight heparinoid ORG 10172 or heparin to rats. Thromb Res 1987;48:549.

157. Van Ryn-McKenna J, Gray E, Weber E, et al. Effects of sulphated polysaccharides on inhibition of thrombus formation initiated by different stimuli. Thromb Haemost 1989;61:7.

158. Van Ryn-McKenna J, Ofosu FA, Hirsh J, et al. Antithrombotic and bleeding effects of glycosaminoglycans with different degrees of sulfation. Br J Haematol 1989;71:265.

159. Fabris F, Fussi F, Casonato A, et al. Normal and

low molecular weight heparins: interaction with human platelets. Eur J Clin Invest 1983;13:135.

160. Fernandez F, Nguyen P, Van Ryn J, et al. Hemorrhagic doses of heparin and other glycosaminoglycans induce a platelet defect. Thromb Res 1986; 43:491.

161. Blajchman MA, Young E, Ofosu FA. Effects of unfractionated heparin, dermatan sulfate and low molecular weight on vessel wall permeability in rabbits. Ann NY Acad Sci 1989;556:245.

162. Levine MN, Hirsh J, Gent M, et al. Prevention of deep vein thrombosis after elective hip surgery: a randomized trial comparing low molecular weight heparin with standard unfractionated heparin. Ann Intern Med 1991;114:545.

163. Hull RD, Raskob GE, Pineo GF, et al. A randomized double-blind trial of low molecular weight heparin in the initial treatment of proximal vein thrombosis (abstract). Thromb Haemost 1991;65 (suppl):872.

164. Prandoni P. Fixed-dose LMW heparin (CY216) as compared with adjusted dose intravenous heparin in the initial treatment of symptomatic proximal venous thrombosis (abstract). Thromb Haemost 1991;65(suppl):872.

165. Ockelford PA, Patterson J, Johns AS. A double-blind randomized placebo-controlled trial of thromboprophylaxis in major elective general surgery using once daily injections of a low molecular weight heparin fragment. Thromb Haemost 1989;62:1046.

166. Pezzuoli G, Serneri GGN, Settembrini P, et al and the STEP Study Group. Prophylaxis of fatal pulmonary embolism in general surgery using low molecular weight heparin CY216: a multicentre double-blind randomized controlled clinical trial versus placebo. Int Surg 1989;74:205.

167. European Fraxiparin Study Group. Comparison of a low molecular weight heparin and unfractionated heparin for the prevention of deep vein thrombosis in patients undergoing abdominal surgery. Br J Surg 1988;75:1058.

168. Kakkar VV, Murray WJG. Efficacy and safety of low molecular weight heparin (CY216) in preventing postoperative venous thromboembolism. Br J Surg 1985;72:786.

169. Bergqvist D, Matzsch T, Burmark US, et al. Low molecular weight heparin given the evening before surgery compared with conventional low dose heparin in prevention of thrombosis. Br J Surg 1988;75:888.

170. Caen JP. A randomised double-blind study between a low molecular weight heparin Kabi 2165 and standard heparin in the prevention of deep vein thrombosis in general surgery. Thromb Haemost 1988;59:216.

171. Hartle P, Brucke P, Dienstl E, et al. Prophylaxis of thromboembolism in general surgery: comparison

between standard heparin and fragmin. Thromb Res 1990;57:577.

172. Fricker JP, Vergnes Y, Schach R, et al. Low dose heparin versus low molecular weight heparin Kabi 2165 in the prophylaxis of thromboembolic complications of abdominal oncological surgery. Eur J Clin Invest 1988;18:561.

173. Leizorovicz A, Picolet H, Peyrieux JC, et al. Prevention of perioperative deep vein thrombosis in general surgery: a multicentre double-blind study comparing two doses of logiparin and standard heparin. Br J Surg 1991;78:412.

174. Samama M, Bernard P, Bonnardot JP, et al. Low molecular weight heparin compared with unfractionated heparin in prevention of postoperative thrombosis. Br J Surg 1988;75:128.

175. Cruickshank MK, Levine MN, Hirsh J, et al. An evaluation of impedance plethysmography and I-125 fibrinogen leg scanning in patients following hip surgery. Thromb Haemost 1989;62:830.

176. Leclerc JR, Geerts WH, Desjardins L, et al. Prevention of deep vein thrombosis after major knee surgery—a randomized, double-blind trial comparing a low molecular weight heparin fragment (enoxaparin) to placebo. Thromb Haemost 1992; 67:417.

177. Turpie AGG, Levine MN, Hirsh J, et al. A randomized controlled trial of a low molecular weight heparin (enoxaparin) to prevent deep vein thrombosis in patients undergoing elective hip surgery. N Engl J Med 1986;315:925.

178. Hoek J, Nurmohamed MT, ten Cate H, et al. Prevention of deep vein thrombosis following total hip replacement by a low molecular weight heparinoid. Thromb Haemost 1992;67:28.

179. Planes A, Vochelle N, Mazas F, et al. Prevention of postoperative venous thrombosis: a randomized trial comparing unfractionated heparin with low molecular weight heparin in patients undergoing total hip replacement. Thromb Haemost 1988; 60:407.

180. Eriksson BI, Kalebo P, Anthmyr BA, et al. Prevention of deep vein thrombosis and pulmonary embolism after total hip replacement. J Bone Joint Surg 1991;73A:484.

181. Estoppey D, Hochreiter J, Breyer HG, et al. ORG 10172 (Lomoparin) versus heparin-DHE in prevention of thromboembolism in total hip replacement—a multicentre trial (abstract). Thromb Haemost 1989;62(Suppl):356.

182. Dechavanne M, Ville D, Berruyer M, et al. Randomized trial of low molecular weight heparin (Kabi 2165) versus adjusted dose subcutaneous standard heparin in the prophylaxis of deep vein thrombosis after elective hip surgery. Haemostasis 1989;1:5.

183. Leyvraz PF, Bachmann F, Hoek J, et al. Prevention

of deep vein thrombosis after hip replacement: randomized comparison between unfractionated heparin and low molecular weight heparin. Br Med J 1991;303:543.

184. Bergqvist D, Kettunen K, Fredin H, et al. Thromboprophylaxis in hip fracture patients—a prospective randomised comparative study between ORG 10172 and dextran. Surgery 1991;109:617.

185. Borris LC, Hauch O, Jorgensen LN, et al for The Danish Enoxaparin Study Group. Low-molecular-weight heparin (enoxaparin) vs dextran 70: the prevention of postoperative deep vein thrombosis after total hip replacement. Arch Intern Med 1991;151:1621.

186. Heit J, Kessler C, Mammen E, et al for the RD Heparin Study Group. Efficacy and safety of RD heparin (a LMWH) versus warfarin for prevention of deep-vein thrombosis after hip or knee replacement (abstract). Blood 1991;739:187A.

187. Prins MH, den Ottolander GJH, Gelsema R, et al. Deep vein thrombosis prophylaxis with a low molecular weight heparin (Kabi 2165) in stroke patients (abstract). Thromb Haemost 1987;58 (suppl):117.

188. Turpie AGG, Levine MN, Hirsh J, et al. A double-blind randomized trial of ORG 10172 low molecular weight heparinoid in the prevention of deep vein thrombosis in thrombotic stroke. Lancet 1987;1:523.

189. Dahan R, Houlbert D, Caulin C, et al. Prevention of deep vein thrombosis in elderly medical patients by a low molecular weight heparin: a randomized double-blind trial. Haemostasis 1986;16:159.

190. Green D, Lee MY, Lim AC, et al. Prevention of thromboembolism after spinal cord injury using low molecular weight heparin. Ann Intern Med 1990;113:571.

191. Turpie AGG, Gent M, Cote R, et al. A low-molecular-weight heparinoid compared with unfractionated heparin in the prevention of deep vein thrombosis in patients with acute ischemic stroke: a randomized double-blind study. Ann Intern Med 1992;117:353.

192. Ofosu FA, Modi GJ, Smith LM, et al. Heparan sulfate and dermatan sulfate inhibit the generation of thrombin activity by complementary pathways. Blood 1984;64:741.

193. Hull RD, Raskob GE, Pineo GF et al. Subcutaneous low-molecular-weight heparin compared with continuous intravenous heparin in the treatment of proximal-vein thrombosis. N Engl J Med 1992;326:975.

194. Prandoni P, Lensing AWA, Buller HR, et al. Comparison of subcutaneous low molecular weight heparin with intravenous standard heparin in proximal deep vein thrombosis. Lancet 1992; 339:441.

195. Albada J, Nieuwenhuis HK, Sixma JJ. Treatment of acute venous thromboembolism with low molecular weight heparin. Circulation 1989;80:935.

196. Bratt G, Aberg W, Johansson M, et al. Two daily subcutaneous injections of fragmin as compared with intravenous standard heparin in the treatment of deep venous thrombosis. Thromb Haemost 1990;64:506.

197. Duroux P, Beclere A. A randomized trial of subcutaneous low molecular weight heparin (CY216) compared with intravenous unfractionated heparin in the treatment of deep vein thrombosis. Thromb Haemost 1991;65:251.

198. Simonneau G. Subcutaneous fixed dose of enoxaparin versus intravenous adjusted dose of unfractionated heparin in the treatment of deep venous thrombosis (abstract). Thromb Haemost 1991;65 (suppl):754.

199. de Bono DP, Simoons ML, Tijssen J, et al. Effect of early intravenous heparin on coronary patency, infarct size, and bleeding complications after alteplase thrombolysis: results of a randomised double blind European Cooperative Study Group Trial. Br Heart J 1992;67:122.

200. Hsia J, Hamilton WP, Kleiman N, et al and the Heparin-Aspirin Reperfusion Trial (HART) Investigators. A comparison between heparin and low-dose aspirin as adjunctive therapy with tissue plasminogen activator for acute myocardial infarction. N Engl J Med 1990;323:1433.

201. Hsia J, Kleiman N, Aguirre F, et al. Heparin-induced partial thromboplastin time after thrombolysis: prolongation magnitude determines coronary patency (abstract). Circulation 1991;84 (suppl II):II-116.

202. Golino P, Ashton JH, Glas-Greenwalt P, et al. Mediation of reocclusion by thromboxane A_2 and serotonin after thrombolysis with tissue-type plasminogen activator in a canine preparation of coronary thrombosis. Circulation 1988;77:678.

203. Golino P, Ashton JH, McNatt J, et al. Simultaneous administration of thromboxane A_2- and serotonin S_2-receptor antagonists markedly enhances thrombolysis and prevents or delays reocclusion after tissue-type plasminogen activator in a canine model of coronary thrombosis. Circulation 1989; 79:911.

204. ISIS-2 (Second International Study of Infarct Survival) Collaborative Group. Randomised trial of intravenous streptokinase, oral aspirin, both, or neither among 17,187 cases of suspected myocardial infarction: ISIS-2. Lancet 1988;2:349.

205. Saltiel E, Ward A. Ticlopidine: a review of its pharmacodynamic and pharmacokinetic properties and therapeutic efficacy in platelet dependent disease states. Drugs 1987;34:222.

206. Di Minno G, Cerbone AM, Mattioli PL, et al. Functionally thrombosthenic state in normal platelets

following the administration of ticlopidine. J Clin Invest 1985;75:328.

207. Gent M, Blakely JA, Easton JD, et al and the CATS Groups. The Canadian American Ticlopidine Study (CATS) in thromboembolic stroke. Lancet 1989;2:1215.

208. Hass WK, Easton JD, Adams HP, et al for the Ticlopidine Aspirin Stroke Study Group. A randomized trial comparing ticlopidine hydrochloride with aspirin for the prevention of stroke in high-risk patients. N Engl J Med 1989;321:501.

209. Balsano F, Rizzon P, Violi F, et al and the Studio della Ticlopidina nell'Angina Instabile Group. Antiplatelet treatment with ticlopidine in unstable angina: a controlled multicenter clinical trial. Circulation 1990;82:17.

210. Arcan JC, Blanchard J, Boissel JP, et al. Multicenter double-blind study of ticlopidine in the treatment intermittent claudication and the prevention of its complications. Angiology 1988;39:802.

211. Balsano F, Coccheri S, Libretti A, et al. Ticlopidine in the treatment of intermittent claudications: a 21-month double-blind trial. J Lab Clin Med 1989;114:84.

212. Janzon L, Bergqvist D, Boberg J, et al. Prevention of myocardial infarction and stroke in patients with intermittent claudication: effects of ticlopidine. Results from STIMS, the Swedish Ticlopidine Multicentre Study. J Intern Med 1990;227:301.

213. Limet R, David JL, Magotteaux P, et al. Prevention of aorta-coronary bypass graft occlusion: beneficial effect of ticlopidine on early and late patency rate of venous coronary bypass grafts: a double-blind study. J Thorac Cardiovasc Surg 1987;94:773.

214. Sakariassen KS, Fressinaud E, Girma J-P, et al. Role of platelet membrane glycoproteins and von Willebrand factor in adhesion of platelets to subendothelium and collagen. Ann NY Acad Sci 1987;516:52.

215. Phillips DR, Charo IF, Scarborough RM. GPIIb-IIIa: the responsive integrin. Cell 1991;65:359.

216. Hynes RO. Integrins: versatility, modulation, and signaling in cell adhesion. Cell 1992;69:11.

217. Kieffer N, Phillips DR. Platelet membrane glycoproteins: functions in cellular interactions. Annu Rev Cell Biol 1990;6:329.

218. Sixma JJ, Sakariassen KS, Beeser-Visser NH, et al. Adhesion of platelets to human artery subendothelium: effect of factor VIII–von Willebrand factor on various multimeric composition. Blood 1984;63:128.

219. Handa M, Titani K, Holland LZ, et al. The von Willebrand factor–binding domain of platelet membrane glycoprotein Ib. J Biol Chem 1986;261:12579.

220. Du X, Beutler L, Ruan C, Castaldi PA, Berndt MC. Glycoprotein Ib and glycoprotein IX are fully complexed in the intact platelet membrane. Blood 1987;5:1524.

221. Sakariassen KS, Nievelstein PFEM, Coller BS, Simma JJ. The role of platelet membrane glycoproteins Ib and IIb-IIIa in platelet adherence to human artery subendothelium. Br J Haematol 1986;63:681.

222. Fressinaud E, Baruch D, Girma J-P, et al. von Willebrand factor–mediated platelet adhesion to collagen involves platelet membrane glycoprotein IIb-IIIa as well as glycoprotein Ib. J Lab Clin Med 1988;112:58.

223. Moake JL, Turner NA, Stathopoulos NA, et al. Shear-induced platelet aggregation can be mediated by vWF released from platelets, as well as by exogenous large or unusually large vWF multimers, requires adenosine diphosphate, and is resistant to aspirin. Blood 1988;71:1366.

224. Weiss HJ, Hawiger J, Ruggeri ZM, et al. Fibrinogen-independent platelet adhesion and thrombus formation on subendothelium mediated by glycoprotein IIb-IIIa complex at high shear rate. J Clin Invest 1989;83:288.

225. Chow TW, Hellums JD, Moake JL, Kroll MH. Shear stress–induced von Willebrand factor binding to platelet glycoprotein Ib initiates calcium influx associated with aggregation. Blood 1992;80:113.

226. Moake JL, Turner NA, Stathopoulos NA, et al. Involvement of large plasma von Willebrand factor (vWF) multimers and unusually large vWF forms derived from endothelial cells in shear stress–induced platelet aggregation. J Clin Invest 1986;78:1456.

227. Peterson DM, Stathopoulos NA, Giorgio TD, et al. Shear-induced platelet aggregation requires von Willebrand factor and platelet membrane glycoproteins Ib and IIb/IIIa. Blood 1987;69:625.

228. Miller JL, Thiam-Cisse M, Drouet LO. Reduction in thrombus formation by PG-1 F(ab')$_2$, an antiguinea pig platelet glycoprotein Ib monoclonal antibody. Arteriosclerosis Thromb 1991;11:1231.

229. Ikeda Y, Handa M, Kawano K, et al. The role of von Willebrand factor and fibrinogen in platelet aggregation under varying shear stress. J Clin Invest 1991;87:1234.

230. Bellinger DA, Nichols TC, Read MS, et al. Prevention of occlusive coronary artery thrombosis by a murine monoclonal antibody to porcine von Willebrand factor. Proc Natl Acad Sci USA 1987;84:8100.

231. Krupski WC, Bass A, Cadroy Y, et al. Antihemostatic and antithrombotic effects of monoclonal antibodies against von Willebrand factor (vWF) in nonhuman primates. Surgery 1992;112(2):433.

232. Hanson SR. Platelet-specific antibodies as in vivo therapeutic reagents: a baboon model. In: Kunicki TJ, George JN, eds. Platelet immunobiology: molecular and clinical aspects. Philadelphia: JB Lippincott, 1989:471.

233. Badimon L, Badimon J, Ruggeri Z, Fuster V. A peptide-specific monoclonal antibody that inhibits von Willebrand factor binding to GPIIb/IIIa inhibits platelet deposition to human atherosclerotic vessel wall (abstract). Circulation 1990;82(suppl III):370.

234. Strony J, Phillips M, Moake J, Adelman B. In vivo inhibition of coronary artery thrombosis by aurin tricarboxylic acid (abstract). Circulation 1989; 80(suppl II):II-23.

235. Plow EF, McEver RP, Coller BS, et al. Related binding mechanisms for fibrinogen, fibronectin, von Willebrand factor, and thrombospondin on thrombin-stimulated human platelets. Blood 1985;66:724.

236. Lawrence JB, Kramer WS, McKeown LP, et al. Arginine-glycine-aspartic acid- and fibrinogen gamma-chain carboxyterminal peptides inhibit platelet adherence to arterial subendothelium at high wall shear rates. J Clin Invest 1990;86:1715.

237. Coller BS, Peerschke EI, Scudder LE, Sullivan CA. A murine monoclonal antibody that completely blocks the binding of fibrinogen to platelets produces a thrombasthenic-like state in normal platelets and binds to glycoproteins IIb and/or IIIa. J Clin Invest 1983;72:325.

238. Coller BS, Scudder LE. Inhibition of dog platelet function by in vivo infusion of F(ab')$_2$ fragments of a monoclonal antibody. Blood 1986;66:1456.

239. Coller BS, Folts JD, Smith SR, et al. Abolition of in vivo platelet thrombus formation in primates with monoclonal antibodies to the platelet GP IIb/IIIa receptor: correlation with bleeding time, platelet aggregation, and blockade of GP IIb/IIIa receptors. Circulation 1989;80:1766.

240. Hanson SR, Pareti FI, Ruggeri ZM, et al. Effects of monoclonal antibodies against the platelet glycoprotein IIb/IIIa complex on thrombosis and hemostasis in the baboon. J Clin Invest 1988;81:149.

241. Gold HK, Coller B, Yasuda T, et al. Rapid and sustained coronary artery recanalization with combined bolus injection of recombinant tissue-type plasminogen activator and monoclonal anti-platelet GPIIb/IIIa antibody in a canine preparation. Circulation 1988;77:670.

242. Gold HK, Gimple L, Yasuda T, et al. Phase I human trial of the potent anti-platelet agents, 7E3-F(ab')$_2$, a monoclonal antibody to the GP IIb/IIIa receptor (abstract). Circulation 1989;80(suppl II): II-267.

243. Yasuda T, Gold HK, Fallon JT, et al. Monoclonal antibody against the platelet glycoprotein (GP) IIb/IIIa receptor prevents coronary artery reocclusion after reperfusion with recombinant tissue-type plasminogen activator in dogs. J Clin Invest 1988;81:1284.

244. Krupski WC, Bass A, Kelly AB, et al. Interruption of vascular thrombosis by bolus anti-platelet glycoprotein IIb/IIIa (GPIIb/IIIa) monoclonal antibodies in baboons. J Vasc Surg (in press).

245. Coller BS. Platelets and thrombolytic therapy. N Engl J Med 1990;322:33.

246. Iuliucci JD, Treacy G, Cornell S. Anti-platelet activity and safety of chimeric anti-platelet monoclonal antibody 7E3 FAB combined with streptokinase and anticoagulant drugs (abstract). Circulation 1991;84(suppl II):II-247.

247. Gold HK, Gimpie LW, Yasuda T, et al. Pharmacodynamic study of F(ab')$_2$ fragments of murine monoclonal antibody 7E3 directed against human platelet glycoprotein IIb/IIIa in patients with unstable angina pectoris. J Clin Invest 1990;86: 651.

248. Kleiman NS, Ohman EM, Keriakes DJ, et al. Profound platelet inactivation with 7E3 shortly after thrombolytic therapy for acute myocardial infarction: preliminary results of the TAMI 8 trial (abstract). Circulation 1991;84(suppl. II):II-522.

249. Cook JJ, Huang TF, Rucinski B, et al. Inhibition of platelet hemostatic plug formation by trigramin, a novel RGD-peptide. Am J Physiol 1989;256: H1038.

250. Huang TF, Holt JC, Lukasiewicz H, Niewiarowski S. Trigramin: a low molecular weight peptide inhibiting fibrinogen interaction with platelet receptors expressed on glycoprotein IIb/IIIa complex. J Biol Chem 1987;262:16157.

251. Ouyang C, Huang T-F. A potent platelet aggregation inducer from *Trimeresurus gramineus* snake venom. Biochim Biophys Acta 1983;749:126.

252. Mellott MJ, Polokoff MA, Bencen GH, Bush LR. Effects of bitistatin, a snake venom peptide and platelet fibrinogen receptor antagonist in a canine model of thrombolysis and reocclusion (abstract). Circulation 1989;80(suppl II):II-216.

253. Shebuski RJ, Stabilito IJ, Stiko GR, Polokoff MH. Acceleration of recombinant tissue-type plasminogen activator–induced thrombolysis and prevention of reocclusion by the combination of heparin and the Arg-Gly-Asp–containing peptide bitistatin in a canine model of coronary thrombosis. Circulation 1990;82:169.

254. Bush LR, Holahan MA, Kanovsky SM, et al. Antithrombotic profile of echistatin, a snake venom peptide and platelet fibrinogen receptor antagonist in the dog (abstract). Circulation 1989;80 (suppl. II):II-23.

255. Yasuda T, Gold HK, Leinbach RC, et al. Enhanced thrombolysis by rt-PA plus kistrin, a short-acting

platelet IIb/IIIa antagonist (abstract). Circulation 1991;84(suppl III):III-277.

256. Chao BH, Jakubowski JA, Savage B, et al. Agkistrodon piscivorus platelet aggregation inhibitor: a potent inhibitor of platelet activation. Proc Natl Acad Sci USA 1989;86:8050.

257. Savage B, Marzec UM, Chao BH, et al. Binding of the snake venom–derived proteins applaggin and echistatin to the arginine-glycine-aspartic acid recognition site(s) on platelet glycoprotein IIb/IIIa complex inhibits receptor function. J Biol Chem 1990;265:11766.

258. Scarborough RM, Rose JW, Hsu MA, et al. A GPIIb-IIIa–specific integrin antagonist from the venom of *Sistrurus m. barbouri*. J Biol Chem 1991;266:9359.

259. Plow EF, Pierschbacher MD, Ruoslahti E, et al. The effect of Arg-Gly-Asp–containing peptides on fibrinogen and von Willebrand factor binding to platelets. Proc Natl Acad Sci USA 1985;82:8057.

260. Ruoslahti E, Pierschbacher MD. Arg-Gly-Asp: a versatile cell recognition signal. Cell 1986;44:517.

261. Gan ZR, Gould RJ, Jacobs JW, et al. Echistatin: a potent platelet aggregation inhibitor from the venom of the viper *Echis carinatus*. J Biol Chem 1988;263:19827.

262. Dennis MS, Henzel WJ, Pitti RM, et al. Platelet glycoprotein GPIIb/IIIa protein antagonists from snake venoms: evidence for a family of platelet-aggregation inhibitors. Proc Natl Acad Sci USA 1989;87:2471.

263. Yasuda T, Gold HK, Leinbach RC, et al. Kistrin, a polypeptide platelet GPIIb/IIIa receptor antagonist, enhances and sustains coronary arterial thrombolysis with recombinant tissue-type plasminogen activator in a canine preparation. Circulation 1991;83:1038.

264. Charo IF, Nannizzi L, Phillips DR, et al. Inhibition of fibrinogen binding to GP IIb-IIIa by a GP IIIa peptide. J Biol Chem 1991;266:1415.

265. Haverstick DM, Cowan JF, Yamada KM, Santoro SA. Inhibition of platelet adhesion to fibronectin, fibrinogen, and von Willebrand factor substrates by a synthetic tetrapeptide derived from the cell-binding domain of fibronectin. Blood 1985;66:946.

266. Hanson SR, Kotze HF, Harker LA, et al. Potent antithrombotic effects of novel peptide antagonists of platelet glycoprotein (GP) IIb/IIIa (abstract). Thromb Haemost 1991;65(suppl 2):813.

267. Strony J, Adelman B, Phillips DR, et al. Inhibition of platelet thrombus formation in an in vivo model of high shear stress by a glycoprotein IIb-IIIa specific peptide antagonist (abstract). Circulation 1991;84(suppl II):II-248.

268. Kessler CM, Kelly AB, Suggs WD, et al. Prevention of embolic stroke by a novel antagonist of platelet GP IIb/IIIa (abstract). Circulation 1991;84(suppl II):II-32.

269. Haskel EJ, Torr SR, Day KC, et al. Prevention of arterial reocclusion after thrombolysis with recombinant lipoprotein-associated coagulation inhibitor. Circulation 1991;84:821.

270. Haskel EJ, Adams SP, Feigen LP, et al. Prevention of reoccluding platelet-rich thrombi in canine femoral arteries with a novel peptide antagonist of platelet glycoprotein IIb/IIIa receptors. Circulation 1989;80:1775.

271. Haskel EJ, Prager NA, Sobel BE, Abendschein DR. Relative efficacy of antithrombin compared with antiplatelet agents in accelerating coronary thrombolysis and preventing early reocclusion. Circulation 1991;83:1048.

272. Lu HR, Gold HK, Wu Z, et al. G4120, an Arg-Gly-Asp containing pentapeptide, enhances arterial eversion graft recanalization with recombinant tissue-type plasminogen activator in dogs. Thromb Haemost 1992;67(6):686.

273. Vu T-KH, Hung DT, Wheaton VI, Coughlin SR. Molecular cloning of a functional thrombin receptor reveals a novel proteolytic mechanism of receptor activation. Cell 1991;64:1057.

274. Vu T-KH, Wheaton VI, Hung DT, et al. Domains specifying thrombin-receptor interaction. Nature 1991;353:674.

275. Hung DT, Vu T-KH, Wheaton VI, et al. Cloned thrombin receptor is necessary for thrombin-induced platelet activation. J Clin Invest 1992;89:1350.

276. Coughlin SR, Vu T-KH, Hung DT, Wheaton VI. Characterization of a functional thrombin receptor: issues and opportunities. J Clin Invest 1992;89:351.

277. Rydel TJ, Ravichandran KG, Tulinsky A, et al. The structure of a complex of recombinant hirudin and human alpha-thrombin. Science 1990;249:277.

278. Vassallo RR, Kieber-Emmons T, Chichowski K, Brass LF. Structure-function relationships in the activation of platelet thrombin receptors by receptor-derived peptides. J Biol Chem 1992;267:6081.

279. Hanson SR, Harker LA, Kelly AB, et al. Hirudin inhibition of arterial smooth muscle cell (SMC) proliferation in baboons (abstract). Circulation (in press).

280. Wilcox JN, Hanson SR, Ollerenshaw J, et al. Thrombin receptor expression in vascular lesion formation. Science (in press).

281. Glenn KC, Frost GH, Bergmann JS, Carney DH. Synthetic peptides bind to high-affinity thrombin receptors and modulate thrombin mitogenesis. Peptide Res 1988;1:65.

282. Carney DH, Mann R, Redin WR, et al. Enhance-

ment of incisional wound healing and neovascularization in normal rats by thrombin and synthetic thrombin receptor-activating peptides. J Clin Invest 1992;89:1469.

283. Ganguly P. Binding of thrombin to human platelets. Nature 1974;247:306.

284. Hamberg M, Svensson J, Sameulsson B. Thromboxanes: a new group of biologically active compounds derived from prostaglandin endoperoxides. Proc Natl Acad Sci USA 1975;72:2994.

285. Moncada S, Vane JR. Arachidonic acid metabolites and the interactions between platelets and blood vessel walls. N Engl J Med 1979;300:1142.

286. Fitzgerald DJ, Catella F, Roy L, Fitzgerald GA. Marked platelet activation in vivo after intravenous streptokinase in patients with acute myocardial infarction. Circulation 1988;77:142.

287. Owen J, Friedman KD, Grossman BA, et al. Thrombolytic therapy with tissue plasminogen activator or streptokinase induces transient thrombin activity. Blood 1988;72:616.

288. Willerson JT, Golino P, McNatt J, et al. Role of new antiplatelet agents as adjunctive therapies in thrombolysis. Am J Cardiol 1991;67:12A.

289. Fitzgerald DJ, FitzGerald GA. Role of thrombin and thromboxane A_2 in reocclusion following coronary thrombolysis with tissue-type plasminogen activator. Proc Natl Acad Sci USA 1989; 86:7585.

290. Yao SK, McNatt J, Anderson HV, et al. Thrombin inhibition enhances recombinant tissue-type plasminogen activator–induced thrombolysis and delays reocclusion. Am J Physiol 1992;262:374.

291. Yao SK, Ober JC, Ferguson JJ, et al. Combination of inhibition of thrombin and blockade of thromboxane A_2 sythetase and receptors enhances thrombolysis and delays reocclusion in coronary arteries. Circulation 1992;86:1993.

292. De Clerck F, Beetens J, de Chaffoy de Courcelles D, et al. R 68 070: thromboxane A_2 synthetase inhibition and thromboxane A_2/prostaglandin endoperoxide receptor blockade combined in one molecule. I. Biochemical profile in vitro. Thromb Haemost 1989;61:35.

293. De Clerck F, Beetens J, Van de Water A, et al. R 68 070: thromboxane A_2 synthetase inhibition and thromboxane A_2/prostaglandin in endoperoxide receptor blockage combined in one molecule. II. Pharmacological effects in vivo and ex vivo. Thromb Haemost 1989;61:43.

294. Ashton JH, Schmitz JM, Campbell WB, et al. Inhibition of cyclic flow variations in stenosed canine coronary arteries by thromboxane A_2/prostaglandin H_2 receptor antagonists. Circ Res 1986; 59:568.

295. Bush LR, Campbell WB, Buja LM, et al. Effects of the selective thromboxane synthetase inhibitor

dazoxiben on variations in cyclic blood flow in stenosed canine coronary arteries. Circulation 1984;69:1161.

296. Yao SK, Rosolowsky M, Anderson HV, et al. Combined thromboxane A_2 synthetase inhibition and receptor blockade are effective in preventing spontaneous epinephrine-induced canine coronary cyclic flow variations. J Am Coll Cardiol 1990; 16:705.

297. Golino P, Rosolowsky M, Yao S-K, et al. Endogenous prostaglandin endoperoxides and prostacyclin modulate the thrombolytic activity of tissue plasminogen activator: effects of simultaneous inhibition of thromboxane A_2 synthetase and blockade of thromboxane A_2/prostaglandin H_2 receptors in a canine model of coronary thrombosis. J Clin Invest 1990;86:1095.

298. Agnelli G, Renga C, Weitz JI, et al. Sustained antithrombotic activity of hirudin after its plasma clearance: comparison with heparin. Blood 1992; 80(4):960.

299. Klement P, Borm A, Hirsh J, et al. The effect of thrombin inhibitors on tissue plasminogen activator induced thrombolysis in a rat model. Thromb Haemost 1992;68(1):64.

300. Yasuda T, Gold HK, Yaoita H, et al. Comparative effects of aspirin, a synthetic thrombin inhibitor and a monoclonal antiplatelet glycoprotein IIb/IIIa antibody on coronary artery reperfusion, reocclusion and bleeding with recombinant tissue-type plasminogen activator in a canine preparation. J Am Coll Cardiol 1990;16:714.

301. Stone SR, Hofsteenge J. Kinetics of the inhibition of thrombin by hirudin. Biochemistry 1986;25: 4622.

302. Bourdon P, Fenton JW II, Maraganore JM. Affinity labelling of lysine-149 in the anion-binding exosite of human α-thrombin with an N^a-(dinitrofluorobenzyl) hirudin C-terminal peptide. Biochemistry 1990;29:6379.

303. Chang J-Y, Ngai PK, Rink H, et al. The structural elements of hirudin which bind to the fibrinogen recognition site of thrombin are exclusively located within its acidic C-terminal tail. FEBS Lett 1990;261:287.

304. Krstenansky JL, Mao SJT. Antithrombin properties of C-terminus of hirudin using synthetic unsulfated N^a-acetyl-hirudin 45–65. FEBS Lett 1987; 211:10.

305. Maraganore JM, Bourdon P, Jablonski J, et al. Design and characterization of hirulogs: a novel class of bivalent peptide inhibitors of thrombin. Biochemistry 1990;29:7095.

306. Maraganore JM, Chao B, Joseph ML, et al. Anticoagulant activity of synthetic hirudin fragments. J Biol Chem 1989;264:8692.

307. Markwardt F. Pharmacological approaches to

thrombin regulation. Ann NY Acad Sci 1986; 485:204.

308. Kelly AB, Marzec UM, Krupski W, et al. Hirudin interruption of heparin-resistant arterial thrombus formation in baboons. Blood 1991;77:1006.

309. Lam JYT, Chesebro JH, Steele PM, et al. Is vasospasm related to platelet deposition? Relationship in a porcine preparation of arterial injury in vivo. Circulation 1987;75:243.

310. Kikumoto R, Tamao Y, Tesuka T, et al. Selective inhibition of thrombin by (2R,4R)-4-methyl-1[N^2-[(3-methyl-1,2,3,4-tetrahydro-8-quinolinyl)sulfonyl]-L-arginyl)]-2-piperidinecarboxylic acid. Biochemistry 1984;23:85.

311. Kettner C, Shaw E. D-Phe-Pro-ArgCh$_2$Cl: a selective affinity label for thrombin. Thromb Res 1979; 14:969.

312. Hanson SR, Harker LA. Interruption of acute platelet-dependent thrombosis by the synthetic antithrombin D-phenylalanyl-L-prolyl-L-arginyl chloromethylketone. Proc Natl Acad Sci USA 1988;85:3184.

313. Lumsden AB, Kelly AB, Schneider PA, et al. Lasting safe interruption of endarterectomy thrombosis by transiently infused antithrombin peptide D-Phe-Pro-ARGCH$_2$Cl in baboons. Blood 1993; 81:1762.

314. Kelly AB, Hanson SR, Henderson LW, Harker LA. Prevention of heparin-resistant thrombotic occlusion of hollow-fiber hemodialyzers by synthetic antithrombin. J Lab Clin Med 1989;114:411.

315. Kotze H, Lumsden A, Harker L, Hanson S. In vivo antithrombotic effects of local vs. systemic therapy with potent antithrombins (abstract). Circulation 1990;82(suppl III):III-659.

316. Krupski WC, Bass A, Kelly AB, et al. Heparin-resistant thrombus formation by endovascular stents in baboons: interruption by a synthetic antithrombin. Circulation 1990;82:570.

317. Lumsden AB, Kotze HF, Hanson SR, Harker LA. Brief topical application of synthetic antithrombin prevents vascular graft thrombosis. Surg Forum 1991;42:320.

318. Bode W, Mayr I, Baumann U, et al. The refined 1.9 Å crystal structure of human alpha-thrombin: interaction with D-Phe-Pro-Arg chloromethylketone and significance of the Tyr-Pro-Pro-Trp insertion segment. EMBO J 1989;8:3467.

319. Kettner C, Mersinger L, Knabb R. The selective inhibition of thrombin by peptides of boroarginine. J Biol Chem 1990;265:18289.

320. Knabb RM, Kettner CA, Reilly TM. Thrombin inhibition with DuP 714 accelerates reperfusion and delays reocclusion in dogs (abstract). Circulation 1991;84(suppl II):II-467.

321. Kelly AB, Hanson SR, Knabb R, et al. Relative antithrombotic potencies and hemostatic risks of

reversible D-Phe-Pro-Arg (D-FPR) antithrombin derivatives (abstract). Thromb Haemost 1991;65: 736.

322. Bagdy D, Barabas E, Szabo G, et al. In vivo anticoagulant and antiplatelet effect of D-Phe-Pro-Arg-H and D-MePhe-Pro-Arg-H. Thromb Haemost 1992;67:357.

323. Fitzgerald DJ, Wright F, FitzGerald GA. Increased thromboxane biosynthesis during coronary thrombolysis: evidence that platelet activation and thromboxane A$_2$ modulate the response to tissue-type plasminogen activator in vivo. Circ Res 1989;65:83.

324. Ginsberg JS, Hirsh J, Gent M, et al. A phase II study of hirulog in the prevention of venous thrombosis after major hip or knee surgery (abstract). Circulation 1992;86(suppl I):I409.

325. Cannon CP, Maraganore JM, Loscalzo J, et al. Antithrombotic and anticoagulant effects of Hirulog, a novel thrombin inhibitor, in patients with ischemic heart disease. Circulation (in press).

326. Kelly AB, Maraganore JM, Bourdon P, et al. Antithrombotic effects of synthetic peptides targeting different functional domains of thrombin. Proc Natl Acad Sci USA 1992;89:6040.

327. Waxman L, Smith DE, Arcuri KE, Vlasuk GP. Tick anticoagulant peptide (TAP) is a novel inhibitor of blood coagulation factor Xa. Science 1990;248: 593.

328. Neeper MP, Waxman L, Smith DE, et al. Characterization of recombinant tick anticoagulant peptide. J Biol Chem 1990;265:17746.

329. Vlasuk GP, Ramjit D, Fijta T, et al. Comparison of the in vivo anticoagulant properties of standard heparin and the highly selective factor Xa inhibitors antistasin and tick anticoagulant peptide (TAP) in a rabbit model of venous thrombosis. Thromb Haemost 1991;65:257.

330. Dunwiddie CT, Thornberry NA, Bull HG, et al. Antistasin, a leech-derived inhibitor of factor Xa: kinetic analysis of enzyme inhibition and identification of the reactive site. J Biol Chem 1989; 264:16694.

331. Nutt EM, Gasic T, Rodkey J, et al. The amino acid sequence of antistasin: a potent inhibitor of factor Xa reveals a repeated internal structure. J Biol Chem 1988;263:10162.

332. Nutt EM, Jain D, Lenny AB, et al. Purification and characterization of recombinant antistasin: a leech-derived inhibitor of coagulation factor Xa. Arch Biochem Biophys 1991;285:37.

333. Tuszynski G, Gasic T, Gasic G. Isolation and characterization of antistasin. J Biol Chem 1987; 262:9718.

334. Dunwiddie CT, Nutt EM, Vlasuk GP, et al. Anticoagulant efficacy and immunogenicity of the selective factor Xa inhibitor antistasin following subcu-

Also, in times of increasing health care cost containment, the adoption and frequent use of novel, expensive therapeutics such as rt-PA and APSAC may not be tenable.

Although plasminogen activators improve a patient's probability of surviving a myocardial infarction, a physician might well hesitate to use them; fewer than 1 in 10 patients dies from the condition, whereas the treatment can cause death in 1 in 50. Indeed, a review of the literature indicates that plasminogen activator therapy is underused in the United States in patients who could benefit from it.[6] The recent flurry of reports indicating that the effects of angioplasty, atherectomy, and thrombus ablation are equivalent to those of plasminogen activators after acute coronary occlusion must reflect a prevailing deep dissatisfaction with plasminogen activator therapy.[7–9] Yet mechanical removal of a thrombus and underlying arteriosclerotic lesion cannot be a practical therapy for most patients with myocardial infarction, if only for reasons of cost and logistics. Catheterization facilities are concentrated in urban areas and presently operate at near capacity, and only a few cities have adequate transportation facilities for moving a patient to an appropriate setting within the time frame required for optimal results. As with the use of novel therapeutics, the use of these very expensive and invasive procedures may be difficult to justify.

If plasminogen activators are an imperfect and dangerous therapy and the mechanical relief of coronary thrombosis is impractical, what are the alternatives? One is to explore better methods for using existing plasminogen activators. In the first trial of the Gruppo Italiano per lo Studio della Streptochinasi nell'Infarto Miocardico (GISSI),[10] which examined the parameters of myocardial infarct size in relation to the time of plasminogen activator administration after the first symptom of coronary occlusion, the earlier the plasminogen activator was administered, the greater was the rate of survival. This observation implies that administering plasminogen activators before a patient's arrival at the hospital in order to reduce the interval between symptoms and administration may increase the therapeutic advantage. The observation also can be extrapolated to suggest that plasminogen activators that work more rapidly—that reduce the interval between administration and reperfusion—may result in greater reductions in infarct size.

Efforts to change the program of plasminogen activator administration have shown some promise both in effecting earlier reperfusion and in reducing the number of resistant thrombi.[11] Coadministration of t-PA and urokinase-type plasminogen activator (u-PA) is believed to combine the benefits of earlier reperfusion (a characteristic of a thrombus-selective plasminogen activator such as rt-PA) with inhibition of rethrombosis (which is associated with nonselective plasminogen activators such as u-PA).[12–14] Adjunctive agents, such as inhibitors of thrombin or platelet aggregation, may be useful both in reducing the number of vessels that are not reperfused and in preventing rethrombosis.[15–17] However, with the exception of aspirin, none of these agents has as yet had its efficacy proven in the required large multicenter trial. And all of them are likely to be associated with an increased risk of bleeding.

A plasminogen activator that would be used more widely (and probably displace the currently available agents) would have the following characteristics: greater potency in lysing resistant (probably platelet-rich) thrombi, earlier clot lysis, and selectivity for coronary thrombi in contrast with thrombi in other vessels (which would reduce the risk of bleeding). A drug with all these properties does not exist at present. My purpose is to trace a potential evolution in research that could allow development of such an agent.

Current Hypotheses of Interest

Existing Plasminogen Activators Can Be Improved Through Genetic Engineering

The last decade has seen incredible activity, both in university laboratories and in the commercial sector, directed at modifying plasminogen activators by recombinant DNA methods. The aim has been to increase potency, improve pharmacokinetics, and increase the resistance of plasminogen activators to inactivation by inhibitors. The present discussion does not afford space in which to review these efforts adequately. Yet in summing up a great deal of work, it has become apparent that single or multiple residue mutations and deletions or alterations in glycosylation patterns have not increased plasminogen activator potency. Sequence changes have lengthened the plasma half-life of plasminogen activators, but this improvement has usually come at the cost of a reduction in potency. A t-PA mutant with a longer duration of action is presently undergoing clinical trial.[18]

Madison et al.[19,20] attempted to improve t-PA by studying alterations to its structure that markedly increased resistance to inactivation by plasminogen activator inhibitor 1 (PAI-1) while having little effect on catalytic activity. Although results for the t-PA mutant were impressive in vitro, the thrombolytic rates of the mutant and native t-PA were indistinguishable in vivo.[21]

Among the many attempts to fuse parts of two different plasminogen activators, perhaps one of the most successful is a molecule consisting of amino acids 1 to 3 and 87 to 274 of human t-PA and amino acids 138 to 411 of human single-chain urokinase-type plasminogen activator (scu-PA).[22] This compound appears to be more potent than its parents and is presently under consideration for clinical trial.

Thrombus Selectivity Results in Enhanced Potency and Specificity

The development of t-PA was buoyed by the concept that a highly fibrin-selective agent would be more potent, resulting in more rapid and complete thrombolysis, and more selective, conserving fibrin and other proteins important for hemostasis and thereby eventuating less bleeding by avoiding a "lytic state." Initial studies comparing t-PA with SK did indeed suggest that reperfusion occurred more rapidly with t-PA.[23] Subsequent larger trials did not, however, show a difference in patient survival between those treated with t-PA and those treated with SK,[2–4] that is, until the aforementioned report of the GUSTO Trial.[5]

Although in animal models t-PA administra-tion was followed by substantially less loss of fibrinogen than was SK administration, the doses of t-PA required for fibrinolysis in clinical practice often did produce a lytic state. In one large multicenter trial (GISSI-2),[2] the incidence of cerebral hemorrhage was no different between groups treated with SK or t-PA, whereas in another trial (ISIS-3, Third International Study of Infarct Survival),[4] significantly more cerebral hemorrhage was observed in the t-PA–treated group. The design of both trials was criticized[24] by leading advocates of fibrin selectivity, who were sufficiently convinced of inherent methodologic problems to undertake another very large trial, GUSTO,[5,25] to test t-PA against SK again.

The highlights of the GUSTO presentations at the annual meeting of the American Federation for Clinical Research on April 30, 1993 can be summarized as follows.[5] In a comparison of 10,377 patients receiving streptokinase and intravenous heparin with 10,344 patients receiving an "accelerated" t-PA regimen (administration of t-PA over a period of 1½ hours—with two-thirds of the dose given in the first 30 minutes—rather than the conventional period of 3 hours[5]) with intravenous heparin, 30-day mortality among streptokinase patients was 7.4% whereas that among t-PA patients was 6.3%, a significant difference. This difference was more pronounced in patients with anterior infarction (streptokinase mortality, 10.5%; t-PA mortality, 8.6%) than in those with infarction at other sites (streptokinase mortality, 5.3%; t-PA mortality, 4.7%), and it was more pronounced in those patients treated within the first 4 hours of symptoms than in those treated later. On the other hand, there was no significant difference in total strokes between patients receiving tPA and those receiving streptokinase, although primary intracranial hemorrhagic strokes occurred more frequently in the t-PA group. Despite the increased incidence of stroke, however, there was a net clinical benefit to those patients who received t-PA. There was also no significant difference in severe or life threatening bleeding at other sites. It is of interest that the incidence of reinfarction (4%) was identical in the t-PA and streptokinase groups,[5] and that reocclusion, by comparison of 90-minute with 5- to 7-day angiograms, was not very different (streptokinase group, 6.0%; tPA group, 5.9%).[26] Perhaps the most significant conclusion to come from this trial is that there was a correlation between 90-minute coronary arterial patency and 30-day survival, providing a physiologic basis for the improved survival observed with t-PA.

The outcome of the GUSTO Trial allows for a cautious acceptance of the hypothesis that more potent and more thrombus-specific thrombolytic agents could have an advantage in the treatment of acute coronary occlusion. Because the differences between t-PA and SK are small, one could argue that t-PA is not the optimal thrombus-selective agent and that other approaches to thrombus selectivity should be explored. Therefore, I next discuss naturally occurring plasminogen activators that appear to be more selective than t-PA and the engineering of antibody-plasminogen activator fusion molecules that are capable of targeting specific components of the thrombus.

NATURALLY OCCURRING FIBRIN-SELECTIVE AGENTS

Staphylokinase

Staphylokinase, a plasminogen activator secreted by *Staphylococcus*, has properties similar to those of SK yet appears to be highly fibrin-selective. Like SK, staphylokinase forms a stoichiometric complex with plasminogen that activates the enzyme according to Michaelis-Menten kinetics. It is this complex that becomes the plasminogen activator. The critical difference between the SK-plasminogen complex and the staphylokinase-plasminogen complex is that SK-plasminogen is inhibited by α_2-antiplasmin in the vicinity of thrombi, whereas staphylokinase-plasminogen is not.

In plasma in the absence of fibrin, the staphylokinase-plasminogen complex (like the SK-plasminogen complex) is rapidly neutralized by α_2-antiplasmin, thus preventing systemic plasminogen activation. In the presence of fibrin, however, the lysine binding sites of the plasminogen-staphylokinase complex are occupied, and inhibition by α_2-antiplasmin is retarded, thus allowing preferential plasminogen activation at the fibrin surface.[27] The net result is effective clot lysis

with sparing of fibrinogen (and, presumably, of other proteins contributing to hemostasis). In a venous thrombosis model in the baboon, staphylokinase was shown to have a thrombolytic potency similar to that of SK.[28] In addition, staphylokinase was less immunogenic and less allergenic than SK, and staphylokinase did not induce resistance to lysis upon repeated administration. In comparison with SK, staphylokinase was significantly more efficient in the dissolution of platelet-rich arterial graft thrombi.[28] Early clinical trials of staphylokinase are in progress.

Bat Plasminogen Activator

A potent, highly fibrin-selective plasminogen activator was isolated from vampire bat saliva, its cDNA was cloned,[29,30] and it was subsequently expressed by recombinant DNA methods.[31] Unlike t-PA, bat plasminogen activator (bat-PA) exhibits a strict requirement for polymerized fibrin before it manifests enzymatic activity,[32] and it is essentially inactive in human plasma (also in contrast with t-PA, which, at sufficient concentrations, is capable of fibrinogenolysis in plasma).[33]

Gardell et al.[34] evaluated the efficacy and fibrin selectivity of bat-PA and compared it with that of t-PA in a rabbit model of femoral artery thrombosis. Bat-PA was equipotent with t-PA in restoration of blood flow, but the time to reach maximal flow with bat-PA was approximately half that with t-PA. In contrast with an equimolar infusion of t-PA, bat-PA brought about reperfusion without fibrinogenolysis and with only slight decreases in plasma levels of plasminogen and α_2-antiplasmin. Nonetheless, bat-PA and t-PA prolonged template bleeding times equally. Thus, although these experiments suggest that bat-PA has the potential for more rapid thrombolysis, they do not indicate a potential for reduced hemorrhagic complications.

Mellott et al.[35] extended these bat-PA studies to a canine arterial thrombosis model with substantially similar results, and Witt et al.[36] confirmed them further in a rat pulmonary embolism model. In comparison with t-PA, vampire bat salivary plasminogen activator (bat-PA) was more potent and at the same time more selective; after administration of bat-PA, there were no reductions in plasma fibrinogen and plasminogen concentrations.

ANTIBODY-TARGETED AGENTS

An alternative strategy for building specificity into a molecule entails linking an enzyme to an antibody. Here the goal is to increase the local concentration of the enzyme at a desired site. For example, with an antibody-targeted enzyme, a plasminogen activator can be concentrated at the site of a thrombus in order to enhance the local production of plasmin,[37] thereby restricting the action of this powerful and nonselective protease to a location where it is required.

Fibrin-Targeted Plasminogen Activators

Reasoning that it was essential that the antigen-combining site be specific for a component of the clot and not cross-react with soluble serum proteins or antigens present on endothelial cells, my research group selected fibrin as a target because it has antigenic epitopes that differentiate it from fibrinogen, its precursor in circulating plasma. Monoclonal antibody 59D8,[38] which is specific for an epitope exposed when thrombin catalyzes the conversion of fibrinogen to fibrin, is the cornerstone of our work in this area. Another monoclonal antibody of similar specificity, 64C5, was used in some of our initial studies.[38–40]

Antibody 59D8 (as well as 64C5) was raised in response to immunization with a peptide of the sequence GHRPLDK(C), which represents the seven amino-terminal residues of the beta chain of fibrin combined with a carboxyl-terminal cysteine for cross-linking to keyhole limpet hemocyanin. The amino terminus of the beta chain appears to be conformationally protected in fibrinogen, as evidenced by the fact that there is essentially no cross-reactivity between fibrin and fibrinogen when tested with this antibody. Another important consideration in selecting a target on the thrombus is whether the epitope recognized by the antibody persists during clot dissolution. We have shown that, contrary to some reservations, the epitope recognized by 59D8 is lost

from the clot (during in vitro fibrinolysis) at a rate identical to the rate of clot dissolution.[41] Thus epitope availability is sufficient for antibody binding throughout the course of fibrinolysis.

Holvoet et al.[42] have confirmed the utility of targeting fibrin in their experiments with monoclonal antibodies that have little reactivity with fibrinogen but react with fragment D of non-cross-linked fibrin or fragment D-dimer of cross-linked fibrin.

My research group first showed that a conjugate of two-chain urokinase-type plasminogen activator (tcu-PA) and antifibrin antibody 64C5 substantially enhanced in vitro fibrinolysis in comparison with tcu-PA.[39] We then showed that tcu-PA conjugated to the 64C5 Fab' was equally active[40] and that scu-PA could be used in a plasminogen activator-59D8 Fab' conjugate.[43] Because the antigen for 59D8 and 64C5 is a hapten, it was possible to demonstrate unequivocally that the enhancement of fibrinolytic potency was solely due to the antigen-antibody reaction: A sufficient concentration of peptide GHRPLDK reduced the fibrinolytic activity of the conjugate to that of its u-PA parent.[39]

Even the activity of t-PA, by itself fibrin-selective, could be enhanced by coupling it to a fibrin-specific antibody.[44] In vivo results for a t-PA–59D8 conjugate in a rabbit venous thrombosis model were very encouraging.[45]

Following these preliminary demonstrations of the feasibility of forming bifunctional molecules by cross-linking methods, we constructed fusion proteins containing an antibody combining site and a plasminogen activator catalytic unit by recombinant DNA methods.

We built on the pioneering work of Neuberger and coworkers.[46,47] Our first recombinant fusion protein combined the activities of t-PA and antifibrin antibody 59D8.[48,49] The protein was assembled by joining the gene coding for the 59D8 immunoglobulin heavy chain to the gene coding for t-PA and transfecting this chimeric construct into a hybridoma cell capable of producing only immunoglobulin light chain. The resulting cell line produced a bifunctional protein with domains for activating plasminogen and attaching to cross-linked fibrin.

A second, more effective bifunctional protein was made by using antibody 59D8 and a part of the gene coding for scu-PA.[50] scu-PA has significant advantages as a partner for a fibrin-specific antibody because of its resistance to inactivation by PAI-1 and α_2-antiplasmin. As it traveled through plasma, a fusion protein containing scu-PA might resist circulating inhibitors and remain incapable of activating circulating plasminogen until it reached the plasmin-rich environment of the thrombus, where it would become active through cleavage of the plasmin-susceptible Lys_{158}-Ile_{159} peptide bond.[51]

To reduce the mass of the chimeric protein to essential components, we decided to include only the Fab part of the antifibrin antibody. In a similar vein, we omitted the u-PA kringle and growth factor regions and used the sequence of low-molecular-weight (32 kDa) scu-PA as described by Stump et al.,[52] which is reported to be as active in fibrinolysis as the intact molecule. We also had initially included the CH3 domain of the antibody heavy chain as a spacer between the antibody and the plasminogen activator; later experience (S.-Y. Shaw, unpublished observations) indicated that this was not necessary.

The fusion protein contained antibody 59D8 heavy chain from residues 1 to 351 and, in contiguous peptide sequence, residues 144 to 411 of low-molecular-weight scu-PA.[50] We included the 3' untranslated region from β-globin because it enhanced protein expression levels in plasma cells.

To assemble a heterodimer that included this fusion protein and an immunoglobulin light chain, we transfected the fusion protein expression plasmid into heavy-chain loss variants. SDS gel electrophoresis, immunoblot analysis, and DNA sequencing showed that the product, scu-PA (32 kDa)–59D8, was a disulfide-linked 103-kDa heterodimer consisting of an immunoglobulin light chain linked to the fusion protein heavy chain.

The K_m of scu-PA (32 kDa)–59D8 was 16.6 μM; that of tcu-PA was 9.1 μM. Fibrin binding also was similar between the recombinant protein and its parent. In an in vitro plasma clot assay, scu-PA (32 kDa)–59D8 was 6 times more potent than scu-PA, with considerably diminished fibrinogen degradation and α_2-antiplasmin inactivation in the supernatant. In vivo, in the rabbit jugular vein model, scu-PA (32 kDa)–59D8 was 20 times more potent than scu-PA (Fig. 30-1). It should be noted that some of this enhancement in in vivo activity must, in part, have been related to a fivefold increase in the half-life of scu-PA (32 kDa)–59D8 (in comparison with scu-PA) in the rabbit.

M. S. Runge (unpublished observations) has since studied the in vivo activities of scu-PA (32 kDa)–59D8, scu-PA, and t-PA in a baboon model that allows comparison of both thrombolytic potency and inhibition of thrombus deposition in relation to the plasma concentration of each plasminogen activator. scu-PA (32 kDa)–59D8 was approximately 8- to 10-fold more potent than t-PA and 15- to 20-fold more potent than scu-PA in the lysis of thrombi and about 11-fold more potent than scu-PA in the inhibition of thrombin deposition.

Of equally great interest is the observation

FIGURE 30-1. Thrombolysis in vivo with scu-PA (dotted line) and scu-PA (32 kDa)–59D8 (solid line). Data represent the means of values from between 3 and 8 animals at each point. The 20-fold increase in potency derived for scu-PA (32 kDA)–59D8 was calculated by comparing the percentage lysis curves in plasma clot and rabbit jugular vein assays, which were fit using a two-parameter exponential function.[44] (From Runge MS, Quertermous T, Zavodny PJ, et al. A recombinant chimeric plasminogen activator with high affinity for fibrin has increased thrombolytic potency in vitro and in vivo. Proc Natl Acad Sci USA 88:10337, 1991.)

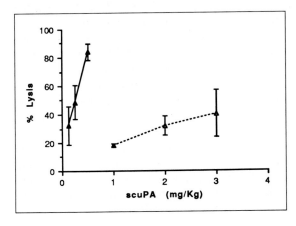

that at equipotent thrombolytic doses, template bleeding times for scu-PA (32 kDa)–59D8 in the baboon were unchanged, whereas those for t-PA and scu-PA were significantly prolonged. Since bleeding time prolongation seems to reflect the risk of clinical hemorrhage,[53] it would be of interest to determine whether scu-PA (32 kDa)–59D8, in addition to being more potent, also might be safer.

Holvoet et al.[54] have further refined this concept by constructing an M_r 57,000 single-chain chimeric plasminogen activator consisting of a 33-kDa fragment of scu-PA and an Fv derived from a fibrin-specific antibody directed at a cross-linked epitope of the D-dimer. This single-chain molecule was expressed by baculovirus-infected cells of the insect *Spodoptera frugiperda*. The recombinant molecule showed high affinity for binding the fibrin D-dimer fragment (essentially identical to that of the parent antibody molecule) and a very similar Michaelis-Menten constant for activating plasminogen. When tested in the lysis of a plasma clot in vivo, the recombinant single-chain molecule was 13 times more potent than low-molecular-weight scu-PA.

In a hamster pulmonary embolism model, a critical comparison among two scu-PA conjugates made with different antifibrin antibodies, scu-PA, and t-PA showed that the two antibody–scu-PA conjugates were equal with respect to thrombolytic potency, whereas both were 40 to 60 times more potent than scu-PA and 6 to 10 times more potent than t-PA.[55] Yet, despite this clear increase in thrombolytic potency, the maximal rate of clot lysis and delay prior to initiation of clot lysis did not significantly differ among the four plasminogen activators. If these findings are confirmed with recombinant molecules, the likely conclusion will be that although it is possible to realize an increase in potency with antibody targeting, it may not be possible to realize an increase in the rate of clot lysis.

Platelet-Targeted Plasminogen Activators

Arterial thrombi contain a high concentration of activated platelets, and it is likely that platelet-rich thrombi are particularly resistant to thrombolysis.[56] Highly platelet-rich thrombi may be a major reason for the failure to obtain reperfusion after thrombolytic therapy, and the accumulation of platelets at thrombi may lead to reocclusion.[56] Platelet aggregation is mediated by fibrinogen binding to the membrane-bound glycoprotein (GP) IIb-IIIa receptor.[56] An antibody specific for this receptor, 7E3, has been shown to enhance the speed of reperfusion and reduce the rate of reocclusion in animal models of arterial thrombosis.[57,58] Most recently this antibody was studied in a clinical trial of coronary angioplasty and was shown to reduce death, nonfatal myocardial infarction, unplanned surgical revascularization, or repeated angioplasty by 35%.[59] It was of interest to determine whether the targeting of a plasminogen activator to the GPIIb-IIIa receptor through 7E3 would enhance the antibody's ability to accelerate clot lysis. We reasoned that a conjugate of 7E3 and u-PA, in addition to blocking the GPIIb-IIIa receptor's access to fibrinogen by virtue of 7E3 binding to GPIIb-IIIa, also would produce a high local concentration of plasmin that could lyse the bound fibrin molecules responsible for aggregating the platelets.

Using chemical cross-linking, we conjugated high-molecular-weight tcu-PA to 7E3 Fab' to produce, after fractionation, a 100-kDa molecule that was predominantly a 1:1 complex of Fab' and tcu-PA.[60] The tcu-PA–7E3 Fab' conjugate bound purified GPIIb-IIIa and intact platelets and exhibited plasminogen activator activity. Figure 30-2 compares the activity of tcu-PA–7E3 Fab' with that of tcu-PA in an in vitro clot lysis assay with platelet-rich plasma clots (14×10^6 platelets/mm^3).

At the concentrations tested, tcu-PA showed very little activity against the clots, whereas the conjugate was 970-fold more active. An equimolar mixture of tcu-PA and 7E3 was no more effective than u-PA alone. The rate of lysis related to the concentration of platelets in the clot, and no enhancement in lysis by the conjugate over u-PA was apparent in clots containing few platelets. Thus u-PA targeted to GPIIb-IIIa by conjugation to the antibody accounted for an improvement in fibrinolytic potency that was substantially greater than that achieved by u-PA and the antibody alone.

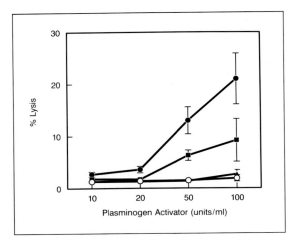

FIGURE 30-2. Plot of lysis of platelet-rich plasma clots containing approximately 14×10^6 platelets/mm³. Lysis at 4 h (filled squares) and 18 h (filled circles) is shown for the u-PA–7E3 Fab' conjugate. Lysis at 18 h is shown for an equimolar mixture of u-PA and 7E3 (Fab')₂ (filled triangles) and u-PA (open circles). Each point represents the mean of three independent experiments. Error bars represent SD. (From Bode C, Meinhardt G, Runge MS, et al. Platelet-targeted fibrinolysis enhances clot lysis and inhibits platelet aggregation. Circulation 84:805, 1991, with permission.)

Dewerchin et al.[61] also have studied several other antibodies to the ligand-induced binding sites on GPIIb-IIIa in conjugates with recombinant scu-PA. They extended our observations by showing that the conjugates were more effective than scu-PA in the lysis of platelet-rich thrombi in vivo in a hamster model of pulmonary embolism. There is little doubt that the next refinement to platelet targeting will require the construction of a recombinant molecule that contains both a binding site specific for activated platelets and a plasminogen activator catalytic site.

The disadvantage of using 7E3 as a targeting antibody is that it interacts with GPIIb-IIIa on both activated and resting platelets and thus does not target specifically to the thrombus.[56] Some of the antibodies described by Dewerchin et al.[61] may be more selective for activated platelets.

Is Targeting to the Coronary Thrombus Possible?

Many of the plasminogen activators discussed in this review are, in one way or another, targeted to

some property of the thrombus. They may have specific affinity for a component of the thrombus such as fibrin (in the case of staphylokinase, vampire bat plasminogen activator, and antifibrin antibody–scu-PA constructs) or platelets (antiplatelet antibody–scu-PA and antiplatelet antibody–tcu-PA constructs). Targeting of this kind may well increase a plasminogen activator's potency with respect to lysis-resistant thrombi and also may accelerate thrombus dissolution. If there is to be a favorable effect on the incidence of hemorrhagic complications, the mechanism of benefit must be through avoidance of a lytic state. The lytic state is characterized by the presence in the circulation of plasmin that is unopposed by α_2-antiplasmin. This situation is widely believed to result only in a loss of fibrinogen, a deficiency not important in the genesis of spontaneous bleeding. What is often forgotten is that plasmin is a promiscuous proteinase capable of destroying a variety of soluble as well as cell-associated proteins.[62–64] By keeping the fluid phase and cellular components of the hemostatic system intact, it may be possible to prevent spontaneous hemorrhage.

Spontaneous hemorrhage that occurs in the absence of a prior breach in vascular integrity must be differentiated from hemorrhage that occurs at a site of surgical intervention or injury, such as a peptic ulcer. However, the thrombus that has stopped bleeding at a site where blood vessels have been disrupted is no different from the thrombus that occludes a coronary artery. All the sophisticated targeting mechanisms discussed here cannot discriminate between these two types of thrombi. Perhaps the only attribute that can effect a significant differentiation is the age of a thrombus. As thrombi age in vivo, platelet epitopes are lost.[65,66]

Sudden and severe chest pain is the hallmark of coronary occlusion. Because thrombolytic therapy is best used shortly after the onset of symptoms, it follows that the objects of this therapy are very recently formed thrombi. By probability alone, other thrombi present in the patient (e.g., clots that beneficially prevent bleeding from sites of vascular injury) are likely to be older than the coronary thrombus. If a strategy could be devised to target a component of the thrombus that was rapidly degraded with time, the coronary thrombus would be attacked, while the older thrombi would be spared. One could envision an antibody-targeted plasminogen activator in which the target was a platelet surface protein that was rapidly degraded. This protein should be present on the surface of platelets only during the early phases of the clotting process; on older thrombi it would be absent. The search for this ephemeral protein may well initiate the next chapter in selective targeting.

REFERENCES

1. AIMS Trial Study Group. Effect of intravenous APSAC on mortality after acute myocardial infarction: preliminary report of a placebo-controlled clinical trial. Lancet 1988;1:545.
2. Gruppo Italiano per lo Studio della Sopravvivenza nell'Infarto miocardico. GISSI-2: a factorial randomised trial of alteplase versus streptokinase and heparin versus no heparin among 12,490 patients with acute myocardial infarction. Lancet 1990; 336:65.
3. The International Study Group. In-hospital mortality and clinical course of 20,891 patients with suspected acute myocardial infarction randomised between alteplase and streptokinase with or without heparin. Lancet 1990;336:71.
4. ISIS-3 (Third International Study of Infarct Survival) Collaborative Group. A randomised comparison of streptokinase vs tissue plasminogen activator vs anistreplase and of aspirin plus heparin vs aspirin alone among 41,299 cases of suspected acute myocardial infarction: ISIS-3. Lancet 1992; 339:753.
5. The Global Utilization of Streptokinase and Tissue Plasminogen Activator for Occluded Coronary Arteries (GUSTO) Investigators. An international randomized trial comparing four thrombolytic strategies for acute myocardial infarction. N Engl J Med 1993;329:673.
6. Doorey AJ, Michelson EL, Topol EJ. Thrombolytic therapy of acute myocardial infarction: keeping the unfulfilled promises. JAMA 1992;268:3108.
7. Grines CL, Browne KF, Marco J, et al. A comparison of immediate angioplasty with thrombolytic therapy for acute myocardial infarction. N Engl J Med 1993;328:673.
8. Zijlstra F, de Boer MJ, Hoorntje JCA, et al. A comparison of immediate coronary angioplasty with intravenous streptokinase in acute myocardial infarction. N Engl J Med 1993;328:680.
9. Gibbons RJ, Holmes DR, Reeder GS, et al. Immedi-ate angioplasty compared with the administration of a thrombolytic agent followed by conservative treatment for myocardial infarction. N Engl J Med 1993;328:685.
10. Gruppo Italiano per lo Studio della Streptochinasi nell'Infarto Miocardico (GISSI). Effectiveness of intravenous thrombolytic treatment in acute myocardial infarction. Lancet 1986;1:397.
11. Wall TC, Califf RM, George BS, et al. Accelerated plasminogen activator dose regimens for coronary thrombolysis: the TAMI-7 study group. J Am Coll Cardiol 1992;19:482.
12. Morris JA, Muller DW, Topol EJ. Combination thrombolytic therapy: a comparison of simultaneous and sequential regimens of tissue plasminogen activator and urokinase. Am Heart J 1991;122: 375.
13. Kirshenbaum JM, Bahr RD, Flaherty JT, et al. Clot-selective coronary thrombolysis with low-dose synergistic combinations of single-chain urokinase-type plasminogen activator and recombinant tissue-type plasminogen activator: the pro-urokinase for myocardial infarction study group. Am J Cardiol 1991;68:1564.
14. Califf RM, Topol EJ, Stack RS, et al. Evaluation of combination thrombolytic therapy and timing of cardiac catheterization in acute myocardial infarction. Results of thrombolysis and angioplasty in myocardial infarction-phase 5 randomized trial: TAMI study group. Circulation 1991;83:1543.
15. Popma JJ, Topol EJ. Adjuncts to thrombolysis for myocardial reperfusion. Ann Intern Med 1991; 115:34.
16. Ellis SG, Bates ER, Schaible T, et al. Prospects for the use of antagonists to the platelet glycoprotein IIb/IIIa receptor to prevent post-angioplasty restenosis and thrombosis. J Am Coll Cardiol 1991;17(suppl B):89B.
17. Imura Y, Stassen JM, Bunting S, et al. Antithrombotic properties of L-cysteine, N-(mercaptoacetyl)-D-Tyr-Arg-Gly-Asp-sulfoxide (G4120) in a hamster platelet-rich femoral vein thrombosis model. Blood 1992;80:1247.
18. von Essen R, Neuhaus K-L, Markreiter M, et al. Double bolus of r-PA in the dosage finding. Results of the GRECO-II study (abstract). J Am Coll Cardiol 1992;19:274A.
19. Madison EL, Goldsmith EJ, Gerard RD, et al. Serpin-resistant mutants of human tissue-type plasminogen activator. Nature 1989;339:721.
20. Madison EL, Goldsmith EJ, Gerard RD, et al. Amino acid residues that affect interaction of tissue-type plasminogen activator with plasminogen activator inhibitor 1. Proc Natl Acad Sci USA 1990;87:3530.
21. Li XK, Lijnen HR, Nelles L, et al. Biochemical and biologic properties of rt-PA del (K296-G302), a recombinant human tissue-type plasminogen activa-

tor deletion mutant resistant to plasminogen activator inhibitor-1. Blood 1992;79:417.

22. Collen D, Nelles L, De Cock F, et al. K1K2Pu, a recombinant t-PA/u-PA chimera with increased thrombolytic potency, consisting of amino acids 1 to 3 and 87 to 274 of human tissue-type plasminogen activator (t-PA) and amino acids 138 to 411 of human single chain urokinase-type plasminogen activator (scu-PA): purification in centigram quantities and conditioning for use in man. Thromb Res 1992;65:421.

23. The TIMI Study Group. The thrombolysis in myocardial infarction (TIMI) trial. N Engl J Med 1985;312:932.

24. Sobel BE, Collen D. Questions unresolved by the third international study of infarct survival (editorial). Am J Cardiol 1992;70:385.

25. Topol EJ, Armstrong P, Van de Werf F, et al. Confronting the issues of patient safety and investigator conflict of interest in an international clinical trial of myocardial reperfusion: global utilization of streptokinase and tissue plasminogen activator for occluded coronary arteries (GUSTO) steering committee. J Am Coll Cardiol 1992;19:1123.

26. The Global Utilization of Streptokinase and Tissue Plasminogen Activator for Occluded Coronary Arteries (GUSTO) Angiographic Investigators. The effects of tissue plasminogen activator, streptokinase, or both on coronary-artery patency, ventricular function, and survival after acute myocardial infarction. N Engl J Med 1993;329:1615.

27. Lijnen HR, Van Hoef B, De Cock F, et al. On the mechanism of fibrin-specific plasminogen activation by staphylokinase. J Biol Chem 1991;266:11826.

28. Collen D, De Cock F, Stassen JM. Comparative immunogenicity and thrombolytic properties toward arterial and venous thrombi of streptokinase and recombinant staphylokinase in baboons. Circulation 1993;87:996.

29. Gardell SJ, Duong LT, Diehl RE, et al. Isolation, characterization, and cDNA cloning of a vampire bat salivary plasminogen activator. J Biol Chem 1989;264:17947.

30. Kratzschmar J, Haendler B, Langer G, et al. The plasminogen activator family from the salivary gland of the vampire bat Desmodus rotundus: cloning and expression. Gene 1991;105:229.

31. Kratzschmar J, Haendler B, Bringmann P, et al. High-level secretion of the four salivary plasminogen activators from the vampire bat Desmodus rotundus by stably transfected baby hamster kidney cells. Gene 1992;116:281.

32. Bergum PW, Gardell SJ. Vampire bat salivary plasminogen activator exhibits a strict and fastidious requirement for polymeric fibrin as its cofactor, unlike human tissue-type plasminogen activator: a kinetic analysis. J Biol Chem 1992;267:17726.

33. Gardell SJ, Hare TR, Bergum PW, et al. Vampire bat salivary plasminogen activator is quiescent in human plasma in the absence of fibrin unlike human tissue plasminogen activator. Blood 1990;76:2560.

34. Gardell SJ, Ramjit DR, Stabilito II, et al. Effective thrombolysis without marked plasminemia after bolus intravenous administration of vampire bat salivary plasminogen activator in rabbits. Circulation 1991;84:244.

35. Mellott MJ, Stabilito II, Holahan MA, et al. Vampire bat salivary plasminogen activator promotes rapid and sustained reperfusion without concomitant systemic plasminogen activation in a canine model of arterial thrombosis. Arterioscler Thromb 1992;12:212.

36. Witt W, Baldus B, Bringmann P, et al. Thrombolytic properties of Desmodus rotundus (vampire bat) salivary plasminogen activator in experimental pulmonary embolism in rats. Blood 1992;79:1213.

37. Haber E, Quertermous T, Matsueda GR, Runge MS. Innovative approaches to plasminogen activator therapy. Science 1989;243:51.

38. Hui KY, Haber E, Matsueda GR. Monoclonal antibodies to a synthetic fibrin-like peptide bind to human fibrin but not fibrinogen. Science 1983;222:1129.

39. Bode C, Matsueda GR, Hui KY, Haber E. Antibody-directed urokinase: a specific fibrinolytic agent. Science 1985;229:765.

40. Bode C, Runge MS, Newell JB, et al. Thrombolysis by a fibrin-specific antibody Fab'-urokinase conjugate. J Mol Cell Cardiol 1987;19:335.

41. Chen F, Haber E, Matsueda GR. Availability of the Bb(15–21) epitope on cross-linked human fibrin and its plasmic degradation products. Thromb Haemost 1992;67:335.

42. Holvoet P, Stassen JM, Hashimoto Y, et al. Binding properties of monoclonal antibodies against human fragment D-dimer of cross-linked fibrin to human plasma clots in an in vivo model in rabbits. Thromb Haemost 1989;61:307.

43. Bode C, Runge MS, Schönermark S, et al. Conjugation to antifibrin Fab' enhances fibrinolytic potency of single-chain urokinase plasminogen activator. Circulation 1990;81:1974.

44. Runge MS, Bode C, Matsueda GR, Haber E. Conjugation to an antifibrin monoclonal antibody enhances the fibrinolytic potency of tissue plasminogen activator in vitro. Biochemistry 1988;27:1153.

45. Runge MS, Bode C, Matsueda GR, Haber E. Antibody-enhanced thrombolysis: targeting of tissue plasminogen activator in vivo. Proc Natl Acad Sci USA 1987;84:7659.

46. Neuberger MS, Williams GT, Fox RO. Recombinant antibodies possessing novel effector functions. Nature 1984;312:604.

47. Williams GT, Neuberger MS. Production of antibody-tagged enzymes by myeloma cells: application to DNA polymerase I Klenow fragment. Gene 1986;43:319.

48. Schnee JM, Runge MS, Matsueda GR, et al. Construction and expression of a recombinant antibody-targeted plasminogen activator. Proc Natl Acad Sci USA 1987;84:6904.

49. Love TW, Runge MS, Haber E, Quertermous T. Recombinant antibodies possessing novel effector functions. In: Langone JJ, ed. Methods in enzymology, Vol 178: Antibodies, antigens, and molecular mimicry. San Diego, Academic Press, 1989: 515.

50. Runge MS, Quertermous T, Zavodny PJ, et al. A recombinant chimeric plasminogen activator with high affinity for fibrin has increased thrombolytic potency in vitro and in vivo. Proc Natl Acad Sci USA 1991;88:10337.

51. Declerck PJ, Lijnen HR, Verstreken M, et al. A monoclonal antibody specific for two-chain urokinase-type plasminogen activator: application to the study of the mechanism of clot lysis with single-chain urokinase-type plasminogen activator in plasma. Blood 1990;75:1794.

52. Stump DC, Lijnen HR, Collen D. Purification and characterization of a novel low molecular weight form of single-chain urokinase-type plasminogen activator. J Biol Chem 1986;261:17120.

53. Gimple LW, Gold HK, Leinbach RC, et al. Correlation between template bleeding times and spontaneous bleeding during treatment of acute myocardial infarction with recombinant tissue-type plasminogen activator. Circulation 1989;80:581.

54. Holvoet P, Laroche Y, Lijnen HR, et al. Characterization of a chimeric plasminogen activator consisting of a single-chain Fv fragment derived from a fibrin fragment D-dimer–specific antibody and a truncated single-chain urokinase. J Biol Chem 1991;266:19717.

55. Holvoet P, Dewerchin M, Stassen JM, et al. Thrombolytic profiles of clot-targeted plasminogen activators. Parameters determining potency and initial and maximal rates. Circulation 1993; 87:1007.

56. Coller BS. Seminars in medicine of the Beth Israel Hospital, Boston: platelets and thrombolytic therapy. N Engl J Med 1990;322:33.

57. Yasuda T, Gold HK, Fallon JT, et al. Monoclonal antibody against the platelet glycoprotein (GP) IIb/IIIa receptor prevents coronary artery reocclusion after reperfusion with recombinant tissue-type plasminogen activator in dogs. J Clin Invest 1988;81:1284.

58. Gold HK, Coller BS, Yasuda T, et al. Rapid and sustained coronary artery recanalization with combined bolus injection of recombinant tissue-type plasminogen activator and monoclonal antiplatelet GPIIb/IIIa antibody in a canine preparation. Circulation 1988;77:670.

59. The Evaluation of 7E3 for the Prevention of Ischemic Complications (EPIC) Investigators. Use of a monoclonal antibody directed against the platelet glycoprotein IIb/IIIa receptor in high-risk coronary angioplasty. N Engl J Med 1994;330:956.

60. Bode C, Meinhardt G, Runge MS, et al. Platelet-targeted fibrinolysis enhances clot lysis and inhibits platelet aggregation. Circulation 1991;84: 805.

61. Dewerchin M, Lijnen HR, Stassen JM, et al. Effect of chemical conjugation of recombinant single-chain urokinase-type plasminogen activator with monoclonal antiplatelet antibodies on platelet aggregation and on plasma clot lysis in vitro and in vivo. Blood 1991;78:1005.

62. Hoffmann JJ, Janssen WC. Interactions between thrombolytic agents and platelets: effects of plasmin on platelet glycoproteins Ib and IIb/IIIa. Thromb Res 1992;67:711.

63. Hamilton KK, Fretto LJ, Grierson DS, McKee PA. Effects of plasmin on von Willebrand factor multimers. Degradation in vitro and stimulation of release in vivo. J Clin Invest 1985;76:261.

64. Rick ME, Popovsky MA, Krizek DM. Degradation of factor VIII coagulant antigen by proteolytic enzymes. Br J Haematol 1985;61:477.

65. Woolf N, Carstairs KC. The survival time of platelets in experimental mural thrombi. J Pathol 1969;97:595.

66. Savage B, Hunter CS, Harker LA, et al. Thrombin-induced increase in surface expression of epitopes on platelet membrane glycoprotein IIb/IIIa complex and GMP-140 is a function of platelet age. Blood 1989;74:1007.

INDEX